Community mental health nursing

AN ECOLOGICAL PERSPECTIVE

Community mental health nursing

AN ECOLOGICAL PERSPECTIVE

JEANETTE LANCASTER, R.N., Ph.D.

Associate Professor, School of Nursing,
The University of Alabama, Birmingham, Alabama

with 31 illustrations

The C. V. Mosby Company

ST. LOUIS • TORONTO • LONDON   1980

Printed in the United States of America

The C. V. Mosby Company
11830 Westline Industrial Drive, St. Louis, Missouri 63141

Library of Congress Cataloging in Publication Data

Lancaster, Jeanette, 1944-
  Community mental health nursing.

  Includes bibliographical references and index.
  1. Psychiatric nursing. 2. Community mental health
services. I. Title.
RC440.L36   610.73'68   79-26185
ISBN 0-8016-2816-4

GW/M/M 9 8 7 6 5 4 3 2 1   03/D/380

Contributors

JUDITH M. ATLEE, R.N., M.S.N.

Assistant Professor, College of Nursing,
University of Oklahoma, Oklahoma City, Oklahoma

MARY LOU BOND, R.N., M.S.N.

Associate Professor, Harris College of Nursing,
Texas Christian University, Fort Worth, Texas

DONNA BLAIR BOOE, R.N., M.S.

Doctoral student in Medical Anthropology,
Southern Methodist University, Dallas, Texas

LYNN W. BRALLIER, R.N., M.S.N.

Director, Stress Management Center of Metropolitan
Washington, Independent practice of psychotherapy and
biofeedback, Washington, D.C.

JUDY BRETZ PRINCE, M.S.S.W., A.C.S.W.

Private practice, Birmingham, Alabama

JOHN G. BRUHN, Ph.D.

Associate Dean for Community Affairs and Professor of
Preventive Medicine and Community Health, School
of Medicine, University of Texas Medical Branch,
Galveston, Texas

CECILIA H. CANTRELL, R.N., Ph.D.

Chairman, Department of Nursing,
Georgia State University, Atlanta, Georgia

LINDA COLVIN, R.N., M.S.

Formerly Assistant Professor, Harris College of Nursing,
Texas Christian University, Fort Worth, Texas

F. DAVID CORDOVA, R.N., Ed.D.

Associate Professor of Allied Health Services,
School of Allied Health Services, University of Texas
Medical Branch, Galveston, Texas

BARBARA S. HENTHORN, R.N., Dr.P.H.

Associate Professor of Nursing, Central State University,
Edmond, Oklahoma

BETTIE S. JACKSON, R.N., Ed.D., E.T.

Adjunct Associate Professor, Montefiore Hospital,
New York, New York

ANN KNECHT KIRKHAM, R.N., M.S.

Assistant Professor, Harris College of Nursing,
Texas Christian University, Fort Worth, Texas

PAT KURTZ, R.N., M.S.

Assistant Professor, Texas Women's University,
Dallas, Texas

JEANETTE LANCASTER, R.N., Ph.D.

Associate Professor, School of Nursing,
The University of Alabama, Birmingham, Alabama

WADE LANCASTER, Ph.D.

Assistant Professor, School of Business,
University of Alabama, Birmingham, Alabama

ANNE LANGSTON LIND, R.N., M.S.

Assistant Professor, Harris College of Nursing,
Texas Christian University, Fort Worth, Texas

ELIZABETH MORRISON, R.N., M.S.

Associate Professor, School of Nursing,
University of Alabama, Birmingham, Alabama

ELAINE ORTMAN, R.N., M.S.

Chief, Family Functioning Unit, Family Resource and
Counseling Center, Upper Mountain Mental Health Center,
Salt Lake City, Utah

SUSAN REESEMAN STEVENS, R.N., M.S.

Doctoral student, Community Mental Health Nursing,
University of Alabama, Birmingham, Alabama

SHERRY YOWELL, R.N., M.S.

Associate Professor, Department of Nursing,
University of Southern Colorado, Pueblo, Colorado

Preface

With increasing numbers of individuals seeking psychiatric treatment the need for prevention cannot be disregarded. Primary prevention of mental disorders is described as biological, social, or psychological intervention to promote emotional well-being and reduce the incidence and prevalence of mental illness in a given population.

According to Caplan's (1976) model of primary prevention, the rate of mental disorder in a community is related to the interaction of both long-term and short-term factors influencing the adaptive capacities of its members. Thus mental illness occurs in a community context, and the resources for helping are provided in the community. The short-term component refers to crisis intervention, whereas the long-term component includes providing ways in which the physical, psychological, and sociocultural needs of the community can be met.

By definition psychiatric nursing is directed toward "both preventive and corrective impacts upon mental illness and is concerned with the promotion of optimal mental health for society, the community and those individuals and families who live within it" (American Nurses' Association, 1973). For nurses charged with promoting preventive health, a conceptual approach directed toward understanding the man-environment relationship is imperative. Too often a conceptual approach is ignored in favor of busy action for action's sake. One's conceptual framework shapes nursing efforts in an organized rather than random manner. One conceptual framework, the ecological perspective, is used in this text in relation to widely divergent theories of human interaction.

The ecological framework or perspective holds that man's health status is the result of the dynamic interaction between his internal environment and the multiple external environments in which he exists. Man's responses to the environment comprise his attempts to maintain homeostasis. The complexity of these adaptive efforts is seen when it is realized that each human organism responds to the total environmental impact. Man cannot sort out certain components of the environment and respond only to those designated aspects. Rather, he reacts in one way or another to the total environmental impact.

Human ecology does not possess a body of knowledge; it is a synthetic science uniting concepts from the natural and behavioral sciences into a holistic approach for viewing man. Its principal value lies in the way in which it views the man-environment system. Human ecology dramatically points out that the whole of the man-environment relationship is considerably more than the sum of its parts. According to Hanlon, "Human ecology sees man at the interface of his two basic environments, the biophysical and the sociocultural, being at once in both, interacting reciprocally with both, affecting and being affected by both" (1969, p. 9). The result of this ecological interaction determines man's place in the health-illness continuum.

The following chapters provide an overview of nursing approaches directed toward the prevention of mental illness. Each chapter calls attention to a specific strategy for improving man's relationship to his environment. In this book environment refers to both internal and external forces influencing human adaptation and behavior. The focus is directed primarily toward psychosocial factors, although the intent is certainly not to disregard the physical effects of the environment on human functioning. Ecology has a keen interest in the effect of the physical environment on the human animal, in that health is determined by the interaction of all forces acting on man.

A wide array of treatment approaches is discussed; they seek to define methods for promoting mental health. Each chapter was written specifically for this book by a health care provider with expertise in the selected topic area. The book is divided into five parts. Part one briefly traces the development of human ecology in the social sciences both to describe its similarity to the development of community mental health nursing and to provide background for the sections on an ecological perspective and ecology as a model for nursing. In essence Part one comprises the theoretical background for each of the sections that follow.

The chapters in Parts two to five assume the framework in Part one and make no attempt to repeat this content. Rather, each provides clinical application relevant to either a specific population or a treatment approach.

Part two presents chapters concerned with three age groups that represent high-risk populations: infants, children, and older adults. Target or high-risk populations are dealt with in this section rather than in Part three in that their developmental stage predisposes them to heightened psychological stress.

Each of the chapters in Part three describes an approach for preventing mental illness in an identified high-risk population. In this section prevention moves from a focus on primary care to include aspects of both secondary and tertiary prevention. While the hope in community mental health nursing is always that of preventing the onset of psychological disruption, in reality many clients come to the attention of mental health clinicians following an episode or life pattern that militates against mental health. Four chapters deal with studies of victims, whereas the remaining four relate to problems of adjustment to changing life situations.

Part four is devoted to nurse-client interactional approaches that can be easily utilized in community mental health nursing. Each therapeutic approach is described by a nurse who has utilized the specific framework in nursing practice. Examples are interspersed throughout each chapter to allow readers to transfer the content to additional treatment settings.

Part five contains two chapters that focus on community mental health nursing from a health systems approach. A business administration emphasis calls attention to the urgent need in health care delivery, especially community mental health, to become increasingly responsive to the specific needs of any given sector of the total population. Health care services can become cost effective only if they meet the needs of the consumer or client group being served. The final chapter summarizes the current status of community mental health nursing by addressing key issues and highlighting crucial roles implicit in this broad, yet highly specialized, area of nursing. An ecological approach serves as the organizing theme for looking at both the breadth and depth of community mental health nursing.

Many individuals have played influential and supportive roles in the development of this text. I would like to express particular appreciation to former teachers as well as colleagues who have encouraged new ideas, raised questions, and challenged assumptions. Special thanks must go to my family—Wade, Jennifer, and Melinda—who patiently waited while I worked on the text and supported this project from its inception.

Jeanette Lancaster

Contents

Part one
THE NEED FOR A CONCEPTUAL BASE FOR COMMUNITY MENTAL HEALTH NURSING

1 Nature and scope of community mental health nursing, 3
Jeanette Lancaster

2 An ecological perspective in community mental health nursing, 9
Jeanette Lancaster

3 History and development of human ecology, 16
Jeanette Lancaster

4 The ecological perspective in a nursing model, 22
Susan Reeseman Stevens

Part two
PREVENTIVE MODELS FOR SPECIAL AGE GROUPS

5 Pregnancy: maternal and fetal perspectives, 33
Mary Lou Bond
Anne Langston Lind

6 Human development program: facilitating the child-environment relationship, 40
Jeanette Lancaster

7 An ecological view of gerontological mental health, 50
Barbara S. Henthorn

Part three
PREVENTIVE MODELS FOR HIGH-RISK POPULATIONS

8 Dealing with the emotional needs of persons undergoing transsexual surgery, 79
Judith M. Atlee

9 Substance abuse: nursing implications for prevention and health promotion, 88
Sherry Yowell

10 A systems approach to spouse abuse, 103
Judy Bretz Prince

11 Nursing intervention in child abuse, 115
Elaine Ortman

12 Epidemiology of rape, 123
Ann Knecht Kirkham

13 Rape as a crisis, 134
Jeanette Lancaster

14 Coping with nonterminal loss, 140
Cecilia H. Cantrell
Bettie S. Jackson

15 Continuity of care program: discharged psychiatric patients, 151
Jeanette Lancaster

Part four
INTERACTIONAL FRAMEWORKS APPLICABLE TO AN ECOLOGICAL PERSPECTIVE

16 Activities as therapy, 163
Jeanette Lancaster

17 Family therapy as prevention, 170
Elizabeth Morrison

18 Therapeutic intervention with children through art, 179

Donna Blair Booe

19 Reality therapy: one approach to enhancing man's relationships, 200

Linda Colvin

20 Wholeness and integration: Gestalt theory and practice, 209

Lynn W. Brallier

21 Holistic health practice: expanding the role of the psychiatric–mental health nurse, 219

Lynn W. Brallier

22 Transactional analysis: dealing with the man-environment relationship, 229

Pat Kurtz

Part five
CLIENT–HEALTH CARE SYSTEM INTERFACES

23 The application of marketing concepts to community mental health nursing, 245

Wade Lancaster

24 An ecological approach to the practice of community mental health nursing, 256

John G. Bruhn
F. David Cordova

Part one

THE NEED FOR A CONCEPTUAL BASE FOR COMMUNITY MENTAL HEALTH NURSING

■ Controversy rages within the nursing profession as to whether there is a science of nursing or whether science exists in nursing. Those who speak of the science of nursing refer to the "body of verifiable knowledge that will be derived from nursing practice" (Andreoli and Thompson, 1977). In contrast, science in nursing denotes the body of identified knowledge found within nursing that was originally derived from either the natural or social sciences or the humanities. Hence, this view describes nursing as a synthetic discipline whose unique contribution is made possible through the organization of knowledge gained from other disciplines as a guide for its practice.

Debate also is ongoing as to the status of human ecology. Is ecology a science or a perspective from which to view situations? Ecology, like nursing, is synthetic in that it borrows content from the established scientific fields. The uniqueness in ecology lies in its organization of a paradigm for the "borrowed" information. Ecology does not possess a unique body of knowledge; its principal value lies in the way it looks at man-environment interaction. Ecology focuses on an examination of the whole organism not just of isolated parts of the whole. One way to approach human ecology is through a systems approach. In essence, systems theory provides the model for the use of ecological concepts to examine principles about the way living and nonliving things exist together.

The commonalities between nursing and human ecology are numerous. Both focus on holism by emphasizing man-environment relationships. Further, both consider man as more than an accumulation of parts: man is described as a biopsychosocial being. One identified goal of both nursing and human ecology is to foster high-level wellness. Each urges that health is dynamic and results from a myriad of influencing forces.

Not only is the relation of science to nursing questioned but considerable attention has been focused on whether or not theories of nursing exist, and if so, whether or not the level of theoretical development is currently at the conceptual stage. It is generally acknowledged that a profession needs a conceptual basis. A conceptual model provides perspective, or a way of looking at phenomena. The model thus serves as a representation of reality (Reilly, 1975).

Models vary in their level of abstraction. The first level refers to pictorial models that try to reproduce the significant aspects of an event. The second level is that of descriptive models, which present the pictorial features as well as the relationships that exist among the components (McKay, 1969). The ecological model, or perspective, of community mental health nursing serves as a model of the second level. Such a conceptual model uses systems theory schema to describe reality. The model is largely synthetic in origin; its main benefit lies in its acknowledgment of the importance of the interaction that occurs among system parts.

By definition, a system refers to a "whole which functions as a whole by virtue of the interdependence of its parts" (Rapoport, 1968). General systems theory seeks to examine the objects or components of a given system by identifying how their distinguishing properties interact. In other words, a systems approach focuses on relationships.

The purpose of the first part of the text is to provide a conceptual base for the provision of community mental health nursing activities. The premises are held that ecology contributes to an awareness of system relationships, and that the crux of community mental health nursing is to intervene at system junctures so as to enhance mental health. While it is hoped that a considerable emphasis in community mental health nursing is placed on primary prevention, in reality attention must also be given to "at risk" populations that may seek intervention following a mental health crisis.

In Part I the nature and scope of community mental health nursing is described in order to provide the reader with an understanding of how the principles of ecology may clarify and expand the role of community mental health nursing. Further, the history and evolution of human ecology is documented to explain its current status in the social sciences. Third, an ecological perspective is set forth—a perspective that has direct applicability to community mental health nursing and that establishes a background for the last chapter in this section—the delineation of an ecological model for nursing.

References

Andreoli, K., and Thompson, C.: The nature of science in nursing, Image **9**:32-37, June 1977.
McKay, R.: Theories, models and systems for nursing, Nurs. Res. **18**:393-399, 1969.
Rapoport, A.: Foreword. In Buckley, W., editor: Modern systems research for the behavioral scientist, Chicago, 1968, Aldine Publishing Co.
Reilly, D.: Why a conceptual framework? Nurs. Outlook **23**:566-569, 1975.

CHAPTER 1

Nature and scope of community mental health nursing

JEANETTE LANCASTER

Only in recent years has psychiatric nursing espoused an orientation toward community mental health. In the past, psychiatric nursing has largely considered its practice domain to be within the confines of hospital walls. The development of a role in community mental health nursing closely follows the historical evolution of mental healing.

ORIGIN OF MENTAL HEALING

The origins of mental healing date back to ancient and prehistoric times. Primitive man viewed disease as an evil spirit that took possession of the body as a punishment for an offense against the spirit world. The primitive art of mental healing consisted of driving hostile spirits away. This mode was dominated by fear and superstition and was carried out through the use of restraints or actual physical rejection of the individual from the community gathering.

From the fifteenth through the seventeenth centuries handling of the mentally ill took on a more forceful and punitive character. People who would be described as mentally ill according to today's standards were legally prosecuted and burned as witches. The inhumane treatment of mentally ill individuals during this era was determined by the underlying belief that they represented a threat to the welfare of the community.

FORERUNNER TO HUMANITARIAN TREATMENT

The eighteenth century witnessed practices that were the forerunner for humanitarian treatment of mentally ill patients. At Bethlehem in London, for example, the custom was to chain the patients' arms and legs together as they lay on the floor. During this period patients usually were restrained, at least during the night.

The period of enlightenment began in the late eighteenth century with the work of Philippe Pinel in France. Pinel removed the chains from mentally ill patients at Salpetriere and Bicêtre in 1793 and put patients to work on farms owned by the hospital. At about the same time, William Tuke, a Quaker, established the Retreat in York, England, which is credited as the first hospital to regard mentally ill persons as having a disorder that required scientific treatment. Although no iron manacles were used to restrain patients at the Retreat, seclusion, leather belts, and strait coats were used.

HUMANITARIAN TREATMENT

A major change occurred during the nineteenth century in the type of care afforded mentally ill persons. The model for care became "custodial care." Mental illness at this time was considered to be a permanent affliction, and deranged individuals were placed in jails and county poor homes to protect society from them. For a fortunate minority of the mentally ill humane treatment was available in private and public hospitals.

Humanitarian reform was first seen in the United States in the work of Benjamin Rush. Called the "father of American psychiatry," Rush began a humane treatment program. He is described as the leader of a transitional period in American history in that his treatment represented humane care intermingled with remedies including bloodletting, purgatives, and a torturelike device called "the tranquilizer," which today are not considered humane.

Beginning of state hospitals

Having observed the beginning success of "humane" or "moral" treatment, an energetic New England schoolteacher, Dorothea Dix, carried on the work of Rush by vigorously exposing the sordid conditions in which mentally ill individuals were kept. In an extremely progressive crusade she recommended that each state assume responsibility for its own mentally ill population. Her work resulted in the establishment of 32 state hospitals, most of which were in rural areas. Three advantages dominated the choice of rural sites for the establishment of state hospitals: (1) land was readily available at a low price, (2) rural locations were sufficiently removed from the mainstream of life such that patients did not threaten other citizens, and (3) it was thought that the country with its fresh air and tranquility would promote mental health restoration.

As the population of the United States increased, mental hospitals were built at a steadily increasing rate until 1900. During the years after 1900 the population continued to grow, but the growth of state hospitals reached a plateau. This trend soon led to overcrowded living conditions, which began to reverse the humane effects of the mental hospital movement. Thus, Dorothea Dix's dream of the state hospital providing protective and healing functions was disrupted. While her hopes were not fully realized,

she did influence greatly the treatment of mentally ill individuals.

Nursing role during "custodial care" era

During the custodial care era of psychiatric care the primary responsibility of the nurse was to guard the patients. Mental illness was viewed as a disease process, and the goal of "treatment" was to keep the patients in a safe place. It was during this time that the field of psychiatric nursing began to evolve. The first psychiatric training school for nurses was established in 1882 at the McLean Hospital in Belmont, Massachusetts (Sills, 1973). A variety of obstacles impeded the development of psychiatric nursing. Foremost was the lack of demand for "asylum-trained" nurses. As late as 1916 only one half of American mental hospitals operated training schools for their nurses. Hospitals without schools chose to employ attendants at a low wage to "care" for the patients.

During this period the belief was held that if nurses needed to know about mental illness, then nursing education should be held in a psychiatric hospital. This idea later led to the concept of affiliations in nursing education. During an affiliation the students went as a group to live for 6 weeks to 3 months in a dormitory at a state hospital. This approach, however, encouraged a dichotomy between illness of the mind and that of the body. The total patient system was not presented, but rather education focused on one component of patient functioning.

Innovations in care

The care and treatment of the mentally ill continued to go downhill until Adolf Meyer took up the banner Dorothea Dix had once waved. Meyer vigorously championed for increased and innovative care of the mentally ill. He was actually the first person to espouse the basic concepts of community mental health. Speaking to delegates at the International Congress of Medicine in 1913 he recommended the establishment of mental disease clinics that would serve first the patient and second the administrative system as well as the study of disease processes to develop new treatment approaches. He contrasted his proposal with the "wholesale handling of patients"; he also suggested that follow-up studies be made of discharged patients and that preventive efforts be developed outside the hospital (Central State Griffin Hospital, undated). Adolph Meyer clearly was foresighted in his vision of mental health services.

GOVERNMENTAL INVOLVEMENT IN PSYCHIATRIC CARE

The federal government first entered into health care in 1935 with the passage of the Social Security Act. Concern developed during the depression, and the proposition was put forth that if a community could not take care of its sick, then the federal government should make provisions to do so. World War II accelerated governmental involvement in psychiatric treatment when approximately 875,000 of 15 million draftees were rejected from military service on the basis of mental or neurological disorders (Snow and Newton, 1976).

In 1946 the United States Congress enacted the National Mental Health Act, which provided grants to the states for the development of mental health programs outside the state hospitals. This act was responsible for radically altering the treatment for mentally disturbed Americans. Although the intent was to apply a public health approach to mental illness, in actuality individual psychotherapy rather than prevention was supported.

Establishment of National Institute of Mental Health

The National Institute of Mental Health (NIMH) was established in 1949, as specified by the guidelines of the National Mental Health Act. The NIMH, organized as the headquarters for the new federal mental health program, em-phasized research into the cause and treatment of mental illness. The Institute also supported training programs for needed mental health personnel and aided states in improving their programs.

Shifts in psychiatric nursing: consistent with national trends

Concomitant with national mental health trends, the focus of education in psychiatric nursing shifted from that of custodial care to emphasis on the treatment of patients. The decision was made in nursing education to integrate knowledge of psychiatric concepts into all areas of nursing care. Nursing education began to include specific content related to psychopathology as well as general concepts of medical-surgical care.

Goffman (1961) presented the view that mental illness is a social process rather than a disease. He graphically described the effect of institutional treatment on patients and declared that hospitals were designed more for the convenience and management of the staff than for the care of the patients. Also, during this period the concept of the therapeutic milieu, which originated in England with the work of Maxwell Jones, was adopted in several American hospitals. The therapeutic milieu concept emphasized open and direct communication between patients and staff including patient participation in planning efforts. At this point psychiatric nursing became actively involved in defining the role of nurses within the therapeutic milieu, or therapeutic community. A shift was seen in the orientation of nursing care toward the recognition of the importance of treating the individual within the context of the total patient group. The belief was held that the informal group process influenced each individual and that treatment must look at the total patient experience during the hospitalization period. The notion of therapeutic milieu represented a significant milestone on the journey toward community mental health.

Joint Commission's report on mental illness and health

In 1955 Congress enacted the Mental Health Study Act, which created the Joint Commission on Mental Illness and Health. The Joint Commission was made up of representatives from 36 organizations and agencies, the members selected by the NIMH. The Commission's report was submitted to Congress in late 1960 and published in 1961 as Action for Mental Health. The 338-page report recommended increases in training and education as well as early, intensive treatment for acutely disturbed patients in outpatient clinics, in psychiatric units in general hospitals, and in regional state hospitals of not more than 1000 beds.

COMMUNITY MENTAL HEALTH ERA

Following publication of the Commission's report, President John F. Kennedy appointed a cabinet-level committee to review the report and make recommendations regarding federal action. Based on the work of this committee President Kennedy sent to Congress in 1963 the first message that any President of the United States had ever sent on behalf of mental health. The presidential message called for a new type of health facility that would upgrade mental health services by providing a full complement of services in the local community and at the same time focus on prevention. These new facilities were to be known as community mental health centers.

Community Mental Health Centers Construction Act

After 8 months' deliberation of the Commission's report the Eighty-eighth Congress enacted Public Law 88-164, the Mental Retardation Facilities and Community Mental Health Centers Construction Act of 1963, which authorized federal matching funds of $150 million over a 3-year period for states to use in constructing comprehensive community mental health centers.

Regulations for use of this money were is-

sued in May 1964. They specified that to qualify for federal construction funds a community mental health center must provide at least five essential services: (1) inpatient service, (2) outpatient service, (3) partial hospitalization, (4) emergency care on a 24-hour basis, and (5) consultation and education to community agencies and professional personnel. Adequate treatment in community mental health centers were to consist of the five essential services plus five additional components. The following additional programs were recommended: (1) diagnostic, (2) rehabilitative, (3) precare and aftercare, (4) training, and (5) research and evaluation.

The original community mental health legislation provided federal funding for centers for 8 years on a declining percentage formula. During the 8 years, in nonpoverty areas, federal support decreased from 80% to 25% subsidy. In poverty areas the federal proportion began at 90% support and decreased to 30% in the eighth year. As the federal percentage decreased, many centers had difficulty continuing their range of services because of insufficient local funds (Landsberg and Hammer, 1977).

Community Mental Health Centers Amendments of 1975

The Community Mental Health Centers Amendments of 1975, Title III, Public Law 94-63, extended funding to community mental health centers. These amendments reiterated the intent of the original legislation as well as specified essential services (Community Mental Health, 1977). They were criticized because they limited the flexibility available to centers in designing programs to meet the needs of the local community.

President's Commission on Mental Health

Early in 1977 President Jimmy Carter organized the President's Commission on Mental Health. One of the 5 mental health professionals on the 20-member Commission was a nurse.

The President's general charge to the group was to identify the mental health needs of the nation. Specific focus was to be on the extent to which the mentally ill were served, methods of dealing with stress, and governmental support for mental health including research and increased coordination among agencies.

After a 1-year study period the Commission released its final report, which contained 117 recommendations. The principal recommendation called for the establishment of a

new federal grant program for community mental health services to encourage the creation of necessary services where they are inadequate and increase the flexibility of communities in planning a comprehensive network of services (MH-MR Report, 1978).

In general the report addressed the items within the original Presidential charge. While the Commission did not ask for massive funding increases, it did request a redistribution of monies so as to focus on prevention, accessibility and better distribution of services, and insurance coverage in any future national policy; to emphasize the chronically mentally ill population; and to research into the cause and treatment of mental illness, mental retardation, drug abuse, and alcoholism.

IMPACT OF COMMUNITY MENTAL HEALTH ON NURSING PRACTICE

The mental health legislation of the early 1960s set into motion some major alterations in the modus operandi of psychiatric nursing. This area of nursing was challenged to design new patterns of care for patients with emotional problems as well as to become actively involved in the prevention of mental illness. The work environment of the psychiatric nurse moved from the confines of the institution walls to the horizons of the community. As the environment changed, so did the role and the title of the nursing care giver. Over the decades the titles referring to nurses working in the psychiatric–mental health area have ranged from psychiatric nurse, to community psychiatric nurse,

to psychiatric mental health nurse, and finally to community mental health nurse.

Role differentiation in psychiatric–mental health nursing

Osborne (1973) differentiates among four titles pertaining to the psychiatric–mental health nurse by contrasting the meanings of psychiatry and mental health. Psychiatry refers to a specialty area designed to deal with disorders of the mind. The goal of psychiatry is to provide treatment, whereas mental health connotes wellness rather than dysfunction. Services designated as mental health are directed toward prevention of illness so as to promote and maintain health. Mental health action "relates to identifying and supporting populations at risk and modifying interpersonal and societal impacts found to be injurious to the mental health of the population" (Osborne, 1973).

The term "psychiatric nursing" refers to care provided typically within an institution and directed toward treatment of individuals designated as "ill." The community psychiatric nurse extends treatment into the community. A public health approach is used, and nursing activities include home visits and group and family treatment as well as consultation and education. The aim in community psychiatric nursing is prevention of mental disorder.

In contrast, in community mental health nursing there is no individual client. The focus centers on populations at risk. To provide nursing services to the community, the nurse must stand back and look at the entire community as a system. Assessing community needs as well as resources is a prerequisite to community planning activities.

Community perspective of mental health

Criticism has been leveled against the community mental health movement because of its inability to meet the original goals that had been established to justify federal funding. Critics contend that the site of treatment should not be moved from the hospital to the community without a concomitant change in focus. Blame for the shortcomings in the implementation of community mental health is attributed to the tendency to transplant psychiatric treatment to a new setting. Indeed it may be that the movement has been more community psychiatric treatment than community mental health.

A community orientation toward mental health indeed requires an adjustment in focus. One approach to a new focus is to define mental health services as occurring on a continuum from wellness to illness:

Wellness ——— Stress ——— Coping ——— Illness
Interpersonal   *Dysfunction*
adequacy

The goal of community mental health nursing includes providing care to individuals on both ends of the continuum, although attention is centered on keeping individuals on the wellness side. The underlying premise in a community orientation is that each individual experiences stress and has problems in coping with daily living. Dysfunction occurs when the amount of stress exceeds the coping capacity of the individual.

A community approach to mental illness focuses on prevention, which begins by identifying high-risk populations and providing services before effective psychological functioning is disrupted. The aim is to strike a balance between the internal or external stressors and the available coping abilities. Community mental health identifies the root of most emotional disorders as occurring within a network of interacting systems. A major element of the community mental health nursing role is directed toward identifying populations at risk and seeking interventions that decrease stress and reduce the incidence of mental disorder.

An ecological perspective is used as an organizing framework for describing ways in which the community mental health nurse can provide services to high-risk populations. Such a perspective is built on a systems theory base and integrates concepts of prevention to set forth a holistic approach to mental health. An ecological perspective is described by tracing ecology's development, its current status, and the implications for a conceptual model adaptable to nursing.

References

Central State Griffin Hospital: Historical background of community mental health movement, Normal, Okla., Central State Griffin Hospital. (Undated.)

Community Mental Health Services Support Branch: A citizen's guide to the Community Mental Health Centers Amendments of 1975, Washington, D.C., 1977, U.S. Government Printing Office.

Landsberg, G., and Hammer, R.: Possible programmatic consequences of community mental health center funding arrangements: illustrations based on inpatient utilization data, Community Ment. Health J. **13:**63-70, 1977.

MH-MR Report: A Morris Associates report from Washington, **15:**1-8, May 5, 1978.

Osborne, O.: A theoretical basis for the education of the psychiatric–mental health nurse, Nurs. Clin. North Am. **5:**699-712, 1970.

Sills, G.: Historical developments and issues in psychiatric mental health nursing. In Leininger, M., editor: Contemporary issues in mental health nursing, Boston, 1973, Little, Brown & Co.

Snow, D., and Newton, P.: Task, social structure and social process in the community mental health center movement, Am. Psychol. **31:**582-594, 1976.

CHAPTER 2

An ecological perspective in community mental health nursing

JEANETTE LANCASTER

Historically the progression of culture has marched through the Stone, Bronze, and Iron ages. The terms "industrial revolution" and "space age" relate to the societal advances made from the late nineteenth century to the midtwentieth century. The second half of the twentieth century will no doubt be recorded in history as the "environmental age," with individuals experiencing the most varied and intense life stresses in the history of mankind. Tremendous advances made during the twentieth century in transportation, science, technology, education, and communication are affecting family and other group structures. Not only the magnitude but the rapidity of change is influencing the man-environment relationship.

Not all societal changes are having a positive and growth-producing impact on the health status of the American people. One of the most well-fed, well-cared-for, and affluent societies in history shows serious signs of illness, as evidenced by an alarming increase in mental illness, crime, and suicide rate, as well as a frightening chemical abuse problem. Moreover, in spite of a great expertise in sanitation and an understanding of its effect on man's health, major lakes, streams, and oceans are becoming more and more polluted. Each attempt to make life more convenient leads to new sources of pollution and subsequent stress for living organisms.

Man is not effectively dealing with the rapidly changing times; the onslaught of societal

change is affecting both physiological and psychological coping mechanisms. Hanlon (1969) notes that "present man-induced drastic alterations and disturbances in his total environment are resulting in insults, excitants, and stresses which necessarily evoke responses from the human organism." Through his responses man seeks to maintain homeostasis. The complexity of this homeostatic mechanism should not be minimized in that it includes the total human organism in its relationship to the total environment.

Past models for dealing with factors influencing health and illness are no longer effective for the complex health problems of the twentieth century. The reductionist approach for dealing with discrete, separate problems is ineffective for promoting and maintaining health for the total person. While some degree of water pollution may not be harmful in itself, when added to a bearable amount of air pollution, coupled with a tolerable quantity of noise, congestion, and intrapsychic stress, the resulting cumulative impact can produce an unhealthy environmental state for an organism attempting to maintain homeostasis.

A new conceptual approach emphasizing a holistic view of man is required. Such an approach must spring from a synthesis of many disciplines to provide a framework for the study of cause and effect relationships. The need for a synthetic framework is based on the belief that

9

man is a total unit, not a compilation of parts, in ongoing interaction and reaction with a constantly changing environment.

WHAT IS AN ECOLOGICAL PERSPECTIVE

The framework, or perspective, that allows health care providers to look at the total man-environment relationship is in essence the application of ecological principles to the human condition. Such an approach is based on a recognition that man's health status results from the dynamic interplay between two ecological universes: his own internal environment and the external multienvironments in which he exists (Hanlon, 1969).

Human ecology is concerned with the broad conception of man and his environment, that is, with the total group of human adaptive processes including physical, cultural, technological, social, and behavioral. Another definition refers to human ecology as the "branch of human biology that deals with the interactions between men and their environment" (Hinkle, 1965). The man-environment relationship, traditionally conceptualized as biological in scope, extends to disturbances in mood, thought, and behavior as well as disorders of adaptation and chronic degenerative diseases.

The ecological view suggests that man and his interactions with the environment must be changed. It is no longer sufficient to rely on "conquering disease in the environment"; prevention must assume a significant role in health care. An ecological approach to health care delivery emphasizes the roles of change and adaptation as ongoing processes.

The term "ecology" was first proposed by the German biologist Ernst Haeckel in 1869. The word "ecology" is derived from the Greek root *oikos* meaning house. Thus, ecology literally means the study of organisms at home. As such, ecology is concerned with both the structure and functioning of the organism and pays attention to the surroundings as well as to

that which is surrounded. Since all objects in the environment are interrelated and interdependent, the study of human ecology is action oriented, which implies that a difference exists between studying "what is," "what has been," and "what can be." Ecology focuses on what can be (Kartman, 1967) and is described from the standpoints of a definition, a set of principles, and an attitude. As mentioned, by definition ecology refers to the study of the interrelationships between man and his environment as well as among men as they seek to maintain themselves within their environment. The principles of ecology, which describe ways in which men live with one another, are derived from the physical, social, and behavioral sciences. The ecological attitude refers to a respect or an appreciation for all parts of the universe.

In human ecology man is viewed as an open-ended system constantly interacting with his environment so as to maintain life and to function as a member of the species. His responses to environmental forces are attempts to maintain homeostasis. The complexity of one's adaptive responses is explained by considering that man cannot pick and choose certain components of the environment toward which his responses are directed; rather he responds to the total environmental impact.

Concept of ecosystem

According to Odum (1972) the concept of ecosystem is "not only the center of professional ecology today, but it is also the most relevant concept in terms of man's environmental problems." An ecosystem is defined as the sum total of all existing subsystems. In studying ecosystems it is necessary to consider man as a part of, not separate from, a life-support system composed of "the atmosphere, water, minerals, soil, plants, animals and microorganisms that function together to keep the whole viable" (Odum, 1972). Translating the ecosystem concept from its biological origin to an interactional focus represents a synthetic, not an analytic, approach based on concepts from systems theory.

The ecosystem concept emphasizes the functional relationships of organisms to other organisms as well as to their physical environment. Ecosystems include both a place and a way of life; in general, the more complex the ecosystem, the more stable is its functioning. The size and characteristics of ecosystems may vary considerably, ranging from a conceptualization of the entire earth as an ecosphere to a consideration of complex microscopic organizations. In human ecosystems the organizational unit is generally intermediate in size and most often refers to families or communities (Wilkinson and O'Connor, 1977). Human ecosystems tend to be complex in that they include the sociocultural as well as the physical and biotic dimensions of the environment (Hoyman, 1971).

A systems theory approach is particularly applicable to the study of complex problems because it involves an organization of information in which the whole is broken down into components in a manner that facilitates examination of the relationships between parts as well as minute study of the components. Although initially the focus is on analysis, the ultimate goal is synthesis, or a reordering of the parts, to consider each aspect of the interaction.

Characteristics of living systems

Systems differ in the nature of their interaction with the environment; that is, systems may be open or closed. A closed system does not exchange matter, energy, or information with the environment. On the other hand, an open system is sustained by a continuous exchange process with the environment. Few examples of closed systems exist: for example, a chemical reaction confined to an enclosed vessel constitutes a closed system. All living organisms are open systems. Throughout his life span, man constantly exchanges materials with the environment, which results in ongoing adaptation.

The system seeks to maintain a steady state characterized by some degree of stability.

Additional system characteristics include a conceptualization of both subsystems and suprasystems. Every order of systems except the smallest has subsystems, and all but the largest systems have suprasystems. The study of any specific system is conducted within the framework of both its subsystems and its suprasystems. For example, man as a system is described in terms of his subsystems such as his respiratory subsystem as well as in regard to his suprasystems, which include family and community.

Additionally, each system has both a boundary and an environment. Boundaries form dividing lines between system components and the external environment. In living, or open, systems, boundaries are semipermeable and serve to regulate the flow of information into the system as well as the flow from the system into the environment.

All open systems are characterized by an exchange of input (information, energy, or matter absorbed by the system), which is processed, or transformed, and subsequently expelled back into the environment as output. One way in which the exchange of information with the environment occurs is through feedback control mechanisms whereby a portion of the output is reintroduced into the system as input.

Feedback loops are channels through which both positive and negative information enter and leave the system. Positive feedback comprises data that lead to change, whereas negative feedback tends to maintain system stability. Negative feedback is the process through which the system continually adjusts its level of activity to decrease the distance between the ideal and actual state of functioning.

Because systems are continuously involved in the processes of input, transformation or handling of incoming data, and output, they tend to be in a constant state of disorganization or disequilibrium. Each system attempts to achieve balance among the various forces operating within and on it. Following any disturbance a system attempts to reestablish its steady state. The concept of equifinality functions in a manner similar to that of steady state. Equifinality means that for each person there is a typical state toward which he aspires. Illness disrupts an individual's pursuit of equifinality as it interrupts his steady state.

Chin (1961) describes three ways in which a system reacts to outside impingements. The system may initially resist the influence of a disturbance by refusing to acknowledge its existence. For example, families often ignore the problems of one of its members. The myth seems to be "If we don't talk about the problem then it must not exist." Systems also can resist disruption by utilizing internal regulatory processes to re-create some semblance of balance. For example, if one family member has a problem the solution would be to discuss the situation in such a way as to convince the member that he "really" does not have a problem; it is only a mistaken perception on his part. In the third mechanism the disturbance leads to a new equilibrium when family members acknowledge that one member has a problem and then as a group discuss the situation, identify alternatives for action, and move toward a resolution of the problem.

CONCEPTUALIZATION OF MAN AND ENVIRONMENT

Since human ecology is concerned with the man-environment relationship it is necessary to discuss the concepts man and environment. Men are as different as are their thumbprints. No two have the same physical or emotional traits. Each is unique and strives to fulfill his needs and life goals in specific ways. The fulfillment of these needs and goals may extend and add quality or quantity ot his life, or they may destroy and decrease the existing quality of his life.

Man is primarily a social animal, conforming to the general norms of the culture and to the specific standards of the subculture and face-to-face groups of which he is a member. The concept of culture refers to the learned behavior shared by the members of a particular society. Culture arises in, and is transmitted by, the group. Thus any attempt to promote mental health and intervene in the onslaught of rapid change must be considered in a societal context and must emphasize the preventive rather than merely the curative components in the psychological field.

Environment refers to the entire spectrum of climatic, adaptive, and biotic factors that act on an organism or on an ecological community, whose form and mechanism for survival they ultimately determine. Environment also includes the aggregate of social and cultural conditions such as customs, beliefs, laws, language, religion, and political organizations that influence the individual.

Implicit in any examination of the man-environment relationship are the concepts of territoriality (niche) and adaptation. In ecology the belief is held that everything has its niche, or unique setting, for its existence. In terms of the physical environment, niche refers to a place or setting. With man the niche is also equated to roles. The scope of territoriality includes both structure (place) and function (role). One's niche is constantly changing in an attempt to adapt and maintain some sense of homeostasis.

Consider, for example, promotion of the head of a family that includes relocation to a different geographic region. Such a common occurrence illustrates the structural and functional aspects of a niche. As the person being promoted into a new position seeks to learn what is expected of him, each member of the family system is affected. Moreover, the actual move affects each member as the family's social and physical environments change. For any organism to survive it must adapt; family relocation calls for immense adaptational efforts. Nothing remains fixed in a changing system. Further, each person in the family responds to the changes differently, which in turn adds to the cumulative effect on each member.

The history of medicine has witnessed three uniquely different approaches to an assessment of the effect of the environment on man's well being. Originally disease was thought to be solely determined by a disturbance of the individual's internal environment. With the formulation of the germ theory attention shifted from emphasizing the internal to closer scrutiny of the external environment. Currently the pendulum regarding causation of disease has swung to a midpoint position that acknowledges the influence of both internal and external environments (Cheroskin and Ringsdorf, 1971). It is now recognized that health disruption also comes from environmental challenges. However, whether an individual succumbs to environmental insults is largely determined by his resistance quotient or the ratio between the environmental impact and the individual's coping ability.

Even when strong environmental forces are evident, each individual has a choice whether or not to succumb. Also, a considerable portion of a person's environment is generated by his behavior. Learning plays a significant role in the behavior of the human animal in terms of his response to the environment.

According to Moos (1976) the environment exerts its effect on man in one of five different ways: The environment may (1) be actively stressful and directly cause disease, (2) limit the individual, (3) select some organism that it seeks to favor, (4) serve as a releaser of man's capacities by offering support, or (5) be an active and positive force in personal development and thereby facilitate growth. The ecological perspective in community mental health nursing focuses on the fifth environmental context.

ECOLOGY'S VALUE TO COMMUNITY MENTAL HEALTH

Ecology's value to community mental health lies in the way it views the man-environment system. Ecology forces health care providers to examine the whole human organism, not just its organs and organ systems. Ecology describes human systems and communities that of necessity include the individual. One viewpoint considers the individual an arrangement of organs, thoughts, and feelings surrounded by a boundary known as his body. The converse view believes that the individual is only one aspect of a larger system—society.

In applying an ecological approach it is essential to recognize that complex problems are not generally solved by simple solutions. In the search for solutions the whole of the situation is separated into component parts for assessment of each part. Providers must be made aware of the ecological view and that it includes all dimensions of the system or they will create more havoc than cure. The great moral principle that is derived from an ecological view is that "we can never do merely one thing" (Hardin, 1970). Often the solution to one problem leads to even greater problems, as seen in the many attempts to overcome the limitations of nature.

From the ecosystem perspective psychopathology exists when groups lack sufficient resources to meet the emotional needs of the members or to foster an even distribution of resources (O'Connor, 1977). The roots of mental illness reside not only in disturbances within the individual but also within the larger system.

In the mental health area the concept of single causation is no longer tenable. Community mental health must conceive of mental health and illness as resulting from a "concentric network of interconnected determinants with the individual at the core but in a constant state of dynamic interaction" with the family, groups, and community (Marmor, 1975).

Health is thus defined and measured in terms

of the adaptive capacity of the individual to environmental circumstances and forces. According to Sargent (1972) health and illness are polar phases in the life sequence continuum. When adaptability is successful, the individual is described as healthy; when adaptability fails, he is ill. From this perspective health is not the absence of all disease but "the ability of the organism to function effectively within a given environment" (Sargent, 1972).

An application of ecological principles to community mental health embodies concepts of prevention. It is no longer adequate to think only in terms of cure for mental illness; the emphasis must shift toward prevention. An orientation toward the role of prevention in community mental health necessitates a new understanding of mental disorders. Basic to this orientation is the belief that all individuals experience stress; the potential for ecosystem disruption is inherent in daily living. Stress is generated in a family and/or community context; hence provisions for prevention of overwhelming stress must come from the community. The focus of community mental health is on the support of effective mental and social functioning in order to prevent illness. It is essential to identify populations that are especially at risk for disruption so that support can be provided.

An understanding of the concept of community is a prerequisite to the application of ecological principles to community mental health. The term "community" refers to a group of people living in close proximity and having some dependency on each other. Community encompasses the place where people live, work, raise children, and in general carry on the activities necessary for daily living (Poplin, 1972; Warren, 1972). A given community is composed of individuals who are engaged in some degree of social interaction within a defined geographic area and who have one or more common ties. The community is the social

environment in which hazards are experienced and supports are provided.

Activities to promote and enhance mental health can be described in accordance with Caplan's (1974) levels of primary, secondary, and tertiary prevention. In primary prevention the rate of mental disorder in a community is related to the interaction of both long-term and short-term factors that influence the adaptive capacities of its members. Short-term refers to crisis intervention, whereas long-term includes providing ways in which the physical, psychological, and sociocultural needs of the community can be met. Physical resources encompass food, shelter, adequate living space, sensory stimulation, and opportunities for exercise, sleep, and dreaming. Psychosocial resources comprise stimulation of a person's intellectual and emotional development through interaction with significant others. Sociocultural resources refer to the influence on personality and functioning exerted by the customs and values of the culture and the social structure (Caplan, 1974).

Preventive psychiatry, or promotion of mental health, refers to reducing the incidence of mental disorder in a community (primary prevention), decreasing the duration of a significant number of the disorders that do occur (secondary prevention), and decreasing the impairment that may result from psychological stress and disruption (tertiary prevention).

Primary prevention of mental disorders is specifically described as biological, social, or psychological intervention that promotes emotional well-being or reduces the incidence and prevalence of mental illness in populations. Primary prevention attempts to lower the rate of new cases of mental disorder by counteracting and preventing harmful circumstances. The focus is on the community as a whole. Stress factors are continuously monitored so that intervention can be provided before disruption commences.

Focusing on the community as client does not imply neglecting the needs of individual members. Rather, a community focus demands a broader approach that acknowledges both those individuals currently seeking health care intervention as well as those who may eventually need intervention if certain deleterious circumstances continue.

Secondary prevention seeks to reduce the prevalence of mental disorder by providing intervention that decreases the number of stressors and shortens the duration of disequilibrium. Secondary prevention is accomplished by encouraging and assisting in early referral as well as by reducing barriers to treatment through the provision of efficient screening, diagnostic services, and effective treatment.

Tertiary prevention refers to measures undertaken in a community to reduce the level of social defects that result from mental disorder. This type of prevention often includes rehabilitation and readaptation to the environment.

SUMMARY

An ecological approach is suggested as a viable method for community mental health nurses to use in assessing the needs of a specific community. Such an approach calls attention to the impact of the environment on both the physical and psychological functioning of the residents. In the face of rapidly changing environmental structures, individuals cannot be viewed and treated apart from their internal and external environmental support systems. Each man is a part of a life-support system whose components have unending effects on his functioning. An ecological approach can be applied at each of the three levels of prevention in an attempt to maximize adaptation.

References

Caplan, G.: Support systems and community mental health, New York, 1974, Behavioral Publications.

Cheroskin, E., and Ringsdorf, W. M.: Predictive medicine. (Part 3). An ecologic approach, J. Am. Geriatr. Soc. **19:** 505-510, 1971.

Chin, R.: The utility of system models and developmental models for practitioners. In Bennis, W. G., Benne, K. D., and Chin, R., editors: The planning of change: readings in the applied behavioral sciences, ed. 2, New York, 1969, Holt, Rinehart & Winston.

Hanlon, J.: An ecologic view of public health, Am. J. Public Health **59:**4-10, 1969.

Hardin, G.: Everybody's guilty: the ecological dilemma, Calif. Med. **113:**40-47, November 1970.

Hinkle, L.: Studies of human ecology in relation to health and behavior, BioScience **15:**517-520, 1965.

Hoyman, H.: Human ecology and health education (Part 2), J. Sch. Health **41:**538-546, 1971.

Kartman, L.: Human ecology and public health, Am. J. Public Health **57:**737-750, 1967.

Marmor, J.: The relationship between systems theory and community psychiatry, Hosp. Community Psychiatry **26:**807-811, 1975.

Moos, R.: The human context: environmental determinants of behavior, New York, 1976, John Wiley & Sons, Inc.

O'Connor, W.: Ecosystems theory and clinical mental health, Psychiatr. Ann. **7:**63-77, July 1977.

Odum, E.: Ecosystem theory in relation to man. In Weins, J., ed.: Ecosystem structure and function, Corvallis, Ore., Oregon State University Press.

Poplin, D.: Communities: a survey of theories and methods of research, New York, 1972, The Macmillan Co.

Sargent, F.: Man-environment problems for public health, Am. J. Public Health **62:**628-632, 1972.

Warren, R.: The community in America, Chicago, 1972, Rand McNally & Co.

Wilkinson, C. B., and O'Connor, W.: Introduction and overview, Psychiatr. Ann. **7:**10-15, July 1977.

CHAPTER 3

History and development of human ecology

JEANETTE LANCASTER

Although the term "ecology" was proposed in the early twentieth century, ecological concepts can be traced to the earliest written history. Evidence exists of a Chinese calendar dating to 700 BC that recorded biological events (Bruhn, 1970). A number of academic disciplines seek to assume credit for originating the conceptual basis for human ecology. Its historical development is most clearly identified in biology and sociology; geography, anthropology, and psychology each provide additional historical content for the student of human ecology. Further, the language of human ecology is noted in economics, archeology, and epidemiology.

DEVELOPMENT OF HUMAN ECOLOGY IN THE BIOLOGICAL SCIENCES

The term "human ecology" was first used in biology by Ernst Haeckel in 1869 when he attempted to devise a systematic framework for the study of human life (Dunham, 1968). The word "ecology" derives from the Greek *oikos*, or house, and literally means the study of organisms at home. Haeckel proposed a separation of those disciplines concerned with internal environments from those concerned with the relationship between man and his external environment. He also pointed out that both structure and function of organisms are significantly affected by their living together.

Tracing ecological concepts through the bio-logical sciences, Malthus was one of the first to describe a relationship between man and the environment on which man depends for his existence. His concern dealt with the ratio of supply and demand of material resources. Malthus questioned how long populations could increase without outgrowing the food sources on which they were inescapably dependent (Bruhn, 1970).

Darwin is credited with the first in-depth analysis of biological and environmental interaction. Darwin's theory of "survival of the fittest" discussed the idea that individuals with high levels of physical and psychological abilities could adapt more readily to the environment and would thereby have a greater chance to survive than less well-endowed persons.

In the first edition of the journal *Ecology*, Moore (1920) said that "all life is controlled by two great forces, heredity and environment, and ecology is the science dealing with the environment. It therefore covers practically the whole field of biology and is related in one way or another to every science which touches life." Moore, therefore, saw ecology as being broader than biology.

The theory of homeostasis was first discussed by Bernard (1957) when he spoke of the internal and external environment of the human organism. He explained that the function of the body was that of maintaining a stable state (homeostasis) between the internal functioning of the organism and the external environment. Cannon (1932) spoke also of the effect of environmental stressors on the emotional functioning of the individual and the subsequent disequilibrium that could result. Selye (1950) elaborated on these theoretical positions by proposing that the quality of an individual's adaptation depends on his ability to mobilize defenses against environmental stressors.

Over the past four decades Eugene Odum has made significant contributions to the field of ecology within the biological sciences. In 1940 when he was a young instructor, Odum suggested that a course in ecology be included in the core curriculum for science majors. His idea found a cold reception. Since then he and his brother Howard Odum have written a text that has become a classic to the field of ecology. In his book, *Fundamentals of ecology* (1971), Odum sets forth two propositions that initially were considered revolutionary: (1) content moves from the whole to the components with consideration given to the ecosystem level as the guiding concept and (2) energy is the common denominator for integrating biotic and physical components into functional wholes. Possibly Odum's most significant contribution to ecology is his description of the ecosystem, which views man as a part of his biotic environment. The term "ecosystem" can be applied to a single cell, organ, individual, family, community, or population.

ECOLOGY'S HISTORICAL DEVELOPMENT IN SOCIOLOGY

In sociology Park (1953) is credited as the founder of human ecological thought. Park, a former reporter who was well acquainted with the city of Chicago, used human ecology to study cities in terms of the man-environment relationship. He saw the city as a group of concentric circles radiating out from the center, or inner city. Each circle was characterized by a different man-environment relationship. Work-

ing with Ernest Burgess and borrowing concepts from plant and animal ecology, Park extended the definition of human ecology to encompass not only the physical but also the social and cultural environments of man (Dunham, 1968).

The term "human ecology" appeared in sociology in 1921 when Park and Burgess established a center for ecological research at the University of Chicago. Park (1952) defined human ecology as an attempt to examine the ways by which the biotic balance and the social equilibrium are maintained as well as the process by which, when the biotic balance and the social equilibrium are disturbed, the transition is made from one relatively stable order to another.

The body of ecological theory developed in the 1920s and 1930s by Park and Burgess is considered "classical human ecology." According to the classical view the basic process in human interaction is competition occurring from a struggle for space (Theodorson, 1961). The classical viewpoint also divides society into biotic and cultural levels. The term "biotic" is defined as "basic, nonthoughtful adjustments made in the struggle for existence" (Theodorson, 1961). In contrast, the cultural level, based on communication and consensus, is seen as a superstructure resting on the biotic level. The biotic level is referred to as community; the cultural level, as society. The biotic level of human organization is considered the proper field of investigation for human ecology, and cultural factors are excluded from ecological investigation. The classical approach is criticized for the dichotomy it creates between the biotic and cultural levels.

Park conceived of human ecology not as a branch of sociology but rather as a perspective or method for scientifically studying the social aspects of living. While recognizing ecology's derivation from biology and geography, Park contrasted its focus from the relationship of man and his habitat to the relationship of man to man (Wirth, 1945). He envisioned human ecology as serving as a method for studying the relationships between men as they are affected by the environment.

McKenzie (1968) extended the classical view, although he did attach more significance to the importance of cultural forces on human ecology than Park did. McKenzie defined human ecology as "a study of the spatial and temporal relations of human beings as affected by the selective, distributive and accommodative forces of the environment." He further described the spatial and sustenance relations in which men are organized as continuously affected by environmental and cultural forces. McKenzie emphasized that the fundamental interest of human ecology is the effect of position: both the position of one community in relation to others and the place of the individual in a selected community are considered to be the core of human ecology. The concept of position in the sociological view is dynamic since ecology is concerned with the process of change as human beings respond to the environment.

The Chicago school of ecological thought dissolved with the onslaught of criticism leveled against their disregard for cultural factors. Actually, human ecology as conceived by Park is more like a perspective for viewing the whole.

Following the classical approach of Park and Burgess, the "neo-orthodox view" led by Quinn and Hawley emerged. They agreed that human ecology should not be concerned with spatial distribution per se but only as it reflected patterns of community structure. Hawley (1944) described ecology as being concerned with the ways in which organisms maintain themselves in a constantly changing yet restricted environment. Hawley further noted that the interrelatedness of living organisms suggests that adjustment and adaptation are mutual or collective phenomena. Thus the neo-orthodox view considers the community to be the

subject of ecological inquiry. The individual enters ecological investigation only in relation to the aggregate.

ECOLOGICAL CONCERNS IN GEOGRAPHY

In geography ecological concepts are seen in the early maps of Flanders dating back to 1537. In 1807 "Pinkerton argued that the landscape is a product of man's activity, and consideration of the physical aspects of the environment should follow instead of precede the consideration of cultural features" (Bruhn, 1974).

The emphasis in geography on the study of regions is reflected in the current method of census taking. By 1900 the country was divided into five regions for the U.S. Census; later it would be expanded to nine. These regions were regarded as homogeneous physically, economically, and socially (Bruhn, 1974).

ANTHROPOLOGY'S ROLE IN THE DEVELOPMENT OF HUMAN ECOLOGY

The approach in geography of viewing the region as a physical and social unity is similar to the "culture area" concept in anthropology. Wissler (1929) examined the concept of whether the environment influences the formation of discrete cultural areas because of their ability to produce selected foods. Steward (1936), an influential proponent of cultural ecology, was particularly interested in the interaction between behavior and environment. Steward's theory coincides with the proposition of Karl Wittfogel that an interplay exists between economics and the environment.

ECOLOGICAL THOUGHT IN PSYCHOLOGY

While ecology did not develop as a special area of study in psychology, as it did in several of the social sciences, the idea that environmental factors affect man's behavior, attitudes, and moods is seen as a recurring theme. Certainly Freud's emphasis on the dynamic and intrapsychic causes of human behavior had an ecological flavor.

The ecological strand in psychology was also strengthened by Murray's (1938) theory of personality. Murray developed a complex theory of personality, which includes both the concept of individual needs and the notion of "environmental press." He stated that the press, or force, of the environment affects the individual's needs, which are one component of the internal environment.

In tracing ecological development in psychology attention must also focus on Lewin's (1935) concepts of "life space," or "psychological field." Lewin considered all psychological happenings to result from the life space, which is made up of the individual and the environment as a constellation of interdependent forces. He described behavior as a function of the total field that exists at the time the behavior takes place. He conceived of the life space as being comprised of the person (P) and of the psychological environment (E). He further said that people have needs and the environment has "valences" that may or may not satisfy these needs (Lewin, 1935).

Wright and Barker in 1950 identified the term "psychological ecology" by describing its task as that of accounting for the impact of the physical-biological environment on psychological functioning. They coined the term "behavior setting" to refer to any part of the nonpsychological milieu that group consensus holds appropriate for certain kinds of behavior. For example, some aspects of the milieu are appropriate for parties and other social gatherings, whereas others are not.

More recently Wohlwill (1970) identified the area of environmental psychology. He described three areas of environment-behavior relationships that have been studied in psychological ecology. These include the study of the environment as a source of (1) affect and attitudes, the (2) approach and avoidance responses as determined by environmental attributes, and (3) adaptation to environmental qualities as a function of prolonged exposure.

Currently psychology is evidencing a growing interest in human ecology as attention focuses on the environmental impact on mental health. Similarities exist between the psychological view of ecology and the perspective in medicine that defines health as the maintenance of a delicate balance between the agent of disease, the organism, and the environment. Disease results when the balance is disrupted. From the psychological standpoint the term "mental health" is defined as "a congruent exchange between an individual's needs and abilities and the ecosystem's resources and requirements" (O'Connor, 1977).

From an ecosystem perspective, psychopathology occurs when insufficient resources are available in the environment to meet the needs of the human inhabitant within the limits of expected behavior. The purpose of psychotherapy is to influence or motivate a patient so that he can modify his interaction with the ecosystem and experience a positive outcome rather than continue to have dysfunctional encounters.

HUMAN ECOLOGY IN MEDICINE

Human ecology from the perspective of medicine initially tended to be medical ecology and focused on the environment's relationship to disease (Dunham, 1968). From this perspective health was seen as resulting from a delicate balance between the disease agent of transmission, the receiving organism, and the environment. Initially the focus of human ecology in medicine was of an epidemiological nature. Hippocrates believed that a direct causal connection existed between elements of the physical environment and health and disease in man. Thus he presented notions from the ecological era far before it was generally accepted.

Gregg (1956) divided medical history into

three major developmental eras that led into the present stage of ecology. The first era was described by Gregg as that of authority, which included the span of history from antiquity to the beginning stages of medical science. During the second era, research, experimentation, and treatment of specific diseases were in the forefront for medical science. The modern era, that of ecology, views the whole patient as well as the community in which he exists as the focus for medical attention.

During recent years the interest in the relationship between man and his environment has extended to disturbances of a psychological nature. As noted in Chapter 1, Tuke established at York, England, a hospital in which he not only emphasized an atmosphere of kindness and consideration toward hospitalized psychiatric patients but also fostered improved man-environment relationships through exercise, a healthy family environment, and productive use of one's abilities.

In America Samuel Woodward, superintendent of the Worchester, Massachusetts, State Hospital, believed that insanity resulted from the impact of social and cultural forces on the individual. He instituted moral treatment, which emphasized that the provision of a psychologically healthy environment was in itself curative of mental disease (Grob, 1966).

Human ecology has become established as an integral component of public health by virtue of its emphasis on looking at the whole rather than assessing only components of human functioning and adaptation. Dubos (1968) pointed out that much of history has been the result of accident or blind choice. He urged the development of strategies for prediction and early detection of stress-producing circumstances on the environment. One approach for actuating Dubos' suggestion is to apply a systems approach whereby parts of a system are analyzed to understand the functioning of the whole. In other words, often analysis precedes the ultimate goal of ecology, which is synthesis, or putting together all of the parts and examining their relationship to understand the whole.

Human ecology has developed as an illusive concept with a different meaning for each of the disciplines concerned with the development of man. In health care delivery areas, human ecology refers to man-environment interaction, implying that a balance must be maintained for health; disease results when the man-environment relationship is disrupted.

References

Bernard, C.: An introduction to the study of experimental medicine (Green, J. C., trans.), New York, 1957, Dover Publications, Inc.

Bruhn, J.: Human ecology in medicine, Environ. Res. **3:** 37-53, 1970.

Bruhn, J.: Human ecology: a unifying science, Hum. Ecol. **2:**105, April 1974.

Cannon, W.: Wisdom of the body, New York, 1932, W. W. Norton & Co., Inc.

Dubos, R.: So human an animal, New York, 1968, Charles Scribner's Sons.

Dunham, W.: Epidemiology of psychiatric disorder as a contribution to medical ecology, Int. J. Psychiatry **5:**124-125, 1968.

Gregg, A.: The future health officer's responsibility—past, present and future, Am. J. Public Health **46:**1384-1389, 1956.

Grob, G.: The state and the mentally ill: a history of Worchester State Hospital in Massachusetts, 1830-1920, Chapel Hill, N.C., 1966, University of North Carolina Press.

Hawley, A.: Ecology and human ecology, Soc. Forces **22:** 398-405, 1944.

Hinkle, L.: Studies of human ecology in relation to health and behavior, BioScience **15:**517-520, 1965.

Lewin, K.: A dynamic theory of personality: selected paper, New York, 1935, McGraw-Hill Book Co.

McKenzie, R.: On human ecology, Chicago, 1968, The University of Chicago Press.

Moore, B.: The scope of ecology, Ecology **1:**3-5, 1920.

Moos, R.: The human context: environmental determinants of behavior, New York, 1976, John Wiley & Sons, Inc.

Murray, H.: Explorations in personality, New York, 1938, Oxford University Press.

O'Connor, W. A.: Ecosystems theory and clinical mental health, Psychiatr. Ann. **7:**363-372, 1977.

Odum, E.: Fundamentals of ecology, ed. 3, Philadelphia, 1971, W. B. Saunders Co.

Park, R.: Human communities, New York, 1953, The Free Press.

Park, R. E., Burgess, E. W., and McKenzie, R. D.: The city, Chicago, 1925, The University of Chicago Press.

Selye, H.: Stress, Montreal, 1950, Acta, Inc.

Steward, J.: Economic and social basis of primitive bands. In Lowie, R., ed.: Essays in anthropology, Berkeley, Calif., 1936, University of California Press.

Theodorson, G. ed.: Studies in human ecology, New York, 1961, Harper & Row, Publishers.

Wirth, L.: Human ecology, J. Sociology **50**:483-488, 1945.

Wissler, C.: An introduction to social anthropology, New York, 1929, Holt, Rinehart & Winston.

Wohlwill, J. F.: The emerging disciple of environmental psychology, Am. Psychol. **25**:303-312, 1970.

Wright, H. F., and Barker, F. G.: Methods of psychological ecology, Lawrence, Kan., 1950, University of Kansas Press.

CHAPTER 4

The ecological perspective in a nursing model

SUSAN REESEMAN STEVENS

A perspective may be defined as a view, or vista, depicting the relationship of the various aspects of a subject to each other and to the whole (Morris, 1973). The term "perspective" most aptly fits the intent of ecology. Ecology ventures beyond holism and systems theory and casts light not only on parts of a system or on the whole system but also on the interfaces and interrelationships among all levels of organization of that system.

The ecological perspective asserts that "living organisms and their environment are inseparably interrelated and interact upon each other" (Odum, 1971). Ecology's broad perspective can be particularly useful as a unifying framework for existing theories as well as a springboard for the development of new and comprehensive theories, ideas, and approaches to treatment. This chapter explores one way in which the ecological perspective can be incorporated into a model of nursing and provide a framework for theories and treatment modalities used in nursing.

THE ECOLOGICAL PANORAMA

Every theory of the course of events in nature is necessarily based on some process of simplification and is to some extent, therefore, a fairy tale.

Sir Napier Shaw
In Odum, 1971

Shaw's observation of the limitations of theory is apropos to the formation and usefulness of ecology as a representation of nature. Ecology developed historically out of concerns that the specialization and compartmentalization that characterized scientific thought resulted in an inadequate understanding of phenomena. Despite the need for a juncture in the view of life, man, and environment, ecology initially "drew pursed lips from the purists, those to whom research meant learning more and more about less and less" (Darling, 1970).

Ecology's goal is the study of the organism in relationship to its environment as well as of the relationships between communities of organisms of like or different kinds. Ecology is characterized by a readiness to cross boundaries and to find correlations, contrasts, and differences. Odum (1977) describes ecology as a tool to combine holism with the reductionistic tendencies of science. Such a combination requires a systematic, interdisciplinary, and collaborative effort, because the cause and effect interrelationships of human behavior and environment should not be broken into pieces (Bruhn, undated).

While ecology may appear to lack a boundary because it encompasses many sciences and theories, it actually orders those theories into a focus on the system as it operates in conjunction with other biotic (living) and abiotic (nonliving) components of the biosphere. The ecological focus as envisioned by Odum (1971) is depicted in Fig. 4-1. Odum (1971) describes the biosys-

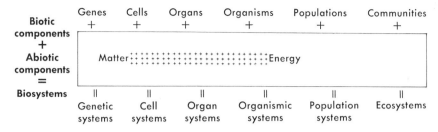

Fig. 4-1. Levels of organization in ecology. Note that ecology focuses on the right side of the spectrum, that is, the levels of organization from organisms to ecosystems. (Modified from Odum, E. P.: Fundamentals of ecology, Philadelphia, 1971, W. B. Saunders Co.)

tem as combining abiotic and biotic components into a related whole, for example, genes plus matter and energy equals the genetic system. However, while acknowledging microsystems such as cells, organs, and genes, the focus of ecology is on higher levels of organization—from organisms to ecosystems.

Ecology facilitates prediction of the consequences of environmental manipulation and can facilitate prescription for treatment of problematic interaction between the organism and the environment (Proshansky, 1970). Ecology serves to integrate the disciplines to solve complex problems such as population overload, pollution, and intersocietal aggression. The synthetic nature of ecology facilitates a more comprehensive description and explanation of phenomena and suggests action where other theories fall short (Revelle and Landsberg, 1970).

TOWARD UNIFICATION

What we need is first approximation to a scheme which will enable us to represent physical, psychological and social events within one system of denotation.

Grinker, 1956

Grinker (1956) described the efforts of a group of behavioral scientists to develop a unified model to order the proliferation of theory and to ensure a thorough examination of phenomena. The group thought that such a model would stimulate a totally new approach to studying the complex relationships between the mind, the body, and social events. The scientists worked toward a framework that would result in simultaneous consideration of the individual and his surroundings, both in health and in illness. The group believed systems theory would assist them in developing a unified perspective (Grinker, 1956).

Riehl and Roy (1976) examined the usefulness of a unified theory of nursing to facilitate communication, and to serve as a structure within which the nurse functions. Bergersen (1971) identifies four purposes of a unifying theory: (1) rationally and logically linking together information essential to nursing, (2) providing new insights into and further elucidation of nursing, (3) explaining nursing, and (4) reliably predicting nursing. The proliferation of new knowledge and the need for understanding that new knowledge in the context of existing knowledge underscore the need for a unifying structure. Recognition that factors that appear to be disparate are actually interrelated or analogous and that problems arise from compartmentalization of knowledge, provides additional justification for a unified framework (Bergersen, 1971).

Donaldson and Crowley (1978) highlight the need for the development or clarification of a unique nursing perspective that can direct the format and focus of nursing research and practice. While a number of nurses recognize the need to provide a synthetic framework to clarify nursing and to cope with the massive proliferation of data, they also see the disadvantages of a unified framework.

One disadvantage stems from the fact that nursing is just developing its own theories and models. Perhaps it is premature to select one model when we have not explored the entire realm of possibilities. A representation of the reality of the nurse-client relationship may be influenced by the singular experiences, values, and attitudes of the model builder as well as by the nonnursing theorists whose concepts are not completely applicable to, or representative of, a realistic model of nursing. Until we have a number of appropriate representations of nursing from which to choose or to merge into an eclectic model, the selection of one model of nursing may inhibit creativity and confine the nurse to a premature, set structure (Riehl and Roy, 1976). Bergersen's (1971) suggestion is to use pluralistic rather than unified approaches so nursing can continue to expand and identify boundaries of knowledge pertinent to nursing.

ECOLOGY AND NURSING

A compromise is proposed that may mitigate some of the disadvantages of a unified model of nursing and at the same time profit from the advantages of such a model. Human ecology as a unifying, synthetic perspective appears to support the broadest view of the client and can direct nursing's attention to a comprehensive number of interrelated variables.

Two difficulties remain with the use of the ecological perspective in a model of nursing. One difficulty, arising from the incorporation of such a broad, complex view of phenomena into a nursing model, is that it is not easy to clearly define the boundaries or limitations of nursing. An additional disadvantage results from using a perspective developed outside of the profession rather than one that is developed for nursing through observation and validation of actual nursing practice.

Yet, ecology should be explored as having the potential to unify the growing theories related to man and the environment and to assist in a representation of nursing. Ecology appears also to correspond with the historical development of nursing's focus. Nightingale (1859) described the function of the nurse as facilitating the reparative process of the sick and maintaining health of the well through environmentally related activities. Nightingale demonstrated the effects of the environment on the health of her clients. Rogers (1970) would later utilize components of ecology in the development of her theoretical basis of nursing. It is the rare nurse who does not believe that nursing should attempt to treat the "whole client." Ecology proceeds one step further to define the whole client as part and parcel of his inner and outer environment.

Ecology represents a valuable resource for nursing. Nurses such as Nightingale and Rogers focused their work toward between-system phenomena, rather than within-system phenomena. Peplau (1970) describes physicians as addressing themselves to "within-person phenomena—to dysfunctions, deficits, defects, and the like in relation to the organism." The focus on inner space has absorbed medicine for centuries and still does despite recent attempts by preventive and environmental branches to refocus the discipline. Although nursing has been influenced by the medical model's "within-person" tradition, the focus on the whole client interacting within his environment has persisted.

Nursing attends to the interfaces between systems—to the client as he responds to an environmental disturbance, for example, rather than to the direct effect of a pathogen on the cellular level. The community mental health nurse functions not as a psychoanalyst who primarily relies on client descriptions of inner-space phenomena but as a participant-observer in the client's network of family, significant others, and milieu. If the client's mental and physical health is to be maximized, the nurse must investigate milieu effects such as color, light, sounds, crowding, and intensity of sensory inputs.

It is obvious that the nurse must be aware of subsystem structure and morphology, but the central concern of the nurse is more closely related to the relationship between systems than to subsystem genetic, cellular, or organ levels of organization. Conversely, the central concern for much of medicine continues to be the inner space of the body, particularly those subsystems affected by illness.

ECOLOGICAL MODEL OF NURSING

Ecological concepts and principles developed by Odum (1971) and used by Rabkin (1970) are included in this model of nursing and furnish a framework for the integration and development of concepts and theories that reflect the complexities of nursing. Rabkin incorporates ecological concepts in his description of the relationship between inner and outer space. Inner space consists of lower levels of organization within the self. Outer space is made up of the network of people, places, objects, time, and space that comprise the environment in which the individual exists. Rabkin encourages open exploration into the merger of inner and outer space, which affects each individual.

Ecology offers principles that describe, explain, and predict the interrelationships between inner and outer space. New principles concerning interface dynamics may be expected as research continues. The following are the ecological principles identified by Odum (1971):

1. The whole is greater than the sum of its parts.
2. The environment changes its inhabitants.
3. Inhabitants change the environment.
4. An ecosystem resists outside forces that could change its balance of subsystems.
5. Both over- and undercrowding are limiting to the ecosystem.
6. New systems are more competitive than cooperative.
7. Systems live together in varying degrees of competition and cooperation.
8. All living things have rhythm.

Ecological concern with stimulus levels, territoriality, temporal relationships, and effects of abiotic factors on individuals has relevance for nurses in any setting. Because of the intensity of the interpersonal relationship in nursing, the nurse must be constantly aware of the nature of the client system in which the nurse and client interact. Odum (1971) notes that biotic and abiotic components merge into biosystems. Use of Odum's observations of the interrelationship between levels of organization (see Fig. 4-1) with abiotic and biotic components reveals the client system's structure:

Client + Biotic components +
                Abiotic components = Client system

Biotic components include higher levels of organization such as the community (if the client is an individual or small group) as well as lower levels of organization such as the individual's organ or cellular systems. Abiotic components include inanimate components of the client's outer space such as objects in the home or air pollution. The nurse enters, affects, and is affected by the client system. The nurse and client interaction, therefore, includes not only the individuals involved, but all the biotic and abiotic components of the client system. The model of the nurse-client system transaction, which incorporates the ecological perspective, is depicted in Fig. 4-2.

The ecological model of nursing highlights not only nurse and client interaction but the transaction between the nurse and client as well as those biotic and abiotic components that comprise the client system. All components merge to produce a unique circumstance. The nurse's observations and actions must incorporate knowledge of the multitude of variables affecting the client's health. Ecology expands those variables under scrutiny.

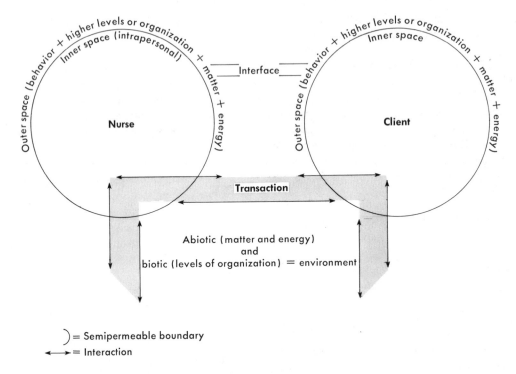

) = Semipermeable boundary
←——→ = Interaction

Fig. 4-2. Model of nurse-client system transaction.

A model of nursing is a representation of reality and serves to structure the available nursing knowledge and to direct nursing practice (Nursing Development Conference Group, 1973). A model may direct and order the type of conceptual framework used in practice, education, and/or research. The ecological model of nursing requires the nursing profession to consider the client and the environment simultaneously. The nurse must consider the biotic and abiotic components of the client system as they are bound together into a whole rather than each in separate compartments. The ecological perspective refocuses attention from subsystem compartments to the interfaces and interrelationships of systems.

Beliefs

Any model is affected by the beliefs of the model builder. These beliefs are reflective of that individual and also reflect the perspective taken by the model builder. Thus, beliefs about the client, about nursing, and about models of nursing influence the development of the model. The ecological perspective implicit in this model is a natural outgrowth of these beliefs and in turn influences the formation of the beliefs.

BELIEFS ABOUT THE CLIENT

1. The client is an autonomous entity.
2. The client and the environment are inextricably entwined.

3. The client participates in all client system shifts.
4. Since the client is autonomous, collaboration is the integrating theme in the nurse-client relationship.

BELIEFS ABOUT NURSING

1. Nursing is a facilitative and sustaining process (doing with, not for or to, the client).
2. Nursing respects the client's autonomy over that client's inner and outer space.
3. The nurse is influenced by and influences the client system.
4. Nurses are knowledgeable, autonomous, and creative professionals.

BELIEFS ABOUT MODELS OF NURSING

1. Models of nursing should view the client and the environment as an entity.
2. Models of nursing should include a depiction of the nurse.
3. Models should be unified, simple, and flexible.
4. Models should not dictate all theories to be used but should allow for the development and incorporation of new theories pertinent to nursing.

Nursing is a profession in transition and is buffeted by a proliferation of knowledge both within and without the profession. Nursing's success in its struggle for autonomy over the profession requires a definition of its own perspective, which differs from that of other health professions. This requires a model that will facilitate a framework for knowledge and provide the vista that will depict the interrelationships between the nurse, the client, and the environment.

Nursing transaction

Nursing has been described as an interpersonal event that consists of a functional closeness between the nurse and client (King, 1971). By synthesizing information about the inter-personal involvement of the nurse and about the interrelationships of individuals and the environment, it is possible to define nursing. Nursing is a transaction between a facilitator and a client system resulting from a potential or actual shift in that system. At least three assumptions underlie the definition:

1. The intrapersonal affects the interpersonal.
2. Shifts in the client system affect health.
3. The client is inseparably interrelated and interacts with biotic and abiotic components within the client system.

Identification of nursing actions may be derived from the model and the definition of nursing. The nurse does the following:

1. Identifies client system shifts.
2. Determines the positive, neutral, or detrimental nature of the client system shift with the client.
3. Facilitates the client's identification, avoidance, minimization, amelioration, or elimination of detrimental shifts.
4. Facilitates the client in identifying, promoting, sustaining, developing, or creating positive shifts.
5. Sustains the client through shifts in the client system, whether the shifts are reversable or nonreversable, detrimental, neutral, or positive.
6. Evaluates outcomes of facilitative and sustaining activities.

The role of the nurse as a facilitator in the interpersonal relationship implies that ''doing for'' is not necessarily to be valued in the nursing act. Rather, the nurse helps to make easier or less difficult the client's actions. When the client cannot act for himself the nurse's role may convert to sustainer. Since any shift in the environment is assumed to affect the client, the nurse acts on the client's responses to environmental shifts. For example, the nurse might assist the client in identifying the source of anxiety experienced during a client system shift. The nurse might also act to protect the client from dangers in the environment that he may not notice because of his high level of anxiety.

The ecological perspective in a model of nursing acknowledges the importance of intrapersonal, interpersonal, and environmental factors. However, these factors are inseparably interrelated. The study of one factor in isolation from the others yields spurious nursing data. Such compartmentalization fosters loss of perspective. For example, an attitude (intrapersonal) may not be fully comprehended until it is understood in the light of interpersonal and environmental contexts.

The nature of client system shifts may be detrimental, neutral, or positive. Shifts in client systems are constant and a part of the life process. The nursing facilitation process involves not only helping the client to overcome or ameliorate shifts caused, for example, by emphysema but it also involves helping the client eliminate factors that lead to detrimental system shifts and increase factors that enhance positive shifts. The nurse also plays a role in sustaining the client through shifts that are healthy. For example, a child's health may be enhanced through open heart surgery directed toward correcting a congenital defect. Yet the child might have difficulty in dealing with the change from a dependent "ill" state to an independent "healthy" state. In this situation the nurse needs to work with the child and significant others in the child's system to sustain the child through the shift. Abiotic components such as toys, stairs, athletic equipment, space, time, and stimuli are likely to be important considerations.

Factors relating to health and illness have long been recognized as complex and multifaceted. Recently increased attention has been paid to the environmental causation of cancer, occupationally related diseases, and mental illness. However, environment alone cannot provide all the answers. Rather, the complex interaction between inner and outer space must be recognized in research, education, and practice. Since the nurse generally participates in a client system more intensively than any other health professional, the nurse is more likely to assess accurately and deal with client system shifts.

IMPACT

A model of nursing using an ecological perspective to unify theories related to inner and outer space influences education, research, and practice. Nursing curricula should focus not on subsystems themselves but on the complex transaction among individuals and the biotic and the abiotic environment. Traditional subsystem courses such as anatomy should expand to include human ecology. Nursing courses can be devised to assist the nurse in identifying and dealing with client system shifts. Since the nurse enters the client system (in contrast to the traditional view of the "client entering the health care system"), the nurse needs information about the client system as well as the impact that the nurse and nursing activities will have on the client system. Facilitative and sustaining techniques unique to nursing can be developed and taught within the ecological perspective. Interface energies and strains brought about by the encroachment of the health care system and personnel on the client system should be identified.

Theories that highlight the complex interrelationship between inner and outer space and that reflect the complexity of nursing practice fit into the ecological model of nursing. The fine line between interpersonal and intrapersonal theory becomes superfluous. The ecological perspective eschews compartmentalization, and nursing activites need not be compartmentalized. Rather, the nurse's focus is toward enhancing positive client system shifts and ameliorating detrimental shifts. Community mental health nurses are best supported by theories that recognize the importance of both inner and outer space to the health of the client.

Many research questions are generated by the ecological perspective. For example, which biotic and abiotic components of a client system are facilitative of health and which are not? This question is particularly important at a time when iatrogenic disease sometimes results from ignorance of which treatment is truly health promoting and when substances in the environment are increasingly hazardous to health.

Some other questions generated by the ecological perspective include the following:

1. How is the mind-body continuum affected by the environment?
2. What is the effect of over- or undercrowding on the healing environment?
3. What variables affect treatment settings?
4. How do changes in the treatment setting affect the interaction between the client and nurse?

One investigation in progress is the use of an ecological model of nursing to generate an ecological assessment tool for children's emergency treatment settings (Stevens, 1978).

> There are more things in heaven and earth, Horatio,
> Than are dreamt of in your philosophy.
>
> *Shakespeare, Hamlet*

The ecological perspective in nursing demands that theoretical underpinnings of practice incorporate into a unified whole knowledge about the client, the nurse, the environment, and the transactions between them. Nursing's unique position vis-à-vis the client portends well for enhancement of the value of ecology to the profession and to the society it serves. The concern about the effects of the environment on the client, reflected in Nightingale's (1859) *Notes on nursing,* is at least as crucial today as it was a century ago. Community mental health nurses, always involved in the complexity of interpersonal relationships and their practice milieu can only profit from extension of that vista to include the complex interrelationship of the "more things" that Hamlet foretold and to which ecology adds perspective.

References

Bergersen, B. S.: Adaption as a unifying theory. In Murphy, J.: Theoretical issues in professional nursing, New York, 1971, Appleton-Century-Crofts.

Bruhn, J. G.: The history of human ecology in the behavioral sciences, (unpublished paper), Oklahoma City, University of Oklahoma Medical Center. (Undated.)

Darling, F. F.: A wider environment of ecology and conservation. In Revelle, R., and Landsberg, H. H.: America's changing environment, Boston, 1970, Beacon Press.

Donaldson, S. K., and Crowley, D. M.: The discipline of nursing, Nurs. Outlook **26:**113-120, 1978.

Grinker, R., ed.: Toward a unified theory of human behavior, New York, 1956, Basic Books, Inc.

King, I. M.: Toward a theory for nursing, New York, 1971, John Wiley & Sons, Inc.

Morris, W., ed.: The American heritage dictionary of the English language. Boston, 1973, Houghton Mifflin Co.

Nightingale, F.: Notes on nursing, Philadelphia, 1946, J. B. Lippincott Co. (Originally published in 1859.)

Nursing Development Conference Group: Concept formalization in nursing, Boston, 1973, Little, Brown & Co.

Odum, E. P.: Fundamentals of ecology, Philadelphia, 1971, W. B. Saunders Co.

Odum, E. P.: The emergency of ecology as a new integrative discipline, Science **195:**1289-1292, 1977.

Peplau, H.: Changed pattern of practice, Wash. State J. Nurs. **42:**4-6, November-December, 1970.

Proshansky, H. M., Ittelson, W., and Rivlin, E.: Environmental psychology: man and his physical setting. New York, 1970, Holt, Rinehart & Winston.

Rabkin, R.: Inner and outer space: introduction to a theory of social psychiatry, New York, 1970, W. W. Norton & Co., Inc.

Revelle, R., and Landsberg, H. H.: America's changing environment, Boston, 1970, Beacon Press.

Riehl, J. P., and Roy, C., Sr.: Conceptual models for nursing practice, New York, 1976, Appleton-Century-Crofts.

Rogers, M.: An introduction to the theoretical basis of nursing, Philadelphia, 1970, F. A. Davis Co.

Stevens, S. R.: An ecological assessment tool for children's emergency treatment settings, (unpublished paper), Birmingham, Ala., 1978, University of Alabama.

Part two

PREVENTIVE MODELS FOR SPECIAL AGE GROUPS

■ A major facet of the community mental health nursing role focuses on identifying populations that are likely to be ''at risk'' for emotional disruption. Populations considered to be at risk are those containing a sufficient number of individuals who have experienced sufficient stress to interrupt their state of emotional equilibrium. Frequently crises lead to an ''at risk'' state. Crises provide a turning point in the lives of individuals. Responses to crises determine the adjustment individuals are able to make during these episodes of disequilibrium. A crisis represents a life situation that presents stresses demanding solutions often new to the individual.

Two types of crises occur that lead an individual to be designated as at risk for emotional disruption. Developmental crises occur spontaneously throughout his life cycle as an individual progresses to new stages of growth. These crises, regarded as stages of the normal life cycle, result from physical, psychological, and social changes. In contrast, situational crises external to the individual are often sudden and accidental and have unfortunate effects on functioning (Robischon, 1967).

Part two describes strategies for providing support during developmental crises. Primary preventive efforts are exerted to help individuals and families respond to naturally occurring crises in an adaptable manner. Primary prevention involves counteracting mitigating circumstances before they have an opportunity to disrupt adaptation. From an ecological point of view intervention means providing nursing support prior to the onset of an emotional problem. The environment is manipulated in an attempt to promote health and prevent unnecessary stress.

Three populations are identified in this section as high risk. The selection of these populations is not intended to be comprehensive but rather to examine groups that have a high incidence of stress at specific developmental periods. Actually the entire area of family life presents opportunities for primary prevention because of the rapid pace of life and the multitude of changes impinging on families.

The developmental crisis precipitated by the birth of a child necessitates an alteration in the family system. With the introduction of a third person the initial dyadic relationship is altered. Each additional child similarly affects the existing family constellation. The goal of nursing intervention with expanding families is to promote growth and adaptation in the face of change.

Not only the birth of a child but the whole area of parenting and child development provides opportunities for community mental health efforts. Although raising children consumes a significant amount of time, only in recent years has attention been focused on education for parenthood. Whether nurses subscribe to a specific approach or use an eclectic technique, the opportunities for promoting mental health abound.

While each developmental stage poses unique stresses, both early and later stages present a multitude of psychological hazards. Considerable attention has been directed toward the increasing elderly population in the United States. The whole area of change has a potentially disruptive impact on the coping capacity of the aged. Using an ecological approach nurses in community mental health direct attention to helping clients utilize their innate resources to cope with the many changes that beset them.

Reference

Robischon, P.: The challenge of crisis theory for nursing, Nurs. Outlook **15:**28-32, July 1967.

CHAPTER 5

Pregnancy: maternal and fetal perspectives

MARY LOU BOND and ANNE LANGSTON LIND

Pregnancy, childbirth, parenthood—these are terms that evoke feelings, precipitate behaviors, and influence relationships. In a narrow yet vital interpretation, the being who is conceived can be viewed both as the recipient in utero of the life-giving bounty of the mother and as the giver of joy or sadness to his parents after birth. In a broader interpretation the effect that this person will have on his sociocultural group and society at large may be that of an Einstein, a criminal, or just an average contributing citizen.

The mother, provider of its environment (herself the recipient of multiple changes and adjustments during pregnancy), affects the development of the fetus and assists the growing child in acquisition of personality and developmental tasks. Both while pregnant and as a mother, she experiences physical and emotional adjustments and growth, and has an influence upon the members of her family system as well as the community.

This discussion will consider (1) the evolvement of the family, (2) the influence of the cultural group, (3) preparation of the family for pregnancy, (4) pregnancy as an internal and external process, (5) the tasks and concerns of the pregnant woman, (6) the effect of pregnancy and birth upon society, and (7) factors contributing to a positive outcome.

Not so many years ago the excitement of the birth of a baby highlighted the obstetrical experience; management of the antepartum period was somewhat routine, with emphasis on the prevention of physiological complications. Today there is an increasing focus on the concurrent psychosocial alterations occurring during pregnancy as well as on the entire developing family unit as it prepares to receive the new member. The external environment with its imposing demands is recognized to influence the manner in which the pregnant woman copes, adapts, and responds to her ever-changing physiological and psychological self.

Pregnancy and birth, like other critical life periods, contain inherent possibilities for personal gain or loss. Developmental tasks for the mother include establishing a bond with the new individual who is developing as a part of her and at the same time still unknown to her, developing identity as the mother of a child, and nurturing present relationships with significant others.

Careful exploration of the childbearing experience requires much more than assessment of the expectant couple at the time of labor and delivery. Adequate consideration of childbearing involves study of the prospective parents: where they exist in the larger society, what they bring to their combined life together, what they plan for their future, and what is possible or achievable for them as individuals or in a group.

At some moment in time a person decides

to relate to another person in a way that ultimately results in a unit of society called the family. This organizational component is a vehicle for the continuation of development of the original couple. These people do not begin their combined life in a chemistry laboratory where there is certainty that chemical elements with certain properties will combine to make exact compounds with different but predictable actions.

Rather each is a unique person who comes to that critical moment of "family beginning" with years of learned responses to stimuli: the impact of multiple environmental bombardments such as air, water, noise, people, food, illness, and stress. These stimuli have acted and reacted upon both of them, but each possesses different biological characteristics. Two very different individuals, strangers to one another and to the role they are assuming, decide to combine their lives and become a family.

THE FAMILY: HISTORICALLY AND TODAY

Hundreds of years ago the family unit was one of mutual protection and survival. Life was a short experience, with death often occurring early. Planting, cultivating, and preserving food were necessities in some cultures. In other groups hunting for game and making clothing from animal skins were the way of life. Few, if any, processed foods or manufactured goods were available. The potential dangers to life were hostile groups of people, wild animals, and the elements. Little was known about treating or curing injury or illness; help was given by treating the symptom and providing comfort. Survival required the combined efforts of a group of people, often encompassing several generations.

Since the infant death rate has been extremely high throughout most of man's history, and birth control not only mysterious but seldom desired, most families had large numbers of children. These children learned while very young to participate in the work of the family. As the children matured, married, and had their own families, they tended to remain nearby, often living on the home property. Thus the larger family could continue to combine their efforts for their mutual benefit.

The family, in addition to survival and procreation, was the educational and social facility for the members. The family shared abilities, teaching one another crafts and occupational skills. The isolation of most families because of limited travel and communication caused them to develop their own resources. They provided entertainment for one another by reading, singing, playing games, or participating in holiday festivities. Basic academic techniques such as reading and arithmetic were taught by older family members, since schools and qualified teachers were in scarce supply.

Various types of families have evolved over the years. Communal families exist today (Jensen et al., 1977). Groups of same-sex persons make up homosexual families. Large, extended families combining several generations are still valued by some cultural groups. Single-parent families, having one adult member by chance or by choice, provide the family structure for some children. The nuclear family, consisting of one male and one female who are married and may have a child or children is still the most common family type in the twentieth century. It is this traditional nuclear family unit that will be the basis of this discussion.

Families residing in the United States today represent diverse cultural groups. Four "ethnic groups of color"—the Afro-American, the American Indian, the Chicano, and the Oriental—were federally defined as a result of the civil rights movement of the 1960s in the United States (Leininger, 1977).

Many other peoples, however, have migrated to North America: with the exception of the American Indian, all other residents of this country or their ancestors have found their way from some other country of the world. The majority of the white population came from Europe. Puerto Ricans, Cubans, Filipinos, and Vietnamese are but a few of the people who have more recently come to the United States seeking a new way of life. With them they have brought their values, their beliefs, and their customs, so that today, varying degrees of traditional customs are apparent in each group.

Within the broad cultural framework of any group there are often specific practices related to childbearing. Nurses, as members of a specific cultural group, have their own cultural frame of reference, which determines in part the attitudes and beliefs that they hold about childbearing and childrearing. When the childbearing patient and the nurse come from different cultural backgrounds an additional variable is inherently present in the assessment of needs and the subsequent care that is given.

Further diversity is found between rural and urban families. Historically the United States was a rural society in which the extended family was the major source of support among its members. The pregnant woman's immediate and extended family members were a source of support in times of need and its women taught the tasks of womanhood. These feminine models were representative of a given culture and its set of values and customs.

Rubin (1967a, b) studied the way in which the maternal role is acquired. She identified five processes that were operative in the subjects who were pregnant either for the first or for subsequent times. Mimicry, one process described to occur throughout pregnancy, makes extensive use of models—those individuals after whom a behavior is copied. A "circular process of introjection-projection-rejection" encompassed the listener's (pregnant woman) consideration of the selected model's behavior, with subsequent rejection or acceptance of approach, and was evaluated to be more selective and discriminatory than mimicry (Rubin, 1967a, p. 242).

Rubin found that the models most commonly used by the woman preparing to be a mother were her mother, older sisters, peers "in contemporary or advanced stages of role acquisition" and self (in other than first pregnancies) (Rubin, 1967b, p. 343). The absence of this female support system during pregnancy has been suggested to be a potential singular index of high-risk pregnancy.

Over the past 50 years, along with a gradual migration of the population from rural to urban areas, there has been a corresponding spatial separation between generations. It is interesting that many of the minority groups such as Mexican-Americans, the American Indians, and the American blacks still maintain an extended-family living pattern in the midst of urban dwellings. But the masses of expectant families, apart from their extended families, have had to learn their new roles and cope with family crises in new ways as living situations have changed.

Health professionals have become more and more intimately involved in the care and nurturance of the expectant family. This care has taken the form of health maintenance as well as prevention of disease, instruction for childbirth and parenting, and support in times of stress (Howells, 1972).

PREGNANCY: A STRESSFUL PHYSIOLOGICAL PERIOD

Physiological changes throughout pregnancy are massive, with alterations occurring in almost all of the body systems. These changes, being brought about to meet the increased demands of pregnancy, are transient in nature and are responsible for the symptoms experienced by the woman throughout the three trimesters of pregnancy.

First-trimester symptomatology, sometimes vague, frequently consists of fatigue, nausea, and vomiting. Shifts in the intricate hormonal interplay are partially responsible for headache and lethargy, which are frequent first-trimester accompaniments. Feelings of disappointment and depression may be present instead of the expected feelings of elation and excitement associated with the idea of becoming pregnant.

As pregnancy progresses, changes in the body systems become more apparent—some only to the woman herself, some to those about her. Uterine enlargement for accomodation of the fetus is most notable externally and is responsible for displacement of other organs in the internal surrounding structures. Moving gradually upward out of the pelvic cavity, the uterus becomes a transient abdominal organ, eventually pushing upward on the diaphragm causing dyspnea and digestive problems. Finally, close to delivery, the fetus descends into the pelvic cavity (lightening) and permits the mother to breathe more naturally and comfortably. She exchanges this discomfort for another, however, as the weight of the gravid uterus places increased strain on ligaments and muscles of the thigh and back, thus causing the low back ache and leg cramps frequently associated with late pregnancy.

Cardiovascular changes are manifested in the increase of total body water, the 25% to 40% increase of blood plasma and blood volume, the subsequent increased cardiac output, and the physiological cardiac displacement and murmurs found during pregnancy. Hemodilution is responsible for decreased hemoglobin, while the red blood cell mass is actually augmented by 10% to 15% after the eighth week of pregnancy, resulting in a "pseudoanemia" of pregnancy (Jensen et al., 1977).

Changes in the endocrine system, in the gastrointestinal system, in the urinary system, and in the metabolism are equally as dramatic, requiring adaptation while providing for increased fetal demands.

Labor, the physiological process by which the products of conception are expelled from the uterus and vagina, is involuntary and represents expenditure of both muscular and psychic energy. The new mother comes to the postdelivery experience fatigued both biologically and emotionally.

It is significant that the new mother comes to a new role (motherhood) with a new set of tasks and expectations, and with no time period of physiological or psychological rest. Encounters with her infant during the ever-shortening hospitalization period are frequently brief and accompanied by new responsibilities for which she may have little preparation or experience. During the difficult and critical period following dismissal from the hospital, there is a notable absence of professional help for the new mother.

PREGNANCY: A PSYCHOLOGICAL PHENOMENON

Consideration of the biological phenomenon of childbearing alone tends to dismiss the massive internal psychological, experiential nature of pregnancy. Pregnancy, often viewed as a transitional state superimposed upon an individual's existent life style, has been described both as a crisis and as a developmental process.

Viewed as a crisis, pregnancy places in delicate balance the interaction between physiological and psychological functioning. These activities are influenced by the woman's personality as well as by the sociocultural and economic forces present. Caplan (1957) suggests that the success with which these forces are balanced may have a lasting effect in "any area of functioning of the mother and her family and may determine to a large degree the quality of her mental health as well as that of her baby, her husband and her other children" (Caplan, 1957, p. 25).

Pregnancy is inherently disruptive and may temporarily impair the individual's usual capacity to cope with changing environmental stresses.

Viewed as a developmental process, pregnancy carries with it tasks that assist the woman to take on her new role as mother of a child. Caplan (1976) suggests two tasks of the pregnant woman: (1) acceptance of the pregnancy and (2) perception of the fetus as an individual.

Clark (1976) identifies four tasks of pregnancy: (1) pregnancy validation, (2) fetal embodiment, (3) fetal distinction, and (4) role transition. Fetal embodiment involves the "incorporation of the fetus into the body image," while fetal distinction involves "viewing the fetus as an individual being, separate from self."

Such massive psychological tasks are indeed extensive, as are the biological changes of the maternal body, yet they are only infrequently given planned emphasis by health care personnel. These maternal tasks, which Rubin (1975) calls "pregnancy work," facilitate the attainment of the maternal role—a "continuous process of which the underlying motive is the wish or the intent to become." Maternal tasks described by Rubin (1975) are (1) "seeking safe passage for herself and her child," (2) "ensuring the acceptance of the child . . . by significant persons in her family," (3) "binding-in to her unknown child," and (4) "learning to give of herself" (Rubin, 1975). These intertwining, cognitive, nonsequential tasks involve seeking prenatal care, protecting herself and her unborn child from external threats, and the complex process of establishing a relationship with her child. Additionally she assists significant others to accept this unknown being.

In considering the tasks of pregnancy, as described by several authors, both similarities and differences are noted. Within the framework of the tasks of pregnancy, what are the concerns of the pregnant woman as she begins a pregnancy, gradually grows into the role of mother, and gains knowledge of herself and her baby?

When a woman first suspects or wonders about a possible pregnancy she faces many feelings and emotions. She may be happy or sad at the prospect of being pregnant. She may be confident of her ability as a prospective mother or terrified of the responsibilities to be

faced. Whatever the reaction, she works through the acceptance of the pregnancy and/or child to some resolution during the pregnancy. It is of primary importance to her that others recognize and accept her pregnant state also. The approval of the father of the child has considerable influence upon her own emotional state. His pleasure or disapproval of the idea of the child that they have conceived reflects personally upon the woman's acceptance of the pregnant state. Dependent upon his reaction, the woman may be proud of "their" pregnancy or ashamed of the situation "she" has provoked.

Early in the pregnancy the woman seeks confirmation of the pregnancy from a professional health care giver. She then places herself in a rather dependent position for a period of time in a relationship with a physician, nurse, and/or midwife. The choice of health care provider may be the result of careful consideration of qualifications, convenience, or indifference. Once under professional health supervision the concerned mother-to-be does the recommended things: she maintains nutrition to meet the needs of the developing fetus; guards her own health, which directly influences the well-being of the infant; and takes prescribed medications while avoiding others to gain optimum development of the baby. She maintains close contact with the health supervisor, making regular visits and watching for any indications that all is not progressing normally. The expectant mother also protects her pregnancy by behaving as a pregnant woman should—in ways acceptable to her cultural group. She may limit social activities, for example, if pregnant women are viewed as less social by her group.

The focus upon the fetus as a being separate from the woman herself begins about mid-pregnancy with the perception of fetal movement. The sensation of quickening emphasizes to the woman that *someone else* is causing movement within her own body. This someone may be perceived as an aggressive intruder or as a welcome boarder in the uterus. This stranger may be desired, but the process of getting acquainted must take place initially. The woman becomes accustomed to the pattern of movement of the fetus and to the response of the baby to her levels of activity or to stimuli from the environment. Generally this period of prenatal acquaintance hastens postnatal attachment or bonding. The fetus gradually becomes, in her mind, first "a" child, then "her" child, and finally "their" child. Another concern of the woman, as the pregnancy progresses, is her ability to have a "good" pregnancy. This ability includes staying healthy while carrying out her usual pattern of life—job, housework, and attention to her husband. Her success with these multiple roles aids in her growing acceptance of her situation and the approval of significant others, particularly her husband. With acceptance and approval, the woman tries to ensure that the child will be welcomed, with the reservation that the child is as expected: right sex, right weight—perfection.

While the woman undergoes many psychological adjustments in her pregnancy, she also experiences many physical adjustments. Her own internal environment becomes the fetus or baby's external environment. She actually shares her body systems. The food that the mother consumes provides the essential nutrients for the fetus. The very air breathed by the mother provides oxygen for the fetus. To transport this food and oxygen, the circulatory system of the mother is required to expand and circulate to the uterus and thus to the baby. Not yet is the baby satisfied: he also requires that his wastes be eliminated through her circulatory system. Enormous demands are made upon the endocrine system for changes and adjustments in hormone production.

In addition to the support systems providing the fetus with life itself, space is required from the mother. The pregnancy requires that she share her body in a very intimate way. This is not a brief, momentary sharing as in sexual intimacy. Rather, it is a sharing of her body and its functions for almost a year.

Pregnant women often describe a sense of inner peace or equilibrium as a balance of mutual needs (hers and those of the fetus) is established. A feeling of complacency, sometimes of isolation, is not uncommon. The labor and delivery process, however, interrupts the status quo of the pregnant state. Reserve energy is called upon as the muscular action of the woman delivers the infant. With the delivery, the woman gives up the pregnancy, which may have become the center of her life. She must now share the baby with others. The loss of the pregnancy and fetus as a part of herself is described by some mothers as leaving them with a feeling of emptiness and sadness.

After birth the new mother has different concerns as she adjusts physically and psychologically to a new state of being. She must share her time as her sleep, activities, and routines are interrupted. If she is breastfeeding, she shares her body again. The baby moves into her home, perhaps into her room, even into her bed. Her ability to give of self is again taxed. Her energy, her space, her emotions—all are demanded of the woman who has just experienced massive physical changes. Pregnancy, childbirth, and now involution cover a time span of about 12 months of continual and different changes. Physically depleted and emotionally drained, she must meet the needs of this child who is once again dependent upon her for his very life needs. Others may need her as well. Her husband, her other children, or her parents may have need of her. Economics or need for success or recognition may require employment, another dimension of concerns.

SUMMARY

The focus of this discussion has been the inward aspect of pregnancy as the mother views herself and her pregnancy with its personal impact upon her and her immediate family system. Millions of pregnancies and births have a further impact upon society and the future of mankind.

Another view that might be explored is the effect that society has upon each pregnancy and birth. Discussion on the future of society can only be conjectured as we try to shape the factors that contribute to a positive outcome. The following factors are of importance:

1. The parents of any child should be healthy, both physically and mentally. The genes that combine to create a new person should be as free as possible from predictable disorders. Many people believe that a gene pool truly free from defects does not exist. The health of the mother is especially important since she becomes the major part of the fetus' external environment. Her mental health is significant both prenatally and postpartally as it influences her care and the nurturance of the baby before and after birth.

2. The parents of any child should live in a safe environment. The environment should provide for essentials such as food, air, water, and a shelter that is not only adequate but free from pollution, overcrowding, and pathological levels of stress.

3. Prenatal care, including health supervision, is essential for all pregnant women. There is some disagreement as to what constitutes satisfactory prenatal care and what method of health care elivery is most effective. As the criteria of care are established and provided, these questions of the health care giver may be answered.

4. Education of the public regarding the rights of childbearing parents and their infants is a major task. There is continued increase of our information on the health-illness continuum as well as on treatment of pathological conditions. Prenatal diagnosis of various fetal conditions is now a reality. Geneticists and philosphers engage in theoretical discussions relating to such topics as in vitro fertilization even as it is becoming realized.

Nurses, as health care givers and members of society, have a role to play in assisting the pregnant woman and her developing family to meet their goals and to make a contribution to society. Many of the changes and tasks of pregnancy are internalized and can be achieved only by the woman herself or within her immediate family. Nurses can assist by providing support and environmental controls within their scope and power of function. Contact time with the expectant family has been limited and sporadic, providing little opportunity to develop long-lasting, effective, supportive relationships. Acute care by nurses during labor, delivery, and the immediate puerperium has been the best-defined role and relationship. Follow-up care during the critical first month after delivery has been almost nonexistent. If the scope of health care is to provide preventative health maintenance and nurses are to participate in such health care, then nursing goals, responsibilities, and functions must also expand to include these concerns.

References

Caplan, G.: Psychosocial aspects of maternity care, Am. J. Public Health **47:**25-31, 1957.
Caplan, G.: Psychosocial aspects of pregnancy. In Clark, A. L. and Affonso, D. D.: Childbearing: a nursing perspective, Philadelphia, 1976, F. A. Davis Co.
Clark, A. L., and Affonso, D. D.: Childbearing: a nursing perspective, Philadelphia, 1976, F. A. Davis Co.
Howells, J. G.: Childbirth is a family experience. In Howells, J. G., ed.: Modern perspectives in psycho-obstetrics, New York, 1972, Brunner/Mazel, Inc.
Jensen, M. D., Benson, R. C., and Bobak, I. M.: Maternity care: the nurse and the family, St. Louis, 1977, The C. V. Mosby Co.
Leininger, M.: Cultural diversities of health and nursing care, Nurs. Clin. North Am. **12:**5-18, March 1977.
Rubin, R.: Attainment of the maternal role. Part 1. Processes, Nurs. Res. **16:**237-245, 1967a.
Rubin, R.: Attainment of the maternal role. Part 2. Models and referrants, Nurs. Res. **16:**324-346, 1967b.
Rubin, R.: Maternal tasks in pregnancy, Maternal-Child Nurs. J. **4:**143-153, 1975.

CHAPTER 6

Human development program: facilitating the child-environment relationship

JEANETTE LANCASTER

PREVENTION: A COMMUNITY MENTAL HEALTH CONCEPT

The application of primary prevention concepts relative to mental and emotional health have been described, applied, and criticized since the early 1950s. Two major national programs have generated enthusiasm for and support of community mental health. In 1963 President John F. Kennedy's endorsement of a "bold new approach to bring psychiatry back into the mainstream of medicine and community life" (Rubins, 1971) led to the allocation of a vast amount of financial support for community mental health.

Subsequently in 1978 the Report of the President's Commission on Mental Health highlighted the still prevalent need for primary prevention particularly to underserved, vulnerable populations. The principal recommendation of the Report called for the establishment of a new federal grant program for community mental health services to encourage the creation of necessary services where they are inadequate and increase the flexibility of communities in planning a comprehensive network of services (MH-MR Report, 1978).

Specifically the Commission selected children as the population with the greatest need regarding primary prevention.

While few mental health care providers would disagree that primary prevention is an important component of a total community-based program, the actual implementation of effective, viable programs has received tremendous criticism. The most common criticism of primary prevention is that only the setting has changed. Critics contend that a one-to-one clinical ideology has merely been translated from a secondary to a primary setting.

If primary prevention is going to "stand up and be noticed" as an essential mode of effecting mental health, then high-risk populations must be identified so that preventive services can be instituted before mental health is disrupted. The goal is to strike a balance between the level of stressors and the supports available to each individual.

Community mental health acknowledges the root of most emotional disruption as occurring within a network of interacting systems. A systems approach to mental health holds that each person's health status is determined by the interaction between the internal environment and the external multienvironments in which he lives. Since each human being is an open system in continuous interaction with the environment, components of the social system such as school, work, church, and family play a significant part in emotional development.

In order to establish an effective program for

primary prevention it is essential to seek a marriage between public health and mental health concepts. Public health ideology calls attention to the importance of environmental factors in the adaptation of individuals within a given population. To intervene in environmental factors, efforts need to be instituted prior to the onset of disease or health disruption to detect vulnerable or at-risk populations and subsequently either avoid the stressors or build coping resistance. The classical epidemiological triad graphically depicts the role of the environment in health promotion. In this model, environment includes physical, biological, and sociocultural forces.

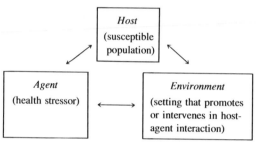

Epidemiological triad

An array of explanations provides support for focusing primary preventive efforts toward children from birth until adolescence. The changing character of the American family imposes a number of potential stresses on the developing child. The annual rate of family mobility dictates that, yearly, approximately 20% of American families will need to adapt to new external environments. Generally a family move means a new job for one or both parents, a new school for the children, and new friends and social groups for the entire family. Mobility may also necessitate adjustment to a different climate and size of community as well as new customs and beliefs within the peer groups.

Also as more mothers move into the labor force children are affected. The mother's work may influence the foods served, quantity of after-school and daytime attention, as well as the number of chores the child is expected to accomplish. While none of these factors necessarily has a negative effect, their onset does represent a change when the mother has not previously been employed. These same factors may occur when parents divorce. The family changes that occur subsequent to a divorce may include additional emotional stress as each family member attempts to adjust to a new role.

Any program that seeks to provide primary preventive community mental health services must provide an opportunity for the target population to learn new ways of responding to environmental stressors. Below a preventive ap-

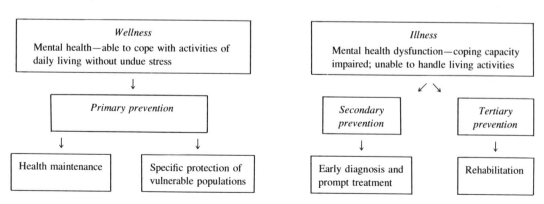

Wellness-illness mental health continuum

proach is depicted that promotes positive emotional development by strengthening the wellness component of the wellness-illness continuum through the creation of a system change in the area of interpersonal communication. According to Caplan (1974) primary prevention is described as

reducing the incidence of new cases of mental disorder in the population by combatting harmful forces which operate in the community and by strengthening the capacity of people to withstand stress.

Specifically, primary prevention is directed toward aggregates of people, not individuals. Each primary prevention program should seek to accomplish a specific goal for a designated population or aggregate. Caplan (1974) describes the mental disorder rate in a given population as being related to the interaction of both long-term and short-term forces impinging on the adaptability of members. The short-term component is illustrated by crisis intervention strategies, while the long term aspect refers to providing physical, psychological, and sociocultural resources. Physical resources include food, shelter, and clothing; psychosocial resources serve to stimulate both intellectual and emotional development through interaction with significant others; values, beliefs, and customs of the social group influence human development and thus constitute sociocultural resources. One group interaction format, the Human Development Program (HDP), provides primary prevention to children via psychosocial and sociocultural resources.

HUMAN DEVELOPMENT PROGRAM: OVERVIEW

The HDP is considered ecological in scope in that it provides organized, sequential opportunities for children to practice interactions with the human and nonhuman environments.

In the HDP children practice productive ways of responding to others.

The HDP was developed because psychologist Harold Bessell (1973) in La Jolla, California, noted that the adults he worked with had a core of basic deficiencies: lack of awareness of motives influencing behavior; absence of self-confidence, and limited understanding of how and why people react to each other. He wanted to develop a preventive program to assure normal, healthy emotional growth, just as a preventive diet program ensures the development of children who are physically healthy. Working with educator Uvaldo Palomares, Bessell developed a program focusing on the areas of awareness (knowing one's thoughts, feelings, and actions), mastery (knowing one's abilities and how to use them), and social interaction (knowing other people). Bessell believed that adults in need of therapy ask, and answer for themselves, three questions: "Will I get hurt?" (Yes), "Will I fail?" (Yes), and "Will I be accepted?" (No). Rather than being realistic appraisals, these pessimistic answers are learned (Bessell, 1973).

The personality-development theory of Horney (1950) is foundational to the HDP. Horney describes man as having an inherent drive toward the mastery of tasks and subsequent approval for his performance. She emphasizes that the competent, accepted child has the ability to develop a positive self-concept. The HDP also integrated Sullivan's (1947) description of the "delusion of uniqueness" into its theory base. Sullivan states that each person thinks he is different from, and inferior to, other people. In HDP groups, known by the children as Magic Circle, each child has an opportunity to carefully consider and discuss how he is similar to, or differs from, every other person.

The program is based on the idea that positive human interactions can be a powerful force in making life meaningful and that a certain amount of structure can be employed to guide and enhance the interactions (Ball, 1974).

The aim of the program is to prevent emotional problems by developing in each person a set of positive adaptive skills to cope with stressful situations (Bessell, 1972).

The HDP provides a vehicle for aiding the enhancement of a healthy self-concept through the leader-student relationship. The curriculum is designed for daily use to teach affective vocabulary by helping children name and discuss their feelings and by identifying the behaviors of others (Nadler, 1973).

MAGIC CIRCLE

The Magic Circle, or circle session, provides the ''core of the HDP.'' The leader and from 7 to 15 children sit in a circle so that each person can see everyone else. The circle was named ''Magic Circle'' after an enthusiastic participant described a session by declaring, ''Gee, this is just like magic'' (Ball, 1974). An atmosphere of acceptance and active listening prevails throughout the 20- to 30-minute session.

Regardless of setting—school, day care center, or residential living area—the format remains the same. Participants are encouraged to share their feelings as they learn to listen and give their attention to each other.

The role of the leader is to begin the session by explaining the topic for discussion and by taking a turn speaking on the topic. The leader may go first and talk until a child speaks up or may take a turn later. After each child who wishes to do so speaks, the leader begins the review, summarizing what has been learned in the session. As with the first, or participant, phase the leader begins by encouraging input from each child. As the sessions continue the leader becomes a less active participant encouraging the children to assume more responsibility.

Circle sessions are conducted in a structured environment. Seven specific guidelines must be followed for the session to be considered a Magic Circle:

1. Everyone gets a turn to respond to the daily topic.
2. One can skip a turn if he wants to.
3. There are no put-downs, interpretations, or analyses of responses.
4. Time is shared equally.
5. The speaker is listened to.
6. Everyone stays in his own space (floor or chair).
7. No gossip is permitted (Human Development Training Institute, 1976).

The program is based on the concepts that positive human interaction can be a powerful force in making life meaningful and that a certain amount and type of structure is useful in guiding the quality of interactions that occur. To facilitate these concepts, the HDP follows a defined structure for implementation.

As a curriculum the HDP presents a series of sequentially developed topics relating to issues of everyday living. The program capitalizes on the desire of children to speak and to seek attention, to win approval, and to gain a better understanding of themselves and their world (Ball, 1974). Enough structure is provided to assure that important concepts are dealt with systematically in an atmosphere where the ground rules are understood. The curriculum is designed for 6-week units, which alternate the three basic themes of awareness, mastery, and social interaction (Henri, 1972). Participants are encouraged to speak from their own experience. What each one says is accepted; no one is supposed to be probed, criticized, or confronted in any way, and no one moralizes to anyone else. In this way each person is valued either for speaking or for listening during the session. The structured group process carried out in the circle differs from other types of groups, such as sensitivity, psychotherapy, or encounter groups, in that negative criticism, acting out, or damaging interaction is prohibited (Henri, 1972).

The HDP believes that behavior and attitudes are learned and that each person needs to be listened to and understood to promote growth and emotional development.

THEORETICAL BASE

The HDP is based on the theoretical assumptions that each person needs to get attention, to be listened to, and to understand the reason for doing what he is asked to do (Human Development Training Institute, 1976). The need for attention is met during the initial phase of each circle session when the curriculum's topic for the day is discussed; the need to be listened to is met specifically during the second, or "review" phase of the session when each child tries to explain what another participant has said. If the children do not listen during the participating, or initial, phase, the review session is ineffective. During the third phase of each session, the summary, the need to understand the reason for doing what he was asked to do is met.

The program describes each person's need for appreciation, acceptance, approval, and affection. It is anticipated that these needs can be met in the circle session once the children are comfortable with one another. Initially participants seem self-centered and unable to relate to one another effectively; each child works to meet his own needs and often fails to recognize or listen to others.

The content of the HDP relates to three theoretical areas: awareness, mastery, and social interaction.

Awareness

Awareness is considered a vital component of mental health. People who are aware usually know a great deal about what is going on inside themselves as well as in the world around them. According to Gordon (1961), the psychologically healthy person is one who is "in touch with himself and is aware of his feelings, attitudes, values, and beliefs. This person is more in communication with himself than is the psychologically unhealthy person."

Often a person is aware of what he thinks but is much less aware of his feelings. For some, negative feelings are unacceptable, whereas positive feelings are highly acceptable. The HDP attempts to demonstrate experientially to children that all people have positive and negative feelings and that these feelings are not to be judged as either bad or good (Ball, 1974).

By sharing experiences, each child has an opportunity to observe that others think, feel, and behave in similar ways. A child can learn that others in the group are much more like him than they are different from him (Bessell, 1968). Some children handle feelings in ways that run counter to that which society expects of them or in ways that are harmful. For example, an angry child may hit another person, back away, and feel anger and resentment; he may on the other hand learn to talk with the recipient of his anger. The circle provides a place where children can practice positive ways of handling feelings and impulses and of observing how others react. Positive reinforcement is received through successes at every session (Bessell, 1968).

At age 6 children typically are open and expressive with their thoughts and feelings; soon after entering first grade many learn to bury or mask thoughts and feelings. They observe in school that most people do not talk about fantasies, dreams, and wishes, and they subsequently decide that it is better if some things are left unsaid.

Awareness objectives in the curriculum teach children a language that can be used to express thoughts and feelings. The children also practice listening to what others say. Moreover, a child who learns at an early age about his secret thoughts, feelings, and fantasies is less likely to act them out (Helfat, 1973). One cue, "something that I am afraid of," is particularly useful for both awareness and social interaction: one child thinks of his fear but does not state it aloud, and another child tries to guess what his friend actually fears.

Additional awareness cues include the following:

1. Having good feelings
2. Something that caused me to feel bad
3. If I could do (have) anything I wanted

Mastery

Effective people have an ample amount of self-esteem and a feeling of mastery; they often perceive themselves as being "okay." They are willing to try new experiences and do not strongly anticipate or fear failure. Generally a person who believes in himself and appreciates his abilities succeeds, with each success leading to further self-appreciation.

The HDP calls the belief in oneself a feeling of "I canness," and it is the goal of the mastery sessions to provide each child with a feeling of accomplishment. The task itself is not the focus; rather it is a vehicle designed to give children "deserved-positive feedback" immediately after a success experience and at an important time — when his peers are present. In these sessions each child is encouraged to share with the group his accomplishments and successes that occur outside the session. Children talk about "when I had a hard time choosing between," "what happened when I did not use self-control," "something I just learned how to do," and "I made a promise and kept it." Cues focus on times when mastery had both positive and negative impacts.

Social interaction

Relating effectively to others is a challenge constantly facing each person. Some children are able to relate effectively by perceiving the moods of others and responding accordingly. The units on social interaction familiarize each child with the basic issues in interpersonal relationship and communication. Children learn about causality in human relationships when they talk about "I made a promise and kept it (but did not keep it)," "someone did something that I liked (did not like)," and "I got help

that I did not want." In order to learn, the child usually turns to the adults in his environment as the source of knowledge regarding the shoulds and should nots. The program stresses that each child has an innate potential for both aggression and nurturance. During a circle session children can test ways of dealing with aggressive as well as with positive and nurturant feelings.

Consistent with the concept that each child needs attention and recognition, the seating arrangement in the circle provides an opportunity for each child to face the others, thereby improving both verbal and nonverbal communication. A child needs acceptance if he is to function effectively in social interactions. On the premise that acceptance implies the absence of evaluative judgments, the HDP emphasizes recognition of each child as a unique individual and acceptance as such. A third need having a direct influence on social interaction is approval. A child needs to receive approval for the acceptable things he does. Frequently people focus on what one does wrong and fail to give notice to the things he does correctly. It is the leader's responsibility to help circle members recognize how they affect others as well as to recognize that each situation provides an opportunity to make choices in behavioral responses.

Children thrive on affection, another integral component of social interaction. A smile, a pat on the shoulder, or a friendly comment conveys a sense of affection. The HDP provides through the circle sessions a structure in which a child can receive attention, acceptance, approval, and affection. Moreover, the child has a safe place in which to discuss with a group which aggressive thoughts and actions are suitable for display and which need to be modified or rechanneled.

The opportunity provided in the circles for children to reflect the feelings of others can help each child develop the ability to identify and articulate feelings (Gerler, 1973). In addition, when a child receives verbal and non-verbal approval for recognizing the feelings of others, his self-confidence may be enhanced.

IMPLEMENTING THE CIRCLES

Not every circle evidences a semblance of "magic." For a variety of reasons some children do not listen, sit still, or respond to the daily cue. Also, the nature of the environment affects the focus of children's attention. If there are present a number of stimulants such as toys, books, or other people in the vicinity, children are more apt to be distracted from the daily topic. The following are some basic guides for implementing circles:

1. Morning hours are generally preferable in that more energy is available for responding to the topic.
2. The group composition should ideally represent a small age span so that children will be at approximately the same developmental level.
3. It helps to avoid having siblings in the same group; they may get involved in arguing about "what really happened."

Although Magic Circle differs from other forms of group therapy in that it avoids such approaches as confrontation or probing, a number of basic group-process skills however are used to facilitate the sessions. The techniques of encouraging active listening, focusing on feelings, providing recognition of the contributions of each member, paraphrasing, reviewing, focusing on similarities and differences, actively involving each member in the session, and transferring leadership from the adult leader to child leaders are clearly useful in these circle sessions.

Active listening

The leader can say, "I hear you," in both verbal and nonverbal ways. When the leader maintains eye contact with the speaker, nods, or leans toward the speaker, he or she conveys the message that the child is heard. The leader may also demonstrate active listening by a smile or pat on the child's shoulder in response to his comments as well as by the verbal techniques of asking open-ended questions that clearly define what was said or by asking the child to elaborate or clarify. Active listening may include *focusing on feelings*. Many children couch feeling responses in between more concrete expressions. A child may also indicate how he feels about a topic by what he avoids saying.

Providing recognition

It is critical for the enhancement of self-concept that the leader learn each child's name as soon as possible. The leader can recognize a member's contribution by a smile, direct eye contact, a gentle pat on the arm, or by verbally expressing appreciation. Recognition of non-verbal responses such as when a child smiles in agreement or frowns in dissent acknowledges that the leader both recognizes and values each response.

Paraphrasing and review

Paraphrasing and review by the leader or preferably by one of the children provide checkpoints for the group and aid in keeping to the topic. Whenever possible, paraphrasing should use some of the child's own words so as to keep the meaning closely related to the original description. Paraphrasing provides the speaker with almost immediate recognition that he was heard.

Initially the leader may do all of the reviewing. As soon as group members become familiar with the review process they can profit from active participation in this process. Reviewing serves as a mechanism to take stock of the group's progress; it often brings digressive discussion back to the original topic.

Involving everyone

Frequently a few children in each circle are significantly quieter and more hesitant than the majority of the membership. Observation of nonverbal indicators can be helpful for drawing quiet members into the group. A child may sit forward when he wants to speak, frown when he disagrees, or smile when he agrees. Often a quiet child can be drawn into active involvement by asking if another member may guess how he would answer the cue. For example, "Joe, may Tom try to guess what makes you feel good?" Once a child agrees to participate in the guessing, he is likely to continue active involvement.

The child who overparticipates needs as much attention as the hesitant one. The leader can acknowledge his contributions and simultaneously note that others would like a turn.

Transferring group leadership

Initially the adult provides circle leadership. Once members become aware of the process of the Magic Circle, leadership can be transferred both informally as well as formally. The leader can first share leadership by asking the members if anyone has questions for someone else and by encouraging spontaneous reactions to what is said. The next step is to formally turn the leadership over to a member during a session. The leader may notice that some children have begun to model leader behavior. Once a child assumes the leadership role it is essential for the leader to recognize his contribution and provide a helpful critique. The leader remains in the circle but intervenes only when a disaster seems imminent.

OBSTACLES TO CIRCLE PROGRESS

Not every circle seems to have "magic." Some days children have a difficult time sitting still because they are tired, irritable, bored, or overly stimulated by the environment. Toys or other people in the immediate area may be distracting. Mornings are preferable to afternoons in that children are less tired earlier in the day. Of course it is unreasonable to expect a group of children to sit perfectly still for any great

length of time any time of day. While it is impossible to think of every potential problem in advance of the sessions, it is helpful to describe some typical disruptive situations so that leaders can anticipate likely responses. A variety of situations that necessitate leader intervention are described.

Copying

Occasionally children are unable to come up with original responses to a particular cue. The daily cue might be "someplace I like to go," and the first four children may say they like to go to the ice cream store. Undoubtedly each one does enjoy such an outing, but the last three may be also saying, "I am afraid no one will like what I think so I'll just use Tommy's comment because everyone liked it." The leader can handle copying by asking the participants to further elaborate on their responses such as, "What kind of ice cream do you prefer?" or "What is it about ice cream that you like—its texture, taste, temperature?" Children may copy the responses of others when they are afraid their comments will be rejected.

Rambling

Some children attempt to retain the group's attention by rambling on, yet actually saying little. These children often desperately want the group's attention but may lack conversational skills. A child may also be afraid that if he relinquishes the focal spot the other members will not notice him again in the future. Each child should be offered a turn during each session although he may repeatedly ask to be passed by.

Nonlistening

Children who listen neither to each other nor to the leader disrupt smooth circle functioning. During each session the leader models listening regardless of who is speaking. Often when a person does not listen to others he is having difficulty focusing on someone besides himself. When nonlistening becomes a pattern for a member, the leader can help the child practice alternative ways of gaining attention. The leader may ask the nonlistener to paraphrase or review the session. Of course the drawback here is that the leader may need to provide him with enough information to accomplish this activity: because of his own excessive talking he may actually have heard very little of what was said. By allowing the talkative child to paraphrase or review, the focus remains on the comments of the original speaker while the leader is simultaneously responding to the nonlistener. Other techniques include responding to the child who is having difficulty listening by providing attention in the form of touching him: the leader may put an arm around him, or if he is small enough, suggest that the child sit in the leader's lap. Since his nonverbal message is, "I feel left out," or, "I only know how to get attention by being disruptive," he requires additional support, although not at the expense of other participants.

Gaining good feelings from unacceptable behavior

Typically in any circle there emerges over time at least one child who describes how he gets pleasure from unacceptable actions towards others, especially siblings. It is not uncommon for a child to respond to the cue "what makes me feel good" by saying, "I really feel good when I hit my sister (or brother)." It is the leader's responsibility to focus on the feeling rather than to encourage elaboration on the unacceptable action. One approach is to ask the child to consider how his sister feels when he hits her. By doing this the child has an opportunity to examine the effect he has on others as well as to consider alternative ways of behaving. The leader can also help the child think about ways to gain power that do not run contrary to societal expectations.

Ignored members

Another problem arises when some members of the group are ignored by the majority. In any social setting such as a school, day care center, or children's residential institution there are those who are considered "low on the totem pole." Children are ostracized for a variety of reasons including their personal appearance, clothes, behavior, or where they live. Others in the group may hesitate to talk with these children lest their own social status be affected. The leader may encourage a member who is both empathetic toward others and highly regarded by the group to clarify what the isolated child says once he risks participating. The leader may need to try particularly hard to involve the isolated child such as by noting his nonverbal responses as a way of drawing him into the conversation.

SUMMARY

Each person defines himself as the result of a multitude of social exchanges. The reflected appraisals of significant other people either enhance or negate a person's self-concept. Participation in Magic Circle sessions seems to serve as an organized and sequentially implemented environment for providing an arena for self-evaluation.

Perhaps the reactions of children aged 8 to 12 in a summer day camp who met three times weekly summarizes the purpose of the HDP. Each child was asked to respond in writing to "Magic Circle is. . . ." Some said it was fun and none responded in a negative manner. One 9-year-old girl said, "Magic Circle is fun because we get to know us." Her contributions during the 2-month, 3-day-a-week circle program had centered largely on events at home and how she had dealt with them. She shared positive behavior as well as instances causing discomfort to family members and feelings of remorse for her. Another 9-year-old girl responded, "Magic Circle is fun because I tell my friends at home about things and all they say is 'so.' I don't care if they don't listen because people listen in Magic Circle.'' A third reaction by a 9-year-old girl was, ''Magic Circle is fun because you talk about things that you need to let out that are in you.''

Magic Circle participation provides an avenue for supporting a positive self-perception; it also provides opportunities for both the leader and the children to intervene in a negative self-evaluation by consistently accepting and reinforcing each contribution.

References

Ball, G.: Magic Circle: an overview of the human development program, La Mesa, Calif., 1974, Human Development Training Institute.

Bessell, H.: The content is the medium: the confidence is the message, Psychology Today **1:**73-76, 1968.

Bessell, H.: Human development in the classroom. In Solloman, L., and Berzon, B., eds.: New perspectives in encounter groups, San Francisco, 1972, Jossey-Bass, Inc., Publishers.

Bessell, H.: Methods in human development, La Mesa, Calif., 1973, Human Development Training Institute.

Caplan, G.: Support systems and community mental health, New York, 1974, Behavioral Publications.

Gerler, E.: The magic circle program: how to improve teachers. Elementary Sch. Guidance Counseling J. **8:**86-91, 1973.

Gordon, T.: Risks in effective communication, Natl. Train. Lab Hum. Rel. Train. News **4:**4, 1961.

Helfat, L.: The gut level needs of kids, Learning **2:**77-80, October 1973.

Henri, S.: Human Development Program Report, Washington, D.C., Office of Education.

Horney, K.: Neurosis and human growth, New York, 1950, W. W. Norton & Co., Inc.

MH-MR Report: A Morris Associates report from Washington, May 5, 1978, **15:**1-8.

Human Development Training Institute: Magic circle/human development program basic training workshop, La Mesa, Calif., 1976.

Nadler, D.: Affecting the learning climates through magic circles, Elem. Sch. Guid. Counsel. J. **8:**107-111, 1973.

Rubins, J. L.: The community mental health movement in the United States: circa, 1970, Am. J. Psychoanal. **31:**68-79, 1971.

Sullivan, J. S.: Conceptions of modern psychiatry, Washington, 1947, William Alanson White Psychiatric Foundation, Inc.

CHAPTER 7

An ecological view of gerontological mental health

BARBARA S. HENTHORN

ECOLOGICAL CONCEPTS

The elderly are an at-risk population for mental health problems. Suicide and mental hospitalization occur between two and four times more frequently for the aged, proof that there is significant stress in old age (Rosow, 1973). The most complex phenomenon that the elderly encounter today is rapid change. Although medical advances have enabled the individual to live longer, change, stress, and technology have taken their toll. Older people have to adapt to new and mostly unfavorable situations at a time in life when the capacity for adjustment decreases. Exposure to new stressful situations as well as the cumulative effect of many stresses and deprivations over a long period of time may lead to psychological breakdown (Kral, 1973; Simon, 1970; Braceland, 1972).

Gerontological mental health can be promoted by using an ecological perspective to identify those mental health environmental resources (physical, psychosocial, and sociocultural) that may be utilized in primary prevention efforts (Caplan and Grunebaum, 1972). The role of the helping professions in the ecological model is to help develop resources and alternatives that emphasize building and supporting the strengths of the individual and community rather than focusing on their deficits

(Rappaport, 1977). This approach is particularly useful for the elderly, many of whom experience increasing deficits in all areas. A focus on strengths and resources facilitates adaptation of older people to changes and losses that occur as part of the aging process (Butler and Lewis, 1977).

Ecological model of aging

In the ecological model aging is seen as an experience that is determined by the interaction of the aging person with his total environment. For an ecological perspective an assessment is made of the elderly person's interactions in five realms of human experience: (1) physiological, (2) physical-environmental, (3) sociocultural, (4) psychological, and (5) spiritual or philosophical (Bircher, 1972, 1973). All of these realms are both interrelated and interacting subsystems of the person's total ecosystem. For the aged, this may be called a gerontological ecosystem (Henthorn, 1975), which may be separated into the above realms for assessment and analysis. Each of these components is discussed in detail in this chapter.

Ecological view of man

The ecological view of man proposed here is based on the belief that man must be viewed in his totality, as an open system in dynamic interaction with his environment. As such, he is a self-regulating, self-actualizing, unique individual (Hoyman, 1971). Each individual is seen as striving to meet a hierarchy of needs, which would, if met, culminate in the attainment of self-actualization (Maslow, 1954). Maslow postulates that there is a universal hierarchy of needs, with the lower needs being the priority needs. Only after the lower needs are satisfied does the individual strive to meet the higher needs of safety, belongingness, self-esteem, and self-actualization. However, because each person is unique, each person's hierarchy may differ. For example, the elderly widow whose sole companion is her aging poodle may spend her limited income on dog food, even at the expense of a well-balanced diet for herself.

This ecological view of man is based on the assumption that each of the environmental subsystems contributes to meeting a basic need or cluster of needs: *physiological* (the survival needs such as oxygen, food, water, temperature, elimination, exercise, and rest), *physical-environmental* (safety and security needs), *sociocultural* (belongingness needs), *psychological* (self-esteem needs) and *spiritual philosophical* (self-actualization needs) (Bircher, 1972, 1973).

To meet these basic needs the individual is continually adapting to changes in his total environment. Successful aging, then, requires adaptation—a dynamic, active process by which the individual constructively copes with those ecological factors within each subsystem that influence the degree to which he meets his needs.

These ecological factors can be classified as adaptors—those agents, factors, or mechanisms that aid in meeting a need, that promote adaptation, or that reduce stress—and stressors—those agents, factors, or mechanisms that cause a change in some environmental factor that hinders the meeting of a need or

intensifies stress. Simply stated, adaptors are environmental resources; stressors are environmental deficits (Luckmann and Sorenson, 1974; Murray and Zentner, 1975).

The relative strength of adaptors and stressors determines the individual's position on an adaptation continuum. In this discussion health is synonymous with adaptation; illness, with maladaptation. Favorable ecological factors (adaptors) tend to push an individual toward health; unfavorable ecological factors (stressors) push him toward illness.

It is important to note that adaptation in this context does not imply a simple adjustment to, and tolerance of, environmental factors; rather it implies a creative, dynamic process. Creative adaptation implies that an individual is not exclusively a passive reactor to his environment but that he also acts upon it. Thus an individual, while shaped by his environment, has the capacity to make conscious and deliberate choices as to how he will adapt to environmental changes in order to meet his basic needs (Murrell, 1973; Dubos, 1978). To a large extent a person can choose whether he will be healthy or ill, adapted or maladapted. He has freedom of choice but is accountable for the choices he makes.

The role of the community mental health nurse is to facilitate psychosocial adaptation by helping the individual to make choices that are creative and adaptive. This requires an assessment in each subsystem of the adaptors and stressors that impinge on mental health. Alternative ways of increasing the number and/or strength of adaptors and decreasing the number and/or strength of stressors can be explored with the client. The client is encouraged to use the problem-solving process to deal with environmental changes.

The goal of the nurse who works with the aged is to maximize gerontological mental health. Gerontological mental health is essentially "a measure of each person's ability to do what he wants to do and become what he wants to become''—the essence of self-actualization (Dubos, 1978; Maslow, 1954).

Ecological principles

The community mental health nurse with an ecological perspective utilizes principles from systems theory to focus on primary prevention and promote gerontological mental health. Trickett and associates (1972) suggest four ecological principles that are useful in assessing and intervening in a particular ecosystem: (1) the principles of interdependence, (2) cycling of resources, (3) adaptation, and (4) dynamic equilibrium and succession.

Principle of interdependence. All components of an ecosystem are interrelated and interdependent. Therefore a change in any component of an ecosystem affects the relationships among all other components. These relationships may be between the living parts of the ecosystem, between the living and nonliving parts, or between the structure and function of ecosystem parts. Some of these relationships or functions are more important than others and therefore have a greater potential for affecting the entire ecosystem. The most important functions are those that are in relatively short supply but in great demand. For the gerontological ecosystem, the most important function may be that of physical health. More than 86% of the elderly have one or more chronic health problems (Butler and Lewis, 1977). Physical health is clearly tied to psychosocial adaptation. Palmore and Luikart (1972) found that self-reported health had a stronger correlation to life satisfaction than any of the other variables investigated (organizational activity, income, internal control, having a confidant, education, and sex). The person's own perception of his health was more important than how his physician rated it.

For some elderly persons, poor health alters relationships in several components of the gerontological ecosystem. Plans to travel or pursue leisure activities with spouse or friends (a way of meeting self-actualization and be- longingness needs) may be thwarted by the residual effects of a cerebrovascular accident. The stroke is an example of the ''limiting factors'' discussed by Trickett et al., which basically can be described by the old saying ''The chain is only as strong as its weakest link.''

The principle of interdependence is used in looking at the sociocultural subsystem to assess the role relationships of the individual. What are the linkages between roles? What is the social network? Which relationship can be used to provide a support system for the elderly? Can new relationships be created?

This principle also implies that one must have a good grasp of the entire ecosystem and its relationships before interventions can be implemented; that is, ''Know the system before you try to change it'' (Rappaport, 1977). Identification of the ''weak links'' in the ecosystem enables the nurse to more effectively promote psychosocial adaptation.

Principle of cycling of resources. Each gerontological ecosystem has a limited number of resources. The functioning of the ecosystem is affected by the way its resources are utilized and divided among the subsystems. For example, money is an environmental resource of the gerontological client. The client must make decisions concerning the expenditure of this money. If medical expenses are so high that most of the income must be spent to meet them, other areas will suffer. There will be insufficient funds to purchase adequate amounts of food, to engage in recreational activities, to meet a pledge to the church, and so forth. Resources are distributed based on the values of the individual.

The role of the community mental health nurse is that of helping the client to mobilize unused resources or to redistribute existing resources. Investigating the eligibility for food stamps or obtaining canned goods from a local church's ''food closet'' are two possible interventions for the client whose food resources are limited.

Principle of adaptation. The survival of an

individual depends upon his ability to creatively adapt to environmental changes. Adaptation is ecosystem specific; that is, behavior that is adaptive in one ecosystem may be maladaptive in another. For example, the nudist in a nudist camp is displaying adaptive behavior; the streaker on a college campus, maladaptive behavior. The ability to behave in appropriate or expected ways has been labeled as "ecosystem competence" (Wilkerson and O'Connor, 1977).

Adaptation is a major concept of the ecological model, and an understanding of its characteristics would guide the community mental health nurse in planning interventions. The following discussion is based on the explication of this concept by Luckmann and Sorenson (1974), Murray and Zentner (1975), Beland and Passos (1975), and Murphy (1971).

Change per se and the rate at which it occurs threaten an individual's psychosocial adaptation. Individuals and groups are able to adapt better to gradual changes than to sudden, rapid ones. In addition, the greater the number of changes occurring within a given period the more difficult it is to adapt.

Change is less stressful when it is at least partially initiated by the individual. The unprepared individual has more difficulty adapting to change than one who is prepared. For example, preparation of elderly persons for admission to a nursing home facilitates their adaptation to that environment (Brudno, 1968).

Creative adaptation can be equated with constructive coping and depends on the individual's ability to use both innate and acquired adaptive mechanisms. These mechanisms may be physiological, psychological, sociocultural, or technological in nature.

Physiological adaptive mechanisms are those compensatory changes occurring within the body in response to stress or increased or altered demands of physiological functions. They include such responses as the homeostatic mechanisms involved in the maintenance of body temperature, the general adaptation syndrome, and body defenses such as immunity. The effectiveness of these physiological mechanisms decreases with age (Shock, 1962).

Psychological adaptive mechanisms are those learned behavioral responses that aid in adjustment to such stresses as developmental crises. Learning, problem solving, and defense mechanisms (denial, projection, rationalization, regression, sublimation, and so forth) are examples of psychological adaptive mechanisms. Butler and Lewis (1977) point out that regression is used in a stereotypical way to explain the behavior of older persons, as in the common expressions "They're like little children" and "He's in his second childhood." In reality, regression may be an adaptive technique for the elderly individual whose limited resources force him into a more dependent role.

Sociocultural adaptive mechanisms include the behavior patterns by which the individual adjusts to the groups, culture, and society of which he is a member. They include adherence to prescribed social norms, role performances, and sets of values (religious, ethical, or philosophical) that guide behavior in a variety of settings. The community mental health nurse promotes these adaptive mechanisms in providing anticipatory guidance for role changes or intervening in those crisis situations that evolve from sudden role changes such as the death of a spouse.

Technological adaptive mechanisms are those scientific and industrial products and innovations by which man has freed himself from the limitations of his environment. For example, air conditioning enables the individual to adapt to a very hot environment; the pacemaker aids the slow heart beat; tranquilizers reduce the impact of emotional stresses; and the hearing aid, by amplifying the declining auditory acuities of the elderly, promotes psychosocial adaptation by decreasing the paranoia that often accompanies a hearing loss.

Individuals who use few adaptive mechanisms are limited in their ability to adapt to new and changing situations. The elderly person who has a varied repertoire of adaptive mechanisms increases his chances of survival. Appropriate crisis intervention by the community mental health nurse helps him to expand his repertoire (Aguilera and Messick, 1978).

Principle of succession. An ecosystem is never stable or static but is in a constant state of flux in response to changing environmental conditions. For the aging individual, this is illustrated by the succession of role changes throughout his life cycle. Life is characterized by a series of role exits and role entrances, such as from the student role to the worker role and from the worker to the retiree role.

If the environmental conditions are known, it is possible to predict the direction in which an ecosystem will change. For example, the adaptation of an individual to retirement can be predicted by the preparations that he has made for retirement, such as savings, pension plans and annuities, development of new skills, and plans for continued involvement in society.

The application of this principle requires looking at the changes in the ecosystem over a period of time. For the gerontological ecosystem this may be achieved by encouraging the "life review" described by Butler and Lewis (1977) in which a person reviews both his history and his current life situation.

Ecological assessment

The effectiveness of using an ecological model depends on the decisions the community mental health nurse makes about how to intervene in a gerontological ecosystem, where to intervene, how abruptly to introduce change, how rapidly to effect the change, and what the side effects may be.

The ecological perspective requires an assessment of each of the gerontological subsystems to identify the adaptors and stressors influencing the psychosocial health of the aging individual. In the following sections each environmental component is described and examples are given of ecological factors that may

interact with the at-risk elderly client and produce mental health problems by limiting his ability to meet his basic needs.

PHYSIOLOGICAL SUBSYSTEM
Physiological changes of aging

Many phsiological changes of aging affect the interaction of the elderly individual with his environment. Changes in physical appearance, decreased sensory acuity, and changes in the cardiorespiratory, neurological, and genitourinary systems have the most potential for affecting psychosocial adaptation.

Physical appearance. Changes in body appearance are the most obvious indicators that one is growing old. Atrophy of the hair follicles leads to graying and thinning of the hair. The skin becomes wrinkled from the loss of elasticity and shrinkage of sucutaneous tissue. There is increased pigmentation of the skin, with the resultant yellow and brown spots so aptly called "age spots" by the layman. Senile warts (seborrheic hyperkeratoses) appear with increasing frequency after 50 years of age. Decreased peripheral blood supply causes fingernails and toe nails to become thicker and more brittle, a condition that is accentuated if a fungus infection develops. The result is the common "ram's horn" toenail of the elderly. Increased fragility of dermal and subcutaneous vessels leads to multiple ecchymoses. Decreased production of sexual hormones increases the amount of facial hair in the elderly female. Between 20 and 70 years there is a height loss of approximately 2 inches, usually from shortening of the vertebral column (Rossman, 1971, 1976; Hayter, 1974; Ahern, et al., 1978).

Because we live in a culture that values the physical attributes of the young, the cumulative impact of these changes in appearance often results in a lowered self-esteem for the aging individual.

Decreased sensory acuity. There are significant changes in hearing and vision. An impaired ability to hear the higher frequencies is apparent by age 50 and accelerates after age 65. Eventually there is a gradual loss in the middle range, the range of speech. The older person has increasing difficulty in discrimination between sounds, particularly the consonants s, t, f, and g. There is increased sensitivity to background noises, which tends to compound difficulties in discrimination. This distortion of auditory sounds may precipitate paranoid ideation (Butler and Lewis, 1977).

The normal vision changes that occur with aging are a decrease in visual acuity, particularly in dim illumination; a decrease in the speed of dark adaptation; loss of lens accommodation; loss of peripheral vision; lessened responsivity of the pupil to changes in light; and decreased size of the pupil (Goldman, 1971). A high percentage (68.6%) of 295 elderly nursing home residents was found by Snyder et al. (1976) to have impaired vision. Of this group 34.6% had low vision (20/100 to 20/70), and 24% were legally blind (20/200 or worse). Interestingly, these results included those residents who were tested wearing glasses. The residents were divided into three groups—adequate vision, low vision, and legally blind. Mean scores on the Mental Status Questionnaire were compared for the three groups: the legally blind group had the lowest scores; the group with adequate vision, the highest. A significant difference ($p = .033$) was found, supporting the authors' hypothesis that mental function and vision are related.

The findings of this study suggest that a primary prevention program for the aged should include vision screening with appropriate referral and followup. Such a program would require a concerted effort to develop community resources, which are vitually nonexistent for low-income individuals in many areas, especially since there is no Medicare reimbursement for eyeglasses.

Impaired taste sensation is caused by a decline in taste bud papillae (from approximately 245 in young adults to 88 in persons aged 70 to 75) and may result in a poor appetite (Shock, 1962). Inadequate food intake accelerates the aging process and adversely affects mental alertness. Vitamin deficiencies—particularly of thiamine, riboflavin, ascorbic acid, and vitamin A—are related to central nervous system dysfunction. More than 10% of older persons have deficiencies in at least three of these important vitamins (Burnside, 1976).

Cardiorespiratory system. At age 75 the heart pumps only 65% as much blood as it did at age 30 (Shock, 1962). The blood vessels elongate, become tortuous, and calcify. There is increased collagen resulting in a loss of elasticity. The lumen may be narrowed by atherosclerotic deposits. As a consequence the blood supply to vital organs is diminished.

Altered distensibility of the rib cage, weakening of the respiratory muscles, and decreased elasticity of the lungs lead to inadequate respiratory exchanges. These changes, coupled with arteriosclerotic changes in the blood vessels, increase the danger of cerebral anoxia in the elderly.

Neurological system. Cerebral anoxia contributes to the organic brain disorders found in approximately 10% of persons over age 65, and in 25% over 75 (Balabokin, 1972). Organic brain syndromes may be either chronic or acute (reversible). Common symptoms are those that typically result in the elderly being labeled as senile: impaired memory, orientation, judgment, and intellectual functions and a shallow or labile effect. The loss of memory for recent events may have both psychological and physiological causes. Current happenings may be too painful or overwhelming and therefore are denied (Butler and Lewis, 1977). From a physiological standpoint, lowered levels of oxygen or increased levels of carbon dioxide interrupt the consolidation process (the formation of a learning trace in the brain). There is increased likelihood of either condition occurring in the aged because of the physiological changes in the respiratory system previously mentioned. The lungs lose some of their elasticity, so that a decreased amount of air is exhaled, resulting in the retention of carbon dioxide. The rib cage becomes more rigid, with calcification of the costal cartilages, and the respiratory muscles become weakened. Therefore less air is inhaled, and less oxygen is obtained. The net effect of these changes is a lower blood level of oxygen and a higher level of carbon dioxide (Leukel, 1976; Rossman, 1971).

Burnside (1976) stresses the importance of differentiating between acute and chronic brain syndrome. Health professionals have a tendency to label all brain syndromes as chronic and hopeless, when many may be reversible. The presence of the following symptoms should alert the nurse to the possibility of reversible brain syndrome: (1) a fluctuation in the level of awareness, (2) hallucinations (especially if these are visual rather than auditory), (3) mistaken identification, for example, the elderly person insists that the nurse is her daughter, (4) increased anxiety and restlessness, (5) loss of remote as well as recent memory, and (6) paranoid ideation. Common causes of reversible (acute) brain syndrome are (1) congestive heart failure, (2) malnutrition and anemia, (3) fluid and electrolyte imbalance, (4) infection, (5) cerebrovascular accidents, (6) drug reactions, and (7) a dull, depressing environment (Butler and Lewis, 1977; Burnside, 1976).

Genitourinary system. Changes in the aging kidney increase the possibility that acute brain syndromes caused by drug reactions will occur. The length of time that a drug remains in the body determines its activity. This period of time is directly related to the rate of elimination, since most drugs are excreted through the kidney (Bender, 1971). Both glomerular filtration and renal blood flow are decreased in the elderly. The kidney receives only 45% as much blood at age 65 as it did at age 30 (Shock, 1962). In addition, there is a decline in the number of functioning nephrons (Rossman, 1971).

Changes in sexual functioning in older people appear to be psychological rather than physiological in nature. Coital frequency declines with age but does not completely cease for many partners. Comfort (1972, 1974) estimates that 15% of married couples over the age of 78 continue having intercourse. He suggests "The only thing age has to do with sex performance is that the longer you love the more you learn." (Comfort, 1972).

Knowledge of the physiological changes occurring with age in both sexes helps to dispel fears of losing sexual functioning. The male has fewer orgasms but no fewer erections. However spontaneous erections are less frequent, necessitating direct stimulation by the partner.

Vaginal dryness may be a problem in postmenopausal women, but this condition can easily be treated with the use of lubricants, such as K-Y jelly or contraceptive creams. Hormonal replacement therapy increases vaginal secretions, sometimes to a greater degree than in the premenopausal vagina. Comfort (1972) cautions that this increased wetness may cause decreased friction for the male partner. Unless he is forewarned, the aging male may interpret the resulting decreased sensations as a sign of impending impotence.

Continued sexual activity helps to maintain sexual functioning. Both lubrication and vaginal flexibility are better in women having intercourse at least once a week than in those having it only once a month. The disuse principle—"Use it or lose it"—applies to both sexes (Ahern et al., 1978).

Implications for nursing

An awareness of the changes in the physiological subsystem of the elderly helps the community mental health nurse to plan more effective interventions. For example, reduction in the incidence of acute brain syndrome can be achieved by careful assessment of the client's diet, fluids, and drug intake and a sensitivity to the signs of impending physical illness. Both the client with a chronic brain syndrome and the client with impaired vision or hearing syndrome may show improved behavior when placed in a therapeutic environment.

The following practical suggestions for interviewing the older client are aimed at compensating for physiological changes (Burnside, 1976; Stone, 1969):

1. Select a setting with quiet surroundings. Carpets, acoustical tile, curtains, and wall hangings help absorb sound and reduce background noise.
2. Sit where the light will shine on your face so that your lips can be readily seen by the client.
3. Use touch freely, both to get the client's attention and to communicate that you care. However, be alert to any nonverbal messages that touching is not acceptable to the client.
4. Assess how well the client can see and hear by moving closer and closer until he can both see and hear you. This may be too close for your comfort, but this should be done when it increases the client's receptivity.
5. Speak slower, lower, and more distinctly. If the client looks puzzled, try to rephrase what you are saying in words that he can understand.
6. Write out all instructions, using white paper and a black, felt-tipped pen.
7. Set aside a longer length of time for the interview than you would normally use for a younger client.
8. Pace yourself, allowing time for the client to perceive and respond.

PHYSICAL-ENVIRONMENTAL SUBSYSTEM

As the aging individual's competence diminishes, he becomes more susceptible to the influence of his physical environment. Faulty perception of the surroundings may precipitate inappropriate behavior. For example, the standard admission kit for a hospital or nursing home contains a blue or green plastic water pitcher. The male patient is also provided with a plastic disposable urinal—of the same color, of course, for a matched set. Is it surprising that an 80-year-old man, vision dimmed by cataracts, mistakes the water pitcher for the urinal? Immediately he is labeled as "senile" or "confused" and thus deficient in some way.

By changing perspective and focusing on the environment rather than on the person, the nurse may discover that the environment is deficient. A simple substitution, perhaps of a red or yellow urinal for the green one, may well change the "confused" behavior. Color vision holds up longer in the aging than visual acuity; therefore colors are more easily discriminated than shapes.

Prosthetic and therapeutic environments

This substitution of colors is an example of providing a geriatric prosthetic environment (Lindsley, 1964). Just as the prosthesis for the amputee helps compensate for his deficit leg, so does a geriatric prosthetic environment compensate for the sensory deficits of the elderly. Lindsley distinguishes between prosthetic environments—those that make provisions to compensate for irreversible deficits—and therapeutic environments—those that facilitate a change in behavior that may be generalized to other settings.

For example, Mr. D., an elderly patient in a nursing home, was progressively losing his sight. He became irritated whenever he could not find his way back to his room from the dining room. As in most nursing homes, there were handrails down each side of the corridors. A sensitive nurse aide decided to tie a large bow at the end of the rail just before his room. When his hand touched the ribbon he knew that he had found the right room. The aide had created a prosthetic environment.

An environment that promotes increased social interaction can be classified as therapeutic. For example, social interaction is increased when chairs are placed in small groupings such as around a table rather than lined up in neat rows around the periphery of the room. Arrangement of chairs in a semicircle compensates for the decreased peripheral vision experienced with aging.

Both therapeutic and prosthetic environmental interventions to promote interaction have been suggested by McClannahan (1973). Locomotion is enhanced when handrails are provided in other areas besides corridors, such as dining rooms, recreation rooms, and patios. Adequate lighting in halls as well as floor and wall coverings that reduce noise levels encourage residents to venture from their rooms. Color can be used to orient patients. One nursing home painted the halls of each of its four wings a different color, so that the resident could recognize that he lived in the "blue hall" rather than, for example, the "yellow hall."

Environmental stimulation

Bright colors in a nursing home not only lessen confusion but provide sensory stimulation. Many gerontological environments are dull and depressing, a condition that Cautela (1972) calls a "Pavlovian basis of old age." He points out Pavlov's findings that monotonous and/or continual stimulation caused his experimental dogs to become drowsy, sleepy, or very quiet. Cautela reflects on the similarities displayed by residents of geriatric institutional settings and proposes that these may be the result of a lack of reinforcement of activity and a limited variety of stimuli.

There appears to be a relationship between the overall amount of stimulation and the activity level. When incoming stimuli drop below a certain level, the brainstem reticular activating system (RAS) does not perform its function of keeping the brain awake. The RAS literally prepares the cortex for incoming sensory input and causes it to attend to stimuli in the environment (Leukel, 1976). An analogy might be that of a small boy and his grandfather waiting to see the Fourth of July parade. Warmed by the

sun, the grandfather dozes off. The grandson keeps stepping off the curb to look down the street. As soon as he sees the red lights of the police motorcycles and the drum major and twirlers of the first band he dashes over and shakes his grandfather: "They're coming! They're coming!" The grandfather is aroused and joins him as the first unit passes by. The small boy can be compared to the RAS, with the stimuli of band and motorcycles sufficient sensory input to activate him to arouse his grandfather. Once awake, the grandfather is not likely to fall asleep again for two reasons: (1) sufficient sensory input will be received from the remainder of the parade to keep the RAS firing, and (2) once aroused, the cortex is more receptive to incoming stimuli.

The problem then is to provide sufficient environmental stimulation to maintain alertness and activity. For the regressed elderly, a program of sensory stimulation increases interaction with the environment (Huber, 1973). Sensory training can be carried out as a structured group experience, with a goal of exercising the five senses. Each session may focus on a single sense or it may be multisensory. A program designed for nursing home residents by three senior nursing students consisted of seven 45-minute sessions. The first session focused on stimulation of taste. As food samples were passed around, each participant was asked to comment on its taste and texture. Contrasting tastes and textures utilized were lemon (sour), crackers (salty), mints (sweet), and orange wedges (fruity). At the end of the session, the group was asked to be aware of flavors and textures in the food they ate the next day. One of the activities during the session on touch involved comparing the texture of a live kitten with that of sandpaper. To stimulate hearing, tape recordings of school children at play during recess and animal sounds (zoo and domestic) were used. The residents were asked to identify the sounds and share the memories that surfaced. For a multisensory session, assorted materials were provided for making a collage. Each participant's collage was hung in his room to provide ongoing sensory stimulation.

These sensory stimulation sessions demonstrated the interdependence of the gerontological subsystems. Altering the physical environment by introducing stimuli for the physiological subsystem created changes in the sociocultural and psychological subsystems. The students noted an overall improvement in social interaction and orientation as the sessions progressed. One resident offered no comments during the first few sessions. By the end of the program the students labeled him as ''the life of the party.'' Another participant initially sat in her chair and grunted. By the final session, she was emitting understandable verbal responses.

Well-meaning family or caretakers may inadvertently reduce the amount of environmental stimuli available by a zealous attack on the ''clutter'' present in many gerontological ecosystems, particularly in the community setting. Many homes contain an accumulation of ''treasures'' gathered over a lifetime. Besides offering the safety and security of being surrounded by familiar things, such clutter may be therapeutic for increasing visual and tactile stimulation (Pastalan and Carson, 1970).

Why do nurses in nursing homes not follow the lead of their colleagues in pediatric and psychiatric units and abandon the white uniforms? Carlson (1972) remarks that white uniforms and caps imply that aging is an illness. Quite a different message would be communicated by staff members wearing street clothes. What a simple way to introduce a variety of sensory stimulation! Clothing changes do not go unnoticed by the nursing home residents, as demonstrated by a conversation between two male residents several years ago. They were bemoaning the change in uniform styles from miniskirts to pantsuits. ''I like to *see* legs,'' one emphatically remarked. ''Yeah,'' the other replied, ''It used to be fun just sitting here watching them nurses go by.''

SOCIOCULTURAL SUBSYSTEM

The assessment of the sociocultural subsystem involves determining the older client's relationship to the society and culture to which he belongs. Two sociological concepts provide a theoretical base for understanding this relationship: age stratification and status/role.

Age stratification

Within a society people form different strata composed of persons of similar age. The age strata change in size and composition through the process of cohort flow, in which successive cohorts (those individuals born in the same period and aging together) form and move through life together and eventually dissolve through death (Riley, et al., 1972). Each cohort can differ in size and composition depending on the number of births and deaths. For example, the cohorts of elderly populations are expected to continue increasing at a rate of 16% to 18% for each decade through 1990 and then to drop sharply for 2 decades as the small cohort born during the depression begins to reach age 65. The baby boom that followed World War II will cause an upward swing again between 2010 and 2020, after which growth will decrease abruptly because of the declining birth rates of the 1960s and 1970s (Public Information Office, 1973).

Age stratification rests on a physiological base—biological aging—and a historical base— those unique historical events that leave an imprint on each generation, affecting knowledge and attitudes (Riley et al., 1972). Thus values and attitudes of one cohort may differ from those of the succeeding cohort because of the different historical events that have occurred during their respective life spans. An appreciation of these differences will help the community mental health nurse to avoid the ''lumping syndrome'' in working with older persons. The lumping syndrome occurs when all older clients are assigned to the homogenous category of ''65 and older'' (Brown, 1978), a maneuver that negates the increasing differentiation that occurs with age. Brown suggests dividing the elderly into two cohorts, the *young-old,* aged 55 to 74, who generally are still independent and physically healthy, and the *vulnerable old,* aged 75 and older, who may still be healthy and independent, but who are more vulnerable to psychological and physical problems caused by biological changes of aging.

The vulnerable old are most likely great-grandparents and have survived such historical events as immigration, the depression, and two world wars plus those in Korea and Vietnam and have seen both the horseless carriage and the spaceship. This cohort remembers the soup and bread lines of the depression days and may equate current nutrition and food stamp programs with these "handouts." Theirs was an era when one was fortunate to achieve an eighth-grade education, when one worked hard for a living (usually at minimal wages), and when one took pride in the ability to "stand on his own two feet." These life experiences fostered an independence that may make it difficult for the vulnerable old to seek or accept the community resources that are available (Brown, 1978).

In contrast, the young-old are grandparents, mostly first-generation Americans rather than immigrants. They are better educated, usually with a high school education, and therefore have had more career options than their parents. Improved economic conditions plus Social Security and pension plans stimulated by union activity have provided them with a increased financial base for retirement. As the generation with the highest percentage of persons voting, they are a strong political force (Brown, 1978).

Life course differences between successive cohorts are caused not only by different historical eras but also by such other factors as the physical environment and the sequence of roles in which they take part.

All cohorts are affected at similar stages of the life cycle (infancy, childhood, young adult,

and so forth) by such environmental factors as the state of public health, child-rearing practices, and the prevailing economic conditions when they enter the labor force. For example, the cohort whose infancy occurred during a period when no polio immunizations were available contains a larger proportion of adults with the residual effects of paralytic polio than does the cohort born in the 1950s and 1960s who received the protection of Salk and Sabin vaccines. The generation reared under the strict child-raising regimes of the 1920s and 1930s differs from those cohorts raised according to Dr. Spock. Similarly, the cohort that entered the labor force during the depression years has a different outlook than the cohort who began work during an economic "boom."

Other factors such as a depression or a recession affect all age cohorts at a particular point in time. However, the effects vary for each cohort, as they are at different stages of the life cycle; all are affected but in different ways (Riley et al., 1972). For example, during the depression some urban families decided to send one or more of their children to live with grandparents back home on the farm in order to ensure that the children would at least be fed. The family who remained in the city subsisted mainly on food from the soup and bread lines. The impact of the depression in this small area of living thus varied for those children who experienced the relative plenty of the farm, as compared to their parents' meager subsistence.

Status/role

The model of age stratification assumes the existence of a social system that contains roles and people who act in these roles. An individual's place in the sociocultural system is determined by his social identity, which is made up of the totality of his roles. Sarbin (1970) proposes three dimensions for assessing social identity: (1) status, (2) value, and (3) involvement.

Status dimension. The term "status" refers to one's position in a social structure and is a collectively recognized category of persons, usually designated by some title such as mother, father, doctor, or nurse. In the ecological model status is synonymous with ecological niche (Wilkerson and O'Connor, 1977). Each ecological niche contains an inhabitant who has certain rights and duties and environmental resources to aid in the performance of these duties. The set of expected behaviors for the occupant comprises his role and is defined and encouraged by the significant others in his sociocultural subsystem.

Status may be either ascribed—granted by society on the basis of such biosocial characteristics as age, sex, or kinship—or achieved—acquired by the individual through his own deliberate efforts. Status can be viewed by the degree of choice involved in entry into a position or status.

The individual gains more power and/or social esteem as he moves toward the achieved end of the continuum. The status dimension of social identity then depends on the performance of roles, which may be located at several different points on a status continuum and which vary in the amounts of power and esteem that accompany them (Sarbin, 1970).

Value dimension. The value dimension is the degree of esteem or respect awarded by society to the occupant of an ecological niche for role performance. This dimension is also a continuum, with a negative end representing low esteem, disrespect, or no respect; a positive end coinciding with high esteem and respect; and a neutral point of zero esteem.

The potential values that may be assigned differ for statuses at the achieved end and for statuses at the ascribed end. Role behaviors for highly achieved statuses, such as that of scientist or writer, may result in rewards of high value such as the Nobel prize. However, failure in performance or poor performance generally receives only a neutral evaluation rather than a negative one. Not all scientific experiments are

successful or fruitful; not all manuscripts are published. Yet the scientist or writer is not negatively valued; indeed they are supported with expressions of sympathy or regret: "Better luck next time." The value range for achieved statuses, then, runs only from the neutral to the positive points on the continuum.

However, the situation differs for role enactments at the ascribed end of the continuum. Little value or esteem is given the customary, minimal performance in such roles as woman, mother, or father; the individual is just doing what is expected. The individual who fails to perform according to societal expectations is often negatively valued and given no respect or esteem. The father who fails to support his children and the woman who rejects heterosexual relationships are scorned by society. Thus the value dimension for ascribed roles runs from the neutral point to the negative end of the continuum. In other words, the individual who performs an ascribed role according to minimal sociocultural expectations receives whatever respect is inherent in the role's position on the status continuum. Nonperformance of the role, however, results in negative sanctions such as disrespect or being treated as a nonperson (Sarbin, 1970).

Involvement dimension. The involvement dimension, also a continuum, represents the degree of participation or involvement in a role. The degree of involvement depends on the amount of time spent in role behaviors of the ecological niche in relation to the time required for other ecological niches, as well as the amount of energy and resources consumed in the enactment. Generally, ascribed statuses such as "parent" require high involvement, while achieved statuses such as "nurse" have varying levels of involvement, usually situational (Sarbin, 1970). For example, one summer a nurse educator observed a young mother and her toddler attending a band concert in the park. Throughout the concert the little boy was constantly dashing off in all directions, with his mother in hot pursuit. She was highly involved in her role as mother. On the other hand, the nurse educator sat listening to the concert; she was relatively uninvolved in her professional role. However, if the mother were to enroll in one of the educator's classes in the Fall, the degree of involvement in their respective roles would be reversed: during the class session the nursing student would be relatively uninvolved in her mothering role, while the nurse educator would be highly involved in her educator role.

Implications for the older client. Roles differ by age groups along the dimensions of (1) the number of different kinds of roles, (2) the number of openings available in each kind of role, (3) the priority given to different roles, (4) the biological constraints on numbers and kinds of roles that can be enacted, and (5) the social evaluation of roles. Mechanisms such as retirement exist for assigning individuals in successive cohorts to appropriate roles (Riley et al, 1972). Compulsory retirement policies make room for entrance into the worker role by younger cohorts.

A progressive loss of roles occurs during the aging process as children move away from home, the worker retires, and spouse and friends die. The social identity of the older client may be transformed in a negative direction (degraded) by such role changes. The degrading of a person's social identity occurs when he is denied the opportunity to occupy positions that have a degree of choice. The more ascribed positions that an individual is occupying, the less opportunity he has to be highly valued and esteemed for his role behaviors (Sarbin, 1970).

An assessment should be made of the current role involvement of the older client. Primary prevention efforts of the community mental health nurse should focus on exploring role alternatives with the older client, particularly those emanating from achieved positions. In addition, younger cohorts should be encouraged to develop a variety of roles in preparation for

aging so that the inevitable role exits do not leave them degraded.

Role alternatives

Despite the loss of roles, there are continuing role alternatives for each cohort. What are the role options for the later years of life?

Family. Roles as grandparents or great-grandparents exist for the 70% of older persons who have living grandchildren and the 40% with great-grandchildren (Atchley, 1972). Older persons with children, grandchildren, and great-grandchildren have a unique opportunity to serve as role models of aging, thus providing the anticipatory socialization for growing old that they themselves may have lacked.

Most older women exit the role of wife to enter the role of widow. Widowhood for women has fewer adverse effects than retirement for men, possibly because the cultural view of retirement, unlike widowhood, carries with it a tinge of failure (Blau, 1972; Cumming, 1968). For a widow, the major factor in continuing involvement in the social culture is the degree to which her various roles were dependent upon her husband (Lopata, 1970). Encouraging women to develop their own identities therefore serves as primary prevention for the depression often associated with widowhood.

Friend. During old age peer friendships become as important as they were during adolescence (Blau, 1972). Friendships are more likely to occur among members of the same age cohort, as they have had similar role sequences, role strains, and historical contexts. Friends provide direct assistance in coping with role entrances, alterations, and exits such as those of spouse to widow and worker to retiree. Once established, friendships endure with only intermittent reinforcement; thus ties may be maintained with old college roommates, army buddies, or former neighbors (Riley et al., 1972).

Citizen. The political role is one that is maintained well into old age. A higher percentage of those in the 80- to 90-year-old group vote than do those in the 20- to 30-year-group. The role of citizen is only slightly constrained by age. There is a minimum age for voting, but no maximum (Riley et al., 1972). Decrease in other role commitments may afford an opportunity to keep up with political affairs and to participate actively in the democratic process (Atchley, 1976). Even physical immobility need not keep the elderly from voting, since absentee ballots may be obtained for most elections, and many candidates offer free rides to the polls.

Association member. Norms exist in our society for the elderly to continue membership in voluntary organizations. Older persons are more likely to belong to these types of organizations (in rank order): fraternal or lodges, church-related or religious, civic or service, veterans, military or patriotic, and social or recreational (Riley and Foner, 1968).

User of leisure. There are indications that the increased leisure time now available in our society is creating a trend toward greater acceptance of a leisure role as a counterpart for the work role (Havighurst, 1973). Leisure activities for the elderly can be categorized into two dimensions: instrumental-expressive and overt/participating-passive/receiving.

Instrumental activities are those that have a goal beyond immediate involvement with an activity and that have the potential to change the participant's situation. Such activities help him learn new ways of living, for example, programs on health concerns. Expressive activities are those activities in which the participant engages for the gratification they provide for the moment, such as making ceramics and the other arts and crafts usually offered at senior centers. Instrumental activities are an important part of the leisure role, for they provide the opportunity to learn competencies to help meet the challenges of the later years (Londoner, 1971).

Overt/participating activities are those that require intellectual and/or physical effort, for example, card playing or dancing. On the other hand, passive/receiving activities require minimal involvement, participation, or effort, for example, watching television or listening to music (Busse, 1956; Kaplan, 1962).

There actually should be a blend of all four types of activities; the proper proportions depends on the status of the individual client. The community mental health nurse needs to be cognizant of community resources providing each type of activity. A senior center may be able to provide instrumental activities such as how to deal with changing roles or how to improve relationships.

Individuals who are approaching retirement should be encouraged to develop leisure skills. Those who lack such skills are more likely to resist retirement (Atchley, 1976).

Retiree. As compared to most roles, the retirement role is more vague and thus more flexible. Perhaps this is a positive aspect, for each retiree differs in physical, mental, and financial status. A vaguely defined role can be interpreted by the individual within the context of his own capabilities and limitations. Each individual is free to negotiate role expectations and behavior for this ecological niche with the significant others in the ecosystem (Atchley, 1976).

Some consider retirement to be a "roleless role" with little agreement about the behavior that should be associated with it. However, Atchley (1972) suggests that there are certain expectations. The retiree is expected to spend more time with family and friends, expand leisure time, drop membership in work-related organizations, get by on a reduced income, and increase involvement in non-work-related organizations.

A previously mentioned characteristic of adaptation, that the unprepared individual has more difficulty adapting to change than one who is prepared, is especially applicable to retirement. Preparation for retirement should begin early in the working years and should include such aspects as financial planning to ensure an adequate income to maintain a desired life-style, development of leisure skills, development of ties with community organizations, and promotion of optimal health (Atchley, 1976). Atchley's discussion of the seven phases of retirement—remote, near, honeymoon, disenchantment, reorientation, stability, and termination—may be used to provide anticipatory guidance for those approaching the retirement role (Atchley, 1976; Burnside, 1976). Retirement cohorts, people who have known each other on the job and who retire together, may also provide a continuity of identification with the work role.

ADJUSTMENT TO CHANGING ROLES

Theorists disagree about the best way to adjust to such role changes as retirement. Activity theorists hold that successful aging means maintaining, as long as possible, the activities and attitudes of middle age. If useful roles are given up, new roles should be substituted (Havighurst, 1961, 1973). Continuity theorists postulate that as an individual ages, he tends to maintain continuity in habits, preferences, associations, and so forth. Therefore the individual increases the time spent enacting the roles he is already playing rather than trying to find new roles (Atchley, 1972). Disengagement theorists assume that withdrawal from roles is a natural, intrinsic, and inevitable process leading to the final stage of life. The gradual withdrawal of the aging individual from his various role-sets prepares him for the only total disengagement—death (Cumming and Henry, 1961; Cumming, 1968, 1975).

The process of disengagement probably begins sometime during middle age when the individual is hit with an awareness of the inevitability of death and the briefness of the time he has left before it occurs. This is the moment when a person senses that there is not enough time left for everything he wants to accomplish. He establishes allocations and

priorities for the future and begins a shift away from the need for achievement and starts the disengagement phase of his life.

The theory of disengagement has been refined by Streib and Schneider (1972), who suggest that there is "differential disengagement": disengagement occurs at different rates and times for different roles.

DISENGAGEMENT AND REINFORCEMENT

There are elements of truth in all three theories, in that each can be used to explain the role behaviors of some of the older population. Both activity and continuity theorists agree that the process of disengagement does occur, but they refute it as a theory of successful aging. Cumming (1975) regrets that these researchers leave the impression that disengagement is the ideal way of aging. Some policy makers, such as politicians and nursing home administrators, interpret the theory in this manner and use it to support negligent practices. If one accepts the premise that the withdrawal from roles seen in disengagement is "normal" and "ideal" aging, then it would be wrong to force engagement by providing opportunities for continued involvement. Many caretakers fail to make the distinction between disengagement that is reversible and that which is irreversible.

The problem, then, is to determine the extent to which disengagement may be related to situational factors (and may therefore be potentially reversible) rather than to aging per se.

One approach is to conceptualize disengagement in behavioral terms as an extinction phenomenon. Disengagement is characterized by withdrawal from social roles. Social roles involve expectations of behavior that are defined, encouraged, and reinforced by the significant persons in an individual's ecosystem. According to learning theory, behaviors that are reinforced will be continued; behaviors that are not reinforced will diminish. When reinforcement stops, behavior will undergo "extinction" and will be emitted rarely, if at all (Skinner, 1974).

Support for a behavioral view of disengagement comes from Lindsley (1964), who describes disengagement as "the abrupt cessation of reinforcement, or extinction." Furthermore, Cumming (1968) remarks that social withdrawal consists of failure to approach others. In behavioral terms, approach behaviors are emitted when one anticipates positive reinforcement (Skinner, 1974).

Two questions are suggested by this conceptualization: (1) Are the role behaviors of the elderly reinforced by the significant others in their environment? (2) If they are not, is the lack of reinforcement of role behaviors a situational factor in disengagement?

The relationship between the degree of disengagement exhibited by elderly persons and the self-reported reinforcement occurring in their lives was explored in a survey of two elderly groups—nursing home residents and community registered voters (Henthorn, 1975). A significant correlation ($p > .001$) was found between scores on a disengagement index and the measures of reinforcement for both groups, indicating that the greater the degree of disengagement, the lower the level of reinforcement (number of reinforcers that the person was "sure" or "pretty sure" he would receive during the next month).

The individuals in this study lend support to the activity theory of aging. The least disengaged person, an 84-year-old community registered voter, was an active participant in 12 clubs and organizations and held current offices in 8 of them. Among the least disengaged of the nursing home residents was a 92-year-old widow who began painting at the age of 72. At the time of the interview she was industriously painting miniature scenes for the annual church bazaar. She was still actively involved in political affairs and voting regularly (and trying to influence the investigator to vote for her favorite candidate in the upcoming election).

Implications for nursing

The application of social learning principles may be a useful tool to retard disengagement and promote engagement of the elderly in the sociocultural subsystem. Relatives, friends, and caretakers can be helped to see how important a part they play in shaping the role behaviors of an elderly person; that is, any behavior that the person exhibits is reinforced, extinguished, or punished. There are no other possibilities.

The elderly themselves can be taught to look at the consequences of their behavior. Knowledge of reinforcement principles may help the older client to regulate and change his own behavior. If family and friends stop visiting, this provides feedback that something may be wrong with his behavior. He then needs to examine his own actions and determine whether they have been positive reinforcers for visits or aversive stimuli discouraging future visits.

Roles are the primary mode of engagement; therefore the engagement of the older person in his sociocultural subsystem can be determined by assessing his level of involvement and participation in social roles. To promote continued involvement, the nurse therapist may need to help the client to evaluate role alternatives. The therapist should enlist the help of "kith and kin" in reinforcing desired role behaviors for both old and new roles.

PSYCHOLOGICAL SUBSYSTEM

If Sullivan's (1953) view of self as "the reflected appraisal of others" is correct, then it is not unusual that many elderly people have a low self-esteem. Our society, with its emphasis on productivity, usefulness, achievement, and independence, does not value its aging citizens.

The concepts of aging that a society holds tend to be internalized as self-concepts of the aged. Expressions of devaluations of the elderly in the United States include numerous misconceptions. Stereotypical thinking holds that most old people are ill, disabled, or senile; rigid and incapable of change; childish; and asexual. The elderly person is not expected to continue learning, to keep up with the times, or to maintain sexual relationships.

Thus ageism—stereotyping and discriminating against people because they are old—has joined sexism and racism as a major prejudice of society. But unlike the racist or sexist, who need not fear a change in skin color or sex, the ageist may some day join the ranks of the aged and become the victim of his own prejudice (Butler and Lewis, 1977).

The Brothers Grimm illustrated this nicely in their tale of the very old grandfather, enfeebled by passing years, who could barely feed himself and spilled most of his food. Disgusted, his son banished him from the table to a stool in the corner and made him eat out of a pottery bowl. One day the bowl slipped from his trembling fingers and shattered. The son's wife chastised the grandfather and thereafter served his meals in a wooden bowl. Some time later, the family observed the young grandson busily hammering together small pieces of wood. "What are you doing, son?" asked the father. "I'm making a bowl," the child replied, "for you and mother to eat out of when *you* grow old."

Self-esteem

Such societal attitudes have an impact on the self-esteem of the older client. An assessment of this important component of the psychological subsystem will determine if interventions are needed to promote psychological well-being. This assessment requires an understanding of the relationship between self-esteem and self-concept.

Very simply, self-concept is the way a person sees himself. It is the sum total of everything an individual can call his own and emerges from social interaction with others.

Self-concept is an accumulation of all one's interpersonal and interactional experiences, but it can change as the person encounters new influences.

Self-concept has two components: one is related to the physical self; the other, to the personal self. The physical self-concept includes an appraisal of the physical body—its appearance, attributes, functioning, sexuality, and wellness or illness. The personal self-concept includes the individual's view of his personality, values and attitudes, conscience, and self-expectations (Roy, 1976).

These two components fuse to form a basic self—a relatively stable and unchanging sense of who one is in the world. In addition, each person has a constructed social self—his image or perception of self in different roles (Kramer and Schmalenberg, 1977).

Self-esteem is the value judgment put on these self-concepts in answer to the question, "How satisfied am I with who I am (physically) (personally)?" To the extent that we are well satisfied with who we are, we will have a high self-esteem. The person who is dissatisfied with his attributes, either physical or personal, will have a low self-esteem. Self-esteem can also be described as the extent to which the person sees himself as competent and able to satisfy his own needs (Korman, 1970; Roy, 1976).

There is a chronic self-esteem associated with the basic self-concept. The individual's level of chronic self-esteem is present in all situations and remains relatively stable. On the other hand, the self-esteem related to the constructed social self varies according to two dimensions—task-specific self-esteem and socially influenced self-esteem (Korman 1970).

Task-specific self-esteem is based on a person's notion of how competent he is in performing the specific tasks associated with a role. For example, the great-grandmother who is babysitting for her first great-grandchild may not feel competent in changing disposable diapers or feeding with a disposable nurser. Neither was available for her mothering tasks 50 years ago.

Socially influenced self-esteem is related to how well one meets the role expectations of others; in other words, it is "reflected appraisal" self-esteem. To the extent that others think that one is competent in enacting a particular role, and to the extent that they communicate that evaluation, socially influenced self-esteem will rise.

The causes for low self-esteem in the elderly are apparent. The physical changes described earlier in this chapter contribute to a low self-esteem of the physical self. Technological changes, such as those in the area of transportation, may make it difficult for the older person to maintain a high level of task-specific self-esteem. Roadways for the model T automobile of the 1920s were considerably less complex than today's interstate highways and six-lane freeways. The younger driver who vents his frustration on the cautious and confused older driver who caused the traffic bottleneck does not increase the older person's socially influenced self-esteem.

Social-breakdown syndrome

Lowered self-esteem of the elderly client increases his susceptibility to the social-breakdown syndrome that is a precursor to poor mental health. Kuypers and Bengston (1973) suggest that the social-breakdown syndrome in the elderly occurs in the following manner.

First, there must be a susceptible individual—one whose self-concept and self-esteem are threatened by the social labeling and value judgments of others. The elderly are a susceptible population because of the role change and societal attitudes previously discussed. Shrinkage of roles leaves the aging individual confused and unsure about the proper behavior of being "old." The vulnerable old particularly have no clear-cut expectations for the role of "old age." The clearly defined roles of earlier

stages of life (worker and spouse) are replaced by those characterized by some degree of ambiguity (retiree and widow). As they are the first cohort to grow old, the vulnerable old lack appropriate reference groups to look to as models of behavior.

Because the older person cannot rely on past experience, he becomes extremely sensitive to the external cues in a specific ecological niche as to what is appropriate behavior. Because of societal attitudes toward aging, the feedback he receives about behavior often indicates that the older person is incompetent, inadequate, and useless. Old people are supposed to be sick and dependent. These are the behaviors that are reinforced when nursing home personnel give a bath or feed a resident who is capable of doing it by himself.

Thus the elderly person may prefer the sick role; he particularly prefers it to being roleless (Blau, 1972). At least the sick role has some specific behaviors associated with it, and the elderly can relate to it from past experience. If the sick role is indeed assumed, coping skills previously possessed will atrophy from disuse. The person eventually begins to believe that in fact he is inadequate, incompetent, and obsolete. This belief renders the individual even more susceptible, and the cycle repeats itself, leading to lesser and lesser degrees of social competence (Kupyers and Bengston, 1973).

Social competence

How can the social-breakdown cycle be broken for the elderly? An assessment of the three components of social competence suggests the points at which ecosystem intervention may be most fruitful.

Effective social-role performance. Social competence can be viewed from a sociological perspective as effective role performance. Four factors affect the performance of major social roles: (1) personal resources, such as health and intelligence, (2) the individual's external support system, (3) opportunities and obstacles encountered during the life course from such factors as age, sex, social class, and historical events, and (4) the individual's commitment and effort on his own behalf (Riley et al., 1972).

Symptoms of possible role insufficiency (ineffective role performance) may be anxiety, depression, unhappiness, grief, frustration, and/or powerlessness (Meleis, 1975). When role insufficiency is diagnosed, two nursing interventions are possible: activating or creating a support system (Hogue, 1977; Garrison et al., 1977) and role supplementation (Meleis, 1975).

Support systems are a psychosocial coping resource that can be mobilized to bolster role performance and to decrease the probability that a sick role will be embraced by the older client. A support system can be defined as all the significant others in a gerontological ecosystem who provide support and guidance to help the aging individual cope with environmental demands. Support systems can be viewed as social networks that provide affective resources for meeting emotional needs or instrumental resources providing help with such tasks as housing, food, and medical care.

Three types of support systems are natural systems (family and friends), nonprofessional, organized systems that are not directed by health professionals (religious organizations, Alcoholics Anonymous, American Association of Retired Persons, and so forth), and health professional systems (nurses, physicians, social workers, physical therapists, and so forth) (Garrison et al., 1977; Hogue, 1977). The types of support systems available to the elderly client should be identified, mobilized, and supplemented as needed.

The nursing intervention of role supplementation is a technique that focuses on increasing the personal resources of the occupant of the ecological niche by teaching both the occupant and significant others about the expected behaviors associated with the role. This tech-

nique is based on the assumption that roles are learned through (1) interactions with significant others, either singly or in groups, (2) rewards for appropriate role behaviors, (3) role modeling, and (4) deliberate role instruction presenting specific knowledge, information, and cues needed to perform a role (Meleis, 1975). Such a technique requires a commitment and effort by the individual involved.

The support groups for elderly persons in the community described by Petty et al. (1976) illustrate both the establishment of support systems and the use of certain elements of Meleis' model: peer reference groups, role modeling and role playing, and deliberate role instruction.

The support group members were recruited from the population screened in a pilot geriatric arthritis program. All were having trouble adjusting to the "old age" role but did not feel that they needed counseling: being unhappy was viewed as "just part of growing old." Therefore the groups were presented to the target individuals as "informal workshops."

A brainstorming session during the first meeting provided opportunity for the members to express the concerns they had about aging. Later sessions focused on such concerns as dealing with faulty memory, adjusting to changes in vision and hearing, improving interpersonal relationships, and making decisions about relocation. The groups provided a model for developing friendships, coping with the stresses of aging, and utilizing community resources (Petty et al., 1976).

Creative adaptation. The ability to cope with, and adapt to, environmental changes is the second component of social competence. The psychologically competent person is able to activate his own support systems when needed and to use a variety of coping mechanisms. If coping skills are inadequate or lacking, when a problem arises, the person will go into a crisis (Aguilera and Messick, 1978).

Anticipatory planning, guidance, and counseling for the maturational crises of old age (retirement and other role changes) are primary prevention strategies that promote creative adaptation. In addition to the traditional crisis intervention focus on increasing the individual's repertoire of coping mechanisms, the therapist needs to look at ways of decreasing such stressors in the gerontological ecosystem as poor health, inadequate income, and substandard housing, which may overtax the older client's adaptive capacities (Kuypers and Bengston, 1973).

Mental health professionals need to remember that coping skills atrophy when the aging individual is institutionalized. If the current trend toward deinstitutionalization—the transfer of older patients from state mental hospitals to such community facilities as nursing homes and room and board homes—is to be successful, there must be adequate preparation for discharge. Prerelease programs should include retraining in those coping skills necessary to survive in a community setting. Plans should be made *before* release for follow-up of clients in the community. The setting and monitoring of standards for community residential facilities that provide aftercare for older clients will ensure that these homes do not evolve into environments sadly reminiscent of the back wards in state mental hospitals (Bachrach, 1976).

Day care centers for the elderly, an alternative to hospitalization, provide support services and the maintenance of coping skills. Oklahoma City's YWCA Daily Living Care Center uses a team approach in assessing clients and prescribing a therapeutic program. A team composed of a nurse, physician, psychiatrist, social worker, and physical therapist meets with each prospective client to determine whether or not he might benefit from the program. They develop individualized programs that provide such activities as speech therapy, physical exercise, health maintenance, sensory awareness, body relaxation, musical expression, recreation, companionship and group interaction, and opportunities for volunteer work.

Community mental health centers are a potential support system for the elderly. In theory, these centers should have provided a considerable increase in mental health care for the older population. In practice, this has not occurred. The elderly comprise only 5% of community mental health center clientele (Butler and Lewis, 1977).

Why are the elderly not served by mental health centers? First, centers are oriented to serve those who ask for help. Few old people ask for help because of a belief that mental health assistance is only for "crazy people." Then, too, in many centers there is evidence of professional discrimination against the aged. Other contributing factors are lack of transportation and insufficient funds to pay for the services (Patterson, 1976; Butler and Lewis, 1977).

Every mental health center should have a staff member who serves as advocate for the elderly. The community mental health nurse with community health experience is well suited for this role. Community mental health centers that use nurses for home visits have discovered that they are more readily accepted by the elderly, particularly when the nurses do not tell the clients that they are from the mental health center until they gain their trust (Patterson, 1976).

For many older persons, the senior center is a significant social outlet that serves to expand their social world, to reduce isolation, and to provide the group support that helps the older person withstand the stresses of aging (Rosow, 1973). The health, societal, recreational, and educational services provided by senior centers aid the senior citizen in developing needed coping skills. The senior center offers an established setting in which the nurse can promote and maintain gerontological mental health by such functions as assessing patterns of coping with crises, providing mental health education, offering consultation services to senior center staff members, and making home visits. The older client may be more willing to take advantage of mental health services if they are provided in the senior center setting in which he feels comfortable.

Personal mastery or ecosystem competence. The third component of social competence includes the feelings that a person has about his ability to influence his environment. When an individual feels that whatever happens is a result of the influence of external forces such as fate, luck, or powerful others, he has a belief in external control. On the other hand, the individual who feels that he controls his own fate and has some power over the environment believes in internal control and has personal mastery over his environment. Such an individual is characterized by autonomy, feelings of power, and responsibility for the results of his actions; he has personal control over what happens (Rotter, 1966).

Intervention strategies designed to increase personal mastery for the older client should focus on ensuring that he does in fact have as much control over his life as is feasible. Whenever possible, the aged client should make those decisions that affect his environment. Nursing homes and housing units for the elderly should be encouraged to establish some type of resident government so that the residents can be involved in decisions that affect their ecosystem.

Decision making was promoted in the community support groups previously described (Petty et al., 1976) during the session on housing and relocation. The group members were given a list of factors to be considered when contemplating a move—factors such as climate, access to stores and health facilities, and proximity to friends and relatives. Additional factors were suggested by group members and then each ranked the list according to personal priorities. The discussion of individual priorities with group members helped each to discover what was important in helping to explore alternatives more effectively.

Assessment of self-esteem

Several techniques are useful for assessing the self-esteem of the elderly client. To use the technique of mirror-reflecting, the nurse asks the older client to look in a mirror (preferably full-length) and describe what he sees. The mirror serves as a trigger for the person to tell about himself. The resulting comments guide the nurse in exploring how the client views himself now, in comparison to the past, and how he sees himself in the future. Such a description can provide clues to the older person's level of physical self-esteem (Butler and Lewis, 1977).

Encouraging the individual to share his life history can be therapeutic as well as diagnostic for self-esteem problems. The life review helps the client to take inventory of what he has become, to evaluate the meaning of his life, and to integrate his experiences into a meaningful whole (Butler and Lewis, 1977). The life review also helps the individual to decide how he wants to spend his final years.

How does one encourage a life review? During a home visit, the nurse can scan the physical environment for such things as pictures, souvenirs, or awards and ask the client to tell about them. The nurse can request that he show his family albums or scrapbooks and suggest that he write a short autobiography or dictate one into a tape recorder. The nurse can ask for a summary of the client's work experiences and his feelings about them. If the client has children, the nurse can encourage him to discuss the experience of parenting.

Reminiscing groups also promote a life review and help the group members to achieve such goals as increased self-esteem and greater awareness of the contributions each has made to society. Ebersole (1976) suggests that specific goals be set for each group in order for the experience to be most beneficial. Questions that need to be resolved before reminiscing groups are initiated include whether the group is to be social or therapeutic, whether it is to be structured or unstructured, and what is to be accomplished for both the clients and the institution or agency in which the groups are held. For example, structured groups can focus on a specific theme such as holiday, food, or toys of childhood. Unstructured groups use freewheeling reminiscing, but, if necessary, the leader can stimulate the group by initiating the discussion and then letting the group take over.

Many families are beginning to realize that reminiscing is as beneficial to the listener as it is to the person doing the reminiscing. As the older family member tells his life history, the rest of the family gain a sense of their heritage. The preserving of this heritage on tape or in a family history or album often provides the older client with a project that will enhance his self-esteem.

SPIRITUAL/PHILOSOPHICAL SUBSYSTEM

The spiritual/philosophical subsystem encompasses religious beliefs and practices, the meaning of life and death, and the striving for self-actualization.

Religion and the aging

The religious beliefs one holds are an important basis of the individual's health behaviors. If one believes that whatever happens is God's will, he is likely to take a passive attitude toward the infirmities of old age and resist rehabilitative efforts. Belief that one is punished for one's sins may cause guilt and worry over past misdeeds, wasting the limited energy resources of the elderly. In this area, the life review may be particularly useful. As the person reminisces over past happenings, he may decide to right past wrongs.

On a more positive note, religious beliefs can give impetus to finding new meaning in life, as expressed by the elderly widow who

thoroughly enjoys her volunteer work in a day care center. "God must have a reason for still having me on this earth," she remarked. "I still can be useful." Belief in an afterlife can help the older client to endure the loss of spouse and friends. Such books as Raymond Moody's *Life after Life* offer a view of death that many find comforting.

Engagement in the religious role continues for most elderly people, although the practice of religious role behaviors may shift from formal church services to more informal modes of praying and reading at home or participating in religious services via television and radio.

Religious groups traditionally have been involved in the care of the elderly, as evidenced by the growing number of church-sponsored nursing homes. In addition, there is an increasing trend toward serving the elderly who are still residing in their homes. A prototype for such a service is the Shepherd Center in Kansas City, Missouri. The center is a cooperative, interdenominational venture of 22 local churches. Older persons share in the programs of the center and work together in meaningful community activity as well. They are not only ministered to but also minister to others: they are encouraged to volunteer and help each other. This multifaceted program provides Meals on Wheels, handyman services, friendly visiting, escort services (such as taking a husband to visit his wife in a convalescent home), health enrichment (blood pressure screening, health teaching, exercise programs, and so forth), crime protection techniques, personal enrichment groups, defensive driving classes, and continuing education classes. It is estimated that 100 to 200 of these people would not be able to remain in their homes if it were not for the services of the center.*

Churches and clergy have a unique contribu-

*The Shepherd Center is described in the film "Volunteer to Live," available from the National Benevolent Association, Christian Churches, Audiovisual Library, P.O. Box 1986, Indianapolis, IN 46206.

tion to make to community mental health (Haugk, 1976). Pastors serve as gatekeepers to the mental health system. A minister is usually the first person who is contacted in a crisis situation such as death of a spouse. A good working relationship with the clergy will promote referral when the expertise of a mental health professional is needed. The church provides a fellowship where belongingness needs may be met and where a support system may be provided when resources are limited. For example, Mrs. S., an elderly widow immobilized by a broken hip, was able to remain in her own home because the members of her church took turns preparing food for her and doing such necessary chores as shopping for groceries and medicines and providing transportation to the doctor.

Many churches tape Sunday worship services and such special events as Christmas programs. The tapes are then distributed to members of the congregation who are homebound or in nursing homes. Listening to the tapes promotes continued involvement not only in the spiritual realm but in the belongingness realm. One nursing home resident particularly enjoyed listening to the usual Sunday morning announcements: "I can keep up with what's going on with my friends," she remarked.

Self-actualization

Self-actualization can be described as the need to find meaning in life, to be somebody. The self-actualizing person is motivated by the desire to "become everything that one is capable of becoming" (Maslow, 1954). This view of humankind holds that man is constantly "becoming," or striving to reach a goal. When one has no goal in life, life loses its meaning. In other words, if a person does not live in a state of becoming he has no purpose in life.

French (1968), in his studies of self-actualization as a variable of mental health, divides the concept of self-actualization into two components—self-development and self-utilization. Self-development is seen as the cultivation of

desired skills and competencies, while self-utilization is the degree to which a person uses his skills and competencies.

Primary prevention efforts should be directed toward providing opportunities for continued self-development of the older client. Many junior colleges offer free courses for senior citizens. A recent curriculum offered by a local junior college included Human Sexuality and Aging; Oral-Dental Health: Tips and Treatment; Ballroom Dancing; Know Your Car; Political Education; Up on Your Toes About Your Feet; and Nutrition: the Dangers of Eating American Style (a variety of both instrumental and expressive activities).

For some older persons, volunteer activities increase the degree of self-utilization, especially those activities that utilize particular competencies. The skills of elderly volunteers in a retired senior volunteer program (RSVP) are matched with community needs. One of the first volunteers in the Oklahoma City RSVP was a model train hobbyist who repaired the collection of model trains housed in a caboose behind a children's convalescent hospital. He then donned his engineer's cap and spent his volunteer hours helping the children to play with the trains.

In Fort Smith, Arkansas, "Love to Share" centers are located in areas with a high incidence of working mothers. These centers are staffed by 44 senior citizens who feed and care for 100 "latch-key" elementary schoolchildren after school until parents return from work (Ellis, 1972). These centers have helped to solve the problem of withdrawal behavior in the children that had been precipitated by entering an empty house at the end of a school day. At the same time, working in the centers has provided a purpose in life for elders, while broadening their ideas and interests.

The Senior Companion Program provides both an opportunity for volunteer activities and a small stipend and other benefits. The senior companions visit older persons with special needs, both those living in their own homes and those in nursing homes. These volunteers provide both companionship and needed services.

Other volunteer opportunities include Friendly Visitor Programs, Foster Grandparent Programs, Service Corps of Retired Executives (SCORE), Peace Corps, Volunteers in Service to America (VISTA), and Green Thumb.

SUMMARY

The central theme of aging can be summarized as a series of losses. The elderly individual's success in coping with these losses will influence his mental health. However, mental health cannot be separated from problems of income, housing, nutrition, physical health, and relationships with significant others. There is need for an ecological perspective in assessing the mental health of the older client— a perspective that considers the adaptors and stressors occurring in the five subsystems of the gerontological ecosystem: physiological, physical-environmental, sociocultural, psychological, and spiritual/philosophical.

Societal and cultural attitudes have influenced the ways in which the elderly have been treated by mental health practitioners. Community mental health nurses must evaluate their biases toward working with the elderly.

Community mental health practitioners must advocate the establishment of preventive mental health services for the aging population. Such services would provide casefinding and treatment of acute crisis situations such as death of a spouse; counseling and guidance about such problems as retirement, use of leisure time, and changes in family relationships; help for families who care for physically or mentally disabled persons; and consultation and collaboration with community agencies serving the needs of the aged. Every effort must be made to keep the older person out of institutions.

The Society of Friends (Quakers) have expressed a summary of the needs of older persons as "somewhere to live, something to do, and someone to care." Do community mental health practitioners really care?

References

Aguilera, D. C., and Messick, J. M.: Crisis intervention: theory and methodology, ed. 3, St. Louis, 1978, The C. V. Mosby Co.

Ahern, C. K., Diekelmann, N., and Panicucci, C. L.: Developmental patterns of interaction. In Jones, D A., Dunbar, C. F., and Jirovec, M. M., eds.: Medical-surgical nursing: a conceptual approach, New York, 1978, McGraw-Hill Book Co.

Atchley, R. C.: The social forces in later life, Belmont, Calif., 1972, Wadsworth Publishing Co., Inc.

Atchley, R. C.: The sociology of retirement, Cambridge, Mass., 1976, Schenkman Publishing Co., Inc.

Bachrach, L. L.: Deinstitutionalization: an analytical review and sociological perspective, DHEW publication no. (ADM) 76-350, Washington, D.C., 1976, National Institute of Mental Health.

Balabokin, M. E.: Health and nutrition, Part 2, Gerontologist **12**:21-28, Summer 1972.

Beland, I., and Passos, J.: Clinical nursing: pathophysiological and psychosocial approaches, ed. 3, New York, 1975, The Macmillan Co.

Bender, A. D.: Drug therapy in the aged. In Chinn, A. B., ed.: Working with older people: a guide to practice. Vol. 4. Clinical aspects of aging, Rockville, Md., 1971, U.S. Public Health Service.

Bircher, A. U.: Mankind in crisis: an application of clinical practice to population-environmental issues, Nurs. Forum **11**:13-33, 1972.

Bircher, A. U.: On quality nursing care, University of Oklahoma College of Nursing, Oklahoma City, April 30, 1973. (Mimeographed.)

Blau, A.: Old age in a changing society, New York, 1972, New Viewpoints.

Braceland, F.: The mental hygiene of aging: present day view, J. Am. Geriatr. Soc. **20**:467-472, 1972.

Brown, M.: The new aged: the young-old and the vulnerable old. In Brown, M., ed.: Readings in gerontology, ed. 2, St. Louis, 1978, The C. V. Mosby Co.

Brudno, J. J.: Experimental approach to services for the ready-to-admit applicant to a geriatric home and hospital, J. Am. Geriatr. Soc. **16**:597-602, 1968.

Burnside, I. M.: Nursing and the aged, New York, 1976, McGraw-Hill Book Co.

Busse, E.: Treatment of the non-hospitalized emotionally disturbed elderly person, Geriatrics **11**:173-179, 1956.

Butler, R. N., and Lewis, M. I.: Aging and mental health: positive psychosocial approaches, ed. 2, St. Louis, 1977, The C. V. Mosby Co.

Caplan, G., and Grunebaum, H.: Perspectives on primary prevention: a review. In Gottesfeld, H., ed.: The critical issues of community mental health, New York, 1972, Behavioral Publications.

Carlson, S.: Communication and social interaction in the aged, Nurs. Clin. North Am. 7:269-280, 1972.

Cautela, J.: The Pavlovian basis of old age. In Kent, D., Kastenbaum, R., and Sherwood, S., ed.: Research planning for the elderly, New York, 1972, Behavioral Publications.

Comfort, A.: The joy of sex, New York, 1972, Simon & Schuster, Inc.

Comfort, A.: More joy, New York, 1974, Simon & Schuster, Inc.

Cumming, E.: New thoughts on theory of disengagement, Int. J. Psychiatry 6:53-67, July 1968.

Cumming, E.: Engagement with an old theory, Int. J. Aging Hum. Dev. 6:187-191, 1975.

Cumming, E., and Henry, W.: Growing old, New York, 1961, Basic Books, Inc.

Dubos, R.: Health and creative adaptation, Human Nature 1:74-82, 1978.

Ebersole, P. P.: Reminiscing and group psychotherapy with the aged. In Burnside, I. M., ed.: Nursing and the aged, New York, 1976, McGraw-Hill Book Co.

Ellis, J.: Love to Share: a community project tailored by oldsters for latch-key children, Am. J. Orthopsychiatry 42:249-250, 1972.

French, J. R. P. Jr.: The conceptualization and measurement of mental health in terms of self-identity theory. In Sells, S. B., ed.: The definition and measurement of mental health, Washington, D.C., 1968, U.S. Dept. of Health, Education and Welfare.

Garrison, J., Kulp, C., and Rosen, S.: Community mental health nursing: a social network approach, J. Psychiatr. Nurs. 15:32-36, 1977.

Goldman, R.: Decline in organ function with aging. In Rossman, I., ed.: Clinical geriatrics, Philadelphia, 1971, J. B. Lippincott Co.

Haugk, K. C.: Unique contributions of churches and clergy for community mental health, Community Ment. Health J. 12:20-8, Spring 1976.

Havighurst, R. J.: Successful aging, Gerontologist 1:8-13, March 1961.

Havighurst, R. J.: Social roles, work, leisure, and education. In Eisdorfer, C., and Lawton, M. P., ed.: The psychology of adult development and aging, Washington, D.C., 1973, American Psychological Association.

Hayter, J.: Biological changes of aging, Nurs. Forum 13: 291-309, 1974.

Henthorn, B. S.: Disengagement and reinforcement in the elderly: an explanatory survey, (unpublished doctoral dissertation), Norman, Okla., 1975, University of Oklahoma.

Hogue, C. C.: Support systems for health promotion. In Hall, J. E., and Weaver, B. R., eds.: Distributive nursing practice: a systems approach to community health, Philadelphia, 1977, J. B. Lippincott Co.

Hoyman, H.: Human ecology and health education II, J. Sch. Health 41:538-547, 1971.

Huber, R.: Sensory training for a fuller life, Nurs. Homes 22:14-15, 1973.

Kaplan, J.: Functions and objectives of a senior citizen's center, Geriatrics 17:771-777, 1962.

Korman, A. K.: Toward an hypothesis of work behavior, J. Appl. Psychol. 54:31-41, February 1970.

Kral, V. D.: Psychiatric problems in the aged: a reconsideration, Can. Med. Assoc. J. 108:584-590, 1973.

Kramer, M., and Schmalenberg, C.: Paths to biculturalism, Wakefield, Mass., 1977, Contemporary Publishing, Inc.

Kuypers, J. A., and Bengston, V. L.: Social breakdown and competence: a model of normal aging, Hum. Dev. 16:181-201, 1973.

Leukel, F.: Physiological psychology: a study guide, ed. 2, St. Louis, 1976, The C. V. Mosby Co.

Lindsley, O. R.: Geriatric behavioral prosthetics. In Kastenbaum, R., ed.: New thoughts on old age, New York, 1964, Springer Publishing Co., Inc.

Londoner, C. A.: Survival needs of the aged: implications for program planning, Aging Hum. Dev. 2:113-117, May 1971.

Lopata, H.: The social involvement of American widows, Am. Behav. Scientist 14:41-51, 1970.

Luckmann, J., and Sorenson, K. C.: Medical-surgical nursing: a psychophysiologic approach, Philadelphia, 1974, W. B. Saunders Co.

Maslow, A. H.: Motivation and personality, New York, 1954, Harper & Row, Publishers.

McClannahan, L. E.: Therapeutic and prosthetic living environments for nursing home residents, Gerontologist 13:424-429, 1973.

Meleis, A. I.: Role insufficiency and role supplementation: a conceptual framework, Nurs. Res. 24:264-271, 1975.

Murphy, J. F., ed.: Theoretical issues in professional nursing, Des Moines, 1971, Meredith Corp.

Murray, R., and Zentner, J.: Nursing concepts for health promotion, Englewood Cliffs, N.J., 1975, Prentice-Hall, Inc.

Murrell, S. A.: Community psychology and social systems, New York, 1973, Behavioral Publications.

Palmore, E., and Luikart, C.: Health and social factors related to life satisfaction, J. Health Soc. Behav. 13:68-80, March 1972.

Pastalan, L. S., and Carson, D. H.: Spatial behavior of older people, Ann Arbor, Mich., 1970, University of Michigan Press.

Patterson, R. D.: Services for the aged in community mental health centers, Am. J. of Psychiatry 133:271-273, 1976.

Petty, B. J., Moeller, T. P., and Campbell, R. Z.: Support groups for elderly persons in the community, Gerontologist **15:**522-528, 1976.

Public Information Office, Bureau of the Census: We the American elderly, Washington, D.C., 1973, U.S. Government Printing Office.

Rappaport, J.: Community psychology: values, research, and action, New York, 1977, Holt, Rinehart & Winston.

Riley, M., and Foner, A.: Aging and society, Vol. 1, New York, 1968, Russell Sage Foundation.

Riley, M., Johnson, M., and Foner, A.: Aging and society, Vol. 3, New York, 1972, Russell Sage Foundation.

Rosow, I.: The social context of the aging self, Gerontologist **13:**82-87, Spring 1973.

Rossman, I.: Clinical geriatrics, Philadelphia, 1971, J. B. Lippincott Co.

Rossman, I.: Human aging changes. In Burnside, I. M., ed.: Nursing and the aged, New York, 1976, McGraw-Hill Book Co.

Rotter, J. B.: Generalized expectancies for internal versus external control of reinforcement, Psychol. Monogr. **80:**1-28, 1966.

Roy, C.: Introduction to nursing: an adaptation model, Englewood Cliffs, N.J., 1976, Prentice-Hall, Inc.

Sarbin, T. R.: A role-theory perspective for community psychology: the structure of social identity. In Adelson, D., and Kalis, B. L.: Community psychology and mental health: perspectives and challenges, Scranton, Pa., 1970, Chandler Publishing Co.

Shock, N. W.: The physiology of aging, Sci. Am. **206:**100-110, 1962.

Simon, A.: Physical and socio-psychologic stress in the geriatric mentally ill, Comp. Psychiatry **11:**242-247, 1970.

Skinner, B. F.: About behaviorism, New York, 1974, Alfred A. Knopf, Inc.

Snyder, L. H., Pyrek, J., and Smith, K. C.: Vision and mental function of the elderly, Gerontologist **16:**491-495, 1976.

Stone, V.: Give the older person time, Am. J. Nurs. **69:** 2124-2127, 1969.

Streib, G. F., and Schneider, C. J.: Retirement in American society, Ithaca, N.Y., 1972, Cornell University Press.

Sullivan, H. S.: The interpersonal theory of psychiatry, New York, 1953, W. W. Norton & Co.

Trickett, E. J., Kelly, J. G., and Todd, D. M.: The social environment of the high school: guidelines for individual change and organizational redevelopment. In Golann, S. E., and Eisdorfer, C., eds.: Handbook of community mental health, New York, 1972, Appleton-Century-Crofts.

Wilkerson, C. B., and O'Connor, W. A.: Introduction and overview, Psychiatr. Annuals **7:**334-336, 1977.

Part three

PREVENTIVE MODELS FOR HIGH-RISK POPULATIONS

■ Part three describes community mental health nursing interventions with four general populations. Prevention occurs with these groups at all three levels, although by virtue of the type of crises each population experiences, most likely secondary prevention is used. Secondary prevention is directed toward reducing the prevalence of mental disorder by providing help that lessens the stressors and thereby decreases the duration of disequilibrium.

Specifically, the clients described in Part three become high-risk populations for mental illness because of situational crises often beyond their control. Both the individual defined as a substance abuser and the client undergoing transsexual surgery are able to exert more control over their life situations than the individuals described as victims of violence, the discharged long-term psychiatric patient, or one who must adjust to an altered body image from a radical surgical procedure.

Although the client populations described in Part three represent a wide array of stressful events and subsequent coping needs, some commonalities exist among the groups. In general the crises presented by members of the populations described are situational. In each case the client has the opportunity to learn new adaptive responses to the environment or to succumb to the stress and be weakened by the situation. The goal of nursing care is to provide support that enhances the client's ability to adapt as he develops new problem-solving skills for responding to both internal and external stress.

Each client population described in Part three can be considered victims. It is easier perhaps to view the battered spouse, abused child, or raped person as a victim than an individual who abuses chemicals, who seeks transsexual surgery, who experiences an altered body image, or who must adjust to a world outside the institution. Indeed each can be considered a victim of the environment and its complex stresses and demands for rapid, often spontaneous change. The goal of nursing intervention is to promote adjustment to societal demands by strengthening the client's coping ability.

CHAPTER 8

Dealing with the emotional needs of persons undergoing transsexual surgery

JUDITH M. ATLEE

Sex reassignment surgery, while not commonplace, is becoming more available and technically sophisticated. Nurses are now more likely to find themselves caring for clients undergoing this surgery, an experience for which few are adequately prepared. Because of inexperience and unfamiliarity with this surgery, the nurse may find it necessary to deal with subjective discomfort, ambivalent curiosity, and even feelings of repugnance when confronted with such patients. Hopefully this chapter will acquaint nurses with the origins and effects of gender dysphoria, and various aspects of sex reassignment surgery, so that they may deal constructively with their clients.

At times nurses find themselves uncomfortable with a particular client for one reason or another. Because of the moral and ethical implications of transsexualism, discomfort is especially likely. To deny this discomfort would be dishonest; to understand its origins and learn to deal with clients frankly, empathetically, and supportively is more effective.

The case history that concludes this chapter serves to illustrate many of the aspects discussed here. This experience and others like it indicate a specific need for nurses who are acquainted with sex reassignment surgery. Nurses need to be knowledgeable about the technical aspects as they relate to the needs of patients and their families as well as about the origins of transsexualism and the kinds of treatment clients encounter before and after surgery.

WHAT IS A TRANSSEXUAL?

Since terms used in discussing transsexuality may be unfamiliar, they should be discussed briefly. Transsexuality is frequently confused with homosexuality and transvestism. Homosexuality refers to one's choice of sexual object, as does heterosexuality. The homosexual has a desire for genital stimulation and maintains a sexual identity that corresponds to his or her anatomy, although cross-dressing in the clothing of the other sex may occur. Transvestism involves deriving erotic excitement from dressing in the clothing of the opposite sex, although the sexual object chosen is heterosexual.

A transsexual is one whose sexual or gender identity does not correspond with his or her anatomical identity. The term "gender dysphoria" is also used to describe this phenomenon; dysphoria refers to the person's pain and conflict at being unable to attain a congruent gender identification. In other words, as many transsexuals say, they feel trapped in the body of the opposite sex.

Adult transsexuals seeking sex reassignment surgery have three characteristics in common: (1) they feel that their bodies are inappropriate, incongruous, and/or grotesque; (2) they believe that changing their roles to that of the opposite anatomical sex will improve their lives; and (3) they are sexually attracted to members of the same anatomical sex, but their interest is of a heterosexual nature (Meyer, 1974). Generally they desire surgery to make the anatomy fit the gender identity. In addition, there are nonsexual reasons such as the individual's need to assume the role of the desired sex in society. Indeed the need to function in society as a member of the sex with which they identify is often far more important than any sexual reasons. The desire and the intensity with which it is pursued is impressive to say the least.

The genitals are usually described by transsexuals with disgust or shame, and even during sexual intercourse or masturbation they may disassociate from them. Dressing in the clothing of the desired sex (cross-dressing) is not a source of erotic stimulation as in the transvestite but is rather an effort to establish a congruence between the person's body and his or her mental self-image. It is this need for congruence that leads to the decision to seek sex reassignment surgery.

ORIGINS OF SEXUAL DYSPHORIA

There is considerable disagreement about the origin of sexual identity, and no one theory seems to answer the question, "How does the individual come to know that he or she is male or female?" The literature suggests that it is a combination of biological and environmental factors.

An individual's behavior may be influenced prenatally by the administration of hormones or at puberty by a spontaneous change in the biological system, but the influence of postnatal rearing and role modeling, as well as the socialization of the individual, play major roles in which sex the individual determines himself or herself to be (Money and Tucker, 1975).

Parents are the primary conveyors of attitudes, prejudices, and expectations of the child's gender role. One hypothesis about gender dysphoria is that one or both parents unconsciously encourage cross-gender behavior, and that the child adopts this behavior to gain parental approval and attention. Conversely, there may be nothing from either parent that might inhibit the child's cross-gender activity (Bentler, 1976). When the reaction of other people to this child makes him aware of his anatomical gender, he also becomes conscious that it is not consistent with his behavior. He or she may become confused and depressed, a fact that is apparent immediately in interviews with transsexuals who inevitably describe painful childhoods in which they often adopted patterns of behavior such as secret cross-dressing at very young ages, while outwardly trying to live up to the behavior expected by their peers and adults. Elements of this kind of sex-role confusion are observed in elementary classrooms where a child may manifest a preference for the activities and dress of the opposite sex and even at an early age may express a wish to *be* a member of the opposite sex. Sex role confusion is common to many young children but where other factors combine to create conditions of sexual dysphoria the confusion persists.

In our society the "tomboy" is more likely to be accepted by peers than the male counterpart who is teased for being a "sissy" and prefers to play with dolls. For the sexually dysphoric child, increasingly hostile disapproval causes much discomfort and discourages him from developing social relationships with peers. Adult transsexuals describe efforts during childhood to reduce role dissonance by adopting roles more congruent with their anatomical sex; that is, male children try to be more aggressive and to take part in games associated with male behavior, while female children take part in doll play with peers and wear dresses—efforts that usually end in failure because their thoughts and feelings are counteractive.

YOUNG GENDER DYSPHORICS

As with many childhood problems, there has been a tendency to let the child "outgrow" this behavior in the hope that the child on reaching adolescence will discover the opposite sex, develop a congruent gender role, and discontinue inappropriate behavior. Some authorities (Money and Tucker, 1975) believe that gender identity is formed during the time the child acquires language. It is apparent, however, that the child's behavior patterns and sexual identity, whatever they may be, become more ingrained as the years pass and that once the gender identity of the transsexual is established neither the weight of societal pressure nor intensive psychotherapy has yet been able to reverse the process.

It may be that sex role stereotyping in our society has a great deal to do with gender dysphoria. Some male-to-female clients relate that their expectations of the future include a wish to be married, not for sexual reasons but rather in the context of the security marriage seems to offer. They wish to be cared for, to be immersed in the stereotype housewife's comfortable life. Independence and sexual pleasure seem equally unimportant to these transsexuals in comparison with the fantasy of the married woman's stable, tranquil life. Some have been married one or more times as men and see the life of a housewife as a haven in which all will be well. It is impossible, apparently, to convince them that this is a fantasy, and they are not interested in lives as independent women.

EARLY TREATMENT

Surgical intervention and administration of cross-gender hormones are generally considered unacceptable procedures prior to the legal age of consent. Adolescents with sexual dysphoria are currently being treated in a number of ways. The nurse's role is supportive and educative, oriented toward helping to make life adjustments less painful for clients and for their families. The nurse plays a part in primary prevention in the community through prenatal and postnatal counseling designed to enhance effectiveness as parents. Preventive efforts also include developing school and community programs that lead to a better understanding of growth and development, teaching recognition and acceptance of one's sexuality, and facilitating communication of thoughts and feelings between family members.

Treatment of the gender dysphoric adolescent has traditionally demanded that the individual engage in behavior congruent with his or her anatomical sex, which included actively pursuing dates and interactions with members of the opposite sex. This approach often reflects the therapist's own discomfort in dealing with problems related to sexual orientation. The therapist's behavior may indicate that the thoughts and feelings of the client are unacceptable and should be modified, with the underlying assumption that changing the outward behavior solves the inner problem.

A more effective approach is to work toward relief of the client's depression, isolation, and lack of self-acceptance by showing a willingness to listen to the client express thoughts and feelings that have been suppressed because of social disapproval. In taking a holistic approach, the therapist examines the person's total lifestyle as well as gender role confusion, thereby assisting the client to explore alternatives instead of focusing all of his energy on maintaining a defensive posture. This approach also encourages the nurse to develop an empathetic attitude toward the adolescent's struggle against isolation and negative criticism from family and peers.

Behavior modification (Green et al., 1972) has been used in an effort to reverse gender dysphoria in early childhood in effeminate boys. While results have been encouraging, long-term effects are not yet known. It has also been suggested that the child undergo psychotherapy with a person of the same sex who can serve as an appropriate gender model. If the parents can openly support and encourage the child's appropriate gender role, their participation would be helpful.

The child who has continually been isolated and criticized by his peers finds adolescence a time of renewed crisis. The appearance of secondary sex characteristics further emphasizes the dissonance between the adolescent's behavior, his fantasy life, and the facts of anatomical reality. He may be curious about, or attracted to, the opposite sex. By this time, estranged from peers, the gender dysphoric adolescent is inadequate to pursue interests of social interaction and formation of intimate heterosexual relationships. Depression and suicidal impulses may be manifested, and the dilemma is intensified by the normal adolescent intolerance of inappropriate sexual behavior. Parents usually become intensely concerned and seek help when they notice behavior that they interpret as overt homosexual activity.

Homosexual activity carries a different connotation for the transsexual than for the homosexual. The transsexual, feeling the sexual impulses of the opposite anatomical sex, is attracted to persons of the same anatomical sex. This of course gives the appearance of homosexual attachment, but transsexuals eventually come to realize that homosexuality is not compatible with what they understand themselves to be. While the transsexual's behavior may indicate overt homosexual activity, denials of homosexual interests and activities are verbalized. The individual feels that he is operating from a heterosexual base. The conflicts inherent in this situation are obvious.

PRESURGICAL TREATMENT

Careful evaluation of surgical candidates is mandatory, since the procedure is irreversible and considered palliative and not curative. The sex change cannot result in a total transformation of person or physique, and while most transsexuals describe improvement in how they feel about themselves after surgery, they still have the same problems and conflicts. Surgery does not change the individual's family, job, or friends. If the person is comfortable living in the desired sex role before surgery, the same will probably hold true afterward.

Since most surgical programs require cross-living for 1 to 5 years prior to surgery, during this time therapy can afford a major source of support for the transsexual in adjusting to this change. It can be a relief for the client to be able to express feelings and discuss gender confusion with a nurse who respects him. Therapy also helps to stabilize the person's gender role before irreversible surgery. Most clients reach their decision for surgery without psychotherapy, counseling, or professional advice, and the requirements of presurgical counseling is often seen by clients as just one more obstacle to overcome before the desired goal can be attained.

Unfortunately, since psychotherapy is often accepted only as a condition to be met before surgery instead of being elected by the client, the outcome is not always positive. A therapeutic alliance with a resistive patient is difficult if not impossible to establish, and the client often suspects that the nurse's purpose in the sessions is to establish grounds for refusing surgery. The client may also sense the nurse's ambivlaence or lack of empathy toward the transsexual's psychophysical rejection of anatomical sexual identity. Some clients have expressed that care givers' lack of understanding causes them to "feel like a freak."

As in other nursing situations, ambivalence may arise when the nurse is confronted with a particularly stressful or "loaded" situation. Just as nurses caring for a dying patient are made acutely aware of their own mortality and the possibility of death, so are the nurses caring for transsexual clients uncomfortably aware of their own sexuality and any existing doubts or anxieties about it. While these feelings may be present in varying degrees, they can be overcome by the nurse who acknowledges that they exist, understands their origins, and frankly tries to establish a trusting relationship with the client by being honest about inherent feelings and conflicts.

For instance, the nurse may be uncertain as to what pronoun to use in reference to the client preparing for sex reassignment surgery. The best course is to acknowledge the question and take one's cue from the client. The transsexual thus feels confident that his feelings are being considered when he becomes aware that the nurse, while feeling some confusion, can deal with it honestly.

HORMONE THERAPY

Endocrine therapy, which induces growth and development of secondary sex characteristics of the desired sex, is instituted at least 1 year prior to surgery. Some transsexuals give histories of obtaining birth control pills or other hormones through clandestine sources before seeking medical intervention. However, all clients should be urged to follow the physician's prescribed endocrine regime carefully, as dosages vary from patient to patient and the proper combination is usually determined over a period of time.

Androgen therapy is generally given to women and estrogen therapy to men, although some physicians prescribe a combination of estrogen and progesterone hormones. Males receiving female hormones experience increased breast size, softening of the skin, and increased subcutaneous fat, which causes a softer curve of the body and atrophy of the testicles. One male-to-female client stated that as her hormone therapy progressed she observed a noticeable decrease in muscular strength, especially of the upper torso. The deep voice is not altered with hormones, but it can be affected by voice training. A tape recorder is often helpful in working toward voice change. The female receiving male hormones experiences beard growth, an increase in body hair, cessation of menstrua-

tion, and sometimes a decrease in breast size and a lowering of the voice.

Almost all clients relate that there is a change in emotions and libido following the course of hormone therapy. They are generally pleased with the increased breast size and softened features or the growth of facial hair and increased musculature but many state that the hormones did not bring about all the hoped-for changes. Evidently there is often a preconceived fantasy that is not completely realized; this fantasy may be similar to the disappointment felt by many women who have small breasts or by men who do not have a full beard or hair on the chest. Additional plastic surgery before sex reassignment surgery is often done in the form of breast augmentation, rhinoplasty, and reduction of thyroid cartilage. Male-to-female transsexuals also require a series of electrolysis treatments to remove unwanted hair.

TRANSITION

Most clients recall painful incidents of rejection and disapproval during the period of transition. It is not uncommon for the presurgical transsexual to find his or her most sympathetic and nonjudgmental friends among the homosexual community. However, once the decision for sex-change surgery is made and becomes known to the person's friends, the homosexuals often exhibit hostility or withdraw from the transsexual.

The transitional need for cross-dressing can produce high levels of anxiety, which necessitates crisis counseling. There is often a real fear of being found out, with such consequences as loss of job, status, and/or friends. The nurse may use a direction-giving approach, which includes helping the stressed client through crises. In extreme cases nursing intervention can include helping the client seek legal counsel, as in the instance of a man dressed in women's clothing who was discovered in a public ladies' room.

In the counseling situation sensitive criticism may be required. Many patterns of behavior are sex coded, and certain manners, gestures, and postures that usually seem insignificant go unnoticed until they are seen out of context. These are things that most heterosexual individuals learn from earliest childhood, but the transsexual is faced with the problem of having to learn these patterns of behavior both quickly and consciously rather than through the usual long process of unconscious acquisition. Transsexual clients are affected by their experience as well as by feedback from others, and in many cases the nurse can help by offering constructive suggestions in an uncritical way. For instance, it is not unusual for a transsexual to overreact to the desired gender role with extreme clothing, gestures, or makeup. A transsexual client pointed out that this may not be recognized by the individual and that it makes him or her unnecessarily conspicuous and vulnerable to being "read" to by others. In addition, the transsexual's friends may be hesitant to offer criticism or indeed may not recognize the extreme mannerisms. Therefore the nurse is in a position to include these aspects of adjustment in the counseling activity.

Another male-to-female transsexual observed that while she had used extreme makeup and clothing when she began cross-dressing, it became less necessary as she became more comfortable in the female role. This may be compared to the need that many people have to interpret their own sexual images through the reactions of members of the opposite sex, a need that usually disappears with maturity and adjustment to one's sexual identity.

In addition to counseling the surgical patient, the nurse plays a major role in the acceptance of the transsexual by hospital personnel (Lark, 1975). If a hospital nursing unit has not had a transsexual client before, team conferences should be called and inservice education given for each shift. The hospital "grapevine" can generate numerous rumors and misinformation,

and the nursing staff needs the opportunity to voice its contents and gain information concerning nursing care for the transsexual patient. Staff members who feel that they cannot accept the patient should not be forced to do so. However, most informed members of the nursing staff, after the initial moment of curiosity, are able to interact with these surgical patients in a caring manner and to treat them with respect due to all patients.

A major problem for transsexuals is financing the treatment process, the cost of which is prohibitive for most. Health insurance plans usually cover few if any of the expenses, and it is not unusual for the doctor and hospital to require cash in advance. Consequently many transsexuals exceed the minimum waiting period by years while trying to get their finances in order. One cannot help being impressed with their persistence and determination to reach their surgical goals.

Many individuals have their gender changed legally; some gender dysphoria clinics are able to facilitate this process by recommending legal counsel sympathetic to the transsexual person. This allows all legal documents to be altered to concur with the person's professed gender. It also allows the individual to enter into a marriage contract. Many clients who have been living as the desired gender for some time are already married or engaged, and this is very important to them.

Prolonged follow-up studies on transsexual clients have been difficult because of their need to establish new identities and disassociate with much of the past. One transsexual summed up the situation, stating, "When surgery and life adjustments are satisfactory the transsexual blends into the general population. It is only the problems you hear about."

ADDITIONAL CONCERNS

Some problems may be related to the transsexual's family. Generally the transsexual has not consulted parents or children about the decision for sex reassignment and is determined to have the surgery regardless of the family's acceptance or nonacceptance. By the time the transsexual announces the decision the family usually knows something is "wrong" but is not aware of the extent of the future change. Responses are varied. Some family members recognize surgery as a resolution of the dilemma; others regard it as a family "skeleton in the closet." Some blame themselves and others renounce the transsexual family member. If the family accepts the decision they may still have some doubts regarding whether to conceal or to disclose the relative's new status. Some choose to edit the story for all but their closest friends. Family acceptance of the transsexual member can contribute to a more favorable adjustment of the transsexual client to his external environment. This requires family members to adapt to new communication patterns and designated roles. The nurse can facilitate this change in the family by giving them support and encouragement as well as information concerning what changes and procedures to expect.

Prior to the surgery, counseling includes orienting the client to the hospital. Even though most are knowledgeable about the surgical procedures and are willing to face the pain and discomfort of surgery, they also experience anxiety and apprehension. Family members can be included in this counseling.

Discharge planning should not be overlooked. Patients should give evidence that they will be able to carry out the prescribed regime for the course of convalescence to prevent postoperative complication. Often a family member will be assisting with the care and should be included in the instruction.

Postsurgical counseling should be encouraged to further ease the client's transition into the community. Prior to surgery the problem of gender dysphoria took much of the client's time and energy to the neglect or exclusion of other aspects of life. After convalescence the client

may take an active role in developing more intimate relationships and change vocation or educational goals. He may pursue the establishment of his own family unit through marriage. The nurse's role is to continue to facilitate the transsexual client's positive interaction with the external environment by helping to decrease stress in his internal environment.

CASE HISTORY

While it is difficult to isolate a "typical" case history, the client described exemplifies in his history and attitudes aspects of the transsexual person that have been described in the chapter. In order to minimize confusion for the reader, the client is referred to as "he" until the decision was made to begin the sex reassignment procedure and as "she" after that point. The history describes a single individual and is taken from interviews after the sex reassignment was complete.

The patient is 44 years old. He lived until the age of 27 in the same town and neighborhood; of middle-class parents, he has a brother 2 years older and a sister 2 years younger. He describes his father as a "hard worker and stern disciplinarian" who wanted a daughter when he was born and to whom he did not feel close until late adolescence. He did, however, feel close to his mother. His father did not accept him as an infant but "warmed up" when the sister was born 2 years later.

He describes himself in school as "scrappy," fighting frequently, and always trying to have girls as friends but being constantly afraid of being called a "sissy" and having to fight to prove his masculinity. Though there were no male children in his neighborhood he was not allowed to join the little girls in play, although he recalls watching them for long periods of time and wanting to play with them. He particularly recalls watching them dress up, and even in elementary school would secretly dress in his sister's clothes, but not for erotic pleasure.

The family was Presbyterian. Through junior high school his main activity outside school was in the Boy Scouts, but his brother excelled in that area and the patient quit because he felt unable to equal his brother's achievements. He did excel in sports, particularly in swimming, but continued to cross-dress in secret. He had a strong desire to participate in high school dramatics but because he felt that acting was inappropriate behavior for a male, he worked instead on stage crews. After completing high school he enlisted in the Navy.

He was discharged in less than a year after being caught cross-dressing in public off the base. The Navy, however, was apparently very discreet in this matter, and the client gave the reason for his discharge as striking an officer, which upheld his masculine image among his friends and family.

He tried to resolve his conflict through marriage, which lasted for 7 years, which produced one son, and which he described as "miserable." He and his wife fought frequently. He had a low sex drive; his discovery of his wife's extramarital affair precipitated the divorce, which gave him custody of their 5-year-old son.

A second marriage, 2 or 3 years later, to a woman with four children, lasted for 10 years. However, after 4 years of marriage, his wife discovered women's underwear in his car and accused him of infidelity. Under the stress of the situation he admitted that the panties were his and sought psychiatric help, feeling that "his world was crumbling around him." In retrospect, he says that he was fortunate to have a therapist who was sympathetic. He was reconciled with his wife and transferred by his company, and he seriously tried to stop cross-dressing. However, he was not able to do this, and eventually the marriage dissolved under the strain of family problems and financial troubles. His wife remained friendly and later was able to voluntarily help him with his cross-dressing. His son joined the military.

By this time he was cross-dressing all of the time except when he was at work, had started taking birth control pills, and had become active in a national organization for transvestites in which he worked as a counselor. He had always considered himself to be a heterosexual transvestite but found that many of his counseling clients were homosexuals engaged in tranvestism. Feeling inadequate to handle these clients, he turned to a local homosexual community church for assistance. A religious person, he subsequently became very active in this church. Through his close association with the gay community he was able to find employment as a woman; about this time he began to consider the possibility that he might be transsexual rather than transvestite. While he was supported and assisted by this community of homosexual individuals, it must be made clear that at no time did he behave as, or consider himself, a homosexual. The associations were religious and social, but not sexual.

He was now living entirely in the role of a woman, and began taking the steps that led to sex-change surgery. (Hereafter the client will be referred to as "she".)

Surgical techniques now in use had not been fully developed at the time of the client's surgery, and she had postoperative complications with vaginal stenosis that necessitated additional surgery after 14 months. During this time she did not date, because she felt that she was "not ready for a relationship with a man"; she was severely depressed, possibly because of the complications. A year after the reconstruction surgery she had breast implants to augment her breasts, because she felt they were too small.

She broke off her relationship with the gay community after surgery, feeling that her new status was threatening to homosexuals and that they did not accept her changed identity although she had been known to them as a woman before. She also left the homosexual community church.

Her name and sex have been legally changed on all her academic and employment records. She notes with irony that her only employment problem after sex reassignment surgery was that there was a marked drop in her income potential as a woman, which presented economic problems. She says that she is comfortable and that she feels her sexual role as a woman is "very natural"; in general she is happy with the change.

She worked again as a part-time counselor after her surgery, and was able to help others making the same change but found that this required that she again lead a "double life," working as a woman at her regular job while counseling in her spare time as a successful transsexual. The fear of being exposed, which would endanger her job and her new social life, led to a decision to "drop out of sight" and build a new life in another part of the country.

Her family's reactions bear describing. Neither of her siblings will have anything to do with her since the surgery. Her father died some years ago. Her mother had difficulty accepting a "new daughter" but since her surgery they have been able to develop a warm relationship. She has remained close to the four children of her second wife, who continue to rely on her for parental guidance and friendship. The second wife, however, who had remained friendly after the end of the marriage, now seems to have developed some hostility, which may arise from the strain of competing with a "second mother."

Her own natural son, who has been on drugs and has had other problems (although apparently not sexual ones) since adolescence, has severed their relationship. In their last encounter, which was during the presurgical transition period, the son expressed great disappointment, saying to a family friend that he had sought the help of his father only to find that instead he "had another mother." She hopes for a reconciliation and plans to remain in contact with her family after she moves.

When asked how she broke the news of her plans to have sex reassignment surgery, she said that she went to the members of her family and told them first that she loved them and cared deeply for them, but that she did not need them. She said she could go on in life without them but, given the choice, she would prefer not to have to do that. She told them about the surgery and what she planned to do, and made it clear that regardless of their acceptance or nonacceptance she would go through with it. The point was that, while she loved them, she had made an important decision about her life and she hoped that they would be able to accept her. But she also made it clear that they would not be able to change her mind.

References

Bentler, P. M.: A typology of transsexualism: gender identity theory and data, *Arch. Sex. Behav.* **5:**567-584, 1976.

Green, R., and Money, J., eds.: Transsexualism and sex reassignment, Baltimore, 1969, The Johns Hopkins University Press.

Green, R., Newman, L., and Stoller, R.: Treatment of boyhood transsexualism, Arch. Gen. Psychiatry **26:**213-217, 1971.

Lark, C.: Nurses' reactions to transsexual surgery, A.O.R.N. J. **22:**743-749, 1975.

Martin, M.: Emergence: a transsexual autobiography, New York, 1977, Crown Publishers, Inc.

Meyer, J. K.: Clinical variants among applicants for sex reassignment, Arch. Sex. Behav. **3:**527-558, 1974.

Money, J., Clarke, F., and Maxur, T.: Families of seven male-to-female transsexuals after 5-7 years: sociological sexology, Arch. Sex Behav. **4:**187-198, March 1975.

Money, J., and Tucker, P.: Sexual signatures on being a man or a woman, Boston, 1975, Little, Brown & Co.

Simone, C.: The transsexual patient, RN **40:**37-44, 1977.

Rekers, G. A., and Lovaas, O. T. Behavioral treatment of deviant sex role behaviors in a male child, J. Appl. Behav. Anal. **7:**173-190, 1974.

CHAPTER 9

Substance abuse: nursing implications for prevention and health promotion

SHERRY YOWELL

Drug abuse, a major social problem in the United States, has been studied in a wide variety of disciplines and from numerous theoretical and philosophical perspectives. The incidence, frequency, and intensity of the impact of chemical use on individual lives, as well as on the American community as a whole, continue to accelerate. Examiners who study drug abuse have identified various rationales for the current failure to curb the problem including (1) lack of individual motivation, (2) irrational legislative practices, (3) the nature of addiction, (4) the innate drive toward altered states of consciousness, (5) lack of ritual in the taking or avoiding of particular chemicals, (6) social and cultural values focusing on the short-term relief of physical and emotional pain, (7) youth's rebellion against a lack of meaning in life, and (8) the medical monopoly. These concepts exemplify the development of a number of theories and perspectives, each logical and applicable given the focus and subject matter of the respective disciplines but limited in terms of relevant application to systematic human functioning.

If spheres of individual, family, or community functioning (for example, biological, interpersonal, spiritual, technological, and economic) were each to be studied and understood in and of themselves, separate from the other spheres, justification for identifying and maintaining distinct boundaries for the utilization of identifiable bodies of knowledge would be evi-

dent. Fortunately, human beings do not function as machines but as complicated entities who act and react holistically. In the course of living people are intricately involved in simultaneous, complicated networks of functioning, which to some extent influence each other; however, data continue to be collected and utilized separately within the various disciplines as though little relationship or interaction existed between these different areas of functioning.

This fragmented pattern of thought and action has become standardized in this country to the point that each of the various theories regarding the nature of drug abuse and routes to its alleviation has at one time or another been discovered as the ''true nature'' of the problem, and each has been received by the populace as such.

However, despite the millions of dollars and exhaustive professional hours spent on the research and development of drug abuse programs of various types and philosophies, drug abuse incidence continues to rise at alarming rates. This, in and of itself, should be an indicator that *what we have done up to this point and what we continue to do is not working;* what is needed is a reevaluation of our basic beliefs related to the issues involved with chemical use and abuse as it affects everyday life. One outcome of this reevaluation may be an increased awareness of the need for collaboration among disciplines interested in investigating this phenomenon so that integrated frameworks may be applied to a multifaceted problem.

Professional nursing has been one of the few human service disciplines that has defined the systematic, integrated nature of human functioning as basic to its theoretical framework for practice. Primarily because of the influence of the integration of basic anthropological concepts with the theory base of nursing, professional nurses are recognizing the value of defining basic belief systems and applying context-based frameworks to the assessment of individual, family, and community health status to plan effective interventions.

Health promotion and education of the general population prior to the development of symptoms is increasingly being recognized as a value that must demand increasing amounts of time, money, and energy from the "health" care system. If any impact is to be made on preventing the destructive consequences of our use, misuse, and mistaken conceptualizations of drugs and the issues related to them and on promoting the positive health status of individuals, then increasing effort must be directed toward facilitating the development of a consumer group that is aware of, and informed on, the issues involved.

MEDICALIZATION OF THE HUMAN CONDITION

Drugs have become in this country a short-cut device for the relief of physical and emotional discomfort. The medicalization of the human condition, which has increased insidiously since the 1950s, reached the point in the 1970s that "about one-third of all Americans between the ages of 18 and 74 had used a psychoactive drug of some kind; less than one-third of the 230 million prescriptions for psychoactive agents written in one year were written by psychiatrists" (Bernstein and Lennard, 1973).

The message is increasingly reinforced in this culture that if a person experiences emotional pain of any intensity—interpersonal struggle,

disillusionment, depression, marital difficulty, or any number of other descriptive terms for what used to be thought of as concomitants of human existence—there is something "wrong" with that individual and he "should" seek help, which usually includes taking something for "it" (Bernstein and Lennard, 1973; Lennard, 1971; Szasz, 1967). The assumption has been made that social intercourse is inherently harmonious and that its disturbance is caused solely by the presence of mental illness: "We have failed to accept the fact that human relations are inherently fraught with difficulties and that to make them even relatively harmonious requires much patience and hard work" (Szasz, 1967). We are taught that we are to be beautiful, happy, successful, popular, happily married, sweet smelling, and blessed with beautiful white teeth and that if we are not the possessors of these attributes it is because we are not consuming the right product, whether it be a specific kind of soup, toothpaste, or tranquilizer.

In the context of current usage, drugs are medical agents whose medical function is the solution of medical problems. Only to the extent that interpersonal and other problems can be construed as medical-psychiatric problems can they be considered appropriate targets for drug treatment (Lennard, 1971).

Bernstein and Lennard (1973) estimate that 60% of the patients who appear in general practitioners' offices do so for vague, nonspecific purposes; they identify two important sets of ideas influencing this high percentage: "One has to do with the ideals of health, normality and functioning that members of our society are expected to live up to; the second is the notion that failure to live up to these can be remedied through the medium of medical practice." This illustrates the assumption often made by Americans that there is a technological solution for every human problem. This common assumption reinforces the view that single cause-effect relationships characterize our thinking and functioning and if one could only identify the specific areas of difficulty (usually referring to separate parts of man's existence and functioning), the appropriate remedy could be identified and administered.

Reinforcement of such thinking is occurring systematically as a result of the interlocking dynamics of a number of health professional groups and business interests and their impact on the consumer. The consumer is continuously being educated, treated, and entertained from a number of significant vantage points and ultimately learns to demand that which he has been taught he needs to function normally. An increased need is thus created by the continuous increase in the production and availability of both prescription and nonprescription drugs. Mental health practitioners, physicians, pharmaceutical companies, legislators, and media promote an image of the personality and accompanying life in America that further perpetuates medicalization and technocratization of human existence. With the idea that any major, minor, or in-between complaint of human existence can be alleviated by taking something or buying something and as long as this idea continues to be mediated by the paternalistic image of the physician and reinforced by significant economic controlling forces in this country, the trend of drug taking, particularly as it relates to "legitimate" drugs, can do nothing but increase.

IMPACT OF LEGISLATION

The cure of drug abuse has been one of the purposes on which not only physicians but members of various disciplines have focused enormous amounts of time and energy. The accepted definition of the drug abuser, as defined particularly by the medical segment, represents an error in definition:

Part of the contemporary medical mythology is that drugs somehow do not exact the same price from the user when they are prescribed by a physician; drug abuse has traditionally referred to the physiological, psychological and social problems associated with illegal, excessive use of drugs and *non-medical* purposes (Lennard, 1971).

The term "drug abuser" refers to the user of illegal or black-market drugs; the "good" drugs (psychoactive drugs referred to above—primarily the amphetamines and barbiturates), which are prescribed by a physician, despite the extensive use of these chemicals, are not included in the definition and scope of the problem. The same is true of the 'nondrugs' (alcohol, nicotine, and caffeine) whose consumption is not only legitimized but encouraged, and whose chronic use results in devastating physical and psychological consequences.

"Being medicated by a doctor is drug use, while self-medication is drug abuse . . . a plea for legitimizing what doctors do because they do it with good (therapeutic) intent, and for illegitimizing what laymen do, because they do it with bad, self-abusive (masturbatory) intent" (Szasz, 1977). Weil (1972) has rephrased the commonly asked question regarding why people take drugs: "We are spending much time, money and energy trying to find out why some people are taking drugs, but in fact, what we are doing is trying to find out why some people are taking drugs *we disapprove of.*" The issues of approval and disapproval and of how we culturally define what a drug is and which of these drugs are to be sanctioned for consumption by the population or specified segments of it are critical to understanding drug abuse in this country. Szasz (1977) identifies many of the consequences of our drug-taking behavior as resulting from a lack of clarity of the basic frameworks or categories that we use to discuss and define the problem; we emphasize the scientific (medical) aspects while the religious (moral) aspects are basic.

The important differences between heroin and alcohol or marijuana and tobacco, as far as drug abuse is concerned are not chemical (medical or scientific) but ceremonial (religious or moral). In other words, heroin and marijuana are approached and avoided not because they are more addictive or more dangerous than alcohol and tobacco, but because they are more holy or unholy as the case may be (Szasz, 1977).

Szasz identified the medical perspective on moral conduct (that is, personal conduct is not volutional but reflective; human beings are not subjects but objects, not persons but organisms) as a critical influencing force on the readiness of the American consumer to find chemical solutions to a wide variety of human problems.

The impact of legislative policy, which ultimately has defined what makes a substance a drug and what makes it a good one or a bad one, has been studied at length by the editors of *Consumer Reports,* and their exhaustive study is documented in Brecher's (1972) *Licit and Illicit Drugs.* From study of the historical perspective presented, the concept of "dictated deviance" becomes a valuable framework for assessing sources of the drug problem. The observation is made that in each generation, respectable society itself dictates the direction that much of the deviance will take. Strict law enforcement has contributed to the drug abuse problem by helping to create addict subcultures. Beginning with the Harrison Narcotic Act of 1914, which cut off altogether the supply of legal opiates to addicts, the withdrawal of the protection of the food and drug laws from the users of illicit drugs has been one of the significant factors in reducing addicts to their present status: "It was the criminalization of addiction that created addicts as a special and distinctive group, and it is the subcultural aspects of addicts that gives them their recruiting power" (Goode, 1972).

A review of the literature since 1956, carried out by the editors of *Consumer Reports,* shows that almost all of the deleterious effects ordinarily attributed to opiates have been effects of the narcotics acts themselves: "By far the most serious deleterious effects of being a narcotic addict in the United States today are the risks of arrest and imprisonment, infectious disease

and impoverishment, all traceable to the resulting excessive black market prices for narcotics" (Brecher, 1972).

Szasz (1977) summarizes the mechanisms that are thus created by the controlling powers for legalized drug use: having successfully deprived vast numbers of persons of the legitimate use of drugs to which they have become accustomed (or in which they have become interested), the governments of the leading nations of the world now satisfy the unquenchable craving of their people for ceremonial drugs in one or more of these three ways:

1. Legitimizing certain drugs by defining them as not drugs at all and by encouraging their consumption, for example, alcohol and tobacco
2. Tacitly fostering an illicit trade in prohibitive drugs, for example, heroin and marijuana
3. Aggressively promoting the use, through medical prescriptions, of certain types of new nontraditional mood affecting drugs

The Consumer Union report also carried out an extensive research effort on the effects of the chemicals that are currently described as legitimate and therefore assumed to be less dangerous than those toward whose control greater efforts have been made. The following summarizes their major findings (Brecher, 1972):

A. Nicotine
   1. Tobacco is one of the most physiologically damaging substances used by man.
   2. From the 1600s until today, no country that has ever learned to use tobacco has given up the practice.
   3. Of those who smoke more than one cigarette during adolescence, approximately 70% continue smoking for the next 40 years.
   4. Cigarette smoking is for most smokers an *addiction* to the drug nicotine. Both physical dependence and tolerance to nicotine have been documented.

5. Conclusive evidence indicates that cigarette smoking is by far the most important cause of lung cancer and is also a major factor in deaths from coronary heart disease, chronic bronchitis, emphysema, and other diseases.
6. Anticigarette laws and campaigns early in the century were among the significant factors popularizing the cigarette; the prohibition served as a lure.
7. Nearly four male smokers out of five consume fifteen or more cigarettes per day, roughly one or more per waking hour.

B. Alcohol
1. Alcohol is treated as a nondrug. It is on sale in multidose bottles at some 40,000 liquor stores. More than $250 million is spent each year on advertising alcohol.
2. Alcohol addiction is second only to nicotine addiction in incidence and prevalence in the United States. A conservative estimate is that 5 million Americans are alcoholics, but figures as high as 7 to 9 million alcoholics and problem drinkers are also cited.
3. Alcohol addiction, unlike morphine addiction, is physiologically and psychologically destructive to the human individual.
4. One of the most powerful arguments in favor of alcohol prohibition is rarely advanced—that it is useless to prohibit other drugs, even heroin, so long as alcohol remains freely available. Many heroin addicts, deprived of heroin, promptly turn to alcohol instead and become alcoholics.

C. Caffeine
1. The desirable effects of caffeine are remarkably similar to those of cocaine and the amphetamines.
2. Investigations have reported that the ingestion of 0.5 grams of caffeine (3 to 4 cups) may increase basal metabolic rate an average of 10% and occasionally as much as 25%.

3. Caffeine unquestionably produces withdrawal effects at some dosage levels.
4. Overindulgence in xanthene beverages may lead to a condition that might be considered chronic poisoning; CNS stimulation results in restlessness and disturbed sleep; myocardial stimulation is reflected in cardiac irregularities, especially in premature systoles and in palpitation and heart rate.

The widespread use of alcohol, nicotine, and caffeine throughout American society cannot be underestimated as a factor contributing to their being overlooked as chemicals and being classified as "nondrugs," despite their abusive and destructive potentials. These drugs, along with the physician-prescribed "good" drugs, are therefore not seen as legitimately related to the drug abuse problem in this country. This "oversight" also makes it difficult for consumers, individually and collectively, to become aware of the consequences these unnoticed drug-taking patterns have in the long run, which may be irreversible in their impact on our society.

QUESTION OF MOTIVATION

Drug abuse is generally defined in American society as the use, usually by self-administration, of any substance in a manner that deviates from the legitimized medical or cultural patterns. Drug abuse has become a major illness in industrial society, and following the cue of medical inquiry characteristic of an industrial society, one major focus is the search for causes. Based on the well-established precedent whereby behavior varying from the norm automatically becomes synonymous with deviant personality types, research efforts have focused on attempts to describe the personality of the offender, his inadequate coping mechanisms, his low tolerance for stress, his weak ego structure, his escape from reality, and other psychological concepts offered to explain the behavior of those taking a chemical substance without medical supervision.

One example of the outcome of early research efforts identified four specific personality characteristics of drug abusers, all of which are based on a need for personal control: a desire (1) to control the level and experience of stimulation, (2) to control the metabolic processes, (3) to modify social role and status, and (4) to modify experiences of time and distance, particularly in relation to other people (O,Connor, 1977).

The use of chemicals can aid a person in fulfilling this need for personal control. By selecting the appropriate drug, one can speed up, feel pleasure, be awakened, or be anesthetized to pain, alienation, or almost any other experience. Time and space can be modified so that one is isolated from, or in touch with, at varying levels, everything in one's surroundings (Yowell and Brose, 1977).

At first, analysis of these characteristics appears to be a key to understanding the drug abuser and why he does what he does, and therefore ultimately the key to controlling drug abuse. On careful examination of these characteristics, however, it becomes evident that the need for personal control is common to all people, not just to drug abusers (O'Connor, 1977). We all make attempts to control such things as how much television we watch, what and how much we eat or drink, how much we smoke, how much exercise we get, and the kind of activities in which we participate. Most people try to choose people with whom to spend time as well as to regulate how closely they become involved with others and on what levels.

Recent inquiries have recognized the futility of singling out the individual and are directing more energy toward a reanalysis of the basic belief systems relating to drug-taking behavior. Weil (1972) suggests that the problems we have with drugs are inherent neither in the individual nor in the drugs, but in our ways of thinking about them. Given the negative consequences of drug use, he identifies two possibilities basic to further consideration of the drug problem: (1) altered states of consciousness are inherently undesirable; or (2) altered states of consciousness are neither desirable nor undesirable of themselves, but can take bad forms, in which case the drive to experience them should be channeled in some "proper" direction. Weil proposes that the drug question be restated as a question about methods rather than goals: Are drugs the right or wrong means to a desirable end? His major premise is that it may be an innate human need or drive to experience periodic episodes of nonordinary consciousness and that by trying to deny people these important experiences we maximize the probability that they will obtain them in ways harmful to both themselves and society.

Szasz (1974) takes a similar position in that he identifies as basic, and second only to the organismic need for the satisfaction of the biological requirements for survival, the need to experience communion with our fellow human beings, and sometimes with the forces of nature, the universe, or a godhead, "and to satisfy this need, we use, among other things, certain substances that affect our feelings and behavior."

OBSERVATIONS FROM A CROSS-CULTURAL STUDY

The cross-cultural study of drug use has aided the understanding of drug-taking behavior, particularly as it relates to sources of motivation. The experiences that result from the ingestion of hallucinogenic agents have been described as one of the most subjective experiences available to man, yet recent anthropological investigation into the drug-taking patterns of traditional societies indicates general trends or themes common both among members of a given cultural group and between the various cultures studied. These patterns are atypical of the idiosyncratic patterns of drug effects common in an industrial society, where specific cultural traditions of drug use, which could serve to effectively program these experiences, are lacking. Various studies have shown how cultural variables such as belief systems, values, attitudes, and expectations structure not only the taking and avoiding of certain drugs but also the individual's experience while under the influence of these drugs (DeRios, 1977; DeRios and Smith, 1977; LaBarre, 1975; Rubin, 1975; Weil, 1972; Castanada, 1972, 1974; and Harner, 1973). Of particular interest here are those societies that make extensive use of certain types of hallucinogenic agents to alter awareness but appear to have few of the problems associated with the use of these or similar agents in an industrial society:

People in these societies do not take drugs to rebel against parents or teachers, to drop out of the social process or to hurt themselves. Neither is the drug use linked in any way with antisocial patterns of behavior, and since the drugs in many cases are the same ones tied to antisocial patterns of use in industrial society, the differences cannot have much basis in pharmacology (Weil, 1972).

DeRios (1977) has extensively studied drug use in traditional societies and has specifically linked psychoactive drug use with belief systems in these societies. Cross-cultural research on altered states has indicated that 90% of the societies had one or more institutionalized, culturally patterned forms of altered states of consciousness, most of which were aided by the use of psychoactive plants. As a result of her investigations, she concludes that the conceptualizations of drug abuse in traditional societies of the world do not exist as they do in an industrial society; in fact, these patterns of ritualistic drug use are generally considered destructive by most industrial societies. Weil (1972) also suggests that the "success" of these societies in regard to the outcomes of their drug taking has to do with the ways they think about drugs and about states of consciousness as well as with certain principles of drug use that they have discovered.

The role of ritual characterizing drug use in traditional society has been identified as the most critical factor underlying its apparent lack of abuse. The preparation of drugs for ingestion, rules surrounding the ingestion, who is present, the time of day or night, and the length of the ceremony exemplify the parameters guiding use specifically outlined by the cultural context. A basic belief described by Weil (1972) is that these societies recognize the normality of the human drive to experience altered states of consciousness periodically for specific, culturally defined reasons; they admit to themselves that their world contains many substances with the potential to trigger altered states of consciousness (for the primary purpose of achieving communication with the supernatural). They do not try to eradicate these substances or prevent people from using them. In addition, drug-induced states are usually entered into for positive reasons, not for negative ones such as escape from boredom or anxiety. Blum (1959) also reports from his investigations that drugs are not used for escape in traditional society but are used to reconfirm the integrity, values, and goals of a culture. Other objectives that are cited include expansion of cosmic consciousness, enhancement of feelings of religiosity, and attempts to gain better self-understanding in both individual and group content (DeRios, 1977).

Accompanying the well-defined motives for using the drugs, a common pattern found was the role of a guide or navigator of the experience. Rarely were drugs taken alone by an individual for personal or introspective reasons, which is a common characteristic of drug-taking behavior in an industrial society. In traditional societies the shaman most frequently performs this valuable function (DeRios, 1977; Weil, 1972; LaBarre, 1975). In the hands of the shaman drugs are used to serve the specific cultural objectives defined and the shaman in most cases is responsible for assuring that the appropriate cultural context is set, as dictated by these objectives. Such navigation (by a guide) is necessary to structure the experience so as to make it as culturally meaningful as possible. A guide's role "is to produce musical accompaniment to bridge two worlds of consciousness as a means of controlling, and neutralizing evil spirits that may appear to the drug user during a session, as well as to evoke culturally expected visions" (DeRios, 1977).

Weil (1972) has identified a final factor that he sees as important in limiting the amount of abuse that occurs in these traditional societies. The chemicals they use are natural; they make no attempts to refine these substances into pure, potent forms or to extract active principles from natural drugs. By contrast, most of the drugs used in industrial societies are highly refined and often synthetic: "It is a striking empirical fact that the difficulties individuals and societies get into with drugs appear to be correlated with the purity of potency of substances in use; the more potent the drug, the more 'trouble' associated with it."

NURSING IMPLICATIONS

If, as has been suggested, a significant portion of the chemical abuse problem in this country relates to the drugs obtained through legal and formal channels, the nursing profession, as an integral part of a system that legitimizes these channels, may inadvertently reinforce the beliefs and attitudes that have been identified as influential in sustaining the cycle of chemical (symptom) response to problems. It is critical that nurses begin to articulate specifically their basic assumptions, their basic epistemological beliefs, and the values on which personal and professional behavior is based, as well as to assess on an ongoing basis the consistency between these basic values and interventions with clients. If we believe in holistic health approaches, nursing implications for action in this area go beyond a discussion of specific chemical substances and their effects on specific individuals. Needed is an identification, and re-evaluation if necessary, of the values that are

inconsistent with our emerging conceptualizations of human functioning.

The following summarizes assumptions underlying present responses to issues of drug use and abuse:

1. Sadness, loneliness, grief, anger, and rage are negative human emotions to be denied and hidden when experienced: they result, particularly if intense, from not living up to accepted cultural standards of performance.

2. Human relations are inherently harmonious: disturbance in this area indicates emotional instability or mental illness.

3. Illegal chemical substances are abused (bad drugs): physician-prescribed drugs are used to treat specific medical symptoms (good drugs): culturally sanctioned drugs are bad habits (nondrugs).

4. Altered states of consciousness are undesirable and synonymous with illicit drug use.

5. Consequences of drug use result from the deviant personality characteristics of the user or from the specific pharmacologic effects of the substances used.

The following exemplifies an alternative epistemological base:

1. Sadness, loneliness, grief, anger, and rage are human emotions: they are neither positive nor negative; they accompany human existence.

2. Human relations are not inherently harmonious: learning how to relate to yourself and others requires patience, hard work, and satisfying results from your efforts.

3. Any chemical substance can be abused regardless of its source, social or legal sanction, or chemical composition.

4. Altered states of consciousness are neither desirable nor undesirable: pursuit of states of nonordinary reality may be an innate human drive.

5. Consequences of specific patterns of drug

use result from the interactions occurring between the individual and the social/cultural system in which he participates.

With the identification of an alternative value framework, nursing action that is directed toward achievement of systematic, holistic responses to the issues discussed here can then be developed. The following section outlines nursing actions in the areas of research and legislation, consumer self-help groups, and educational focuses as well as guidelines for the nurse/client relationship.

Research and legislation

The role of legislation in defining parameters for the trends of drug use in this country has been discussed at length. Legislation reflects both the existing social and cultural beliefs representative of the general population and the legitimizing of these beliefs through definition of legal response to various types of drug-taking behavior. The significance therefore of organized nursing input into the formation of these policies cannot be overstated, as they determine to a large extent the scope of nursing practice in relationship to these issues. Nurses should be encouraged to participate in special interest groups within local and national nursing organizations and to participate actively in nursing research in this critical social area. For example, possible actions include the following:

1. Lobbying for the reclassification of chemical substances so that all drugs regardless of source and social sanctions are defined and treated as such. This may aid in increasing recognition of the far-reaching individual and social consequences not only those of defined as illicit substances but also of culturally sanctioned drugs.

2. Influencing policy regulating dissemination of information to the public of both licit and illicit drugs and minimizing campaigns based on scare tactics. These programs have been identified as significant in the encouragement rather than discouragement of use because of the widespread emphasis and attention drawn to selected substances through publicizing efforts.

3. Studying the cumulative effects on the body of chemicals used on a long-term basis as well as the interactive effects of chemicals administered simultaneously. Research continues to focus on the isolated actions of individual drugs regardless of the well-established practice of prescribing multiple drugs simultaneously, often for periods of years at a time. One alarming consequence of this limited line of research has been the recent linking of irreversible neurological damage known as tardive dyskinesia to the long-term use of the phenothiazine derivatives (Bernstein and Lennard, 1973).

4. Studying the effects of the long-term administration of psychotropic drugs on social participatory patterns, decision-making ability, and interest in the environment. Often the assumption is made that a progressive, decreasing level of functioning in these areas results from the natural course of the illness rather than possible impact of years of chemical intervention on the individual's cognitive abilities and his relationship with the environment.

5. Identifying relationships between lifestyle, pace of living, and the types of chemicals selected for individual use as well as emphasizing possible connections between patterns of drug use and the development of carcinogenic and other debilitating physical illnesses. Multiple causation theories of illness, including elements of life-style, have yet to be identified as priority areas for medical research with the continued dominance of the single cause-effect theories of etiology and symptom response intervention.

Consumer self-help groups and educational focuses

Increased consumer responsibility for health maintenance prevention and illness care monitoring is becoming more of a necessity as specialization and health care fragmentation increase. If the trend continues of a nursing discipline that identifies health promotion and maintenance as key priorities, it is essential to develop a consumer population knowledgeable about factors that are identified as significant in impacting the overall health status. This places a great demand on health care practititioners to develop mechanisms for the effective transmission of knowledge to the consumer group to serve as a basis for increasing consumer-defined action and decision making. Nurses, comprising the largest health care profession, could have significant impact on what and how information is made available to consumers regarding drug use and abuse and its related issues, as well as on facilitating independent self-help skills in this area. As an illustration of this role, nurses could be more active in the following areas:

1. Developing consumer and nursing groups to monitor advertising campaigns that advocate use of chemical substances known to be destructive to human beings. The mass media such as radio, television, newspapers, and billboards are employed extensively to encourage use of chemical substances, particularly the socially sanctioned ''nondrugs.'' Professional journals are supported in part by advertisements from industries that profit from increased numbers of prescriptions obtained legitimately through the health care system.

2. Sponsoring consumer self-help groups that increase the level of awareness of the extent of chemical use in characteristic life-styles with identification of the ways consumers may intervene to make desired changes in their own lives. Socially sanctioned chemical use and abuse, because they are normative and therefore acceptable, are often not recognized by the general population as ''drug use'' much less as abusive in the sense of having a negative impact on their overall health status.

3. Providing training and supervisory sessions for individuals in the community to staff switchboards, hot lines, rap centers, and crash pads as well as defining communication networks for publicizing procedures and resources for responding to negative or harmful drug reactions on the street. Nurses can prepare themselves for these activities not only by learning the specific pharmacological properties of commonly used chemicals and reviewing the literature that describes drug use and abuse from an ecological perspective but also, and more important, by listening and learning from individuals who have had personal experience with various chemical substances and altered states of consciousness. Theories and attitudes regarding drugs and the individuals who use them taught in formal educational settings are at best experienced as irrelevant and can be perceived as condescending and therefore counterproductive to an individual who needs to be understood. The establishment of trust is critical, particularly where the youth drug culture is concerned; providing appropriate responses to the needs of individuals whose life-style is centered around the use of drugs is more effective if individuals within the same peer group participate in the provision of these services. Intervention prior to involvement with the official health care system may also decrease the likelihood of consequences resulting from hospitalization or other forms of institutional response. For example, a person's experience of a panic reaction after ingestion of a hallucinogen may only be intensified if brought by police or parents into an active, loud, and otherwise stimulating emergency room. Also, unless indicated for immediate life-saving measures, drugs administered to counterbalance the effects of a drug (or drugs) already taken often intensify the emotional and physical reactions.

4. Developing and participating in educational programs that expand the scope of discussion to include all potentially abusive substances including prescription drugs, over-the-counter products, chemicals used in food processing and preservation, alcohol, nicotine, caffeine, and the illegal drugs. Many educational programs present only negative or socially disapproving reactions; this may increase rather than decrease continued experimentation because informal communication networks provide counterinformation that emphasizes only the positive or pleasurable qualities of the drugs in question, casting doubt and mistrust on the validity of the other information made available through more formal channels. Both are ineffective methods of drug education in that they are presenting the incomplete, emotional, and biased viewpoints of those transmitting the information. It is therefore difficult for individuals to make well-informed decisions based on a thorough presentation of information available about drugs and their probable consequences.

It is also important in these programs to discriminate between the effects of the drugs themselves and the characteristic life-style of the users of the various chemicals, as they are often confused. Stress should also be placed on discussion of drugs known to produce physical dependence (nicotine, barbiturates, alcohol, and heroin). Many individuals may begin using these substances with the idea that they can stop whenever they choose; the suffering that accompanies the alcoholic dilemma is a constant, visible example in this society of the complicated nature of addiction; it has yet to be described in a way that would allow for the development of successful intervention approaches.

5. Initiating general health education courses for consumers that emphasize the development of chemical-free alternatives to life situations that are characteristically responded to with chemical or medical intervention. This is a critical area for the prevention of debilitating emotional difficulties with accompanying drug dependence and may include classes on stress management; on problem-solving and decision-making models, and on issues related to life changes, growing older, and developing ways of tapping the unlimited, unused resources of the aging population. Other areas include discussions on the impact of loss through separation, divorce, death, or geographical relocation and on value differences on an individual's physical and emotional functioning. Functional patterns of family living, parenting, preparation for marriage, relating as partners, and single-adult parenting and alternative family styles may also be considered.

6. Incorporating into educational programs a discussion of drug use in other cultures that use similar substances with no apparent abuse. The intent here is not to suggest adoption of drug-taking practices observed cross-culturally, as this obviously implies taking specific behavior out of the intricate social and cultural context within which the behavior occurs. Rather the intent is to reinforce the idea that outcomes of drug-taking behavior vary in different cultures and that the ways in which the culture conceptualizes drug use to a large extent determines the consequences of use. This idea may add a new dimension for the analysis of drug-taking behavior in our own culture. The following characteristics have been identified from cross-cultural studies as significant factors that lessen the potential for abuse of chemical substances: (1) avoiding substances that are known to have physical or psychological addictive properties, (2) utilizing natural substances in natural ways rather than those that have been refined or synthetically developed, (3) describing altered states of consciousness as a valued and positive individual and cultural experience, (4) sanctioning use only for positive reasons rather than as a method of coping with stress, (5) surrounding the use in ritual, and (6) educating persons in how to use particular substances and then only in the presence of a guide or navigator—someone with personal experience of drug use and the altered states of consciousness that may accompany it.

7. Supporting and developing programs that emphasize the search for chemical-free methods of achieving altered states of consciousness. This implies acknowledgment of the hypothesis that experiences of nonordinary reality may be an innate human need. If so, then the encouragement of participation in chemical-free alternatives that are not accompanied by the negative consequences of drugs is a viable option for meeting this need. These alternatives may include regular physical exercise and activity, prayer and religious experiences, ritual, sexual experiences, carefully selected dietary patterns, massage, and travel. Sensitivity training, encounter therapy, transcendential meditation, Zen Buddhism, yoga, music, art, dance, and nature study have also been identified as important facilitators of this type of experience.

8. Correcting misinformation and rumors publicized regarding the effects of illicit drugs. The Consumer Union report identifies a number of points that are commonly discussed in drug education programs, which were assessed as being false based on the results of investigations for the report. The following summarizes major findings of the study, which may dispel common misconceptions (Brecher, 1972).

a. Overdose deaths have been linked to shooting an opiate while also drunk on alcohol or a barbiturate; heroin overdose has not been documented as the cause of death among heroin addicts.

b. It is easier to become dependent on cigarettes than on alcohol or barbiturates.

c. Frequent relapse among chronic users of heroin, barbiturates, alcohol, and nicotine has little to do with motivation or will power; it relates to the fact that these are addictive chemicals.

d. Methadone maintenance itself does not change people's lives; the change results from the economic and social life-style changes that occur when the source of the drug is legitimized.

e. Abrupt withdrawal of both alcohol and the barbiturates can be fatal.

f. Legal prohibition of socially disapproved drugs does not work.

g. Cocaine addiction differs from opiate, alcohol, or barbiturate addiction in that

physical effects are minor; psychological depression is severe.

h. Compulsive patterns of LSD usage rarely develop; the nature of the drug is that it becomes less attractive with continued use and in the long run is almost always self-limiting.

i. It was a change in the laws rather than a change in the drug or in human nature that stimulated the large-scale marketing of marijuana for recreational use in the United States.

j. Heavy use of sedatives (alcohol and barbiturates) rather than marijuana has most frequently preceded heroin use.

k. The amount of harm done to the human body by nicotine and alcohol vastly exceeds the physical harm done by all other psychoactive drugs put together.

l. The ritualization of certain types of drug use in American society may have decreased the dangers in using the drugs.

m. All psychological effects of marijuana turn out to be common features of altered states of consciousness unassociated with drugs.

n. Caffeine can be a dangerous drug.

o. The damage done by the arrests and imprisonments of children for glue sniffing during the 1960s far exceeded damage done by glue sniffing during the decade and served to popularize rather than discourage the practice.

Nurse-client relationship

The context and quality of the relationship developed between the nurse and client is the key factor in determining how successfully mutually defined goals will be achieved. This necessitates broadening the focus of assessment beyond the individual client and his specific "drug problem" to utilization of the nursing process in all nursing situations in a manner that recognizes the systematic relationships existing between drug use and other areas of individual functioning. Equally important is a focus on the nurse's own attitudes and values. Application of this perspective to utilization of the nursing process includes the following.

1. Routinely incorporating into health assessment activities a thorough review of chemical substances used by the client and providing information about these substances. An important area of discussion is identification of factors that may influence the outcome of using a specific substance including individual metabolic makeup and personality, reason used, frequency of use, mood at the time taken, anticipated drug effects, specific pharmacological actions, persons and objects present during the experience, knowledge of the drug and its effects by those present, and previous experience with drugs or other forms of altered states of consciousness. Within the hospital or clinic setting, providing clients with complete data about their prescribed drug regime facilitates an increased awareness of individual responsibility for management of what they choose to put into their bodies. The following information should be included: rationale for use; relationship to medical diagnoses; actions, specific and general; side effects; addictive potential; contraindications; toxic effects; and data known regarding long-term usage.

2. Identifying values in oneself as a professional practitioner that may influence or bias interactions with clients. Being educated and practicing within a health care system guided by the assumptions previously identified, nurses may behave in ways that perpetuate these assumptions. Of particular significance are those assumptions related to the experience and expression of basic human emotion. The following questions may serve as a guide for an initial self-inventory:

a. Do you experience discomfort and tension when someone is expressing intense emotion or make consistent attempts to calm someone who is crying?

b. Do you support the administration of psychotropic drugs to persons experiencing intense feelings of grief and loss?

c. Do you support the administration of psychotropic drugs to older persons for purposes of calming or quieting their behavior?

d. Do you deny these feelings in yourself or attempt to hide them from others?

e. Do you automatically assume something is "wrong" when you or someone else is experiencing intense feeling?

f. Do you think that experience or expression of these feelings is symptomatic of an emotional disorder or label emotional expression with a psychiatric description?

g. Do you acknowledge, accept, and allow these feelings within the context of your relationships with your clients, or do you refer to a "specialist"?

h. Do you support the administration of tranquilizers and phenothiazine derivatives to hospitalized clients prior to considering alternative chemical-free treatment approaches?

i. Do you support the administration of additional drugs to counterbalance the effects of other drugs given?

j. Do you support short-term chemical relief of emotional pain over responses that may be more time consuming?

k. Do you support the client's right to refuse chemical intervention?

3. Developing counseling guidelines for one-to-one relationships with clients based on holistic, interactive models of human functioning:

a. Inventory your own areas of functional and dysfunctional communication patterns, unresolved emotional issues, decisionmaking skills, impact on others, perceptions of self, satisfaction with present life situations, beliefs about drug use and abuse and the individuals who use them; the influence of chemicals on your life-style and pace, and thoughts about the relationship of drug dependence to the larger cultural context.

b. Identify your values relating to human

emotions and their expression, how individuals develop and maintain mutually satisfying relationships with others, standards for professional and personal behavior, and beliefs about guidelines for facilitating the therapeutic process.

c. Assess the impact of drug use in the client's life on the level of stress, stress management, functioning in the areas of perception, judgment, memory, problem-solving, activities and patterns of daily living, descriptions of work activities and relationships, relationships with family members and peers, expressive movements, emotional tone, verbal responses, attitudes toward self and others, and sexual feeling and expression.

d. Review the client's philosophy relating to the use of drugs, history of specific and patterned drug use, intended use, expectations of outcomes, knowledge of specific pharmacological effects of substances used, short-term and long-term outcomes, potentials for abuse, addictive properties, decision-making process involved in the selection of particular chemicals for use, reasons for taking, and awareness of consequences of use.

e. Identify the client's perceptions of past and present, supportive and disruptive relationships; satisfaction level with these relationships; awareness of specific expectations and needs from others; awareness of the relationship between unidentified, unmet needs and the experience of frustration; and resource networks available.

f. Contract for specific time parameters and goals following a thorough nurse-client assessment of priorities and problem areas, development of alternative action behaviors for the client to alter his present relationships with himself and others in environment to meet stated goals.

It is apparent that attempting to develop effective preventive approaches to substance abuse in this industrial society requires a critical emphasis not only on the consequences of drug-taking behavior or the individuals identified as our abusers but also critical study of the social and cultural conditions that structure the behavior of individuals. It is from this perspective that the values that form the basis for normative behavior become clarified, and thus more amenable to change.

References

Barker, R. G.: Ecological psychology, Stanford, Calif., 1968, Stanford University Press.

Bateson, G.: Steps to an ecology of mind, New York, 1972, Ballantine Books, Inc.

Bateson, G.: Breaking out of the double bind, Psychology Today **12**:42-51, August 1978.

Bernstein, A., and Lennard, H.: The American way of drugging, Society **10**:14-25, May/June 1973.

Blum, R. et al: Drugs and society, San Francisco, 1959, Jossey-Bass, Publishers, Inc.

Brecher, E., ed.: Licit and illicit drugs, Boston, 1972, Little, Brown & Co.

Castaneda, C.: Journey to Ixtlan, New York, 1972, Simon & Schuster, Inc.

Castaneda, C.: Tales of power, New York, 1974, Simon & Schuster, Inc.

Crosbie, Q.: The environment of a community drug program for youth: resources, use and benefits, (unpublished doctoral dissertation), Lawrence, Kans., 1972, The University of Kansas.

DeRios, M.: The wilderness of mind: sacred plants in cross-cultural perspective, Beverly Hills, Calif., 1977, Sage Publications, Inc.

DeRios, M., and Smith, D.: Drug use and abuse in cross-cultural perspective, Hum. Org. **36**:14-21, Spring, 1977.

Dunn, H.: High level wellness, Arlington, Va., 1961, Beatty Publishers.

Goode, E.: Drugs in American society, New York, 1972, Alfred A. Knopf, Inc.

Hanlon, J.: An ecologic view of health, Am. J. Public Health **59**:4-11, 1959.

Hanna, J.: Coca leaf use in Southern Peru: some biosocial aspects, Am. Anthropologist **76**:281-296, 1974.

Harner, M., ed.: Hallucinogens and shamanism, New York, 1973, Oxford University Press.

Kartman, L.: Human ecology and public health, Am. J. Public Health **67**:737-750, 1967.

LaBarre, W.: Anthropological perspectives on hallucinations and hallucinogens. In Siegel, R. K., and West, L. J., eds.: Hallucinations: behavior, experience and theory, New York, 1975, John Wiley & Sons, Inc.

Lennard, H.: Mystification and drug misuse, New York, 1971, Harper & Row, Publishers.

Lieber, C.: The metabolism of alcohol, Sci. Am. **234:**25-33, 1976.

Lutes, S.: Alcohol use among the Yaqui Indians of Potan, Senora, Mexico (unpublished doctoral dissertation), Lawrence, Kans., 1977, University of Kansas.

Lynch, R., ed.: The cross cultural approach to health behavior, Rutherford, N.J., 1969, Fairleigh Dickinson University Press.

Murry, R., and Zentner, F.: Nursing concepts for health promotion, Englewood Cliffs, N.J., 1975, Prentice-Hall, Inc.

O'Connor, W.: Ecosystems theory and clinical mental health, Psychiatr. Anal. **7:**63-77, 1977.

Odun, E.: The emergency of ecology as a new integrative discipline, Science **195:**1289-1293, 1977.

Rubin, V.: Cannabis and culture, The Hague, 1975, Mouton Publishers.

Smith, D.: The trip, Emerg. Med. **1:**90-93, December 1969.

Szasz, T.: The myth of mental illness. In Scheff, T. J., ed.: Mental illness and social processes, New York, 1967, Harper & Row, Publishers.

Szasz, T.: Ceremonial chemistry, Garden City, N.Y., 1974, Anchor Press.

Szasz, T.: The theology of medicine, New York, 1977, Harper & Row, Publishers.

Weil, A.: The natural mind, Boston, 1972, Houghton Mifflin Co.

Weppner, R., ed.: Street ethnography, Beverly Hills, Calif., 1977, Sage Publications, Inc.

Yowell, S., and Brose, C.: Working with drug abuse patients in the ER, Am. J. Nurs. **77:**82-85, 1977.

CHAPTER 10

A systems approach to spouse abuse

JUDY BRETZ PRINCE

Spouse abuse is an increasing social problem requiring the intervention of nurses and other health care professionals. It has in the past been hidden from public view, and only recently has it begun to be studied carefully. For the purpose of this chapter, spouse abuse is defined as any physical attack by a spouse, ranging from a slap to homicide. Its etiological roots will be examined within the context of the interplay between internal and external multienvironments.

Currently health care professionals are being asked to respond to spouse abuse through medical emergencies via the provision of "patch-up" treatment for the victims in families as well as through psychological curative measures such as the development of services to prevent stress for those identified as being caught in dysfunctioning, abusive family systems. Medical treatment of injuries can bring immediate relief for physical suffering; family therapy can improve the quality of interpersonal relationships. Tangible community support for battered family members (for example, emergency shelters and day care centers) can help meet survival needs and promote individual comfort for those who choose to leave their homes. However, utilization of only these secondary and tertiary preventive interventions may distract persons involved in the dilemma from recognizing the seriousness of the total situation.

A systems approach to spouse abuse holds that the dynamics of abuse are broad and complex, with changing causation. It explores the pattern of relationships and reciprocal transactions between the individual, the couple, and the environment to aid in effective intervention at a primary prevention level.

This chapter presents the multidimensional dynamics in spouse abuse. The purpose is to give the professional a body of knowledge that is somewhat broader than that which is now being utilized in addressing the problem. I shall describe the kinds of conflicts and conditions, increasingly prevalent throughout the country, that in combination result in spouse abuse; present a specific case example; and consider several postures that nurses might assume in confronting the problem in a holistic manner.

A MULTIDIMENSIONAL PROBLEM

A characteristic feature of our day is that the family is being blamed for various social ills while it is simultaneously being confronted with dehumanizing social institutions that are no longer reliable as emotional support systems. The family also faces social changes and cultural norms that increase the frustrations and aggressiveness of its members and inhibit family solidarity. Additional crippling factors for family systems actively engaged in spouse abuse are societal myths, situational crises, and residual early-life stresses that reinforce their vulnerability.

Dehumanizing support institutions

Historically our institutions of church, school, work, and hospital or clinic have not only served the family by satisfying spiritual, educational, financial, and medical needs but have also served as supports to the family in meeting social and emotional needs. Five basic human needs—stimulation, power, intimacy, interdependence, and "anger outlets"—are discussed to give perspective to the lack of supportive interplay between the individual and these institutions.

The church presently provides some psychic stimulation, a sense of worth (power), some feeling of closeness, and a sharing of philosophical truths for those individuals who choose to become members of the organization. In recent years maintaining itself as an institution has resulted in spending less energy in ministering to the human needs of nonmembers. In addressing anger it has always encouraged control or denial rather than viewing outlets for anger as viable human resources.

The school, especially in urban areas, is unable to successfully meet any of these five basic needs, largely because of inadequate financial resources. The classroom is generally a lonely and boring place with opportunities for sharing and experiencing a sense of worth often being relegated to performance on verbal or written examinations. When expressing anger, a student risks being expelled or referred to a health care professional (many times for tranquilizers or for written assurance that the student will not openly display aggressiveness in the future).

Work as an institution currently cannot be relied on to assist in promoting a sense of power based on achievement, although most employees have been conditioned to expect this for themselves. While many continue to hold sacred the "climb-or-be-climbed" philosophy, the world economy no longer permits such upward mobility. Such pressures for occupational achievement have been directly related to causative factors in spouse abuse (Downey and Howell, 1976). Additionally, workers have resorted to labor unions and "out-of-the-shop" conferences in order to have meaningful experiences in stimulation and joint participation with others. Current job shortages and demands for better access to employment opportunities by various minorities make it risky to express anger within the institution of work.

The hospital or clinic shares the school's dilemma in that its limited funding makes it almost impossible to provide comprehensive service delivery with attention to human needs. In receiving service it is thus difficult for the individual to feel a sense of worth or to be a participant with the professional. If one experiences frustrations in an encounter with this institution (for example, a low-income mother having to lose a day of work each time a different child becomes ill to process an application for reduced medical costs), it presents a problem for the individual and for the professional. They may both be far removed from the decision makers who established the guideline that created the particular stress factor. The individual's expression of anger, then, is met with sympathetic listening, defensiveness, or avoidance of the issue, which ultimately may result in reinforcing a sense of powerlessness within both the individual and the health care practitioner.

Rather than supporting the family, these institutions seem to be contributing to conditions or reinforcing situations that are dehumanizing. Certainly these entities are not advancing an attitude that encourages appreciation of the significance of the total person and his multienvironments. When individual human needs are not being met through traditional channels and when individuals are limited in their appreciation of the past and have little trust in the future, they often turn inward for instant gratification of their needs. This can in turn lead to "epidemics" such as drug abuse (Ball et al., 1975) or illegitimate pregnancies, or there may be massive outward expressions of anger either in the street or in the home. When individuals feel powerless already, they have very little to lose by crushing others. Unfortunately, when there are large-scale crises or epidemics, the helping persons are usually called upon for a prompt resolution of the surface problem. It is often difficult to utilize thoughtful processes for planned intervention: the demands of the moment thus result in "Band-Aid" treatment, making it impossible to establish a comprehensive approach that addresses the need for systematic change.

Social changes

Even if the individual within the family system is understood and/or supported by other systems, social changes present additional stresses on family life. The women's liberation movement, the sexual revolution, the rootlessness of society in general, and the rapidity of change will be examined in relation to their impact on spouse abuse.

The women's movement to provide women with the freedom to seek power on an equal basis with men places a new stress on marriages for two reasons. Many men are programmed during childhood to use physical aggressiveness to demonstrate their masculinity (Martin, 1976). Also men are supported by society in using force when their power position in the family is threatened (Goode, 1971). The conflict between changing roles and cultural norms may therefore result in an increase in violent behavior in marriages until men are able to subscribe to an equalitarian rather than male superiority norms (Whitehurst, 1974).

A theme in much of the literature on spouse abuse is that husbands who exhibit violent behavior are those who are characteristically deficient in societally ascribed masculine resources or in certain status characteristics relative to wives (for example, lesser education or job status) (Gelles, 1977; O'Brien, 1971). Through the women's movement men stand to lose some of the advantages they have had in, for example, the development of personal traits and the securing of material goods and services. Women are simultaneously being presented with increased opportunities, thus elevating wives to the status of adults (instead of being

"dependent children") and giving them options other than the wife and mother roles for investment of their energies. As these changes occur between men and women within the larger society, the family may increasingly become a battleground, since men are unlikely to relinquish passively their culturally sanctioned positions of power in the home.

The women's movement has fostered a climate that is less tolerant of abuse. The issue of spouse abuse and its prevention has become a growth-producing, solidifying force for some women (Viano, 1978); for others who are not that conscious of the social and political dynamics of the issue, however, this movement creates turmoil within their interpersonal relationships and increases the potential for abusive confrontations.

Closely linked to the women's movement is the sexual revolution, which presents a threat to some men as well as to their superior position in marriage. Sexual freedom, combined with better access to the world outside of the home for women, seems to shift somewhat the double standard in sexual behavior. Jealousy and possessiveness have been given as causative factors in some physical assaults on wives (Shepard, 1961); it is evident that increasing sexual freedom, or providing more opportunities for multiple relationships, could increase violence in marriages. An additional pernicious aspect of social change is the loss of a close-knit community base for the family. Largely as a result of family members' quest for economic progress, many couples no longer live near their parents and grandparents, their extended families or their long-time friends (Kopernik, 1964). Geographic mobility results in isolation, loss of social controls, and a sense of rootlessness. These characteristics in and of themselves become additional social indicators for spouse abuse.

The rapidity of social change makes it difficult for any individual to maintain an intellectual perspective or "a feeling knowledge" (Perlman, 1966) of what the world is like for others. It is especially hard for the elderly who have in past generations been not only a source of wisdom for the young but also the stabilizing force for married couples.

This rapidly changing society has also brought about new stresses for racial minorities who lived through the transition period in history that resulted in their becoming more aware of opportunities in the marketplace. This new awareness has brought additional frustrations because while it is in fact a possibility for some, for most it continues to be difficult to achieve. This employee has problems understanding just what, if anything, he has gained and frequently does not wish to share this disillusionment with the other family members. The internal turmoil can thus consciously or unconsciously spill over into family life and result in violent explosions around unrelated issues.

Cultural and environmental factors

Although some of the cultural norms affecting spouse abuse have been briefly mentioned earlier, additional factors will receive elaboration here. One is the contradiction of characterizing the family as a nonviolent institution (Steinmetz and Straus, 1974) while marital violence is legitimized in the legal system, in literary expressions, in everyday discourse, and implicitly within the family itself (for example, glorifying aggression as a means of control in the discipline of children) (Straus, 1973). With such a broad sanction of violence, students of family violence have classified a marriage license as "a hitting license" (Straus, 1976). The literature on the importance of observational learning in the acquisition of aggressive behavior indicates that children who are physically punished by their parents for their aggressiveness are actually being aided in developing violent responses to stressful situations (Kaplan, 1972). Therefore the family is not only supported by external forces in its sanction of violence, but through its own internal socialization and interactive processes it establishes itself as "a breeding ground of violence" (Kopernik, 1964).

The aspect of sex role stereotyping of men as "tough" and "powerful" has reinforced either their development of these traits or their feeling of worthlessness if they are unable to project such images. During both the ongoing reciprocities and the conflicts in marriages, husbands consistently appear to have more power than wives. Superior strength and a readiness to exhibit it explain why violence remains "a clandestine masculine ideal in Western culture" (Toby, 1966) and may deprive men of opportunities to appreciate their capacity for intimate love and harmony.

As previously mentioned, women are shifting from viewing themselves as appendices of men and becoming more self-assertive. However, it is a real struggle and requires pushing for equal rights; families will not become more equalitarian spontaneously. This transition period is bringing a temporary increase in violence as conflicts arise over substantive issues (Straus, et al, 1976).

Societal myths

Literature on spouse abuse states that some providers of services to abusive families have helped perpetuate the myth of the nonviolent family by classifying these individuals as "sick," of low-income status, or as "criminals" (Field and Field, 1973; Edmiston, 1976). This has resulted in their focusing treatment on aggressive male drive and female masochism (Straus, 1977). It also resulted in depending on the legal system for remedies (Miller, 1975) and a subsequent neglect of comprehensive planning for prevention at the primary level. Further, the research indicates that, while a few individuals involved in spouse abuse may evidence psychopathology, this is not universal (Steinmetz and Straus, 1973; Gelles, 1972). Several factors inherent in the status of poor people (including both the direct stress of poverty and structural deficits in their relationship to community systems) are observed to be prevalent among abusive couples (Giovannoni, 1971); however, spouse abuse is reported in families of all socioeconomic levels (Hendrix et al., 1978). Currently most of the statistical data on the problem come from the criminal justice system; since middle-class families do not use the criminal justice system as frequently as do low-income families, and since not all cases of abuse are reported even in lower income families, it is difficult to measure the extent of spouse abuse within the total population. Spouse abuse is not a manifestation of criminal or abnormal behavior; recent studies indicate that family members abuse each other far more often than do unrelated adults (Steinmetz and Straus, 1973). Stark and McEvoy (1970), in their analysis of the National Commission on the Causes and Prevention of Violence, found that one fifth of all Americans approve of slapping one's spouse on "appropriate" occasions and that abuse actually occurs in one fourth of all families. Thus it is important to recognize that "normal" families are not free of conflict (Steinmetz, 1977).

Internal stresses

Situational crises (for example, pregnancy, financial strain, unemployment, and a wage earner's disability) can also provide fuel for explosive behavior in marriage. In a study of 80 New Hampshire couples, Gelles (1972) found that in almost one fourth of the violent families the wife was attacked while pregnant. Gelles (1975) postulates that the stress of pregnancy itself is a precipitating factor in spouse abuse. Preexisting stress factors can further complicate this particular situation.

Financial pressures on family members, especially the poor, frequently necessitate struggling with the welfare bureaucracy (for example, repeated visits to the food stamp office), living in overcrowded housing, or losing hours of work to provide transportation for a clinic appointment. From intensive study of family

violence Steinmetz and Straus (1973) found that the crisis of unemployment itself, with its resulting boredom and the lack of a job position as a means of self-esteem, produced more wife battering in middle-class families than in comparable middle-class families in which the husbands remained employed. All or any one of these structural conditions can increase the potential for spouse abuse when they reinforce feelings of powerlessness, hopelessness, or alienation. It is indeed ironic that it is these same feelings that have been identified as presenting psychological barriers for poor persons in utilizing preventive health care services (Bullough, 1972).

The family wage earner's becoming physically disabled also creates a potentially explosive situation if both husband and wife have been performing traditional sex roles. In my limited clinical experience with abused husbands, violence usually occurred in such situations because of the wife's disappointments in her unfulfilled expectations coupled with the husband's nagging behavior, which is a symptom of his depression in relation to loss of physical power. Each spouse thus either consciously or unconsciously reacts to the forced power redistribution in the family. Some individuals bring with them to their marriages a pattern of learned behavior from early life, which, when combined with appropriate environmental stresses, provides a fertile base for spouse abuse. In childhood they were either victims of abuse themselves or they observed one parent abusing the other (Silver et al., 1969; Gelles, 1976). These individuals in their own marriages will pattern the problem-solving responses of the parent of the same sex; if the parent was abusive the child may be abusive later and if the parent was submissive during physical attacks the child may also accept violence when it erupts (Curtis, 1963).

Through this assessment of the family system in its social, cultural, and economic setting and the related analysis of the generative sources of spouse abuse, it is apparent that the family is a highly differentiated social network in which human relationships are, to say the least, precarious and tenuous and affected by wider social processes. A spouse abuse case history can increase awareness of the complexities in the situation for those who must develop and implement services to family members to prevent emotional and physical damage for individuals in the present and the future.

A CASE HISTORY

Each marital relationship is unique and the twists and turns of encounters in the environment have infinite variety. The following case history is fairly typical of the couples whom I have seen for spouse abuse treatment and of the manner in which these types of dysfunctioning systems are reinforced by the depersonalized community environments. It should be noted that inclusion of the battering spouse in treatment is not always possible, even though it did occur in this situation and resulted in growth experiences for both spouses. While focus here is on the dynamics of secondary and tertiary intervention techniques, it is hoped that this example of "after-the-fact" treatment will also help document the need for professionals to address spouse abuse in a more systematic way on a primary prevention level.

George, age 26, and Sandra, age 20, had been married for 3 years when Sandra first officially asked for help in dealing with George's physical abuse. They had one daughter who was 15 months old, and George also had custody of his 4-year-old son. This child's mother, George's first wife, had permanent brain damage as a result of an automobile accident following their divorce.

When George and Sandra first met both were attempting to cope by themselves with their problems. George felt inept in being the sole parent for his son, and Sandra was struggling to complete her high school education while living with her fifth foster family. They needed one another both for their well-being and because of their problems. They formed a quick, intense relationship and were married before Sandra could complete her education.

The couple lived on a moderate income from George's job as a truck driver with a parcel delivery company. He took pride in his performance as an employee and as the financial provider for the family. Most of their social life was centered around George's friends whom he had met at the company. Sandra seemed to have only a few superficial relationships with adults and devoted much of her energy to being with the children. Both George's and Sandra's natural parents lived several hundred miles away and there was little communication with them.

The first incidence of physical abuse occurred during Sandra's pregnancy. At that time she was too embarrassed to tell her physician in the prenatal clinic about the actual cause of her bruises and lacerations; however, following the second beating, a sensitive and sensible nurse in the clinic did not accept "a fall" as the origin of her physical injury. Sandra then told the nurse that George seemed to be under a great deal of pressure at his job, became angry easily, and had actually beaten her the previous night. When the nurse asked if they had considered marital counseling, Sandra said they had not but that she felt sure things were going to get better because George was getting a new supervisor at work. The nurse let her know that if the violence continued the clinic could be a resource for her in getting help. When this aspect of the patient's present functioning was reported to the physician, the nurse was told that, since the bruises were facial ones and not too severe in nature, the clinic should not be quick to get involved in marital friction. In taking this further the nurse learned that this manner of handling abuse was standard in the clinic because of the limited time and also because of the belief that marriage is a personal and private relationship.

The situation stabilized somewhat between Sandra and George, and the third violent explosion did not occur until several months following the birth of their child. The precipitating factor in this incident was George's inability to make payments on a car that he had purchased from a friend. The friend had taken back the car from the parking lot at the company. George, feeling embarrassed and disgusted with himself, that evening hit Sandra with a tire tool, while his son watched and cried. This was the beginning of a series of separations and reconciliations. Each time they separated, George would apologize and explain that he would try to control his anger. When Sandra would threaten to get a job and establish herself as a separate household George would call her a "woman's libber" and make her feel guilty by talking about how hard it would be for him to take care of his son.

Both George and Sandra were ill equipped for marriage. George had frequently observed his father physically abusing his mother, and Sandra was exploited by strange adults in her early life when she was left during her mother's absences. In their early years neither had received support from any member of the extended family because of frequent family moves.

In later years Sandra's numerous foster home placements resulted in her being so mobile that she had little opportunity for forming peer relationships. She became somewhat a loner and out of necessity learned many practical ways of fending for herself. George's adolescent years were spent striving to compete in sports but he could never achieve better than average. Within his family he was considered somewhat of a "mother's boy," which seemed to cause him to try harder than ever in adulthood to be a man. These early victimizations and cultural conditioning experiences, combined with social pressures in the persent, raised the tolerance level for spouse abuse within Sandra's and George's marital union. While George tried to prepare himself for an active life outside the home, he quickly lost patience; he felt wronged and cheated. When he received less respect outside the home than he felt he deserved he was hurt and frustrated. Not knowing how to talk about his feelings, he resorted to violence to overcome his pain of impotence. At other times he would demand sexual intercourse in an effort both to feel some sense of importance and to communicate closeness with his wife.

Sandra sought help from the legal system following one beating but was told that there was no basis for such intervention since she had neither witnesses nor medical documentation to support a complaint of assault and battery. Several weeks later she called an attorney about a divorce but was told that she would need $100 in advance. Sandra later heard on a public affairs television presentation that a community crisis telephone service was available. Through this service she was referred to a counselor who treated her for depression and masochistic tendencies.

Being resourceful, Sandra visited a local day care center to determine eligibility for her children. Through a woman at the center, Sandra located a counselor. Initially in working with Sandra it was important for the counselor to let her know that counseling was not made of magic and that she would have to do a considerable amount of work to change her life stresses. Themes dealt with Sandra's reliance on authority figures including social workers, foster parents, and finally George to make decisions for her. Through counseling, she began to recognize that both as a child and as an adult she had had an innate ability to manage everyday struggles even though she did not consciously recognize this strength.

These explorations helped Sandra build a trusting relationship and examine the need for a separate identity for herself in relation to George. While this approach helped her move toward more independence, sessions simultaneously focused on her safety as well as on maximizing opportunities to make improvements in the marriage.

To provide a safe temporary housing resource for Sandra and the children, the counselor found a volunteer family with a large house in a rural area who allowed Sandra and the children to stay with them. This resource seemed to lend itself well to the spouse abuse dilemma, because it provided an isolated refuge without George's intervention; it also presented Sandra with an option to choose a foster home placement without feeling placed in it; and it linked individuals from rural and urban areas in confronting human struggles.

In offering help for the marriage itself the counselor regularly encouraged Sandra to ask George to come for marriage counseling but he repeatedly refused. However, when Sandra told him one day that she was leaving, and it was not a reaction to a beating, George agreed to go with her for counseling. He recognized that Sandra was changing in her behavior toward him in that he could no longer "make her feel guilty" when she threatened to leave and that she had become more vocal about her unmet needs.

Sandra remained with the volunteer family for a month. She then informed George that she had become too heavily reliant on him and the marriage for her total identity. She asked him to keep the children 3 nights a week while she attended adult education courses. He agreed to do so; in return Sandra agreed to make extra efforts to improve her housekeeping skills. Both used the joint counseling sessions to focus on improving their communication. They were encouraged to tell each other what type of feeling was being generated by a particular interaction so that each would have a better understanding of the other, which would reduce their tendency for violent explosions. This was accomplished through individual sessions helping each "debrief" regarding their past family struggles and present external stresses. George was relieved that he was not condemned for beating his wife. He was able to work through previously unexpressed resentments toward both of his parents and through writing to his deceased father discussing a violent encounter George had witnessed as a child; he was able to discuss his feelings about this behavior. He also visited his mother in an attempt to reestablish a relationship on a more realistic level.

During counseling George committed himself never again to attack physically anyone who was important to him; however, he felt he would continue to use physical force if persons important to him were faced with harm from outside forces. This shifted the counseling to gain some insight into the lack of emotional support that family members received from traditional institutions. George focused specifically on his job situation which was becoming almost intolerable. He was encouraged to confront problems there directly to prevent further buildup of angry feelings; however, he was too afraid of being fired to do so. He ultimately developed the depressive symptoms of a nagging behavior, which was the last straw for Sandra who was now feeling better about her own worth. She announced in a joint session that, although she realized that both of them had tried hard to save the marriage, she was not willing to continue it; she had found a job and would move out of the home with the one child who was hers.

George was left to fend for himself and to provide child care for his son while trying to cope with job stress and the sense of loss related to the marriage. He continued seeing the counselor to work through his grief. He was assisted in finding a foster home for his son for 6 months, during which time George visited him regularly and made plans for their living together. He was able slowly to relieve his job frustration by recognizing that career-striving stress was not necessary to prove his masculinity and that it was self-defeating to hope that the work situation would satisfy his need for a sense of worth. He became more self-reflective and began to write poems inspired by daily encounters with others. By the time his son returned to live with him, George was feeling more confident in his ability to give to another person. He accepted the fact that his marriage had ended but realized that both he and Sandra had grown through the process.

THE NURSE'S INTERVENTIVE REPERTOIRE

It would seem that over the next few years environmentally oriented nurses will explore various ways of participating in the arena of delivering preventive services to individuals in families. Some will actively try different alternatives to alter the potential for violence within marriages.

The dynamics in spouse-abusing family systems clearly emphasize the need for various interventive measures to humanize society. These include maximizing opportunities for meeting human needs through (1) the creation of new arrangements, (2) restructuring of traditional institutions and old social forms, and (3) improvement of public policies affecting family life. Along with the appreciation of diversity and flexibility, nurses will need interventive repertoires that will enable them to respond in the areas of health care institutions, professional organizations, and the community at large.

Creation of new arrangements

In creating new arrangements for promoting health, the professional can support and develop measures to encourage the interdependence of many individuals and service disciplines. Because the health care field has been successful in integrating the expertise of different professionals in delivery treatment services through a team approach, it seems that a primary prevention effort can borrow from this established pattern and expand it to work in a different arena of service to form a new type of service with providers outside the traditional team concept. For instance, focusing on individuals' needs for stimulation could link the nurse with a recreation specialist, an educator, an environmentalist, and a ''street'' or community person who is knowledgeable about resources in a specific locality.

In recognition of the importance of cooperative efforts with other community supporters of the family unit, the nurse through the professional organization may wish to join forces with other professional and citizen groups to address the phenomenon of unmet human needs (for example, intimacy, independence, and stimulation) that is encouraged by geographic mobility. This could possibly result in convincing government and industry to remedy deficiencies created by their practices of transferring families geographically (for example, offering to employees who are transferred fringe benefits that would include frequent visits to extended family members and to significant friends of the employee and family). Other efforts in addressing the crippling effects of social isolation may be to promote a climate within the community that would help family members with the multiple health factors to be considered before accepting transfers to new job locations (for example, the internal stress produced through career striving and the external barriers to developing new community ties) (Skolnick and Skolnick, 1971). This aspect of intervention could also be incorporated within traditional institutions and will be discussed further below.

Because the intricate complexities of causative factors in spouse abuse have made it difficult for those involved to receive comprehensive help through traditional channels, self-help organizations are being started throughout North America to provide integrative services (such as medical, financial, legal, employment, and housing resources). Even though these efforts most often offer only secondary and tertiary intervention, it is important that nurses who have primary prevention skills or the desire to develop such skills join with these grassroots organizations. Through community-based approaches a slow educational process may evolve that could lead to a broader focus including systems intervention at the primary prevention level.

Restructure of traditional institutions and old social forms

While strategies for creating arrangements outside traditional institutions have merit, it is also important to work closely within existing institutions to reshape programs and permit personnel to use their accumulated experience and strength in new directions. In beginning at the patient-nurse interaction level, it may be necessary to seek additional funding to permit

more time to be spent individualizing patients' human needs; in contrast, the nurse who is not knowledgeable might strive to prevent interactional exchanges, which would serve only to reinforce the individual's depersonalized environment.

Additionally, creative mechanisms could be developed to help the individuals receiving care to adjust to the current reshaping of family roles (McBride, 1975). For instance, within the patient-nurse relationship a climate of acceptance could be promoted in males, especially young boys, to express hurt feelings rather than expressing only anger. However, to facilitate this process during a period of transition, when social consciousness has not yet become a part of most adults' socialization experiences, it may be necessary for the health care institution to provide its personnel, including nurses, with continuing education opportunities that would focus on heightening sensitivity to sex-role stereotyping within individuals and society. Kurtz (1978) believes that one approach is to eradicate "the myth of female inferiority" by helping women to have faith in their own equality. Sex-role awareness groups of an educational or therapeutic nature are useful in achieving this end.

In addition to promoting human exchanges between patient and professional, strategies could also be used to assist patients to interact while receiving services. For instance, an intergenerational linkage of persons using hospital or clinic services could reduce isolation and polarization between age groups and thus stimulate a climate for the appreciation of all family members. Such an approach could be promoted through the physical location of patient services and by developing programs that utilize the emotional and intellectual energies of both young and old, thus resurrecting a cross-stimulation process that communities have lost in recent years. An indirect benefit of such interdependence would be to deemphasize the cultural norm of the "privacy" of the family unit and promote the value of "outside supporters" for its members.

Modification within the hospital or clinic programming could also focus specifically on needs of individuals who may be in situational crises that make them particularly violence prone. Within the services of prenatal clinics in particular there could be early intervention, which might include modeling of positive approaches to dealing with anger, emphasis on nonsexist family structures, and promotion of the advantages of evaluating one's personal worth based on internal strengths. Caution must be used in this respect as moral, ethical, and legal questions (for example right to privacy) could potentially bar the extension of such helping services if these are pushed on patients (Bard and Zacker, 1971).

Specific primary prevention programs could be offered either by utilizing multiple referral resources for enrichment and education in healthy family functioning or by broadening the institution itself in its function of offering such services. At any rate, the macroculture conditioning of children's behavior indicates a need for early intervention to prevent conditions that could ultimately produce an abusive adult. Parent discussion groups based on a model similar to that described by Atkenson (1975) could be effectively implemented within pediatric services. Topics discussed could relate to child development and family functioning (for example alternatives to force for resolving problems, the importance of human need exchanges in everyday interaction between family members, and the need to reevaluate normative perceptions of sex-role functioning as a result of the rapidity of societal changes).

Another possible setting for an enrichment program is a family practice clinic. Weekend family meetings in the clinic, or more ideally family retreats with nature as the setting, could be useful in increasing cooperation, interaction, and division of responsibility within the family unit. I have found such a design to be most ef-

fective when it utilizes play as one of the tools and an interdisciplinary team as the means for service delivery. Scheduling such activities for weekends would make it more accessible to low-income and moderate-income families. This type of emancipatory family education could strengthen the family environment from within.

In addition the hospital or clinic could sponsor community forums on topics related to the root causes of spouse abuse and offer enrichment group experiences for men and women who wish to improve their communication skills. New skills in direct verbal expression of anger, hurt, sadness, joy, and other human feelings could become well-integrated personal resources and ultimately assist the individual when confronted with interpersonal conflicts. Through the provision of personal assessment and values clarification sessions, participants would learn to relate everyday pressures to overall life goals.

Both the weekend retreats and the community forums and groups would also provide insight into the complex environmental forces that make the process of "familying" difficult in society today. It would seem that as a result of such experiences some individuals would choose to become involved in broader institutional efforts to strengthen family life in general. Because the problem of spouse abuse is defined as one that involves the functioning of the institutions of society as a whole, it is imperative that any primary prevention solution offer individuals and professionals the opportunity to address broad social structures, which unless confronted may not only continue to create problems but may actually obstruct efforts to solve them. Public policy must therefore be a target for intervention.

Improvement of public policies and practice procedures

The nurse, as a professional and as a citizen, must consider the demands of society. The choice in the public arena is either to be an active participant in the development of laws and social attitudes or to have both health care consumers and nurses helplessly controlled by external forces. If one is to be active in working toward improvements in the primary prevention area of spouse abuse, it is necessary to develop strategies that aim toward alleviating the disasterous effect of being poor in an affluent society. Even though spouse abuse is not limited to any socioeconomic class, the poor have been identified as having a high incidence of spouse-abusing family systems; therefore specific efforts need to be made within the hospital or clinic and the larger community to prevent further alienation, which could ultimately reduce stresses within families and indirectly improve utilization of preventive health services. Within the community at large one approach would be to promote measures that would assure a guaranteed annual income for all families. Within the hospital or clinic, changes in operational procedures (for example, establishment of evening hours for all families would make services more accessible for low-income and moderate-income persons but would not separate them from the total population) and in general attitudes toward low-income patients (for example, recognition that lack of responsiveness to services offered is often a result of general feelings of powerlessness, polarization, and anger toward societal insitituions) would be helpful.

As the nurse becomes aware of the human needs of many different people and of the environmental factors contributing to the problem of spouse abuse, primary preventive activity may result in "social action for the provision of socio-cultural supplies" (Caplan, 1964). This can be effectively achieved through educational procedures to help professionals, administrators, and legislators understand the human dimension of the problem. Once the multiple nature of explanation is acknowledged, the decision has to be made as to the effective allotment of funds. The informed nurse can thus serve as educator for the primary prevention needs of the health care consumer and advocate for, among other things, expansion of services that build on strengths of individuals and families to prevent human suffering and ultimately reduce public health care costs.

All of these suggestions have inherent drawbacks toward achieving such a goal because of the overall policy and resource decisions as well as the specific constraints encountered in a given situation. However, this presentation should be useful in stimulating exploration into the many avenues of creative intervention that are available to the nurse who is clinically and sociopsychologically equipped to meet the challenge of spouse abuse prevention.

References

Atkenson, P.: A parent discussion group in a nursery school, Soc. Casework **56:**515-520, 1975.

Ball, J. C., Graff, H., and Chien, K.: Changing world patterns of drug abuse: 1945-1974, Intl. J. Clin. Pharmacol. Biopharm. **12:**109-113, 1975.

Bard, M., and Zacker, J.: The prevention of family violence: dilemmas of community intervention, J. Marriage Family **33:**677-682, 1971.

Bullough, B.: Poverty, ethnic identity and preventive health care, J. Health Soc. Behav. **13:**347-359, 1972.

Caplan, G.: Principles of preventive psychiatry, New York, 1964, Basic Books, Inc.

Curtis, G.: Violence breeds violence—perhaps? Am. J. Psychiatry **120:**386-387, 1963.

Downey, J., and Howell, J.: Wife battering, Vancouver, B.C., 1976, United Way of Greater Vancouver Social Policy and Research.

Edmiston, S.: The wife beaters, Women's Day, **16:**110-111, March 1976.

Field, M., and Field, H.: Marital violence and the criminal process: neither justice nor peace, Soc. Serv. Review **47:**221-240, 1973.

Gelles, R.: The violent home, Beverly Hills, Calif., 1972, Sage Publications, Inc.

Gelles, R.: Violence and pregnancy: a note on the extent of the problem and needed services, Fam. Coordinator **24:**81-86, 1975.

Gelles, R.: Abused wives: why do they stay? J. Marriage Family **38:**659-667, 1976.

Gelles, R.: Power, sex, and violence: the case of marital rape, Fam. Coordinator **26:**339-347, 1977.

Giovannoni, J.: Parental mistreatment: preperators and victims, J. Marriage Family **33:**649-657, 1971.

Goode, W. Force and violence in the family, J. Marriage Family **33:**624-636, 1971.

Hendrix, M., LaGodna, G., and Bohen, C.: The battered wife, Am. J. Nurs. **78:**650-653, 1978.

How to help the battered female patient, Prac. Psychology for Physicians **4:**11-14, 1977.

Kaplan, H.: Toward a general theory of psychosocial deviance: the case of aggressive behavior, Soc. Sci. Med. **6:**593-617, 1972.

Kopernik, L.: The family as a breeding ground of violence, Corrective Psychiatry J. Soc. Therapy **10:**318, 1964.

Kurtz, I.: All in the mind, World Health **31:**4-7, January, 1975.

Lieberknacht, K.: Helping the battered wife, Am. J. Nurs. **78:**654-656, 1978.

Lystad, M., ed.: An annotated bibliography: violence at home, Rockville, Md., 1974, National Institute of Mental Health.

Martin, D.: Battered wives, San Francisco, 1976, Glide Publications.

McBride, A.: Can family life survive, Am. J. Nurs. **75:**1648-1653, 1975.

Miller, N.: Battered spouses, Occasional papers on social administration, No. 57, London, 1975, S. Bell & Sons.

O'Brien, J.: Violence in divorce prone families, J. Marriage Family **33:**692-698, 1971.

Perlman, H.: Social work method: a review of the past decade. In Trends in social work practice and knowledge, proceedings of the NASW tenth anniversary symposium, New York, 1966, National Association of Social Workers.

Shepard, M.: Morbid jealousy: some clinical and social aspects of a psychiatric symptom, J. Ment. Sci. **107:**687-704, 1961.

Silver, L., Dublin, C., and Lourie, R.: Does violence breed violence? contributions from a study of the child abuse syndrome, Am. J. Psychiatry **126:**152-155, 1969.

Simpson, O., and Green, Y.: Coming of age in nursing: androgynous nurses, Can. Nurse **71:**20-21, December 1975.

Skolnick, A., and Skolnick, J.: Family in transition, Boston, 1971, Little Brown & Co.

Stark, R., and McEvoy, J.: Middle class violence, Psychology Today **4**(6):107-112, 1970.

Steinmetz, S.: The use of force for resolving family conflict: the training ground for abuse, Fam. Coordinator **26:**19-26, 1977.

Steinmetz, S., and Straus, M., The family as a cradle of violence, Society **10**(6):50-56, 1973.

Steinmetz, S., and Straus, M.: Violence in the family, New York, 1974, Dodd, Mead & Co.

Straus, M.: A general system theory approach to a theory of violence between family members, Soc. Sci. Information **12**(3):105-125, 1973.

Straus, M.: Sexual inequality, cultural norms, and wife-beating, Victimology. **1:**54-70, Spring 1976.

Straus, M.: A social structural perspective on the prevention and treatment of wife-beating. In Roy, M., ed.: Battered women, New York, 1977, Van Nostrand Reinhold Co.

Straus, M., Gelles, R., and Steinmetz, S.: Violence in the family: an assessment of knowledge and research needs, paper given before the American Association for the Advancement of Science, Boston, February 1976.

Toby, J.: Violence and the masculine ideal: some qualitative data, Anal. Am. Academy Polit. Soc. Sci. **364:**19-28, 1966.

Viano, E., ed.: From the editor: special issue on spouse abuse and domestic violence, Victimology **2:**417, 1978.

Whitehurst, R.: Violence in husband-wife interaction. In Steinmetz, S., and Straus, M. eds.: Violence in the family, New York, 1974, Harper & Row, Publishers.

CHAPTER 11

Nursing intervention in child abuse

ELAINE ORTMAN

Child abuse and neglect are symptoms of a society in trouble. They constitute situations in which individuals are dehumanized and family units disintegrate. Early abusive experiences have profound, long-term effects on society. Sirhan Sirhan, James Earl Ray, and Arthur Bremer, all major American assassins, were abused as children. The increasing availability of statistics and greater attention to documentation of violence are helping to dramatize the magnitude of the problem.

There are more than 300,000 cases of child abuse and neglect reported nationally each year (Besharon, 1975). Since only 1% to 10% of the suspected cases are usually reported, this figure does not reflect the extent of the problem.

Child abuse is a family tragedy. It is devastating for the child, for the abusing parents, and for society. Grant-funding priorities, state legislation for child advocates, and mandatory reporting laws highlight the nation's concern for society's children. Mass media campaigns have attempted to increase public awareness of the problem. The emotional fervor is justifiable, but as is so often true, moral indignation can cloud judgment and lead to policies that can be equally abusive. Decisions guiding legislation and policies on behalf of children need to be based on a clear understanding of the principles of child development and family relations.

According to Sullivan (1953), Bowlby (1958), and Erikson (1963), the initial patterns of relationships that children establish within their families form the framework for all other relationships. Without the foundation of "tenderness and reciprocal emotions" (Sullivan, 1953), "attachment" (Bowlby, 1958), or "basic trust" (Erikson, 1963), a child's emotional development is impaired.

An abused or neglected child's needs for recognition, stimulation, security, and supervision are entirely or partially unmet. To compensate for this lack, the child may resort to antisocial behavior. Neglect or abuse can impair physical growth and development as well as the normal course of socialization and personality development.

CHARACTERISTICS OF ABUSIVE RELATIONSHIPS

Kempe and Helfer (1972), in their extensive writings, identify significant variables in abusive situations. The major variable appears to be a distortion of the normal mother-child relationship (usually seen as nurturant and protective). Abusive parents raise their children as they were raised. They appear unable to assess stress or change in their environment, in their internal needs, or in the needs of their children. They have deep-seated fears of abandonment and are sensitive to feelings of failure. They have difficulty in establishing trust relationships, in expressing anger or disappointment directly to a significant person, and in asking for help. They may painfully disregard the infant's own needs, wishes, and age-appropriate

115

limitations. When discipline gets confused with expressions of their own inner anger, they commit violent acts against their children. In addition, the high frequency of home changes that the children usually experience adds to the turmoil in their lives. Environmental stress, such as the loss of employment, precipitates a crisis for families with inadequate problem-solving skills. Unfortunately, abusive families are typically socially isolated and do not seek help from social service agencies.

There is also an interactional component to abuse. The abused child's milieu and the parent's perception of the child are critical influences on the child's development. Children who see recurrent expressions of violence in their family and are recipients of that violence grow up to believe that violence is a way of life and a viable problem-solving mechanism. They may identify with the aggressor to gain a measure of self-protection and mastery. Although the children do not originally activate the hostility that is directed against them, they may begin to provide a reciprocal stimulus for the continued abuse by increasingly requesting attention when they perceive high levels of anxiety. The child's demands tend to increase the mother's already elevated level of stress and she may respond with abusive actions.

A delay in the "mothering" process has emerged as a predominant feature in the pathogenesis of child abuse situations. Steele and Pollock (Kempe, 1972) found that since abusive parents had suffered a lack of nurturance themselves they revealed deficiencies in their own "motherliness" or "fatherliness," which interfered with the parent's ability to perform the mechanics of child care. In looking at abused, low-birth-weight premature infants who required extended hospitalization, Stern (1973) found that abusive mothers had difficulty forming attachments to their infants and responded with indifference or rejection, which inhibited the children's abilities to form attachments to their mothers (Rutter, 1974).

Infants and young children need stimulation and socialization for neurological and ego development. Physical growth, intellect, curiosity, language, and learning all require nurturance from a consistent primary caretaker. Erikson (1963) maintains that without the development of basic trust in the maternal figure, the child's personality development has no firm foundation on which to develop autonomy, initiative, and self-esteem. The process of sharing one's inner self with others requires a firm basis of trust and security. Abused children who lack that foundation lag behind normal children in motor skills, play, peer relationships, and socialization skills.

BONDING BEHAVIORS AND CRITICAL DISCRIMINATORS
Normal children

Although no conclusive studies have been done of parent-child attachment, or bonding behaviors, resulting in abuse or neglect, several studies have suggested that a disturbed mother-child relationship exists in abuse cases (Morse et al., 1970; Ounsted et al., 1974). The theoretical premises and research findings of Bowlby (1958) and Ainsworth et al. (1972) are relevant to the interactional pattern of abusive parents and their children. Ainsworth et al. and Bowlby have discussed the attachment, or bonding, relationship between mothers and children. Ainsworth et al. have researched behavioral characteristics of attachment in normal mother-child relationships.

Normal children display a set of behaviors, defined as attachment behaviors, that consistently discriminate between their parents and strangers (Cohen, 1974). Separation anxiety is one aspect of mother-child attachment behavior. Beginning at about the age of 6 months and lasting until about 2 years, normal mother-child separation behavior is commonly identified by the child's demonstrative distress on separation from his mother. The absence of this characteristic pattern of interaction should alert human service personnel to possible problems in the mother-child relationship.

Abused children

There appears to be a critical period for the development of attachment after which bond formation becomes increasingly less likely. Terr (1970) observes that when the primary caretaker is the abusive parent, children are prone to ego defects that interfere with attachment formation. These defects—withdrawal, indifference to the mother, and psychomotor retardation—make it progressively more difficult for mothers to relate to their infants. The absence of expected attachment behaviors in abused children has been observed clinically. Galdston (1965) notes that in the hospital abused children display profound apathy or extreme fright, but not the expected separation anxiety behavior. Silver (1968) observes that abused children, unlike the normal population, do not look toward their parents for assurance in emergency room situations. These children show no real expectation of being comforted by their parents. Silver concludes that abused children learn that their parents are not a source of safety, but a signal for danger. They seek safety by sizing up their situation rather than by seeking out their parents. Ounsted et al. (1974) interpret the "frozen watchfulness" that abused children display as an adaptive response to the unpredictable loving and abusing behaviors of their parents.

CHILD ABUSE AND THE LAW

Reporting and early identification make up the first phase of intervention in child abuse. People who are most likely to come into contact with child abuse situations are physicians, nurses, social service workers, school personnel, police, neighbors, and relatives. In 1971 the Florida Legislature revised the state's child abuse statutes and attempted to make the public more aware of the problem as well as to whom and where to make a report. Only 200 reports of child abuse were made during the year before this revision. In the following year, 19,000 reports were filed (Child abuse and neglect, 1974).

Although persons who report instances of child abuse and neglect are protected by law from liability, the failure to report these incidents prevents many abused and neglected children from receiving protective services. Lynch (1975) estimates that in 1973 reports covered only 1% to 10% of the total number of cases of abuse and neglect. Inadequacies, breakdowns, and gaps in the system make detection and reporting haphazard and incomplete. An estimated three fourths of those children who die as a result of abuse are suspected by, or known to, authorities before their death (Child abuse and neglect, 1974). Class and Norris (1960) identify increasing social mobility and deterioration of social cohesiveness of neighborhoods as additional factors that decrease the visibility of neglect and abuse.

MENTAL HEALTH NURSING AND CHILD ABUSE

Child abuse and neglect is a multidimensional problem that requires a multidisciplinary treatment approach. Child abuse families characteristically display closed, rigid family systems with inconsistent and ineffective feedback mechanisms. This may be one explanation for the fact that abuse seems to be multigenerational. Child abuse is a symptom of a family in crisis. Treatment must therefore include all family members. Therapy may focus on one of the subsystems (for example, parent counseling or mother-child dyads) or on the total family. Regardless of the approach, the goal is to produce a change in the interactional behavior of family members while maintaining the family integrity if at all possible. Children should be separated from their parents only when the situation threatens the children's safety.

The concept of child advocacy provides for the development of a mental health delivery system for children. The basis of this approach is the idea that every child is entitled to the care and assistance that he needs for optimum growth and development. The legal process is involved in adjudication of cases in which abuse or neglect is suspected. The court serves to balance the rights of parents with society's interests in assuring the child's rights. It must weigh the risk of future and increasing injury to the child against the trauma of separation from family and familiar surroundings. This study presents a modified Ainsworth (Ainsworth et al., 1972), paradigm which can help the courts better evaluate attachment and avoid unnecessary traumatic separations. It also provides a training and evaluative tool for foster parents who work with abused children. Placement in foster care is usually made on a temporary basis. The majority of children who are not returned to their parents in the first year of placement are moved around from foster home to foster home throughout their childhood. If an attachment has been formed, each move decreases the child's opportunity for bonding.

Nurses are often in the best position to identify high-risk groups. Because nurses observe the parent-child separation experiences that occur in hospital units, emergency rooms, pediatricians' offices, and public health agencies such as well-baby clinics, they need to have a clear understanding of functional and dysfunctional separation patterns.

In addition, nurses often have an opportunity to influence parents' child-rearing practices. Early intervention can foster mother-child attachment and prevent further distortion in the bonding process. Since the characteristics of infants have a profound effect on mother-infant interactions, adequate evaluation of the infants' emotional and behavioral functions becomes important. By pinpointing particular areas of need, vulnerability, and idiosyncratic response in specific infants, nurses can help mothers be more sensitive to their particular infant's needs.

PARADIGM FOR EVALUATING BONDING

Concurrent with the lack of adequate reporting in child abuse is the lack of adequate research. Problems in the analysis of data stem from the varying definitions of abuse and neglect that do not discriminate between punishment or discipline and abuse. A review of the literature reveals that concepts of child abuse have been value-oriented, highly emotional, and confused with corporal punishment. The focus has been directed toward descriptive reporting rather than the collection of research data.

The following section describes a study that focused on the evaluation of the differences between mother-child relationships in abused and nonabused children. The importance of the study lies in early prevention. If nurses can identify early disturbances in parent-child relationships, then it is possible to prevent further breakdown in the primary relationship between parent and child. This could promote mental health and break the multigenerational cycle of child abuse.

An approach is described that uses a quasi-experimental research model to look at the differences between mother-child relationships in abused and nonabused children. A modification of the Ainsworth et al. (1972) paradigm allows the researcher to study the attachment behaviors of abused and nonabused children during brief separation from and reunion with their mothers and strangers. The essence of the Ainsworth paradigm provides for both separation and reunion experiences to be used in a research design to evaluate attachment behaviors manifested by the children who are studied. Since abuse commonly occurs in children between the ages of 3 and 5 years, it seemed that if differences in the mother-child relationship could be identified at an earlier age (9 months to 2 years) then intervention could be instrumental in the prevention of child abuse. The researcher introduced treatment variables (that is, separation and reunion experiences), scored observations via videotapes of 21 mother-infant dyads (14 abused and 7 non-abused), and noted the significant differences in attachment behaviors manifested by the abused and nonabused children, specifically exploration and locomotion during free play; head-turning, following, crying, and distress with separation; and positive greeting behaviors during reunion. The abused children's lack of attachment behaviors in both separation and reunion appears to be consistent with Ainsworth's (1963) observations of children in the "non-attached" group. This research supports the theory that there is a distortion in the bonding process between mother and child in situations where the children have been abused or neglected.

Discriminating variables

The variable "exploration" was defined as being present when the child made excursions away from the mother and manipulated other objects or people visually, verbally, or manually but returned to the mother from time to time (Ainsworth 1963). "Locomotion" was defined as being present if a child moved his body from one spot to another by crawling or walking. If the child turned his head toward the door after his mother left, the variable "turns head" was considered to be present. "Following" behavior was defined as occurring if the child crawled or walked to the door after his mother left. As in Stayton and Ainsworth's study (1973), "crying-with-separation" was defined as being present if the child cried when his mother or a stranger left the room; if crying had begun previous to departure and increased in intensity at the time of departure or within 10 seconds thereafter, then "crying on departure" was recorded. Conversely, "soothing" was defined as being present if sustained cessation of the child's crying occurred (Harmon et al., 1976).

"Distress," as defined by Harmon et al.

(1976), was considered to be present if the child displayed any fussing or crying behavior beyond minimal or brief whimpering. This was measured on a scale of 1 to 5, with 1 being absence of crying and 5 being cumulative and durational crying.

If the child acknowledged the reentering person by smiling, laughing, bouncing, jiggling, leaning, lifting arms in greeting, or standing up in response to the entering figure, then "positive greeting" was identified as occurring (Ainsworth et al., 1972).

Before videotaping began the photographer greeted each mother and gave her a standardized set of instructions. The sequence had seven specific phases. The first was a 2-minute period in which each mother was encouraged to make her infant comfortable in the playroom setting. The second phase contained 5 minutes of free play in which the infant initiated interaction. These phases provided the investigator with information regarding mother-infant interaction, child temperament, and spontaneous and responsive exploration. The third phase began with a 1-minute period in which the stranger, mother, and child were present. The stranger initiated play interaction with the child. At this point, the mother was directed to say good-bye to the infant as if she were leaving the child with a babysitter and to leave the playroom. In the fourth phase, a 3-minute period of separation followed. During the first minute, the stranger remained available for play with the infant at the infant's initiative. The stranger did not intervene unless the infant appeared distressed. If the infant was not distressed after 1 minute, the stranger took a chair. If distress occurred at any time and the infant could not be soothed, the mother was requested to return. If no distress occurred, the mother came back at the end of the period, at a point when the infant was away from the door so that reunion behaviors could be observed. In the fifth phase, the stranger remained in the playroom for a 2-minute period so that a comparison between the differential interactions with mother and stranger could be made. Then, in the sixth phase, the stranger left for a 3-minute period and returned in the seventh, for 1 minute of reunion.

Results

Clinically the investigator saw evidence of marked inhibition and wariness among abused children. Where the nonabused child showed active pleasure and interest in the play sequences, the abused or neglected child showed lack of responsiveness. A statistically significant difference between abused and nonabused children was found in both absence of exploration and absence of locomotion. A statistically significant difference also occurred between natural abusive parents and foster parents in the children's locomotion during the mother-child sequence and in the children's responsive exploration during free play. One significant finding was that in the normal population the mother separation often elicited distress vocalization, and mother reunion provoked increased frequency and intensity of attachment behaviors. Conversely, the lack of proximity-seeking and proximity-maintaining behaviors, lack of distress with separation, and the lack of reunion behaviors characterized the abused population. Of particular interest was one abused infant who showed no emotional reaction to either his mother's separation or her return but showed mild to moderate distress and search behaviors in response to the stranger's departure and positive greeting on reunion with the stranger. This was not seen in any of the nonabused children.

The relationship between level of distress with mother separation and abuse or nonabuse supports the previously presented data regarding lack of separation anxiety in the abused group. In 10 of 13 cases of abused children distress during separation was absent; cumulative distress, in contrast, occurred in six out of seven nonabuse cases. Since no single criterion of

attachment could serve as a basis for judging whether or not an infant had become attached to his mother, the overall combinations of attachment behaviors were evaluated. Both abuse and nonabuse groups demonstrated attachment behavior specific to their groups. The outstanding feature was that no one pattern appeared in both groups.

Conclusions

This study indicates that there are significant differences between the responses of abused and nonabused children to a time-limited mother separation and reunion. Nonabused children exhibited exploration behavior and locomotion in a free play setting. During separation, nonabused children turned their heads and moved toward the place where they last saw their mother. Mother separation also evoked crying and distress behaviors in nonabused children. Positive greeting behavior was evident in the nonabused children on reunion with their mothers after separation. All of the nonabused children exhibited at least seven of the nine behaviors.

The abused children's responses were demonstrably different. During free play their exploration and locomotion was minimal, if it existed at all. On mother separation the abused children did not turn their heads or they did so briefly. They showed little or no crying and distress and did not follow through with locomotion. On reunion they did not greet their mothers positively. Abused children characteristically exhibited eight of the nine behaviors.

The results of this study indicate that there is a significant difference in attachment behaviors manifested by 9- to 23-month-old abused and nonabused children during a brief separation from and reunion with their mothers. There appears to be a difference in the mother-infant interactional process between the two groups, as evidenced by a distortion in the bonding process between mother and child in child abuse or child neglect situations. These nine behaviors

TABLE 1

Discriminating behaviors

Time period	Behavior	Abused	Nonabused
Free play	Exploration and locomotion	Minimal	Actively present
Maternal separation	Head-turning and following (through locomotion)	Brief or absent	Present
	Crying	Absent	Durational and/
	Distress	Absent	or cumulative
Maternal reunion	Positive greeting	Absent or dis-tress response	Actively present

can be considered essential variables for identifying functional and dysfunctional mother-child relationships (Table 1).

Clinical applications

This research indicates that there are many areas in which clinical evaluation and intervention could be of significant help. This paradigm could be used to assess the parent-child relationship and to work with parents around specific issues. Nurses and other health service personnel could use videotape replays to stimulate discussion and demonstrate important points to the parents.

Mother-child evaluation would further help nurses assess possible therapeutic interventions and disposition of children in child abuse cases. The quality of the relationship as well as the occurrence of abuse could be evaluated. Since abuse can be episodic or occur over a period of time, the incidence of abuse should not be the focus; rather the depth of the disturbance between parent and child should be central to the nursing observation. If the child demonstrates attachment behaviors during separation and reunion, the child should remain in the home and the mother-child relationship should be worked with in an intensive manner. If no bonding is present, then the child should be considered for placement in a foster home so that the child and a foster parent might have the opportunity to attain attachment.

If the nurse decides that the behaviors identified in the study are not consistently present or if only a small percentage are present and if there is no evidence of abuse and/or neglect; then the nurse can help teach the parents ways of increasing their child's attachment. For example, on reunion a positive greeting can be fostered by holding and comforting the child if he appears distressed by the separation but takes no initiative to ask for comforting. Increased eye contact between parent and child when the parent wants to engage the child fosters bonding. Nurses can help parents identify and respond to behavioral cues from their child instead of being intrusive into the child's world. Give-and-take games between parent and child increase trust. Videotape playback of play sessions can be useful by stopping the film at opportune times and asking the parents, ''What do you think Johnny is feeling here?'' or ''What was happening here?'' In this fashion nurses can foster parents' insight into their relationships with their child.

In addition, longitudinal changes in mother-child relationships following intervention could be assessed. For example, this paradigm could be used to study the attachment relationship between foster mothers and children before children are removed from foster care and returned to their natural mother or vice versa. Using this paradigm, the children's behavior with their natural mothers would be compared to that with their foster mothers. Videotapes would also show "remnant effects" of abuse found in children in foster care; they would indicate useful types of intervention and help to teach foster parents specific parenting skills for these children.

Prevention is a community process. It is necessary to incorporate into individual families and community life a greater understanding of family mental health. The learning of family developmental concepts should be a lifelong process against child abuse with booster shots of increased learning in crucial periods of family stress, such as divorce, death, remarriage, or the birth of a new child. Positive self-concept and communication skills can be taught in elementary school, the role of family members can be incorporated into the curriculum in the middle school years, and premarital counseling and parenting can be taught in high school. Society demonstrates by its dysfunctional and often abusive patterns that family-development skills need to be addressed, especially during critical developmental stages.

References

Ainsworth, M.: The development of infant-mother interaction among the Ganda. In Foss, B., ed.: Determinants of infant behavior, New York, 1963, John Wiley & Sons, Inc.

Ainsworth, M., and Bell, S.: Attachment, exploration and separation: illustrated by the behavior of one year olds in a strange situation, Child Dev. 41:49-67, March 1970.

Ainsworth, M., Bell, S., and Stayton, D.: Individual differences in the development of some attachment behaviors, Merrill Q. 18:123-143, April 1972.

Besharon, D.: Building a community response to child abuse and maltreatment. Child. Today, 5:2-4, September-October 1975.

Bowlby, J.: Nature of the child's tie to his mother. Int. J. Psychoanal. 39:350-373, January 1958.

Bowlby, J.: Separation anxiety. Intl. J. Psychoanal. 41: 89-113, November 1958.

Child abuse and neglect (draft), Utah State plan, November 4, 1974.

Class, E., and Norris, D.: Neglect, social deviance, and community action. Natl. Probation Parole Assoc. 6:2, January 1960.

Cohen, L.: The operational definition of attachment, Psychol. Bull. 81:207-217, April 1974.

Erikson, E.: Childhood and society, New York, 1963, W. W. Norton & Co., Inc.

Galdston, R.: Observations on children who have been physically abused and their parents, Am. J. Psychiatry 122:440-443, 1965.

Harmon, R., Morgan, G., and Klein, R.: Determinants of normal variation in infants' negative reactions to unfamiliar adults (unpublished manuscript), 1976.

Kempe, C., and Helfer, R., eds.: Helping the battered child and his family. Philadelphia, 1972, J. B. Lippincott Co.

Lynch, A.: Child abuse in school age population, J. Sch. Health 45:141-147, March 1975.

Morse, C., Sahler, O., and Friedman, S.: Three year follow-up study of abused and neglected children, Am. J. Dis. Chil. 120:439-446, 1970.

Ounsted, C., Oppenheimer, R., and Lindsey, J.: Aspects of bonding failure: the psychopathology and psychotherapeutic treatment of families of battered children, Dev. Med. Child Neurol. 16:447-456, 1974.

Rutter, M.: Maternal deprivation, Baltimore, 1974, Penguin Books.

Schaffer, H., and Emerson, R.: The qualities of mothering: maternal deprivation reassessed, New York, 1974, Jason Aronson, Inc.

Silver, L.: Child abuse syndrome: a review, Med. Times 96:803-820, 1968a.

Silver, L.: Psychological aspects of the battered child and his parents, Clin. Proc. Child. Hospital 24:355-364, 1968b.

Stayton, D., and Ainsworth, M.: Individual differences in infant responses to brief, everyday separation as related to other infant and maternal behavior, Dev. Psychol. 9:226-235, 1973.

Stern, L.: Separation of premature infants and mother may be a factor in child abuse, Hosp. Prac. 8:117-123, 1973.

Sullivan, H.: The interpersonal theory of psychiatry. New York, 1953, W. W. Norton & Co., Inc.

Terr, C.: A family study of child abuse, Am. J. Psychiatry 127:665-671, 1970.

CHAPTER 12

Epidemiology of rape

ANN KNECHT KIRKHAM

In studying health problems, the application of the epidemiological process has been utilized primarily with infectious diseases such as rubella, syphilis, and tuberculosis. Recently, however, the epidemiological process has been successfully utilized in the study of multifaceted health problems. The epidemiological process analyzes the health problem by examining the commonalities in and the relationship between three components: agent (rapist), host (victim), and environment (place, time of day, day of week, month). The researcher utilizing the epidemiological process of investigation concentrates first on commonalities among each of the cases of rape in regard to the rapist, victim, and environment and then focuses attention on the interrelationship of each of the components. Fig. 12-1 depicts the epidemiological triad, the way in which a health problem is conceptualized.

The epidemiological method of studying

health problems is compatible with an ecological perspective. Both deal with the need to comprehensively analyze health problems in relation to the interaction of man's internal and external environments. The rape event represents a unique, dynamic interaction between the internal and external environments of two people. The physiological, sociocultural, psychological, and legal ramifications are evident for each. A review of the literature indicates that the epidemiological method of investigation has never been utilized in the study of rape.

An ecological perspective insists that complex health problems cannot be successfully dealt with by the application of a simple, single solution. Failure to recognize and analyze each component of the problem often leads to a partial solution, which may be more detrimental than beneficial. An example of this may be the harm inherent in teaching women to vigorously fight the assailant. Selkin (1975) states, "It is necessary to stress the fact that playing along with an assailant to calm his anxiety, and then counterattacking with a kick in the genitals may be an invitation to murder." The rapist, frightened by the sudden unpredictability and loss of control over the victim, may become panicky and commit murder in a desperate attempt to regain control.

Inherent in the ecological and epidemiological approach to community mental health are concepts of prevention. While primary prevention involves averting the occurrence of a health problem, secondary prevention involves early

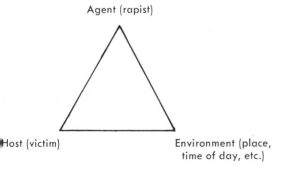

Agent (rapist)

Host (victim)

Environment (place, time of day, etc.)

Fig. 12-1. Epidemiological triad applied to rape.

123

treatment to prevent complications. Tertiary prevention then is aimed at stopping even further progression of the results of the initial health problem (Murray, 1975). In this chapter, the application of the epidemiological process in relation to planning for primary, secondary, and tertiary prevention will be presented.

While nurses may have contact with both rapists and victims, the opportunity to deal with this health problem comprehensively as it relates to the individual, family, and community provides a unique contribution. For example, the role of the police officer is primarily that of securing evidence and apprehending the alleged rapist. Similarly the district attorney focuses on the successful prosecution of the rapist, whereas the volunteer crisis intervention worker applies principles of crisis intervention to enable the victim to cope with immediate and long-term ramifications of the rape. The community mental health nurse, on the other hand, assesses the total health problem and plans for primary as well as secondary and tertiary prevention.

Rape is one of the ugliest of crimes. All too often the subjugation and humiliation do not end with the rapist's attack. If the victim reports the rape, her suffering is frequently prolonged and even increased by police skepticism and tactless comments regarding the victim's role in the attack. This alienation also frequently prevails in the medical care facility, where rape is usually not considered an emergency unless physical trauma is obvious.

Negativism is also inherent in an emergency room case priority-setting system. Some authorities maintain that rape victims should be given triage status next only to life-threatening cases (McCubbin and Scott, 1973). To be binding in court, evidence for prosecution should be collected before the victim bathes, douches, changes clothes, or even urinates or defecates. It seems sadistic to require a woman to wait in this condition for several hours. The soiled and disheveled victim may have to wait many hours for treatment while other people in the busy waiting room gawk at her and speculate about the uniformed police officer who accompanies her. The medical examination may be performed without explanation and medical personnel may make remarks about women who "ask" to get raped. "She leaves the hospital alone, to return home, frightened, confused, dirty and distraught. She was raped in private during the crime; she has now been raped in public" (Brodyaga and Gates, 1975).

Rape is legally defined as natural or unnatural sexual intercourse forced on an unwilling person by threat of bodily injury or loss of life. Usually the rapist is male and the victim is a child, female, or another male; however, some cases of female rapists have been reported. In describing the psychodynamics of rape, the pronoun "she" will be used to denote the victim and the pronoun "he" will be used to denote the rapist.

Rape is not commonly perceived by society as a sexual deviation. Even though the *Diagnostic and Statistical Manual of Mental Disorders* (American Psychiatric Association, 1968) defines sexual deviations as sexual behavior that is carried out under bizarre circumstances, the manual does not list rape as a sexual deviation. Cormier (Resnik, 1972) defines deviant sexual behavior as a harmful sexual act that is performed without the mutual consent of the partners. Eaton (1976) refers to sexual deviation as sexual behavior that is the source of worry, concern, or disagreeable consequences to the participants. A significant variable in differentiating between normal and deviant sexual behavior is the accepted value system of a given culture or subculture. In the United States, it is not uncommon to find people (both male and female) who view rape as a natural phenomenon caused by the lasciviousness of the victim. The tenaciousness and pervasiveness of this myth is thought to be a defense against acknowledging the possibility of one's own rape.

Research regarding the etiology of rape has become available only in the past 5 years. The long-held belief that rape is motivated by a need for sexual gratification has been disproved. It is now clear that rape is performed to satisfy pathological, nonsexual needs. Brownmiller (1975) illustrates how rape has been used throughout history as a weapon to keep people in a state of submission. For example, a principal method of humiliating and breaking the spirit of the enemy during wartime has been the public raping of the enemy's women and girls. In America, rape was used to deliberately crush the black female's sexual integrity, an essential part of the subjugation of black slaves.

This chapter will discuss the internal environment of both the rapist and the victim, the aspects of the external environment that promote or thwart care of the rape victim, and the epidemiology of rape, with emphasis on interventions for primary prevention. Internal environmental dynamics refer to the psychodynamics of individual motivation. This chapter addresses two key questions related to individual motivation: (1) What is going on in his subconscious to cause a person to commit rape? (2) What is it that motivates *some* victims to set themselves up to be raped?

INTERNAL ENVIRONMENTAL DYNAMICS OF THE RAPIST

The following descriptions of four fundamental psychodynamics of rapists are based on the four patterns of rape described by Burgess and Lazare (1976). Although these etiological dynamics may be interwoven in a single assault, one pattern is usually dominant. Other types of rape, such as homosexual rape, gang rape, and child rape, each have unique etiological dynamics but these motivations are less common and will not be discussed in this chapter.

Displaced anger

The rapist who is motivated by displaced anger uses rape to express his rage toward women and to relieve his psychological stress. The psychopathology stems from a lifetime of rejection and/or humiliation at the hands of a significant female. The rapist usually experiences an uncontrollable impulse following a frustrating situation with a significant female. The rape victim is therefore merely a symbol of his repressed resentment and hatred. Frequently the victim is a stranger to the rapist and often she is somewhat older than he. The assault on the victim is usually much more brutal than would be required for vaginal penetration. The primary gain for this rapist is the expression of a long-repressed hatred for a significant female. In fact the rapist frequently requires oral stimulation to achieve an erection. The feeling of revenge and the degradation and humiliation of the symbolic hate object are the rapist's motivation and compensation for the rape.

Feelings of incompetence

The rapist who feels inadequate uses rape to prove to himself that he is strong, competent, potent, and heterosexual. The psychopathology stems from a permeating feeling of worthlessness and vulnerability. Frequently this person is fearful of emerging homosexual impulses. By subduing a woman who symbolizes qualities of weakness and helplessness—qualities that he fears in himself—this rapist gratifies a need to feel powerful, dynamic, and in control. He usually does not physically harm his victim more than is necessary to subdue her. This rapist does not have a need to brutalize or vent hostile feelings toward the victim. Instead, he needs to overpower, control, and assert his manhood. The act of rape also enables the rapist to deny his anxiety regarding homosexual feelings. This type of rapist usually commits assaults over and over, either because "successful" rape does not reduce his anxiety or because he fails in his rape attempt.

Sadistic needs

Both sexual and aggressive needs combine in the internal environment of the sadistic rapist. Because this person is unable to experience sexual arousal without concomitant arousal of aggressive thoughts and actions, he is likely to be impotent unless his sexual partner resists. Therefore he perceives the victim's struggle, terror, and protest as an expression of excitement and pleasure. The sadistic rapist does not confine his abuse to the genital areas of his victim; he may also mutilate the victim's hands, feet, legs, and abdomen by cutting, burning, and biting. In extreme cases, this psychopathological thinking can result in "lust murder." One victim, after several hours of this type of mutilation, pleaded to the assailant to kill her and put her out of her misery.

Antisocial personality disorder

The dynamics of this rapist relate primarily to faulty conscience development. The faulty conscience creates an environment in which any desired goal is determined as acceptable. Thus this person has few or no constraints on his behavior. He is self-centered, opportunistic, and impulsive. He takes what he wants and does what he wants when he wants. His approach to the world is characteristically exploitive. Frequently this person commits rape while engaging in some other antisocial activity such as burglary.

INTERNAL ENVIRONMENTAL DYNAMICS OF THE VICTIM

Based on the literature and an epidemiological study now in progress, the following dynamics appear to play a role in increasing the chances of some women to be rape victims.

"Rapo"

The myth that the victim "asked for it" needs to be carefully and objectively analyzed. The accusing attitude that permeates the atmosphere surrounding the rape victim may be closely tied to this myth. There are cases in which the victim encourages and promotes sexual intercourse but later claims that the act was rape. The motivation for this type of behavior is best explained through transactional

analysis game theory. Briefly, a game is defined as "an ongoing series of complementary ulterior transactions progressing to a well-defined, predictable outcome" (Berne, 1964). Put more simply, psychological "games" are usually played on an unconscious level and consist of the "player" with an ulterior motive making moves toward another person or persons. The ulterior motive, or payoff, fills a psychological need of the game initiator.

The game that is significantly associated with rape is entitled "Rapo." Rapo may be played with different levels of intensity. These levels of intensity are defined by degrees: first-degree, second-degree, and third-degree Rapo. First-degree Rapo is basically the type of flirting that many women have engaged in at one time or another. In first-degree Rapo the woman leads a man on by indicating that she may be sexually available, then politely rejects his passes: her payoff is the pleasure of being pursued.

Rapo to the second degree consists of the same scenario as in first degree; however, the woman leads the man on more intensely. The payoff is the gratification that comes when the woman rejects the man with great indignation.

Third-degree Rapo is a vicious game that usually ends in the courtroom as a result of aggravated rape or murder. Here the woman leads the man into having sexual intercourse with her and then cries "rape." Sometimes, particularly in the case of girls under the age of legal consent, significant others encourage her to charge a lover with rape to save face or to protect the family's standing in the community.

Based on game theory of transactional analysis, some rapes may thus conform to the myth of the provocative, seductive, yet punitive woman. Myths are, after all, based on a fragment of truth. Groth and Cohen (1976) contend, however, that no matter how lascivious, provocative, and inviting the victim is, she maintains the right to change her mind at any point. They argue that they have yet to identify a "real" case of victim-induced rape in many years of treating convicted rapists at the Massachusetts Treatment Center. On the other hand, the following case was described by a police officer. A woman and man were having sexual intercourse in the front seat of a car and the officer investigating the vehicle observed the activity. When the woman—who up to then had appeared to be enjoying the activity—saw the officer, she began yelling "rape."

The woman who for some psychopathological need of her own brings false rape charges against a man is not only hurting an innocent man but is promoting the myth that women desire and "ask for" rape. She is unknowingly, or uncaringly, doing a great deal of harm to other members of her own sex. Since some alleged victims play games like Rapo repeatedly, police officers understandably become disenchanted with apprehending the alleged rapist. But the victim who has been humiliated and frightened for her life deserves protection—not the implied and sometimes explicit message from health and police professionals that she somehow provoked the attack.

If a community has a particularly high number of women who are "chronically" raped the credibility of, and therefore the response to, all rape victims is understandably affected. The attitudes of medical and nursing personnel, particularly in emergency rooms, is generally negative toward the rape victim. A nationwide survey of the care that rape victims receive in the emergency room indicates that victims wait long periods of time (as much as 4 hours).

Naïveté

Unfortunately, in today's society helpful and courteous intentions may be a naïve invitation to rape. In a study of women who were attacked by strangers in Denver from 1970 to 1972, one fourth were responding to the attacker's plea for help (Selkin, 1975). Selkin contends that rapists test their victims before they threaten them. The testing comes in many forms. One rapist might ask to use the victim's phone for an emergency. Another rapist might ask a potential victim for directions. Still another might drive up next to a potential victim at a stop light, tell her she has a flat tire, and advise her to follow him to an isolated street. In each of these cases the rapist tests the potential victim, first to see if she will be helpful and courteous, then to discern her capacity for being intimidated. If she reacts fearfully and submissively when told "Don't scream and I won't hurt you," he knows he has a victim. McDonald (1971) believes that the most important reason a rape attempt is successful is that the rapist is assured in some way that he is able to predict and will be able to control the victim's behavior.

An 84-year-old woman was raped by a young neighbor whom she knew. He came to her home under the pretext of obtaining help for his mother who had "had a heart attack." When allowed to enter her home, he turned on his potential rescuer and raped her while the elderly woman's husband lay nearby helplessly paralyzed.

Some writers theorize that a certain amount of suspicion or paranoia is essential for survival in today's society. In regard to rape, numerous case studies indicate that this theory has elements of truth.

Vulnerability

In the Denver study of rape (1970 to 1972), almost one fourth of the victims were under the influence of alcohol or drugs at the time of the rape (Selkin, 1975). Some rapists report that they look for victims who are retarded, physically handicapped, intoxicated, or in some way vulnerable, such as a sleeping woman.

EXTERNAL ENVIRONMENTAL FACTORS

A complex array of external environmental factors can promote improvement in the care of rape victims. "Rape holds two unenviable records in recent FBI *Uniform Crime Reports:* it is the fastest growing of the Index Crimes against the person; and among these it has the lowest proportion of cases closed by reason of arrest" (Brodyaga, 1975). Mounting national anxiety about all forms of violence may constitute the major thrust to effective intervention in the incidence of rape.

The woman's movement has called attention to the inequities in care of rape victims. Some health professionals believe that the rape problem will become resolved at the same pace that society's attitude toward females changes.

External environmental factors that thwart efforts to prevent the occurrence of rape as well as to improve care of the rape victim relate to myths regarding the victim. Not only broad cultural myths but also specific medical myths influence the care of the victim. A predominantly supported medical myth holds that a healthy adult woman cannot be forcibly raped with full vaginal penetration unless she cooperates to some degree (Amir, 1971). The antithesis to this belief of course is the failure to view the victim holistically and to acknowledge the emotional determinants of the victim's response. Automatic reactions such as submissiveness ensure life. The predominant emotion of the acute (immediate) phase after rape is the overwhelming fear of physical violence and death (Burgess and Holmstrom, 1974).

EPIDEMIOLOGY OF RAPE

In 1975 a comprehensive, nationwide survey of health facilities and criminal justice agencies in regard to the care of the rape victim was accomplished through grants from the National Institute of Law Enforcement and Criminal Justice. The following general observations resulted from this research (Brodyaga, 1975).

1. Cooperation among all institutions dealing with rape victims is relatively rare.
2. No programs in the 39 medical facilities surveyed attempted to look at the medical treatment process and how it related to other organizations.
3. Most institutions have made only superficial changes in programs, not real reform.
4. Only one program has attempted to find nonreporting victims who may need medical assistance and to ascertain why victims do not report rape.

This same nationwide study found a great need for research: "The little research done on rape has been mostly basic social science research; with a few striking exceptions, few studies or evaluations, either completed or underway, are immediately applicable to police work" (Brodyaga, 1975). As discussed earlier in this chapter, a research methodology that lends itself to multifaceted problems such as rape is the epidemiological method.

In dealing with rape it would seem most cost effective to place the emphasis on primary prevention. With some health problems the etiology is diverse or unknown, thus eliminating the possibility of planning for primary prevention. However, utilizing the epidemiological method of research, factors in the external and internal environments that create a high-risk environment for rape in a community can be identified. These high-risk factors can then be taught to the potential hosts (victims). For example, the most common place of rape is identified from an epidemiological study as being the victim's home.

This information can be disseminated to high-risk populations by teaching preventive measures such as discouraging the admittance of strangers into homes and encouraging the validation of repairmen's credentials by a phone call to their company. Public education such as this would intervene between the host and the environment, as depicted in Fig. 12-2. On the other hand, public education regarding methods of thwarting a rape attack would attempt to intervene between the host and the agent, as depicted in Fig. 12-3.

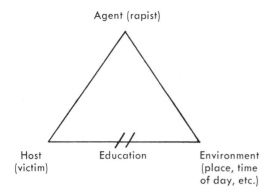

Fig. 12-2. Public education regarding high-risk environment.

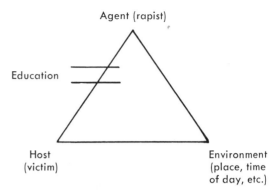

Fig. 12-3. Public education regarding thwart of rape.

Epidemiological investigation is based on the assumption that health problems occur in populations nonrandomly. Determinants of any health problem then lie in relation to host, agent, and environmental factors and their interrelationship. Directly or indirectly, patterns of people's lives are therefore linked to health problems.

Descriptive epidemiology utilizes information about the community that is available through existing sources (medical records, birth and death certificates, and immunization records). These data are then used to describe how the health problem is distributed in the community with respect to time, place, and person. Long-term trends and seasonal variations can be ascertained; high-risk individuals can be described by such characteristics as sex, race, age, and socioeconomic status (Peterson and Thomas, 1978).

Once the data are collected into an orderly arrangement of host, agent, and environment, the chains of inference are laid. When sufficient information about risk factors is available, interventions aimed at decreasing the risk can be formulated.

Epidemiological investigation of rape would address 5 of the 11 top priority research questions deserving study, as determined through the nationwide survey described previously (Brodyaga, 1975):

1. What ways does the rape victim unknowingly contribute to the rape? How can this information be used to help prevent rape?
2. Are there commonalities in victim response to attempted rape and rape? If so, how can these commonalities be utilized in planning for rape prevention?
3. What are the commonalities in rape cases that prosecutors fail to prosecute? Why?
4. Are there commonalities in the convicted rapist? In the unconvicted rapist?
5. Is nonreporting common among particular races or cultures? How can interventions be made to increase the rate of rapes reported and the timeliness of the report?

In 1978 a descriptive epidemiological study was carried out by nursing students in a university of a Southwestern city (Angelo, 1978). Data regarding each of the components—agent, host, environment—were extracted from the city's police sexual offense reports. There were 189 reported rapes and 63 reported attempted rapes for the year 1977. The following data are based on the total of 252 rapes and attempted rapes.

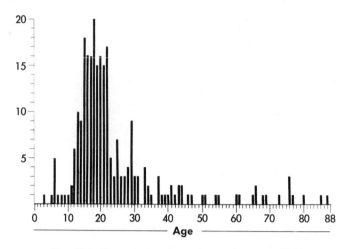

Fig. 12-4. Attempted rapes and rapes by age—1977.

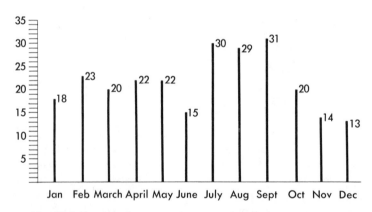

Fig. 12-5. Number of rapes and attempted rapes by month—1977.

Data relating to the host (victim)

Age of the victims range from 3 to 87 years. Fig. 12-4 depicts the ages of the victims. The high-risk age group was identified and educated as to their particular vulnerability. The potential victims were taught ways in which they might prevent being in a vulnerable situation. Also, in the case of rape, the recommended procedure that enables the victim to obtain an accurate medical-legal evaluation at the local hospital was described, for instance, the victim should not urinate, defecate, shower, or change clothes.

Data relating to the environment

Of the three factors (agent, host, and environment), data related to environment were found to be the most abundant. The location of the

Location

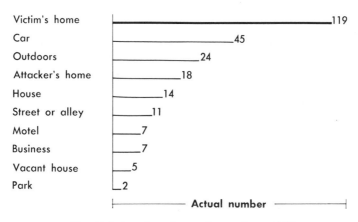

Fig. 12-6. Location of rapes by number—1977.

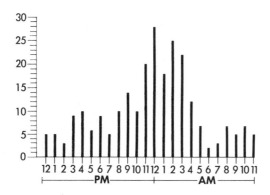

Fig. 12-7. Number of rapes by time of day—1977.

rapes, time of occurrence, day of week, and month were tabulated. Fig. 12-5 shows the high-risk months for rape. This data facilitated planning for rape crisis volunteers. For example, they indicate that more volunteers need to be trained and made available for the summer months. Additional analysis of the epidemiology is needed to isolate those factors that contribute to the summer months' being a high risk for rape. Further defining of the place of rape indicated that the most common site was the victim's home (Fig. 12-6). Whether the rapist gained entry by force or was willingly allowed entrance is a crucial question and data on this are currently being collected and analyzed. Time is also a factor of environment (Fig. 12-7). At least half of the rapes and attempted rapes occurred between 10:30 PM and 4:30 AM.

Fifty-six percent of the rapes and attempted rapes occurred on Friday, Saturday, and Sunday, with Saturday and Sunday having the greater incidence.

To assess geographic locations, each rape was color-coded by month and indicated on a map of the city. A definite pattern began to take shape. Rapes occurred in different parts of the city, depending on the place and type of social functions occurring at the time. This type of information enables police to plan coverage more efficiently and effectively.

Data relating to the agent

Fifty-six percent of the alleged attackers were black. Forty-nine percent of the rapes and attempted rapes were recorded as aggravated. Aggravated rape is defined by the Texas Penal Code as rape that causes serious bodily injury or compels submission by threat of death, bodily injury, or kidnapping. Weapons used in aggravated rape included the rapist's own body, guns, knives, and other weapons. The most commonly used weapon was the rapist's body (41%), second to knives (29%). Guns accounted for 19%, whereas other weapons comprised 11%.

In summarizing the data from the descriptive study, the following risk factors are known. The high-risk person for rape in this city in 1977 was female, white, and between 13 and 22 years of age. The high-risk environment was the victim's home, with the high-risk days of the week being Friday, Saturday, and Sunday, between 11 PM and 3 AM. The high-risk months were July, August, and September. Aggravated rape occurred in one of two reported alleged rapes and attempted rapes. For every three rapes there was one attempted rape.

Descriptive epidemiology utilizes existing data found in health department records, death certificates, special registers, police records, and other similar sources. These data are used to compute rates and to make possible a description of how the health problem is distributed in a population with respect to time, place, and person. This description of the problem frequently provides hints as to possible factors that cause the problem or increase the host's susceptibility.

Analytic epidemiology of rape is the next step in studying this health problem. Analytic epidemiology pertains to the formulation and testing of hypotheses as to specific risk factors that might be determinants of the health problem. This usually entails the collection of data not available from existing records. These data are then imaginatively analyzed. For example, data are currently being collected as to the incident, action, or situation that the victim feels interrupted the attempted rapes. If the data indicate the persistence of a common disruptive action, for example, the victim's screaming, this information could be disseminated to high-risk populations, thus initiating primary prevention (Friedman, 1974).

The correlation of the age of the victim (host) with the place of rape (victim's home, car, or a park) and the rapist's method of gaining entrance would answer the question Are older women more apt to be raped in their own home by a rapist who asks for assistance? If the answer is yes, the intervention of teaching this particular age group about the perils of being a Good Samaritan would be predictably effective.

One method of ascertaining the scope and planning for prevention in a particular community is by assessing the community's rape "profile." The rape "profile" is the pattern of rape unique to the community. For example, if the rape pattern for two cities were studied, a difference might be found in the high-risk age and race of the victim in city A as compared to city B. By the interplay of external environmental factors such as attitudes, mobility of the people, prevading value system, and subcultures, an atmosphere is created that contributes to, or minimizes, particular kinds of rape. The internal environmental dynamics of both the rapist and the rape victim would also be reflected in the rape "profile."

SUMMARY

In this chapter rape as a health problem has been discussed. The utilization of the ecological perspective and the epidemiological approach to the problem has been presented. Care of the rape victim has been enhanced by more effective planning based on a preliminary descriptive investigation of rape. More important, the potential for planning effective primary prevention of rape appears excitingly feasible by the further use of the epidemiological method of investigation.

No profession more than nursing appears to be in a better position to undertake the task of dealing with the prevention of rape in a community. While each profession deals with a unique part of the problem, the nursing profession has the skills and boldness to apply effective research techniques that would enable other professions to deal comprehensively and effectively with rape.

References

American Psychiatric Association, Committee on Nomenclature and Statistics of the American Psychiatric Association, Diagnostic and statistical manual of mental disorders, ed. 2, Washington, D.C., 1968, American Psychiatric Association.

Amir, M.: Patterns of forcible rape, Chicago, 1971, The University of Chicago Press.

Anderson, W. S., ed.: Ballentine's law dictionary, Rochester, N.Y., 1969, The Lawyers Cooperative Publishing Co.

Angelo, C. I., Kirschbaum, L., et al.: An epidemiological study of rape in Fort Worth, Texas (unpublished study), 1978, Texas Christian University, Fort Worth.

Berne, Eric: Games people play, New York, 1964, Grove Press, Inc.

Brodyaga, L., Gates, M., et al.: Rape and its victims: a report, 1975, for citizens, health facilities and criminal justice agencies, Washington, D.C., 1975, U.S. Department of Justice, National Institute of Law Enforcement and Criminal Justice Law Enforcement, Assistance Administration.

Brownmiller, S.: Against our will: men, women, and rape, New York, 1975, Bantam Books, Inc.

Burgess, A. W., and Holmstrom, L. L.: Rape trauma syndrome, Am. J. Psychiatry **131:**981-986, 1974.

Burgess, A. W., and Lazare, A.: Community mental health: target population, Englewood Cliffs, N.J., 1976, Prentice-Hall, Inc.

Eaton, M. T., Peterson, M. H., and Davis, J. A.: Psychiatry, Flushing, N.Y., 1976, Medical Examination Publishing Co., Inc.

Friedman, G.: Primer of epidemiology, New York, 1974, McGraw-Hill Book Co.

Goldstein, B.: Human sexuality, New York, 1976, McGraw-Hill Book Co.

Groth, A. N. and Cohen, M. L.: Aggressive sexual offenders: diagnosis and treatment. In Community mental health: target populations. Englewood Cliffs, N.J., 1976, Prentice-Hall, Inc.

Kneisl, C. R. and Wilson, H. S.: Current perspectives in psychiatric nursing: issues and trends, Vol. 1, St. Louis, 1976, The C. V. Mosby Co.

McCubbin, J. H., and Scott, D. E.: Management of alleged sexual assault, Texas Med. **69:**59-64, 1973.

McDonald, J. M.: Rape: offenders and their victims, Springfield, Ill., 1971, Charles C Thomas, Publisher.

Murray, R. and Zentner, J.: Nursing concepts for health promotion, Englewood Cliffs, N.J. 1975, Prentice-Hall, Inc.

Offir, C. W.: Don't take it lying down, Psychology Today **8:**73-79, January, 1975.

Peterson, D., and Thomas, D. B.: Fundamentals of epidemiology, Lexington, Mass., 1978, D. C. Heath & Co.

Resnik, H., and Wolfgang, M., eds.: Sexual behaviors: social, clinical, and legal aspects, Boston, 1972, Little Brown & Co.

Selkin, J.: Rape, Psychology Today **8:**70-72, January, 1975.

CHAPTER 13

Rape as a crisis

JEANETTE LANCASTER

Although the ultimate goal in relation to rape is prevention of the act, this is not always possible. Rape is described from an epidemiological framework in Chapter 12. The dynamics and a community profile are identified to provide an understanding of the magnitude and ramifications of rape as a social problem as well as a risk factor for mental illness.

Currently rape is one of the most underreported yet fastest growing crimes in America. Primary prevention seeks to reduce the possibility of mental disturbance as a result of the crisis imposed by rape. The goal of crisis intervention with rape victims, using an ecological focus, is twofold. Attention is directed both toward reestablishing equilibrium within the victim and toward attaining some degree of stability in the victim's relationship with components of the external environment. The possible outcomes of the experience of rape are depicted in the following:

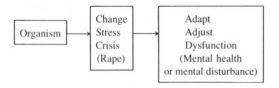

Nursing intervention attempts to help the rape victim deal with the crisis so that she may emerge from the situation with an ability to cope and to continue functioning at a psychologically adaptive level.

Victims of rape are considered a high-risk population for mental illness because of the immense trauma they experience. The impact of the crisis continues, indeed is often compounded, long after the actual sexual assault. Hospital personnel, police, and legal representatives in particular affect the victim's reaction to the assault.

The community mental health nurse typically becomes involved with rape victims through consultation or direct service in hospital emergency rooms as well as in follow-up counseling. Nursing involvement may also include an advocacy component with the goal being to assist the victim in negotiating the legal system with a minimum of psychological trauma. Nursing action seeks first to increase public awareness of the problem of rape. Target populations for education include the staff in hospital emergency rooms and police officers. Informal sessions with these groups serve to (1) increase knowledge of the phenomenon of rape, (2) raise questions regarding attitudes and beliefs about victims, and (3) consider intervention strategies that promote mental health. To provide services to rape victims through consultation, either directly or indirectly, the nurse must understand the emotional aspects of the rape experience.

The aim of this chapter is to present a two-phase prevention approach for victims of rape. To discuss the intervention schema an overview of rape would be helpful, with general comments as to the emotional needs of the client. The first phase entails an acute crisis-oriented approach for the rape victim who seeks treatment in the hospital emergency room. The second phase deals with concepts of crisis intervention that can be utilized by community mental health providers in follow-up counseling.

RAPE AS A MENTAL HEALTH CRISIS

Rape is defined as a forced act of intercourse or coitus involving any penile vaginal penetration without the consent of the woman (Williams, 1973). The phenomenon of rape crosses all socioeconomic and educational boundaries; it frequently occurs without warning and is no respector of geographic setting. While rape is clearly a sexual activity, the underlying motives are not always sexual. Rather, for the rapist the aim is often to relieve anger and rage. The victim may be randomly selected. For the victim rape constitutes an act of violence in which her very existence may be threatened. A significant number of victims suffer bruises and lacerations; many are threatened with a weapon such as a gun or knife.

Even though rape presents a crisis situation for the victim, many do not report the assault because of fear or shame. The myths that "All women want to be raped" and "Anyone can avoid rape if she tries" influence the attitudes of health care providers, victims, and law enforcement officers. Staff members in emergency rooms, for example, may display their bias by comments that are demeaning to the victim or that cast doubt on her account of the incident. Negative attitudes detected by the victim may offset the possibility of a therapeutic relationship. Community mental health consultation is directed toward helping the emergency room staff discuss and examine their attitudes in an atmosphere that encourages expression of negative thoughts and feelings yet that does not directly affect the client. The staff are thus encouraged to talk about their beliefs and personal fears regarding rape in the consultation session rather than repressing their beliefs and feelings but passively displaying them toward clients in subtle ways.

CRISIS INTERVENTION STRATEGIES

Rape is viewed as a legal diagnosis rather than a medical one, which implies a degree of doubt and disbelief in the documentation of the incident. Describing rape as "alleged rape" or "said to be raped" causes increased uneasiness for the victim who already fears what others will think. The first supportive mental health measure is to believe the victim.

Victims who seek treatment should be received without bias or judgment. Guilt is already a predominant feeling and reinforcement of that guilt only leads to emotional trauma. The victim's most predominant need when she seeks care is to feel safe and not to be further threatened by an attitude set, the lack of acceptance, or needless questions, many of which may be irrelevant to the assessment of the trauma.

Whether the nurse working in community mental health actually sees rape victims directly or serves as a consultant to the emergency room staff, it is important to remember that each client responds differently to a particular crisis. Evaluative opinions need to include recognition of individual differences to stress. Some react to a crisis with silence, whereas other victims may talk readily about the experience. The primary reaction to rape is fear; each individual responds to fear in an exaggerated manner but one that largely corresponds to her usual response style.

Immediate intervention strategies

Upon the rape victim's admission to the emergency room, the first nursing intervention is to assure her that a nurse will remain with her at all times. The nurse should answer any questions, for example, about the physical examination, venereal disease, or pregnancy and assist the victim in working out a way to tell her family and friends about the rape.

In a study of all rape victims who presented for treatment over a 1-year period at the emergency ward of Boston City Hospital, Burgess and Holmstrom (1975) identified a two-phase reaction to the crisis imposed by rape. They describe the rape trauma syndrome as consisting of both an acute phase and a long-term reorganization process. During the acute phase an obvious amount of disorganization occurred in the women's lifestyle with concomitant symptoms of physiological stress. Frequently observed somatic reactions to rape included physical trauma caused by the combative nature of the attack; skeletal muscle tension manifested in headaches and wakefulness; gastrointestinal irritability including pain, nausea and lack of appetite; and genitourinary disturbances that included vaginal symptoms of burning, itching, and pain.

The emotional reactions of women varied considerably from one person to another during this stage. The predominant feelings were fear, anger, and anxiety; their manifestation varied from overt expression such as crying, verbalization, or laughing to controlled repression. The therapeutic approach during the acute phase is based on crisis intervention. According to crisis intervention theory, the nurse assumes that the client functioned within normal limits prior to the rape. Immediate problems are thus dealt with; crisis intervention serves to prevent mental disruption.

As mentioned above, each woman reacts to rape in a unique way. Some are able to express openly their feelings of fear, guilt, rage, or helplessness, whereas others are unable to discuss the situation at all. It is essential that the nurse provide the victim with an opportunity to express her feelings. It may be necessary for the nurse to help the woman name her feelings by saying, "You seem . . . ," or "Are you afraid?" Just naming a feeling usually can decrease some of the woman's confusion; it also conveys that at least one other person is aware of her turmoil.

The nurse should listen carefully so as to hear what the victim says as well as to take note of what she does not say. This includes of course listening to her pain and distress. Victims, in discussing the rape experience, may laugh or speak in a tone inconsistent with their actual feelings. When the nurse conveys that she has "heard" the victim's pain, regardless of how it is expressed, the victim often feels less alone and more understood and cared about.

Because of the legal implications of rape a physical examination is required immediately after the incident. Three major purposes of the examination are (1) prevention of pregnancy, (2) prevention of venereal disease, and (3) documentation of physical evidence of trauma, which could be supportive to the victim's case in a legal proceeding. Since the examination presents an additional trauma for a person already in a crisis, supportive nursing attention is essential.

Moreover, in a busy emergency room patients are usually seen according to the assessed medical emergency of their presenting crisis. Medical treatment is likely to be given to someone with a deep stab or gunshot wound or to a person with acute cardiac problems before a rape victim is treated. Generally rape in itself does not constitute a medical emergency when life or death are the alternative reactions.

During any waiting period consideration should be given to providing privacy. Questioning about the rape in a crowded waiting area only reinforces the psychological upset. The attitude conveyed by the interviewer has considerable impact on the victim's reaction and response pattern. A warm, accepting, nonjudgmental attitude often promotes discussion and immediate expression of feelings, whereas a hostile, condemning attitude stifles expression and may reinforce repression of feelings.

During the emergency room phase of treatment arrangements should be made with the victim for her to seek follow-up counseling, at least on a short-term basis. The name of a community mental health nurse with expertise in crisis intervention can be provided. Also it may be helpful to notify the nurse that the victim may call; in the event that the woman hesitates to call for an appointment the nurse may assume this responsibility by calling and offering services.

Follow-up counseling during the reorganization phase

During the reorganization phase of the rape syndrome, the victim begins to realize that the sexual assault was just the beginning of her ordeal. Nursing intervention varies according to the needs of the client. Whether the woman needs to find a new home or job or to talk out her fear or anger, the nurse should make services available in terms of listening, problem-solving efforts, and providing concrete information such as a community resource list, which includes information on medical and legal assistance.

Burgess and Holmstrom (1975) document a set of long-term reactions to rape. While each victim reacts differently, the researchers found several symptoms that were often experienced in the months following rape: increased motor activity, nightmares, and phobic reactions. Increased motor activity included moving, taking trips, changing telephone numbers, and frequently seeking the presence of family members or friends.

In the study population dreams and nightmares were observed in two phases. Initially many women relived the attack and awoke before they could fight off the attacker. In the second dream phase the woman was able to fight off the assailant.

Phobic reactions served as a defensive response to the rape. Commonly observed phobic reactions included fear of going outside; fear of staying inside; fear of being alone, or conversely, of being in a crowd; and fear of being followed; as well as sexual fears related to future relationships.

Rape constitutes a situational crisis in which external events, sudden and unexpected, disrupt the woman's homeostasis. Counseling therefore seeks to maximize the ability to cope with the stress caused by the external event of the rape and to minimize the psychological disruption.

Follow-up counseling for the rape victim conforms to the general principles of crisis intervention. Counseling is here-and-now oriented, designed to deal with current issues, through the utilization of a problem-solving approach. This implies an action-oriented approach whereby the victim examines alternative reactions and is supported as she plans a coping strategy. Crisis intervention keeps the client involved. The approach is based on the premise that each person has an innate ability to help himself. Professional assistance seeks to mobilize the client's resources so that she can make decisions regarding possible actions.

In the early stages of the counseling the nurse should assess the client's level of anxiety to determine the extent to which stress is interfering with her ability to cope. It is important to decide if the client is able to view the situation clearly or if her perception is distorted. Is she responding to the crisis with despair, anger, acceptance, or resignation? Further, it is important to determine whether or not her method of coping with this stressful event is similar to her usual coping pattern. That is, has she previously withdrawn, overtly expressed anger, or become involved in physical activities to dissipate the energy generated by a high level of stress? Another area for observation deals with how the crisis has affected the client's daily activities. Is she able to think clearly or does she find herself mentally reliving the rape trauma?

The nurse needs also to determine who constitutes the woman's support system. Are family members and friends viewed as a support? Whom has she told about the experience? Which, if any, significant friends or relatives do not know about the rape? Nursing assistance may also be directed toward helping the woman talk to others about her experiences. Techniques such as role-playing or psychodrama may be used to practice talking to others. Such approaches help in the initiation of client-environment communication by rehearsing and examining potential problems in a controlled situation.

The following principles can be utilized in a crisis intervention framework for counseling rape victims:

1. The first step is to cease thinking of the woman as the ''victim'' and begin to think of her as the ''client.'' Often in instances of crimes it is difficult for the abused person to move out of the victim role and view himself as a coping person. The counselor should consistently focus on the woman as a client who seeks assistance in coping with a crisis. Reality holds that the crime has already been committed; it cannot be undone. The client's goal therefore is to cope in a way that prevents dysfunction.

2. A person in crisis needs to confront the situation and verbalize its impact. As mentioned, anger, fear, and guilt are often prevalent feelings associated with rape. The emotional wound cannot heal until it is cleaned. Just as a severe burn does not heal prior to debridement, the rape victim needs to debride her psychological wound before healing can occur.

3. The person should be helped to confront the crisis one step at a time, being cautious not to overly dampen its impact. This step implies that the counselor's own feelings about rape should be resolved before any attempts to help the client cope are initiated. Old biases are often hard to acknowledge consciously and they affect the nurse-client relationship. The open expression of feelings can be aided by techniques such as role-playing in which the client tells the assailant all of the things she has fantasized about wanting to say. The gestalt tech-

nique of talking to a chair may help a client express built-up feelings. For example, initially the client portrays herself and talks to an empty chair that is designated as the assailant. After she has said much of what she has been thinking she switches chairs and pretends to be the assailant. As the assailant responds to the woman's comments, she can begin to consider his mental processes.

4. The nurse should help the client gain an understanding of the crisis (Hoff, 1978). Individuals who have experienced situational crises often repeatedly ask themselves and others, ''Why me?'' Such questioning often implies that the person views herself as bad and deserving of such punishment. It is important to face realistically whether or not the client had any responsibility for the attack. If so, the goal then becomes one of examining other ways of behaving so as to avoid such situations in the future. For example, one client went to a local bar looking for some respite from loneliness. She met a man who seemed pleasant and polite; after they left the bar he raped her. Perhaps other alternatives exist for meeting people. In many instances of rape the victim is randomly selected; in others she does not know her assailant although he may have selected her previously. The opportunity to have avoided the attack may have been minimal; if so, feelings of guilt and self-blame are unrealistic.

5. The nurse should help the client to examine alternatives for coping with the problem. The client may have a lowered tolerance for stress following the crisis experience. The tendency to behave impulsively to relieve discomfort may override the ability to weigh the consequences of one's behavior. Nursing assistance should be directed toward helping the client consider what is likely to result

from various behaviors. Anticipatory guidance is needed so that the client will receive support prior to taking action.

Throughout the acute and reorganizational phases of the rape syndrome nursing intervention should be directed toward helping the client make the best possible adjustment so that she can return to her previous level of functioning as quickly as possible. Since the crisis was precipitated by an event external to the client, considerable attention must be given to helping her focus on productive ways to respond to people and events.

References

Burgess, A., and Holmstrom, L.: Rape trauma syndrome, Nurs. Digest **3:**17-19, May-June, 1975.

Hoff, L. A.: People in crisis: understanding and helping, Palo Alto, Calif., 1978, Addison-Wesley Publishing Co., Inc.

Williams, C., and Williams, R.: Rape: the plea for help in the hospital emergency room, Nurs. Forum **12:**388-401, 1973.

CHAPTER 14

Coping with nonterminal loss

CECILIA H. CANTRELL and BETTIE S. JACKSON

The terms "self-concept," "self-esteem," and "body image" are frequently used interchangeably. A differentiation should be made however; body image and self-esteem are really just a part of the overall concept of self. For example, a mentally healthy person might have an intact self-concept while experiencing adaptation to an altered body image. A woman having undergone a mastectomy may return to work and family duties fully recovered from surgery because her self-concept encompasses a sense of responsibility to and involvement with work and family. Yet at the same time her body image—the mental picture she has of herself in her mind—may be undergoing alterations. Her altering body image has not disrupted her overall self-concept.

The concept of self and more specifically body image in relation to the individual, significant others, and legal, ethical, economic, and health care complexes has profound implications for society. The purpose of this discussion is to assist health care providers in facilitating their clients' healthy adaptation to a body alteration. In addressing the realization of this goal, body image is discussed including a definition and origins of the concept; the relationship of the grief process to body image is also explored, as is the interrelationship of society and individuals experiencing body image alterations. Implications for the care of clients undergoing body image change are integrated throughout the discussion with the use of examples.

BODY IMAGE CONCEPT AND DEVELOPMENT OF BODY IMAGE

A primary source of stress is either the actual loss of a loved object or the threat of its loss. The loss is meaningful only if the object is loved or has special meaning. During infancy and early childhood, attachment to significant objects, including parts of the body, develops. To understand why the loss of an object is a stressful event the origins of its significance must be explored.

HISTORICAL PSYCHOANALYTICAL PERSPECTIVE ON ORIGINS OF BODY IMAGE

Psychoanalytical literature is the best resource for theory of the concept of body image, its development, and its significance, as well as reactions to it. The first written accounts date from the sixteenth century, when a surgeon, Ambroise Paré, described the phantom limb phenomenon (Kolb, 1974). Head, in the nineteenth century, was responsible for the description and development of the first basic concepts of the body functioning in relation to motility, to localization of tactile stimuli, and to the phantom phenomenon (Kolb, 1974). It was Schilder (1950); however, who developed the broader concepts used today. He describes body image as the picture of our own body that is formed in our mind. It is the way in which our body appears to us. To Schilder the body image in our mind is a tridimensional unity involving interpersonal, environmental, and tem-

140

poral factors. It includes not only our personal and psychological investment in our body and its parts but also a sociological meaning both for us as individuals and for society. He adds that we have to expect strong emotions concerning our own body: we love it; we are narcissistic.

There is not complete consensus on the origins of the body image. Federn (1952) disagrees with Schilder, believing that the ego is not identical with the body image.

Federn's attitude explains the tenet held by many that children up to 6 years old undergoing pain and body alterations such as amputation have considerably less difficulty adapting; there is also less change in their body image. This adaptive ability is also observed in children born without certain body parts such as hands, arms, or legs.

In a study entitled "The Appraisal of Body Cathexis: Body Cathexis and the Self," Secord and Jourad tested the hypothesis that feelings about the body are commensurate with feelings about the self (Rosen and Ross, 1968). They asked a sample of people to rate their satisfaction with aspects related to their body images and self-concepts. The results of the study showed that satisfaction with the body image and satisfaction with self-concepts are positively correlated (males, 0.58; females, 0.66).

It is not unusual for a person who was once overweight to report that he feels so much better about his body and himself since losing weight. Nor is it unusual for women who have experienced a mastectomy to initially express feelings about body and self together in a self-deprecating or at least doubtful tone.

A discussion of body image development provides the foundation for a discussion of alterations in body image and the effects that the event, especially when occurring under catastrophic circumstances, has on one's behavior, functioning, and adaptive mechanisms.

Some argue that at birth one is devoid of any physical or psychological concept of body image except at a feeling level such as comfort-discomfort, hunger, rage, and pain (Blaesing and Brockhaus, 1972). However, Kolb (1974) points out that even in utero there is a hand-to-mouth relationship, a proprioceptive sensory impression. With increasing mobility, the newborn acquires body knowledge from tactile impressions and explores his body and space with his hands and mouth. Kolb emphasizes that these are processes on which the beginnings of self-awareness, individuality, and a sense of ego are founded. Pleasure and pain stimuli begin to be differentiated as the infant begins to discriminate between himself and the external world.

Many psychoanalysts clearly state that the parents (especially the mother) impart an indelible impression on a child's concept of self, his body, and its functions (Kolb, 1974; Suttie, 1935).

In American culture a great deal of emphasis is placed on cleanliness, including bowel control. Toilet training is highly valued by the mother for the child between 2 and 3 years of age. Through conditioning, a child learns to perform automatically his body functions (bowel evacuation) and to forget that at one time they were a source of pleasure because of the physical feeling evoked and the praise and delight of the mother.

Regardless of one's theoretical position it is possible to appreciate the stress a person experiences when he has bowel or urinary bypass surgery resulting in a colostomy, ileostomy, or urostomy. This stress is compounded when the effluent and its odor are not properly contained. The motion of social isolation becomes a real possibility. The implications for proper nursing care are vast.

Phantom limb

The concept of body image had its origin in the study of the phantom limb phenomenon. Psychiatric and surgical literature is replete with articles on this subject. A phantom limb is just what the term implies: feelings that the missing part still exists despite the fact that one's visual perception confirms that it does not. There seems to be an ongoing disagreement as to whether the phenomenon is of neurophysiological or psychiatric origin.

Schilder (1950) states that we are accustomed to an intact and complete body. The phantom of an amputated person is therefore the reactivation of a given perceptive pattern by emotional forces. Kolb (1974) acknowledges the existence of the phantom as an expected healthy response to the amputation of a limb or body part occurring any time after early childhood. Amputation results in an alteration, perhaps even a distortion, of one's body image, and is therefore experienced as a distortion of the self. Other writers such as Riese, take the attitude that "the phantom is the expression of a difficulty in adaptation to a sudden defect of an important peripheral part of the body" (Schilder, 1950). Many prefer to view the phantom limb phenomenon on a purely neurophysiological basis, explaining that since nerves have been severed it takes time for the sensation to regress. The question regarding origins of the phantom goes unanswered. However, it is apparent in clinical practice that many health care providers base their treatment for this phenomenon on personal attitudes. For example, patients with the same complaint of phantom limb may be treated quite differently—with inattention, mockery, psychotherapy, nerve block, analgesic, or tranquilizers. The phantom phenomenon has been described for every amputated body part, including arms, legs, breasts, and the rectum. In our clinical experiences and in the literature the phantom rectum following abdominal-perineal resection is indeed experienced. Some patients may continue to have the urge to expel flatus or defecate despite the physiological impossibility of this task. The solution for some is actually to sit on the toilet. Healthy adaptation may be measured (1) by the patient's willingness to discuss his disfigurement or dismemberment or functional loss and the phantom and (2) by his ability to accept offers of aid (Kolb, 1974). However, this willingness may take months to be expressed.

Object loss: body part loss or alteration

A discussion of the phantom limb phenomenon provides a connection between the origins of body image and the concept of object loss, which has been described above as the primary basis of a stress. In general, of course, the object may be one of many different things, for example, a body part, internal or external; a loved one; or one's life itself. There is one unifying factor that makes the loss of the object or alteration of it significant: object loss refers to the loss of an object that has special value and emotional meaning to the person and on some level the loss is experienced throughout life. Engel (1963) states that persons, ideals, body functions, and image become part of oneself. They are necessary for effective ego functioning and for a sustained sense of intactness. It is the dependence on these psychic objects that render an individual vulnerable to his loss and imposes the requirement for some kind of adjustment in compensation of which mourning is a familiar response. Meaningful objects to each person are quite individual. One must be careful not to assume hastily, for example, that breasts are of the same importance to all women and hence that losing one carries the same impact for each woman. The loss of a diseased or painful part might bring physical and psychological relief and comfort. Careful, thorough assessment through history taking and observation is essential to better understand the meaning of a client's body part and the potential or actual significance of its loss.

Body image alterations and the temporal factor

Schoenberg and Carr (1970) from their findings while working with mastectomized patients comment that a patient's response to the loss of a body part varies with the specific significance of that part. The emotional impact of a mastectomy has a significance to a woman that transcends functional or cosmetic factors, since a breast, like the uterus, is far more likely to symbolize a woman's femininity.

They add that sudden changes that are the result of trauma or surgery evoke different initial reactions than those that are the result of chronic disease. The anxiety reaction is related to fear of rejection by significant others; the abruptness of the alteration in the body appearance has not permitted formation of a new body image.

A temporal factor is introduced here: having the time to do "worry work" prior to a stressful event such as surgery and having someone—a nurse, for example—to support the patient in this work become vitally important to healthy, successful adaptation.

Hollender (1960) studied female patients admitted to Syracuse Psychiatric Hospital in 1958; in all of these psychiatric patients their illness seemed to be related to their pelvic surgery. Each had had benign tumors, yet their number was almost twice that of women admitted following other kinds of operations. Hollender's subjects were unwilling to discuss sex; results of interviews with them led Hollender to conclude that they felt neutered or castrated, that they viewed the uterus and ovaries in the same context as a man's penis and testicles. They saw sex only from an anatomical-physiological perspective, not a psychological one. Whether or not they had had sexual drives or a desire to have children before surgery bore little relation to the depression these thoughts evoked after surgery.

Knorr (1967) studied 14 patients following pelvic exenteration and ileostomy. Of the 14 patients, 11 were depressed. They refused to verbalize their feelings and were anxious, passive, and submissive and, although friendly, they maintained distant relationships. Their reactions ranged from crying to insomnia and mild depersonalization. Postoperatively for about a week the remaining three were optimistic, cheerful, and eager to talk. During the second week, however, all three became listless, sleepless, and demanding: they asked for more pain medication, felt slighted, and assumed the emotional status of the other 11 patients. All 14 kept their abdomens covered and showed high levels of anxiety and depression after managing their appliance. During instruction periods they turned away, cried, sulked, and directed their anger at the staff instructing them. While they welcomed visitors and their mood improved because of the visitors, they tired quickly. They geared conversation to neutral topics and directed discussions to past accomplishments, which also seemed to improve their mood.

Knorr (1967) followed these women after discharge and concluded that adjustment in the hospital does not correspond to the adjustment made after discharge. There are a number of explanations for this. Many patients try to be "good patients"; they attempt to hide their feelings in order not to burden the staff. Other individuals make conscious and unconscious attempts to push unpleasant thoughts from their minds at times when such thoughts might evoke anxiety that they cannot adequately deal with. In still others it is apparent that the implications of their stressful event have not yet had their full impact.

Many people who have had an ileostomy created following years of struggling with chronic ulcerative colitis and who had become socially isolated by illness and multiple bowel movements each day report an almost immediate rebirth following the operation. They are rendered disease free and for the first time in years are neither ill nor out of necessity socially isolated.

Burn trauma is another crisis in which the threat and stress of object loss occur in a severe form. The burn victim, suddenly and catastrophically hospitalized and separated from his family and work, is in severe pain as well as threatened with changes in his appearance and loss of body parts or even of life itself.

Andreasen et al. (1971) studied long-term adjustments of burn patients from a psychiatric perspective with the objective of determining the incidence of psychiatric complications in a group of "normal" adults burned during the productive years of their lives. He was interested in finding out if psychiatric problems could be foreseen so that steps could be taken to avoid them. Six patients (30%) were found to have emotional problems as a result of the burns. Their problems were not directly related either to the extent of the burn or the resultant deformity; nor did adjustment seem to improve with time. The patients' problems were primarily in the area of interpersonal relations and because of the staring and curiosity of strangers 20% of the burn victims became hesitant about interacting with other people. If they forced themselves to go out in public and meet strangers they reported becoming desensitized with time. The researchers conclude that the prognosis for developing successful adjustment after incurring severe burns is quite good. The burn victims place a new value on nonphysical, internal qualities and emerge from the crisis with renewed self-esteem based on their demonstrated ability to triumph over external limitations.

Alteration of internal body function caused by internal factors

The threat of object loss such as body image may be internal as well as external. Two nurses, Foster and Andreoli (1970), were interested in the behavior of patients following an acute myocardial infarction. They describe overt and subtle reactions in their sample. Anger, hostility, overtalkativeness, crying, fear, and demanding behavior were more obvious than the patients' bad dreams and grinding of teeth while asleep as well as their hyperactivity in bed and projection of feelings to others. Operant here is the threat that a myocardial infarction may disrupt one's total sense of integrity. When

the threat to self-image is too overwhelming one might resign himself to a life of dependency out of fear of additional heart disease and the subsequent further decay of his self-image.

The literature contains little on the loss of an internal organ; however, with the advances that have been made in heart surgery and transplant there is interest in this loss in relation to the body image concept. Blacher (1970) explains that one would expect but could not assume that cardiac surgery would elicit a stronger response than a cholecystectomy. An organ commonly considered psychiatrically insignificant may be important because of previous experiences or fantasies associated with it. Blacher uses the example of a person who was quite anxious over an anticipated splenectomy. His younger sibling had died of a spleen injury and the guilt associated with his sibling's experience was reawakened at the time of his own surgery.

The American Medical Association describes a permanent disability as the effect of any kind of impairment that interferes with gainful employment. It is less an expression of a person's pathological condition than the result of a way of functioning that does not meet the demands of the situation. Reusch and Brodsky (1968) add that a social disability is the end result of any impairment that leads to more or less permanent exclusions.

Of 1,372 colostomates responding to Cunningham's (1969) question, "Do you feel handicapped because you have an ostomy?" 213 said yes; 503, no; and 656, sometimes. Of interest are the results of the same question when asked of 2,092 ileostomates: 143 said yes; 1,186, no; and 763, sometimes.

A pattern becomes apparent in the behaviors and fears of people who experience an alteration in their body's configuration. Body image, a significant part of self-concept, is disrupted. The fear of social isolation, and hence rejection, predominates consciously or unconsciously. Various coping mechanisms, adaptive and maladaptive, are adopted by these people.

BODY IMAGE, OBJECT LOSS, AND THE GRIEVING PROCESS

A proliferation of grief literature related to thanatology has occurred over the last 10 years (Kubler-Ross, 1969; Kastenbaum, 1972; Cantrell, 1974, 1975; Parkes, 1972). Concentration of interest in this literature has been primarily on the grief process related to termination in death. All grief, however, is not related to death but may necessitate a life-long adjustment process to self-loss.

Thus the four-stage or five-stage process most frequently described in the grief literature is not inclusive enough to illustrate the grief process experienced by those who experience "adaptation losses," or a loss that requires an alteration in life-style.

In the discussion that follows, a staging process more applicable to "adaptation losses"—such as chronic illness, divorce, death of a significant other, and body image alteration—is explored.

Caution is always advised when attempts are made to categorize human reactions. Certainly individuals vary from the progression outlined below; the first rule in effectively assisting persons in grief is to be aware of their individuality. Nonetheless research and personal observation of persons experiencing loss suggests that, within limits, a progressive staging occurs during the resolution of grief. With this reservation in mind, following is an exploration of the grief process related to situations resulting in lifetime coping.

Coping with nonterminal grief

Shock and denial. The initial state of grief, regardless of the anticipated consequences, is shock. During this time, the individual is unable to comprehend either the reality of the situation or its significance. Denial is a manifestation of this initial shock and may in some situations result in procrastination seeking health care or acknowledging the correctness of a diagnosis. Frequently, numerous opinions are sought—first from physicians and later from less traditional healers. Delay in accepting a diagnosis may result in greater alterations or necessitate more severe treatment than might originally have been required.

Body alterations that occur rapidly, such as amputation during or immediately following an accident, may restrict the ability of the client to deny his loss because visibility of the loss is present and reacted to by the staff and significant others. This visibility and its subsequent "forcing of the issue" need further study to determine if the denial stage differs in clients experiencing observable loss and those with internal or nonobservable changes.

Denial of disability is possible even when the loss is visible. It is often this aspect of denial that causes a client to attempt unrealistic physical maneuvers or refuse to follow a prescribed regimen. In those coping with lifetime alterations, this aspect of denial may emerge again and again as new abilities are acquired, creating the desire to achieve a prealteration level of function. Health care workers must be alert to the repetitious nature of denial to assist clients.

Emotional release. Following shock and denial the client may experience an emotional release. Outward expression of anguish may occur. Expression of emotion is personal and support should be provided during this time. Traditionally Americans have cherished the stoic reaction to loss (Zborowski, 1952; Phillips, 1965; Mechanic, 1972). Socialized to believe that overt emotional expression indicates weakness of character, clients may hesitate to demonstrate emotion both because they expect this control of themselves and/or because they believe others expect it of them. Providing clients with an opportunity and place for emotional release may allow them to overcome the need for stoic reaction. Health care facilities need areas designed for the private release of frustration; screaming rooms as well as chapels should be available. Encouragement of client emotional release at this stage of the grief process is vital to the successful evolution of the necessary grief work.

Health care professionals can also assist clients during this stage by discouraging the use of sedation. Often it is our own tranquility we seek in giving sedation to clients who might embarrass or frighten us by overt displays of anguish. It is hard to observe another person's grief because of the empathetic process of being human. Our need to deny our own vulnerability often results in an attempt to avoid confrontation with another's grief. Those who undertake to care for the grieving and willingly allow clients to express grief openly accept for themselves a difficult task. Support for these health care providers is vital if they are to remain effective. Staff support is discussed in a later section of this chapter.

Depression. Having expended some immediate emotion, the third stage that clients usually exhibit is depression. Depression for the dying is different than that experienced by survivors of loss. The dying person sees that he is experiencing an end to the grief, no matter how dissatisfactory that end may be. Unlike the dying person, the client faced with body alteration is aware that this is a permanent situation that must be dealt with constantly. The desolation related to the permanency of the alteration seems to increase vulnerability to suicide attempts. Alertness to covert as well as overt indicators of suicidal tendency is vital.

Physiological symptoms. Regardless of whether the initiating trauma is physiological or psychological, physiological symptoms that complicate an already difficult health condition may eventually develop anorexia and/or weight loss, dizziness, gastrointestinal disturbance or even hysterical paralysis or blindness. Manifestations of these grief-related physiological symptoms usually occur within the first 6 months to 1 year of the grief onset.

The clients' significant others may also demonstrate physiological symptoms of their own grief process, need for attention, and/or relief from added responsibilities because of the client's inability to function in previous capacities. Identification of potential problems and effective intervention early in the grief process may reduce many of the physiological reactions to grief. Certainly this is an area of potential prevention that has not received adequate attention.

Anxiety and panic. Closely related to physiological changes, or stage four, is the feeling of panic identified as the fifth stage of grief. Knowledge and awareness increase concerning the pathology of inadequate nutrition from anorexia, or failure to bother with balanced meals. A significant relationship can be identified between extended nutritional deficit and emotional reactions of anxiety and panic (Paykel, 1974; Holmes and, 1974; Mishler and Scotch, 1963; Guillemin, 1977).

Common to this stage of grief is a feeling of the inability to cope and a fear of insanity. These devastating emotions emerge when society begins to expect that the griever should be achieving a "business as usual" attitude. Failure to adhere to the time expectations of society not only frustrates both the client and significant others but often results in client guilt. Clients experience a sense of failure at not being able to cope effectively.

Hostility. The guilt and frustration of panic evolves finally into the sixth stage of grieving—hostility. Various targets for the hostility exist. One or a number of targets may be independent or jointly focused on during this stage. Hostility toward self or another individual may occur if there is a belief that the body alteration was caused by neglect. In addition, persons not having the alteration are often targets of hostility; their wholeness emphasizes the client's loss. Both significant others and the staff require assistance in understanding and coping with client hostility. Failure to dissipate the hostility appropriately can result in reduced support at a time when it is extremely crucial. Assurance that hostility is understandable and accepted must be given to the client—a mandate more easily stated than acted upon.

Languor. Feelings of hostility toward self, others, or God may elicit guilt, thereby compounding the emotional energy expenditure of the client. It is this expenditure of energy during the hostile stage that results in the seventh stage of the grief process—languor. Extreme fatigue, lassitude, general disinterest, and feelings of deep depression characterize this period. For clients who must learn new skills such as ostomy care or use of a prosthesis, this stage is particularly devastating because the physical and emotional energy required to learn are just not available to the client.

Further, society expects by this time that the client will be eagerly attempting to leave the sick or impaired role assigned to him both by himself and others (Mechanic, 1976; Suchman, 1965.) During this stage there is often great discouragement for the client and significant others. Others may at this time begin to suspect that the client enjoys the "invalid" role; often they tend to withdraw somewhat fearing that the client is never going to progress to a more independent, emotionally secure state because of his failure to achieve expected goals and because he seems to be having an emotional setback with recurrence of depression.

Thus rehabilitation attempts may be thwarted, which elevates the frustration levels of all involved. Taxed creativity and genuine concern are necessary to facilitate continued client improvement. Assurance that languor is a normal reaction this far into the recovery phase can help reduce fears that prevous gains will be lost and recovery never achieved.

Anticipation. Following the languor stage most people experience a "bottoming out." It is as though the client is feeling that if things do not improve he will just be too depressed to live. Thus the eighth stage is labeled anticipation. At this time a belief begins to form that in essence indicates that "Just maybe there is something worthwhile for me after all." It is, not to be overly dramatic, a spring following a winter of grief.

While stage eight is emotionally gratifying to the staff, health care professionals must guard against a tendency to reject those who might decide that the glimmer of hope is too dim to sustain the efforts necessary for continued life. Increasingly an individual's right to define life for himself is evolving, necessitating ethical and moral considerations that heretofore did not exist. Clients deserve support regardless of our personal approval of their decisions.

Reentry into society. The ninth and final stage of the grief process for those sustaining permanent lifelong loss is reentry. Reentry into society is dependent on a multiplicity of factors such as societal reaction to the body image alteration and the level of recovery achieved. Exploration of societal influence on the client's adjustment and his reentry into society is considered in the following section of this chapter.

However, before we examine the influence of society on the client's recovery, let us consider why health care professionals need knowledge concerning the stages of grief experienced by persons with body alterations that require readjustment to life.

Issues pertinent to health care professionals

Major emphasis is placed on early education efforts by health care professionals. While this need is not disputed, careful examination of the stages causes one to question how much information can be assimilated at an early stage. Continued research into client readiness and ability to learn during the various stages is needed to assist health care workers in determining effective learning strategies. It is possible that since the grief process takes approximately 3 months to a year to begin readjustment, a client really is not able to absorb adequate information prior to his discharge. Yet the hospital stay for many body-altering surgeries is only a few weeks, and the client goes home before much, if any, psychosocial adjustment evaluation and/or additional teaching can be done.

A second benefit derived from being knowledgeable about the grief process is that the staff can assist in identifying potential health problems related to loss before they occur. Thus considerable illness prevention could be achieved if existing facilities and organizations were oriented toward detection and alleviation of problems prior to their eruption into major concerns. Collaborative inhouse consultation, discharge planning, and effective referrals among the staff in both secondary and tertiary settings, community health nurses, and clients all enhance the continuity of care.

In conjunction with preventing various severe emotional and/or physical reactions, health care providers should be alert to the fact that persons experiencing loss are in a state of decreased judgment acuity. Efforts to adjust to make life "normal" again as quickly as possible often result in inappropriately based decisions, which in turn increase the extant crisis.

The challenge is that as knowledge concerning the grief process increases human needs will be more adequately met in areas frequently overlooked heretofore. Yet we must not expect "superhuman" perceptiveness and therapeutic behavior from providers who deal with those experiencing alteration and/or loss.

Not infrequently health care professionals have been labelled cold, unfeeling, and unemotional by clients and the public. In the recent past an attitude of detachment was encouraged, even demanded, as the acceptable professional response to client misfortune. To achieve detachment, disengagement was probably employed as a defense mechanism against the empathy felt for the suffering. Most health care workers initially enter the health field because of a desire to help alleviate pain. Often encounters with the magnitude of pain and distress human beings are required to face on a nonending basis result in a need to block the realization of this pain if one is to continue to be exposed to it. Emotional withdrawal is not the only alternative. With support and realistic goal expectations staff members can confront suffering in a way that increases their own

job satisfaction while decreasing the clients' trauma.

Extensive effort will have to be made to bring about this desirable situation. The staff will need counseling, education, and relief from intense confrontation with client distress in order to deal effectively with their own as well as the clients' problems. As primary nursing regains popularity as an approach to providing care and nurses (health care workers) more and more are expected to deal with clients and their significant others on a long-term, in-depth basis, demand for staff support will increase (Tinkham, 1972).

One method of assisting the staff in their efforts to cope with legal, ethical, and emotional issues related to caring for clients who are experiencing loss is for institutions to employ mental health nurses as consultants to the staff on specific units. Based on a collaborative effort, an agenda and schedule of contact should be established. The consultant then should meet with the staff to assist with staff coping. Should primary solutions to specific unit problems relate to institutional organization, consultation with the administration may be advisable. Resolution of the problems related to client and staff coping necessitates innovative utilization of existing facilities and health care providers in expanded roles.

Societal reactions to grief

From early childhood, conflicting societal expectations inundate us concerning how, when, where, and for what one is to grieve. For example, the griever must be stoic and yet not too stoic lest an accusation of a lack of feeling be pronounced. Similarly, while one is expected to be functioning shortly after the loss is sustained, functioning too well too soon also can result in criticism. Thus when a spouse is lost and the remaining partner remarries within a period of time under a year there is often criticism regarding the level of devotion, and yet researchers indicate that persons who were happier in the first marriage tend to remarry more quickly than those reporting less contentment with previous relationships. Persons with an altered body image (such as the result of the creation of an ostomy) are expected to return to daily activities after 6 weeks, yet often no provision is made for sexual counseling or activity since society stigmatizes both sex and the body image alteration.

Another societal reaction to loss or grief is that the individual is entitled to assistance to some degree depending on such factors as the type of loss, the reason the loss occurred, and the sex and age of the person (Lewis et al., 1975; Greenley and Mechanic, 1976; Parkes, 1972). The right to assistance carries with it the contradictory demand that the person attempt to achieve independence but not gain too much independence. Thus a blind person is expected to learn to function to some extent; yet most people would hesitate to elect a blind person to a national office.

In attempting to assist those with body image alterations society develops labeling processes, social policies, and social organizations that influence how various alterations and conditions are treated. Some illnesses have more prestige and less stigma than others. For instance, a heart attack still signifies to many hard work and achievement, while cancer is still considered by many to be an unclean affliction.

As the social policies and organizations develop, selfish altruism can be identified. That is, these self-help agencies are organized so that they are self-perpetuating and broad enough in scope to ensure a supply of clients. An excellent example of this self-perpetuation is readily seen when one studies the genesis and evolution of the March of Dimes. Originally set up to eliminate polio, it later expanded its efforts to include birth defects when polio became a manageable problem.

The labeling process is capricious and many clients may find themselves falling between or among organizations with not enough of any one element to merit inclusion in an organization or to receive any of its benefits. Yet when considered as a whole their disability or need may be greater than many who fall clearly into one category or another.

If the agencies are to exist there must of course be clients; thus the labeling and organization evolves for some conditions that earlier were left unorganized. Increasing numbers of groups have emerged for those with terminal illness, for those losing significant others, and for those with a variety of body part losses (for example, ostomy clubs, TOUCH, Make Today Count, and Reach to Recovery). Health care professionals need to be increasingly aware of the developmental process surrounding these self-help groups, the labeling process involved in determining whether or not a client could benefit from one, and the long-term effects of labeling the client in this manner. Careful scrutiny should be given to organizations as they develop to determine their cost effectiveness before they develop accepted status and demand social support. Evaluation of existing and proposed agencies can be enhanced by employing community health nurse consultants to address both client and community needs.

Finally society tends to indicate that persons who experience a loss deserve societal assistance because they are not responsible for their condition. Yet throughout the socialization process another message comes across: the good have good things happen to them and live happily everafter; the bad, on the other hand, are punished for their behavior with a variety of afflictions. This idea of punishment for wrongdoing is frequently a cause of guilt in those who have suffered a loss. Often health care workers hear the question ''What did I do that was bad enough to merit this punishment?''

If we are to assist persons to adjust to their loss, a normal condition of life, we must begin early, before there is a loss to cope with, and teach the inevitability of failure, loss, and sadness in life. This does not necessitate a gloomy outlook, only a realistic one, which allows both for anticipation of some normal unpleasantness and for learned coping mechanisms before the crisis occurs. Someone once said, ''Life is a series of hellos and good-byes.'' This is a process related not only to relationships between individuals, but in the individual's relationship with self. As man ages, various losses and alterations occur. Preparation for these losses and alterations can result in more adequate coping, increased life satisfaction, and a healthier self-concept.

References

Andreasen, N. J. C., Norris, A. S., and Hartford, C. E.: Incidence of long-term psychiatric complications in severely burned adults, Anal. Surg. **174:**785-793, 1971.

Blacher, R. S.: Loss of internal organs. In Schoenberg, B., et al., eds.: Loss and grief: psychological management in medical practice, New York, 1970, Columbia University Press.

Blaesing, S., and Brockhaus, J.: The development of the body image in the child, Nurs. Clin. North Am. **7:**597-609, 1972.

Cantrell, C. H.: An empirical study of the relationship between comparative life satisfaction and death anxiety among aged men (unpublished dissertation) Columbus, Ohio, 1974, Ohio State University.

Cunningham, M. E.: A demographic survey of ostomates, Los Angeles, 1969, The United Ostomy Association.

Engel, G.: Psychological development in health and disease, Philadelphia, 1963, W. B. Saunders Co.

Federn, P.: Ego psychology and the psychoses, New York, 1952, Basic Books, Inc.

Foster, S., and Andreoli, K.: Behavior following acute myocardial infarction, Am. J. Nurs. **70:**2344-2348, 1970.

Greenley, J. R., and Mechanic, D.: Social selection in seeking help for psychological problems, J. Health Soc. Behav., **17:**246-262, 1976.

Guillemin, R.: Endorphines: brain pepticles that act like opiates, New Eng. J. Med. **296:**226-228, 1977.

Hollender, M. H.: A study of patients admitted to a psychiatric hospital after pelvic operations, Am. J. Obstet. Gynecol. **79:**498-503, 1960.

Holmes, T. H., and Masuda, M.: Life change and illness susceptibility. In Dohrenwend, B. S., and Dohrenwend, B. P., eds.: Stressful life events: their nature and effects, New York, 1974, Wiley Interscience.

Kastenbaum, R., and Aisenberg, R.: The psychology of death, New York, 1972, Springer Publishing Co., Inc.

Knorr, N. J.: A depressive syndrome following pelvic exenteration and ileostomy, Arch. Surg. **94:**258-260, 1967.

Kolb, L. C.: Disturbance of the body image. In Arieti, S., ed.: American handbook of psychiatry, ed. 2, New York, 1974, Basic Books, Inc.

Kübler-Ross, E.: On death and dying, New York, 1969, The Macmillan Co.

Lewis, C. E., Lewis, M. A., Lorimer, A., and Palmer, B.: Child-initiated care: a study of the determinants of the illness behavior of children, Los Angeles, 1975, Center for Health Sciences, University of California.

Mechanic, D.: Social psychological factors affecting the presentation of bodily complaints, N. Eng. J. Med. **286:**1132-1139, 1972.

Mechanic, D.: Stress, illness, and illness behavior, J. Hum. Stress, **2:**2-6, June 1976.

Mishler, E. G., and Scotch, N. A.: Sociocultural factors in the epidemiology of schizophrenia, Psychiatry **26:**315-351, 1963.

Parkes, C. M.: Bereavement: studies of grief in adult life, London, 1972, Tavistock Publications, Ltd.

Paykel, E. S.: Life stress and psychiatric disorders. In Dohrenwend, B. S., and Dohrenwend, B. P., eds.: Stressful Life Events: Their Nature and Effects, New York, 1974, Wiley Interscience.

Phillips, D. L.: Self-reliance and the inclination to adopt the sick role, Social Forces **43:**555-563, 1965.

Rosen, G. M., and Ross, A.: Relationship of body image to self-concept, J. Consult. Clin. Psychol. **32:**100, 1968.

Ruesch, J., and Brodsky, C. M.: The concept of social disability, Arch. Gen. Psychiatry **19:**394-403, 1968.

Schilder, P.: The image and appearance of the human body, New York, 1950, International Universities Press.

Schoenberg, B., and Carr, A. C.: Loss of external organs: limb amputation, mastectomy, and disfigurement. In Schoenbert, B., et al., eds.: Loss and grief: psychological management in medical practice, New York, 1970, Columbia University Press.

Suchman, E. A.: Social patterns of illness and medical care, J. Health Hum. Behav. **6:**2-16, 1965a.

Suchman, E. A.: Stages of illness and medical care, J. Health Hum. Behav. **6:**114-128, 1965b.

Suttie, J.: The origins of love and hate, London, 1935, Kegan, Paul, Trench, Trubner & Co.

Tinkham, C. W., and Voorhies, E. F.: Community health nursing evolution and process, New York, 1972, Appleton-Century-Crofts.

Zborowski, M.: Cultural components in response to pain, J. Soc. Issues **8:**16-30, 1952.

CHAPTER 15

Continuity of care program: discharged psychiatric patients

JEANETTE LANCASTER

Prior to 1946 the concept of community mental health was scarcely known. The passage of the 1946 Mental Health Act, which established the National Institute of Mental Health, led to the dawning of a new era marked by a wide array of treatment approaches. The initial thrust of mental health legislation in the post–World War II years was to apply a public health approach to the prevention and treatment of mental illness within local communities. Historically a classical public health approach has focused on population-based problems rather than on treatment of individuals. In the mental health area the primary implementation strategies have been directed toward the individual as client rather than toward family or community as client. The focus on individual treatment continued with the development of large state hospitals, extensive psychiatric services in Veteran's Administration hospitals, and ultimately even in the implementation of community mental health centers.

Even with the many advances in manpower development and mental health research that took place after World War II, little effect was seen in the provision of mental health care to the population at large. In the postwar years psychiatry continued its preference for providing private care, which ultimately resulted in serious inequities in the availability and caliber of care available within the mental health system. Few alternatives were accessible to the general public other than treatment in a state hospital.

Perhaps the most significant event to date in community mental health was the passage of the Community Mental Health Centers Act. This act stipulated that federal support would be provided for both direct and indirect mental health services. In implementing the act the indirect services of community consultation and education were given secondary emphasis when compared to the direct care focus on emergency care, outpatient, partial hospitalization, and inpatient services.

The Community Mental Health Centers Act authorized considerable funding allocations for the construction and staffing of comprehensive community mental health centers. The hoped-for goal in the original community mental health legislation was that centers would decrease the need for long-term hospitalization by providing an array of support systems within the local community. Although the original vision of community mental health was to provide support for the residents of a specific catchment area, it is important to remember that this legislation emphasized direct services with minimal attention to the provision of indirect and preventive services.

Critics contend that the focus of community mental health services to date has largely dealt with decentralization of care rather than the actual implementation of community-based services responsive to the needs and desires of each local community. Zusman and Lamb (1977) hold that many of the criticisms leveled against community mental health are well deserved, especially regarding society's failure to provide care for the many thousands of patients who are discharged from state hospitals following an extensive hospitalization. They accuse society of taking the cheap way out: instead of providing comprehensive community treatment for this often overlooked population, discharged patients are often placed in group settings with minimal attention to reintegration into the community.

In the late 1970s national attention was again directed toward the needs of the mentally ill within the community setting. In the 1978 publication of the Report of the President's Commission on Mental Health, the principal recommendation of the Commission called for the establishment of a "new federal grant program for community mental health services to encourage the creation of necessary services where they are inadequate and increase the flexibility of communities in planning a comprehensive network of services" (MH-MR Report, 1978).

The report recommends that in the future mental health funding priorities be given to unserved and underserved areas; services for children, adolescents, and the elderly; and specialized services for racial and ethnic minority groups and for the chronically mentally ill population. General themes within the report address goals for remedying several of the areas in which community mental health has been described as providing inadequate services. One theme emphasizes the relevance of seeking community support for program development, while mention is also made of the necessity for flexibility in the development of programs unique to the assessed needs of the entire population as well as those of high-risk populations within a specific community. The report calls for further phasing-down efforts of state hos-

pitals. Also, each state mental health authority is urged to develop a case management system coordinated by one agency that would assist the chronically mentally ill population.

The purpose of this discussion is to propose a community-based plan for providing comprehensive services to discharged psychiatric patients. The program is particularly applicable to patients who are discharged following a period of extensive hospitalization and who need to learn of ways for becoming resocialized into the community. In the proposed continuity of care program the role of the nurse is emphasized with recognition that program support and assistance must come from a variety of health care providers.

Prior to discussing the continuity of care program, it is necessary to briefly trace critical legislative and social actions that have to a large extent determined the state of the art in community mental health, especially in regard to treatment of the long-term institutionalized population. Any program that looks to the future must maintain a keen awareness of past events that have affected present patterns.

DEINSTITUTIONALIZATION: LEGISLATIVE MANDATES

In the 15-year interim between the enactment of the Community Mental Health Centers Act and the publication of the Report of the President's Commission on Mental Health, a significant decline in the state hospital population occurred. In a 10-year span, from 1966 to 1976, the inpatient census of public mental hospitals decreased from 490,000 to 215,000. While the notion is widely held that community treatment is frequently as effective if not more so than hospitalization, the failure to establish a network of community services prior to the discharge of such a massive number of patients has elicited a clamor of protest from health providers, patients, their families, and concerned community groups (Becker and Schulberg, 1976).

Legislative decisions

Until recent years the rights of the institutionalized mentally ill population have been limited, or ignored, by law. Recent legislative decisions have called attention to the civil and personal rights of these patients. The 1966 landmark decision, *Rouse vs. Cameron,* in the District of Columbia Circuit Court of Appeals, stipulated that mentally ill persons committed by the criminal courts had the right to adequate treatment (Kaplan, 1973). The rationale behind this decision was that the mental condition of these patients had resulted in a sentence of not guilty by reason of insanity; thus treatment rather than incarceration was indicated. Two years after this decision, in the *Nason vs. Superintendent of Bridgewater State Hospital* case, the right to treatment was extended to persons unable to stand trial for a criminal offense by reason of mental incompetence (Kaplan, 1973).

Subsequently an Alabama federal district court further extended the right to treatment to all involuntarily committed mentally ill persons; this right included persons retained as a result of either civil or criminal procedures (*Wyatt vs. Stickney,* 1971). In the *Wyatt vs. Stickney* proceedings, Judge Frank Johnson declared that Alabama state hospitals were not providing adequate treatment to patients (Becker and Schulberg, 1976). The court ordered the state of Alabama to draft within 6 months a comprehensive plan to provide treatment to patients hospitalized in public mental hospitals. Dissatisfied with the state plan, the court appointed a panel of national experts to provide guidance in establishing criteria for adequate treatment. After the panel submitted its first set of guidelines, the court issued an order (*Wyatt vs. Stickney,* 1972) that established three minimal characteristics of adequate treatment: (1) a humane psychological and physical environment, (2) a sufficient number of qualified staff to provide adequate treatment, and (3) individual plans for patient care (Kaplan, 1973).

Moreover, the appendix to the court order stipulated requirements regarding size of patient units, standards for toilet facilities, heating and cooling, nutrition, personnel per 250 patients, and contents of patients' records.

Both the regulations that addressed improved facilities and those that increased the staff necessitated a dramatic increase in the proportion of state mental health funds that were to be mandated for institutional care. Since each state has a finite amount of funds, an increased focus on inpatient care of necessity affected funding allocations for community-based treatment.

In a further judicial decision, *O'Connor vs. Donaldson,* the United States Supreme Court ruled unanimously that mentally ill patients who are both harmless and capable of survival outside the hospital cannot be held against their will and without treatment. The key issues here relate to definitions of What is harmful to society? as well as What is treatment? The majority of psychiatric patients pose threats neither to themselves nor to others. Similarly a large percentage of these patients can survive outside the hospital. However many are, without considerable support, incapable of caring for themselves in an autonomous fashion that reflects a satisfactory quality of life. Thus in the new era of community mental health several legislative decisions have significantly altered state funding priorities.

Social policy influences on mental health

Since funds are always limited, decisions regarding allocations are based on a set of priorities. Both legislation and general social policies have influenced funding decisions. In the final analysis funding priorities depend on a set of values. Mechanic (1969) identifies two prevailing values that largely determine the provision of mental health services: (1) need is a humanitarian belief based on the premise that the best possible services are a "right" of all mankind; and (2) gain is based on the idea that the range and intensity of services available should correspond to the observed outcome. Public policy generally mediates a compromise between gain and need in planning services for a particular population.

Few would dispute the needs of the chronically mentally ill population. In contrast, limited documentation supports the notion that this group of patients gains a sufficient amount from mental health services. A further consideration, however, revolves around the entire issue of How much gain is enough to economically validate the expenses? The prevailing goal in health care is directed toward cure. Often for chronically mentally ill patients the gain is not directed toward cure but rather toward remission of acute symptoms or improvement of coping capacity.

Mental health providers historically have been less enthusiastic about designing programs for chronically ill patients than for the young, the acutely ill, and more recently the aged population. Lack of staff interest and zeal for initiating innovative programs coupled with the reluctance of this group of patients to demand services has often resulted in their being society's "overlooked or forgotten members." These patients frequently lack assertiveness and sufficient self-confidence to demand quality health care. Adjustment to long-term institutionalization may foster compliant and subservient behavior that is not quickly unlearned (Lancaster, 1979).

The major obstacle to the development and implementation of a continuity of care program is the difficulty in getting one agency to act as the advocate or sponsor for the program. For a program to function effectively the designated staff must maintain responsibility as the patient secures services from a variety of agencies. Patient advocacy is often discussed but rarely implemented. An effective continuity of care program would assist discharged patients in locating housing, obtaining employ-

ment, budgeting and managing their finances, and developing social relations where necessary; the program would also provide instruction and support in readjusting to activities of daily living such as managing clothing or shopping.

A significant obstacle to the development of an effective continuity of care program for discharged psychiatric patients is the paucity of effective and previously tested models. Financial as well as social policy factors influence agency initiative in developing this type of program; thus few comprehensive programs have been funded and implemented.

PROGRAM PLANNING: ECOLOGY'S CONTRIBUTION

As mentioned in Chapter 2, ecology is the science, or perspective, that studies the relationship between organisms and their environment. When human beings become the organism under discussion, then the term "human ecology" is applied to the study and analysis of man-environmental interaction. The relevance of utilizing an ecological perspective for depicting a continuity of care program lies in the tremendous change that occurs both within the social system, which must provide new accommodations, as well as within each discharged person, who must learn new ways of coping with a radically different environment than that provided during hospitalization.

In looking at the social system that encompasses community mental health, an ecological approach for intervention includes "assessing a natural setting and then redesigning the context surrounding a social problem so that a specific community problem is altered as the host environment is changed" (Kelly, 1971). Three ecological principles are described by Kelly (1971) as guiding precepts for use in the planning of community interventions:

1. *Interdependence* means that when a component of any natural system is changed, alterations occur in all other components of the sys-

tem. The system components can be designated as subsystems. For example, consider the state mental health department as a system and each component agency as a subsystem. The closing of state hospitals affected a number of the subsystems as new programs needed to be implemented rapidly to provide community services. Also, the closing of hospitals had system effects on external agencies such as those dealing with law enforcement and community welfare.

2. *Adaptation* implies that for any organism to survive over time it must learn to cope with continual environmental change. This principle is especially applicable to the discharged person who must move out of a relatively sheltered setting where many decisions were made for him by virtue of institutional prerogative and where the majority of his physiological and safety needs were met by the agency. Relocation into the community demands an immediate adjustment to an environment that often contains an array of new or novel components. During a lengthy hospitalization, changes in society occur that may not be obvious in the institutional setting. For example, improvements in technology may have provided new food processing equipment that is novel to a discharged person; in order for him to adapt following discharge from the institution he must be provided with community support.

3. *Succession* deals with community change from the perspective of remembering that change is directional and therefore predictable, that societal change results from physical changes within the community, and that change culminates in a stable ecosystem. The application of the principle of succession to community mental health includes not only the present rate and scope of change, but also the anticipated future rate. For example, the planning of a continuity of care program should take into account that patients who have recently been discharged as well as those who anticipate discharge within the next 3 months. A successful continuity of care program must

actualize the belief that behavior is affected by the environment and that at the same time one's behavior affects the environment. A simplistic principle of ecology postulates that "the environment changes its inhabitants and vice versa." By definition environment includes physical, psychological, and sociocultural components; hence ecology calls particular attention to the attitudinal and value system aspects of the environment. This man-environment interaction is explained by utilizing systems theory concepts as a framework for understanding the man-environment relationship. Each human being is considered an open system who maintains continuous interaction with the environment. As an open system the boundaries are permeable, which permits energy and information to pass from inside out and from outside in. Input is transformed by the workings of the system and subsequently expelled back into the environment as output.

The human ecological approach seeks to understand human behavior in terms of cause and effect relationships, bearing in mind that there is no single causative factor. Mental health and mental illness result from a network of interconnected influences both within and external to the individual including family, friends, social class, and the sociocultural and economic aspects of the community.

Using ecological concepts, the community mental health nurse assists discharged psychiatric patients to attain a steady state, or the ability to maintain homeostasis in the face of environmental stressors. Nursing actions seek either to reduce the onslaught of environmental stress through anticipatory guidance and preplanning activities or to strengthen the patient's coping capacity through repeated successful exchange with the environment. This requires a carefully planned and continuously monitored program that seeks to facilitate mental health through strengthening the person's ability to attain need fulfillment within the confines of the environmental resources, constraints, and require-

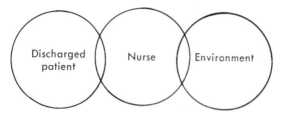

Fig. 15-1. Starting point of continuity of care program in which nurse actively connects discharged patient with environment.

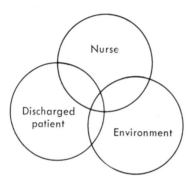

Fig. 15-2. Nursing support when continuity of care program is operational and when discharged patient is able to negotiate with environment in a somewhat autonomous fashion.

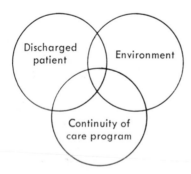

Fig. 15-3. Discharged patient-environment and program interaction once program is operational. Nursing position in Fig. 15-2 and program position in Fig. 15-3 are synonymous. Continuity of care program consists of nursing direction in relation to (1) community acceptance, (2) client advocacy, (3) individual supervision, (4) patient education, and (5) group supervision.

ments. Figs. 15-1 and 15-2 depict the shift in nursing involvement as the discharged person becomes increasingly adept at maintaining productive interaction with the environment.

In Fig. 15-1 the nurse actively links the client with the environment by providing intensive support. Figs. 15-2 and 15-3 depict the use of the continuity of care program in encouraging patient autonomy.

CONTINUITY OF CARE PROGRAM

The continuity of care program focuses on providing support to discharged psychiatric patients so that they can attain a state of equilibrium in their interactions with the environment. Lacking social and rehabilitative abilities, this group of individuals may withdraw from societal interaction, become more psychotic than they were prior to discharge, or fall victim to unscrupulous members of society (Becker and Schulberg, 1976).

Program planning in community mental health can be described in four phases: (1) idea generation, (2) diagnosis and assessment, (3) decision making, and (4) evaluation. In regard to the continuity of care program, social, political, and patient factors have been discussed to support the need for such a program. A community diagnosis should be completed to assess the needs of program consumers as well as to determine the resources available to support and facilitate the implementation of the plan. Community diagnosis begins with an assessment of the number of psychiatric patients who have recently returned to the community as well as those who anticipate hospital release in the near future. Once the target population has been identified it is important to determine community resources. Resources include agencies, health professionals, and community services, as well as family supports available to the patient population. Diagnosis also includes the specific program component of community acceptance.

The next phase, decision making, begins

with the determination of community acceptance including examination of the power structure or style prevalent in the community. The completion of the program component of community acceptance includes an awareness of who makes decisions, how they are made, and what informal sources of power exist within the community.

Program evaluation is described in the last section following specific delineation of the five unique facets of the program: (1) community acceptance, (2) client advocacy, (3) individual supervision, (4) patient education, and (5) group supervision. A nurse with advanced preparation in community mental nursing serves as the program coordinator with public health nurses implementing a considerable portion of the program. Additional personnel include a social worker, vocational counselor, psychiatrist, and psychologist whose services are used on an ''as needed'' basis.

The setting for a continuity of care program varies: patients may be in a group home, in an apartment building housing several discharged patients, in foster homes, or returning to their previous living arrangements. Implementation of the proposal varies according to the location, but the major components remain unchanged.*

Community acceptance

Any program designed to provide community treatment for discharged psychiatric patients must take into account the prevailing attitudes of community residents. Vague expressions of support for the concept of deinstitutionalization are often replaced by adamant resistance when community treatment refers to ''my community.'' Opposition seems to snowball overnight once a particular site is selected for a community program such as a group home. Fears of physical and sexual attack, bizarre behavior, destruction of property and lowering of property values are only a few of the often-expressed concerns (Becker and Schulberg, 1976).

Prior to establishing a continuity of care program for discharged patients, the response of the community must be assessed. Fostering community acceptance of mentally ill individuals is the first step in program development. Citizen acceptance can often be increased by open dialogue, skillful public education programs and support from local radio, television and newspaper resources. Effective citizen acceptance programs start with a determination of community attitudes and fears which is followed by discussion of plans and education regarding the needs of mentally ill individuals in the community. A major problem in attaining citizen acceptance is gaining access to the community. Public meetings are not consistently well-attended; therefore, door-to-door dialogue may be necessary although it is time-consuming and costly. Mental health volunteers such as through the local Mental Health Association can provide an excellent resource for increasing community acceptance by speaking at any public or organizational meetings in regard to community responsibility toward mentally ill residents.

Community residents often fear physical assault, bizarre behavior or decreased property values. In truth, long-term psychiatric patients tend to be withdrawn rather than assaultive. There is some truth in the fear of bizarre behavior in that patients may wear inappropriate clothing or walk down the street hallucinating. Such behavior may not be particularly deviant in light of current dress styles, although mentally ill persons are target populations for criticism.

Moreover, a community's property values may increase with the establishment of a group home in that due to limited funds, generally a house in poor repair is purchased.

---

*Descriptions of the five program components are from Lancaster, J.: Community treatment for mental health's forgotten population, J. Psychiatr. Nurs. Mental Health Serv. **17:**20-27, July, 1979.

Residents and staff frequently attach renovations on the home with zeal and soon change a community "eye-sore" into an acceptable dwelling.

Client advocacy

Since discharged patients do not tend to be assertive, they often need a specific person to serve as an advocate who can help them negotiate the community system. This program component is analogous to the inpatient practice of making rounds. One person, generally a public health nurse, makes regular visits to a specific client caseload to determine needs in relation to obtaining community services. For example, the task of communicating with a public agency may prove overwhelming to this population. Rarely does one telephone call or visit settle a complaint with an agency or organization. Patients often become discouraged with the "red-tape" of requesting services or issuing a complaint and withdraw from the process prior to the resolution of the problem. Nursing intervention in the form of offering direct assistance by providing the correct person to talk with or accompanying the patient may be implemented. Indirect help may be given through role-playing to allow the patient an opportunity to practice needed social-interaction skills.

Individual supervision

As the nurse visits each person in the caseload for the purpose of client advocacy, an assessment is made of physical and psychological needs. Continual attention is given to medication maintenance in that a large proportion of discharged patients are maintained indefinitely on psychotropic medication. Patient compliance with the medication regimen is a continual problem due to lack of funds, inadequate knowledge about the purpose of the medication, as well as discomfort from side effects. Sometimes changing medications decreases both cost and side effects.

The nurse remains constantly attentive to any patient needs which are presented. For example, some patients will take their medications as ordered but fall short of eating nutritious meals; on occasion the services of a dietician may be warranted. Patients are encouraged to discuss any problems which arise; nursing intervention employs a problem-solving approach to help the patient examine his response to either internal or external stressors and to identify alternative ways of responding.

Patient education

Test and Stein (1976) assert that community treatment of discharged psychiatric patients should focus on teaching basic skills of daily living. Their rationale is that the majority of patients admitted to public mental hospitals present a limited array of both social interaction and problem-solving skills. They are, therefore, significantly impaired in their ability to manage outside the hospital.

Four general categories of coping skills include: activities of daily living, vocational skills, leisure time skills and social or interpersonal skills (Test and Stein, 1976). In this proposal the first category is taught via didactic and practice techniques either in the hospital or community setting immediately following discharge. This category includes activities such as grooming and hygiene, room upkeep, laundry, meal preparation, use of public transportation and telephone utilization. Instruction begins with a discussion of the topic followed by a staff modeling session then a practice session by the group. For example, if the topic is hygiene the nurse or psychiatric aide discusses aspects of cleanliness, use of soap and deodorant, hair washing and appropriate dress. This discussion is followed by the nurse actually washing either her face and hair and applying deodorant or asking for a patient volunteer. Last, each patient practices these skills with supervision.

Vocational skills are handled by the vocational counselor and may include testing and training as well as initial placement in a sheltered employment setting. Vocational abilities are continuously monitored to detect problems as well as readiness for change and/or advancement (Hogarty, 1971).

Leisure time and social skills are generally handled during the group supervision component of the program. Group interaction allows for considerably more information to be provided to each patient than a staff member alone could give.

Group supervision

Regular group sessions provide a valuable component of a continuity of care program. The purposes are multiple, ranging from providing an opportunity for patients to talk to one another to exchanging information needed by many patients, and also a time for sharing and recognition that others have similar feelings and fears. A popular format is to vary the group focus from week to week from that of an unstructured "rap" group to providing specific information.

The group sessions provide a controlled milieu in which members can practice the development of social relations. Often the serving of refreshments fosters improved social skills as well as provides a focus for anxiety as members stir coffee or tea.

Topics which readily lend themselves to group discussion include common side effects of psychotropic drugs as well as ways to manage these effects, problems in getting along with others and examination of alternative ways of communicating and acting. It is often helpful to ask guests to attend the group sessions to provide specific information. For example, the vocational counselor connected with the continuity of care program may attend in order to describe vocational rehabilitation opportunities as well as to assess needs and arrange appointments to work with individual members.

The length of the group sessions varies with members' abilities to handle anxiety. Specific objectives often include:

1. Helping patients function outside the institution through support and medication monitoring.
2. Reinforcing strengths already present.
3. Assisting patients to learn in a safe setting how others perceive them and to recognize what they do which causes others to withdraw from them or seek their company (Lindberg and Branch, 1973).

Evaluation

Although a specific evaluative format is not presented for the continuity of care program general comments related to evaluation are set forth, since when possible evaluation should begin at the outset of the plan rather than after the program is operational.

The purpose of evaluation is to ensure some degree of quality control and accountability (Blackwell and Bolman, 1977). Basic to evaluation is the belief that a specification or program goals and objectives is a prerequisite and that the outcome of the care itself provides the ultimate criteria for determination of program effectiveness (Speer and Tapp, 1976).

In general, three quality assessment methods—structure, process, and outcome—constitute the evaluative choices. In the structure approach the guiding principle holds that standards and criteria can be designed to examine the organizational structure's effect on health delivery. This approach assumes that care can be improved by increasing the quality and quantity of the staff as well as by improving the physical facilities.

The process approach assesses the quality of care against a standard that is previously determined. The underlying assumption is that health care providers can decide on what comprises "quality care."

The outcome approach evaluates care by documenting the results of treatment in terms of patient survival, recovery, and remission from symptoms, as well as the patient's own satisfaction with the care he received.

Although quantity of care is the simplest factor to measure, attention to outcomes and quality provide the most useful feedback regarding program effectiveness. In establishing an evaluation program for the continuity of care program, both quantity and quality should be assessed. Records should be kept of how many patients used the services, as well as if more patients needed services than staff could provide, outcome evaluation begins at the outset of the program when nurse and patient mutually determine goals in the form of a treatment contract. Each item on the contract is stated in behavioral terms that can be readily measured. Outcome measures should be simple, concrete, readily observable, and subject to minimal variation in interpretation.

SUMMARY

This chapter has presented a proposal that suggests several components of a continuity of care program for discharged psychiatric patients. The purpose of the proposal is to identify various ways in which patients can be assisted to interact more productively with their environment. Hospitalized psychiatric patients tend to lose their self-identities and become isolated from society in direct proportion to the length of time they were hospitalized. An intensive community reorientation program is suggested to overcome the effects of institutionalization and facilitate adaptation to society with its many demands for flexibility and change.

References

Becker, A., and Schulberg, J. C.: Phasing out state hospitals: a psychiatric dilemma, N. Eng. J. Med. **291:** 255-261, 1976.

Blackwell, B. L., and Bolman, W. M.: The principles and problems of evaluation, Community Ment. Health J. **13:** 175-186, 1977.

Hogarty, G.: The plight of schizophrenics in modern treatment programs, Hosp. Community Psychiatry **22:**197-203, July 1971.

Kaplan, H.: Institutions and community mental health: the paradox in Wyatt v. Stickney, Community Mental Health J. **9:**34-37, 1973.

Kelly, J.: Qualities for the community psychologist, Am. Psychol. **26:**897-903, 1971.

Lancaster, B. J.: Community treatment for mental health's forgotten population, Psychiatr. Nurs. July 1979.

Lindberg, H. and Branch, C. H.: Community health nursing in the changing mental health scene, J. Nurs. Admin. **3:**41-44, November 1973.

Mechanic, D.: Mental health and social policy, Englewood Cliffs, N.J., 1969, Prentice-Hall, Inc.

MH-MR Reports: A Morris Associates report from Washington, D.C. **15:**1-8, May 5, 1978.

Speer, D. C., and Tapp, J. C.: Evaluation of mental health service effectiveness: a start-up model for established programs, Am. J. Orthopsychiatry **49:**217-228, 1976.

Test, M. and Stein, L. I.: Practical guidelines for the community treatment of markedly impaired patients, Community Ment. Health J. **12:**72-82, 1976.

Zusman, J., and Lamb, R.: In defense of community mental health, Am. J. Psychiatry **134:**887-890, 1977.

Part four

INTERACTIONAL FRAMEWORKS APPLICABLE TO AN ECOLOGICAL PERSPECTIVE

■ Part four is founded on the premise that there is no one "right" way to approach or respond to all clients in community mental health nursing. The approach taken by each practitioner depends on personal preferences, educational background, and type of clientele for whom services are provided. In this section, seven nurses each describe the therapeutic approach they use in the practice of community mental health nursing. Each of the following seven chapters is presented from the perspective of a nurse therapist who has actually implemented the theoretical concepts in clinical practice. These chapters discuss the basic premises upon which the nursing approach is based and document with clinical examples and illustrations the application of theoretical content.

Although each of these therapeutic approaches can be used at each level of prevention, the majority are described from the framework of secondary prevention. By definition primary prevention describes activities serving to prevent the onset of a problem or mental health disruption from occurring. While several of the approaches discussed in Part four, especially the practice of reality therapy, holistic health practice, Gestalt therapy, and transactional analysis, lend themselves to primary prevention, individuals do not typically seek the services derived from these approaches prior to the onset of stress or psychological discomfort.

The majority of clinical examples provided in each chapter, with the exception of activity and art therapy, portrays nursing intervention in the arena of secondary prevention, which implies preventing the client's psychological stress or discomfort from progressing. In each approach clients are taught new ways of handling stress so that they have greater emotional responses available for dealing with activities of daily living.

Chapters 17 and 18 describe tools with particular relevance to tertiary prevention. Activity group therapy seeks to facilitate the environmental responsiveness of psychiatric patients who have a long history of hospitalization. This approach teaches individuals to become active rather than passive respondents to the environment in which they are expected to function. It also provides an arena whereby patients can practice new activities as well as learn new patterns for responding to others.

Chapter 18 discusses the use of art with children. This approach has wide applicability: it can be used for diagnostic and treatment purposes as well as to stimulate communication between nurse and client. Although this particular chapter directs the reader's attention toward clinical application with children, the theory, tools, and strategies discussed could be used with adults as well. The section on developmental sequencing in art could well be used as a diagnostic and assessment tool for clients of all ages, particularly when some evidence of regression or fixation at a previous developmental phase seems apparent.

Each chapter in Part four, with the exception of chapter 19, describes therapeutic interventions with individuals. Chapter 19 considers the family as the system presenting for treatment. Many of the concepts discussed in this chapter have applicability and are of interest to nurses whose practice does not include families. The discussions of the levels and development of anxiety, the differentiation of self, the triangle as a basic unit of human interaction, and the multigenerational transmission process are relevent to clients of all ages and in varying settings.

Chapters 21 to 24 present four therapeutic approaches that can readily be used in nursing practice. Each of these approaches (reality therapy, Gestalt, holistic health, and transactional analysis) implies that the client must assume considerable responsibility for any changes he wants to bring about in his life. Moreover each has a unique vocabulary, which necessitates that clients become involved in learning how to help themselves. Each chapter provides clinical illustrations of how clients have been taught to become a comember of the therapeutic team and thereby remain responsible for their own behavior and the degree of change in which they are willing to become involved.

CHAPTER 16

Activities as therapy

JEANETTE LANCASTER

Chapter 15 described the need for a carefully planned continuity of care program for discharged psychiatric patients. The essential purpose of such an aftercare program is to counteract the deleterious effects of long-term institutionalization and provide opportunities that increase each patient's chances of being able to cope with the environment outside the hospital. Whether or not an individual remains outside a hospital largely depends on his ability to negotiate the multitude of complex social systems and encounters with others that present in daily living.

One mode of therapeutic intervention—activity group therapy—is described in this chapter. Activity group therapy, a specific type of group psycho-therapy, is defined as a group situation in which interaction is stimulated by the use of simple tasks such as drawing pictures, reading poetry, and listening to music, as well as engaging in simplistic goal-directed activities. This type of group interaction is likely to be less threatening to many patients than open-ended discussion in that a definite, extrinsic structure is provided by the activities. Moreover, accomplishment of group activities allows individuals an opportunity to recognize their abilities and acknowledge that some tasks are within the realm of achievement.

Activity group therapy provides a medium through which ecological principles can be applied to a selected group of patients. As a therapeutic modality, activity groups can be used during hospitalization as well as in posthospital programs. The goals remain similar regardless of the environment in which the groups are conducted. Although activity groups have applicability at all three levels of prevention, perhaps they most often are used in the area of tertiary prevention. While the ultimate goal in community mental health strives for prevention of psychiatric disorders, in reality a considerable segment of the American population is suffering from some degree of emotional impairment. Once emotional disequilibrium has occurred, preventive efforts are directed toward reducing the duration of the disability (secondary prevention) as well as toward decreasing the resultant degree of impairment (tertiary prevention). As previously mentioned, the goal of mental health intervention is to facilitate the man-environment relationship regardless of the level of prevention. For the purposes of this chapter activity group therapy is described as an application of ecological principles toward the goal of tertiary prevention.

A considerable proportion of patients requiring long-term hospitalization suffer from a psychotic thought disorder, often schizophrenia. Documentation exists that suggests that schizophrenic individuals often possess a limited self-concept and view themselves as incapable and socially inept. Activity group therapy provides a medium through which schizophrenic individuals are afforded an opportunity for success. In this chapter discussion centers around the deleterious effects of institutionalization on the self-concept, the characteristics related to the self-concept of schizophrenic persons, and ways in which activity group therapy can intervene in a negative self-view.

EFFECT OF INSTITUTIONALIZATION

Hospitalization necessitates that patients be removed from their usual surroundings and be required to live in a communal setting. Problems of adjustment are typically encountered as patients forfeit temporarily their daily routine and adapt to one dictated by others. Entry into a psychiatric hospital often results in patients' having to relinquish many of the vestiges of adulthood and independence.

Lack of individuality often characterizes psychiatric hospitalization. Patients tend to be dealt with en masse rather than as individuals. It is not uncommon for psychiatric patients to perceive the problem that required the hospitalization as a major catastrophic event for which no adequate solutions are available.

Schizophrenic persons are particularly susceptible to the effects of institutionalization because of the faulty development of their self-identity. On one hand the inadequate development of a sense of identity makes these patients susceptible to dependency on the hospital, while on the other hand their self-concepts are simultaneously affected by the demands and experiences confronting them during hospitalization. To counteract the effects of institutionalization schizophrenic patients need to be part of an environment that facilitates the enhancement and clear differentiation of self-concept.

Ideally the hospital environment will encourage individual development. If such is not the case, then activity therapy in a continuity of care program can maintain and enhance self-development. When concerted efforts are omitted during hospitalization to assist patients maintain a sense of identity, the task confronting the aftercare program includes a major emphasis toward self-development to assist the individual in his reintegration into the environment outside the hospital.

DEVELOPMENT OF SELF-CONCEPT
Description of the normal self

Each person has an image of himself that differentiates him from every other person. This image is made up of a set of attitudes reflecting what an individual thinks and feels about himself. These attitudes form an abstraction known as the self-concept, which is represented by the symbol "me."

The self-image includes both a physical and a psychological appraisal. Moreover, for each "bad" or negative component of the self-concept a positive aspect is available. Three components of the self have been identified by Jersild (1960). He describes a perceptual component of the self that refers to the way a person perceives himself including his body image and the impression he recognizes that he makes on others. The second component of self, a conceptual one, refers to the person's conception of his unique characteristics, abilities, assets, and limitations. The third component, an attitudinal one, includes the feelings a person holds about himself for the present as well as for future expectations. This component includes feelings of both pride and shame toward the self.

In the development of the self the child learns the norms of his group. These expectations are learned in early interactions between the child and those most important to him. The mother is often the chief instrument in this development. Sullivan (1953) emphasized the concept of the self as first evolving from the approval and disapproval that the mother gives to an infant. From the time of birth an infant has an empathetic relationship with some significant adult, usually the mother. Therefore the earliest attitudes are learned by an infant from the way his mother responds to him. Essentially each child comes to think of himself as "good me" or "bad me" depending on the way his mother responds to him. Experiences in which the mother is pleased with the infant lead to the development of the "good me." The "bad me" results from experiences during which the infant emphathizes that his behavior has aroused anxiety in the mother. As the child grows older he appraises himself by the reflected appraisals of significant people other than his mother.

Wylie (1974) extended Sullivan's formulation regarding the mother as the significant other for an infant to include both father and mother. According to Labenne and Green (1969), what a person believes about himself is related to how he interprets the reactions of others to him. No one can know exactly how others see him; he must infer this from their behavior toward him. His self-concept therefore depends to some extent on what he believes others think about him. An individual's perception of what others think of him thus are the crucial elements in self-concept development (Rosenberg, 1973).

Cooley (1902) described the "looking-glass self" in which an individual imagines how others will react to him and feels either satisfied or ashamed. Mead (1934) also described the self in terms of social interactions. Mead discussed the process by which an individual could become a member of his social group by internalizing the ideas and attitudes of significant people. Each individual, then, comes to respond to himself and develop self-attitudes consistent with those expressed by significant others. If an individual places a high value on himself it is because key people in his life have treated him with concern and respect.

The phenomenological view of self, as defined by Rogers (1959), holds that the "self-concept consists of all the perceptions of self admissible to awareness and contains one's perceptions of his characteristics and abilities." Rogers defines the self-concept as the "organized, consistent conceptual gestalt composed of perceptions of the characteristics of the 'I' or 'me' and as the perception of the relationship of the 'I' or 'me' to others and to the various aspects of life, together with the values attached to these perceptions."

The existential viewpoint also includes the development of the self in relationship with others. Man's meaning occurs in relation to some other person (Marcel, 1962). Even the most self-centered person looks to others for his final definition of self. The other person serves as a mirror to reflect a picture that the individual incorporates into his self-view. Marcel (1962) refers to man as a wayfarer, a "homo viator", in search of himself. Man comes to know himself as he relates to others by participating in small groups, the first and foremost being the family.

Need for a positive self-concept

A positive self-concept is one of the greatest assets an individual can have. If one thinks well of himself it is easier to cope with problems of daily living. Branden (1969) explains that there is no other value judgment more significant than a person's estimate of himself. A person's self-estimate is viewed as the most decisive factor available in psychological development and motivation; one's self-view continually has a profound influence on thoughts, emotions, values, and goals. Combs (1965) defines the self as being the most important influence affecting a person's behavior in that what a person believes about himself influences and alters every aspect of his life.

Stability of self-concept

The self-concept is unique in that "no two people ever hold identical sets of beliefs about themselves" (Purkey, 1970). Not only does a person have countless beliefs about himself, but no two beliefs have the same weight and impact on the individual. Closely held beliefs about oneself are difficult to change. When a potentially new concept appears to an individual and is consistent with his current concept of self it may be accepted and assimilated. Conversely, if the new view seems to have no relationship or relevance to the system of self-beliefs it is generally ignored or if an inconsistent or incongruent concept is proposed it is often rejected or distorted.

Description of the schizophrenic self

According to Sullivan (1953) the schizophrenic person comes to think of himself as ''not me'' during infancy. The ''not me'' personification is marked by uncanny emotion and evolves from experiences resulting from forbidding gestures on the part of the mother, thus bringing about intense anxiety on the part of the child without any cause and effect connection. In this way the development of self comes about from the way an individual appraises the approval or rejection by others of his behavior. Schizophrenic persons are so preoccupied with themselves that they are often unable to share their experiences, which leads them to have fewer situations than most people do on which to judge the reactions of others to them.

Moreover the boundary between the self and the external world is sometimes blurred for the schizophrenic. In descriptions of self-perceptions it is not uncommon for these individuals to mix in components of the external setting such as characteristics of objects or other people.

BENEFITS OF GROUP EXPERIENCES

If the theories that a positive self-concept is necessary for normal adjustment and that one's self-concept is influenced by the reactions of others, then a group experience has the potential for enhancing the man-environment relationship. Adler (1924) perceives man as primarily a social being whose prime motivation is the desire to belong. According to Adler the ability to participate in a group and the willingness to contribute are prerequisites for adequate social functioning; lack of these abilities results in social maladjustment.

Group experiences not only provide a sense of belonging but also help patients realize that they are not alone in having problems. Group situations have the potential for reducing a patient's feeling of stigma related to his illness through discussion and comparison with other members. Further, the ongoing association with others in a group may decrease the person's feelings of inferiority and isolation and increase his feelings of self-worth by providing an experience in which the patient belongs.

Groups can also serve as appropriate situations in which ideas and beliefs can be tested. If an individual's concept of self is determined to some extent by the reactions of others to him, a group situation should provide rewarding opportunities for his obtaining feedback on how others react to what he says or does.

Although the group situation has been found useful for helping chronic schizophrenic patients learn to interact with each other, some schizophrenic individuals have difficulty verbalizing when in a group. Often interaction seems to be easier for these patients when they are participating in some activity. The activity may serve as a stimulus for discussion by providing a starting point for the conversation.

ACTIVITY GROUP THERAPY

As mentioned, activity group therapy uses simple tasks to facilitate both group discussion and practice in learning new behaviors that may ease readjustment to the social environment outside the hospital. In activity groups members are encouraged to direct their attention to a group goal outside themselves. Since patients who have been hospitalized for psychiatric reasons may tend to be preoccupied with themselves, the externalization needed to heed a group goal may in itself be advantageous. Activity group therapy enables members to do things for themselves as well as for one another as they learn to cooperate in carrying out a group goal. Group members can be provided with opportunities that allow for practice in activities of everyday living. For example, members can practice meal preparation including budgeting and shopping as well as the actual cooking and serving of the food.

As members work together both individually and within the activity group they often receive cues from other members as to what impact their communications are having. Members are often better able to accept criticism and sanctions from one another than from the leader.

Activity group therapy may help chronic scizophrenic patients by providing an opportunity for the enhancement of their self-esteem through identification with a successfully functioning group. Mentally ill persons are particularly susceptible to loneliness and alienation; they often feel like a perennial isolate, a marginal man, an outsider. Group members may believe that they have suffered more than any other living person. Identification with others having similar fears and difficulties may help members realize that others have experienced many of the traumas which they have endured. Furthermore, members may recognize some of their own maladaptive behavior patterns by observing similar patterns in other members. While a member may be unable to tolerate direct confrontation because of his low self-esteem, he may gain self-awareness through identification with others in the group.

Activity group therapy meetings usually include from 10 to 12 members who meet for 1 hour a week; there are at least 12 meetings but the group may be ongoing for an extended period of time. The initial step in conducting an activity group meeting is to establish rapport among the members. The leader may introduce himself first and then ask each member to do likewise. It is important for the leader to address each member by his surname to convey respect and to preserve the individual's dignity. After the members are introduced to each other the leader assists the members in focusing their attention on the world of reality. A variety of techniques are available for encouraging the members to think about a selected topic for discussion.

Drawing provides a useful medium for facilitating activity groups. Art is used to help psychiatric patients communicate the fears, anticipations, and experiences of emotional dysfunction. One approach is to provide the members with art supplies and ask them to draw a picture. Next the therapist asks each person to describe and discuss his picture; in order to participate in an activity members must direct their attention to an object outside themselves. If distortions are observed constantly in the drawings it is important to point these out to the member. By so doing reality rather than fantasy is reinforced.

Reading aloud is used in activity group therapy to encourage interaction with others as well as to foster self-confidence and a sense of personal worth. Reading aloud provides the patient with a specific medium for verbalization. For many it is easier to read aloud than to articulate thoughts and feelings. Once the individual begins to verbalize through his reading he may be encouraged to discuss what the passage means or conveys to him. Each positive interaction offers the possibility of further attempts to communicate. In terms of reintegration into the environment individuals are often forced to read rules, conditions, and other stipulations prior to signing agreements essential to daily living. Official documents as well as pleasure reading can be included in group meetings.

Poetry is beneficial as a tool for activity group therapy because of the rhythm and the style in which the words are linked, which tend to be pleasant to the listener. Since the sounds of poetry are different from those of normal speech, poetry tends to capture the individual's attention and interest. Also, patients who read poetry are afforded an opportunity to discuss abstract topics and this provides the leader with some clues as to the degree of concrete thinking present in each individual.

Following the period of activity group therapy that is devoted to the activity, the group leader gets the members to participate in a discussion. The various visual aids used in the first part of the meeting serve as stimuli for this discussion. During this phase of the meeting, the leader uses techniques commonly associated with group therapy such as clarification, verbalization of feelings, and provision of feedback.

ACTIVITY GROUP THERAPY: CASE ILLUSTRATION

The patients in the study described were se-lected from two locked wards of a large psy-chiatric hospital. One ward housed 71 patients; the other, 69. The patients ranged in age from 23 to 83 and had been hospitalized for as short a time as 1 month to as long as 44 years. Twelve patients, 6 from each ward, were selected ran-domly to serve as control subjects; 12 patients were also selected to serve as experimental subjects. Six members of each group were male and 6 were female. The 12 subjects in the ex-perimental group met with the group leader twice a week for 12 weeks for activity group therapy meetings.

All subjects, including the patients in the control group, were asked to respond to Os-good's semantic differential scale for self-con-cept. Participants in both groups were given the Semantic Differential Scale on three dif-ferent occasions: prior to beginning activity group therapy, midway in the series of meet-ings, and following termination of the meet-ings. Activity group sessions were held during early evening and lasted approximately 1½ hours. Attendance was regular and only 4 of the 12 group members missed any meetings. Each patient was encouraged to participate but no one was forced to do so.

At times members of the group selected ac-tivities for the meetings; otherwise the leader chose the activity. Selected activities included drawing, reading short stories and poetry, look-ing at pictures, baking, and listening to one of the members play the piano. At times the dis-cussion centered around the activity; at other times the patients discussed thoughts and feel-ings elicted by the activity.

Early in the series of meetings, selected members took responsibility for various tasks without being asked by the leader to do so. For example, at each meeting the men arranged the chairs around the table and also assisted in carrying supplies to the group room for making coffee. The leader encouraged members who knew how to make coffee to assist other group members in the preparation of the coffee.

The leader encouraged the members to in-troduce themselves to each other and to call one another by name. This attempt was made to combat the lack of self-identity that patients frequently experience as a result of institutional-ization. The leader attempted to set an example by calling each patient by name when she spoke to one of the group.

Initially most of the group members lacked self-confidence and the ability to do things for themselves. Changes were observed in the be-havior of various members who became more self-directive. Throughout the series of meet-ings the leader encouraged members to do things both for themselves and for others. She also assisted members in examining some of their reactions regarding the deprivations that they experienced in the hospital. At first the members did not express negative feelings to-ward the hospital but rather talked about what a nice place it was in which to live. One tech-nique employed by the leader was to point out that she would not consider the hospital such a nice place if what the patients had described actually occurred. The members apparently realized that they did not have to say that the hospital was a nice place in order to be accepted by the leader and several members began to talk about the negative experiences for which they needed to find solutions.

Another therapeutic measure used during the group meetings was clarification. Each member was urged to confront another member when circumstances invited such action. For ex-ample, on occasion group members used such large quantities of cream and sugar in their cof-fee that little was left for others. When this oc-curred the member who felt left out was sup-ported as he discussed his reaction to this lack of supplies. While the leader supported attempts at intervention by members she would not speak for them.

The patients assigned to the control condition did not participate in activity group therapy, nor did the investigator have any formal contact with them other than at times of data collection.

Analysis of the data concerning self-concepts, using a t-test for correlated means, revealed that the self-concept scores for the patients who participated in activity group therapy increased during the group sessions. There was no significant difference on the first test between the group of subjects who participated in activity group therapy and the group who did not. There were significant change score differences within the experimental group but no significant differences within the control group. The lack of a significant difference in the control group suggests that the self-concepts of the control subjects who received custodial treatment and did not participate in activity group therapy were not positively influenced by the daily ward life. These subjects received little if any recognition from ward personnel and other patients. A significant difference in the experimental group from the first to the second test suggests that activity group therapy enhanced self-concept.

IMPLICATIONS

Since schizophrenic patients are frequently described as being "nonverbal, withdrawn, confused and disturbed conceptually and perceptually" (Hogarty, 1971), they can easily get lost in the hospital as well as in the community once discharged. Activity groups provide a sheltered opportunity for individuals to learn and practice interaction as well as the basic skills essential to independent living. While this chapter has focused on the chronically mentally ill, hospitalized patient, group activities such as these have a wide range of transferability.

For an individual to maintain himself external to an institutional setting he must be able to relate to the environment in which he lives. Each one must have the ability to perform a variety of essential activities. Basic to any attempt to reintegrate long-term hospitalized patients into the community is a belief on the part of the patients that they can manage their lives without the support of hospitalization.

Activity groups provide an arena where patients can practice tasks as well as experiment with ways of talking with others. In the group the risk is minimal in that the leader continuously encourages and models acceptance as well as honest information as to how the patient appears to others. The groups furnish a controlled external environment that for many proves to be a transitional setting between hospitalization and increased levels of independence.

References

Adler, A.: The practice and theory of individual psychology, London, 1924, Kegan Paul Co.

Branden, N.: The psychology of self-esteem, San Francisco, 1969, W. H. Freeman & Co., Publishers.

Combs, A.: The professional education of teachers, Boston, 1965, Allyn & Bacon, Inc.

Cooley, C. H.: Human nature and social order, New York, 1902, Charles Schribner's Sons.

Hogarty, G.: The plight of schizophrenics in modern treatment programs, Hosp. Community Psychiatry **22:**197-203, 1971.

Jersild, A. T.: Child psychology, Englewood Cliffs, N. J., 1960, Prentice-Hall, Inc.

Labenne, W., and Green, B.: Educational implications of self-concept theory, Santa Monica. Calif., 1969, Goodyear Publishing Co., Inc.

Marcel, G.: Homo viator, New York, 1962, Harper & Brother.

Mead, G. H.: Mind, self and society, Chicago, 1934, The University of Chicago Press.

Purkey, W.: Self-concept and school achievement, Englewood Cliffs, N. J., 1970, Prentice-Hall, Inc.

Rogers, C.: A theory of therapy, personality and interpersonal relationships as developed in the client-centered framework. In Koch, S., ed.: Psychology: a study of science, Vol. 3, New York, 1959, McGraw-Hill Book Co.

Rosenberg, M.: Which significant others? Am. Behav. Sci. **16:**829-830, 1973.

Sullivan, H. S.: The interpersonal theory of psychiatry, New York, 1953, W. W. Norton & Co., Inc.

Wylie, R.: The self-concept, ed. 2, Lincoln, 1974, University of Nebraska.

CHAPTER 17

Family therapy as prevention

ELIZABETH MORRISON

Systems exist at a variety of levels. There are two general ways to look at systems: one is to define the universe as the system and to put everything else in the perspective of subsystems; the other is to take naturally occurring systems such as societies and define their component parts as subsystems. In the second approach, families are considered the building blocks of society as well as a subsystem of the larger societal system; individual family members are subsystems of the family. If the family is thought of as a building block of society it is placed in an important ecological position. In the last decade an increasing amount of attention has been paid to the family. Although anthropologists have realized for years that the family is the microcosm of society it has taken other disciplines a long time to appreciate this idea.

Families can also be thought of as naturally occurring systems with all systems principles being applicable to the family as a unit. Some of these principles can be stated as follows:

1. All systems have structure.
2. All systems have function.
3. The totality of the system is greater than the sum of its parts.
4. The parts of a system are interrelated.
5. Dysfunction in one of the parts affects every other part.
6. It is the last two principles that are the focus of this chapter.

The parts of a family system are the individual members of that family. Members of a family are assigned roles based on their relationships to one another. The roles shift as the relationships shift. A female member of a family can assume the role of wife, mother, daughter, sister, niece, or aunt depending on the reciprocal role assumption of another family member. Similarly a male family member can become father, son, husband, brother, nephew, or uncle depending on the relationship. Each role assignment carries with it different behaviors and attitudes; therefore it is important to consider that within the context of a family system no one member is ever the same all the time. This can be demonstrated empirically by asking various family members to describe one particular family member. The responses are based on the reciprocal role relationship the individual has with that family member.

Family therapy as a treatment modality emerged in an attempt to make sense out of how people get to be the way they are. Traditional cause and effect thinking stated that when an individual developed a problem the therapist assisted the individual to search for the cause of the problem as well as for a treatment or cure of the problem. Family therapists operating on systems principles are not concerned with cause and effect thinking but rather they pay attention to how the parts of the system interrelate. Dysfunction in an individual is thought to be a signal of dysfunction in the system since all individuals function as part of a family system. A variety of ways exist for describing dysfunction but for the purposes of this discussion dysfunction is defined as emotional disruption in a family—as opposed to structural or functional disruption. In order to further explicate and clarify how emotionality affects the interrelationship of the parts of a system and how dysfunction occurs, selected concepts, their practical application, and preventive implications follow.

ANXIETY

Anxiety is the emotional glue that holds families together; it is the motivating energy in relationships. All systems require some kind of motivating or driving force to function. Some systems operate on electrical energy; others, on chemical energy; and still others, on solar energy. Families operate on emotional energy or anxiety. Without an emotional bond a family might just as well be a collectivity of individuals.

Peplau (1963) delineated four levels of anxiety. At the first level (+) an individual is alert, can see relations and connections, and is able to use problem-solving steps. At the second level (++) the individual's perceptual field narrows and he fails to notice all but details of the immediate focus; yet he is still able to use problem-solving skills surrounding the immediate focus. At level three (+++) the individual's perceptual field is greatly reduced to either a single detail or scattered details; he is unaware of other stimuli in the environment as he focuses on gaining relief instead of on problem-solving. At level four (++++), known as panic, the individual emotionally disorganizes and is unable to attend to anything but minutiae that are distorted out of realistic proportion. At this level his behavior is random and chaotic, focusing on anything that will produce immediate relief.

Most people become aware of anxiety when it reaches unpleasant or uncomfortable levels—++ to +++. The sensation of anxiety is

familiar to everyone although its manifestations vary from one person to another. Anxiety is experienced as sweaty palms, a knot in the stomach, weak knees, or being uptight. At the level of perceived discomfort, the most usual response to anxiety is to do something to make the anxiety go away. Making it go away takes one of two characteristic forms—fight or flight. A third way to deal with anxiety—using it for learning—is not usually employed without conscious effort and intent because the perceived experience of anxiety is so unpleasant. The use of anxiety in the service of learning is one of the goals of family therapy. A family can range from being minimally to being maximally disorganized when the perceived level of anxiety increases. It is therefore important to teach family members about anxiety and its effects as well as to help them investigate what it is that triggers increased anxiety in their family. Further, anxiety can be used by the family members to learn about themselves. In each family issues come up that evoke increased anxiety in its members. The content of the issues is unique to each family although the experience of increased tension is common to all families.

A clue to the content issues in any family is gained from touching on topics that no one will bring up at a family gathering because someone will be "upset." Family secrets are indicative of family issues. Family issues may also include those behaviors that no member dares not to do for fear of increasing the anxiety in the family. Some of these issues are readily identifiable by families, with each member's being consciously aware of them. Other issues are kept out of awareness so that the anxiety surrounding them may or may not be evident to family members. For example, in many families where one member has a drinking problem every member is aware of the problem but no one mentions it to the person who has the problem. In other families in which education is an issue no one dares not to go to college and each member would most likely say he wants to go to college as he is aware of the anxiety involved in not going.

Anxiety can be empathically transmitted from person to person (Sullivan, 1953). In a family, members can experience anxiety about a certain issue, event, or person without ever having first-hand experience with that issue, event, or person. Suppose the father comes home one evening upset over something that happened at work that day. Without his having to tell his wife and children they notice that "something is wrong" and subsequently each responds with anxiety of his own: the mother may burn dinner and the children may forget to feed the dog. While only the father experienced the initial upset the subjective discomfort was communicated empathically in the family.

An operating principle in family therapy is that all families who come for help are anxious. Families generally have tried everything they can think of to solve whatever problem exists before they seek help; they often have exhausted their resources and consider therapy a last resort. It is thus imperative to assess the level of anxiety in the family. Usually that level of anxiety is high enough so that the family can no longer think clearly about the problem. The first step is to assist the family in lowering the operating level of anxiety so that thinking and problem solving can occur. This can be accomplished by asking each family member what he or she usually does to relax when tension is high. Asking specific questions about the problem—how it began, when it began, the context in which it occurred, and what would make it better, what would make it worse, and what they have tried to solve the problem—also aids in engaging the thinking processes and reducing anxiety. Taking a family history and putting the problem in the context of the family system is another way to reduce anxiety to workable levels. Teaching the family about levels of anxiety and how they affect perception, thinking, and functioning is of value not only in the immediate situation but also as a preventive step in helping family members to assess their own levels of anxiety and learn how each responds to increased tension. Regardless of which method of anxiety intervention is selected it is essential that the therapist remain calm in the presence of an anxious family. He must be aware of the empathic nature of anxiety as well as the issues that evoke his own anxiety in order not to become caught up in the prevailing atmosphere. Once the therapist's own level of anxiety reaches a certain point, work with the family becomes ineffective.

At the same time that the therapist is assessing the anxiety quotient in the family it is also helpful to assess the amount and number of stressors to which the family has recently been subjected. Some families seem to be able to cope with considerable stress before problems become apparent in the system; others seem to tolerate very little stress before dysfunction occurs. Questions about births, deaths, job changes, geographic moves, divorces, and marriages should be asked to evaluate stress factors in the year or two before the current problem developed. The variation in stress tolerance in different families can be accounted for by the level of differentiation operative in the family.

DIFFERENTIATION OF SELF

Differentiation of self is a concept developed by Bowen (1976) and can be thought of as being roughly equivalent to emotional maturity. In essence differentiation involves the ability to separate the logical processes such as thinking from the emotional processes of feeling and to take personal responsibility for one's own behavior. According to Bowen, two major forces tug at an individual: one is the force for togetherness—a force that compels a person to be part of a group, to go along, and to be liked and accepted; the other is the force for individuation and compels a person to be an individual, to stand on his own, to make rational decisions.

When an individual is born into a family, he becomes an automatic part of an ongoing sea of togetherness; the sea of togetherness is the emotional system in the family. Every newborn needs care and nurturing and is dependent on others to meet survival needs. It is not too long, however, before the individual begins to assert a developing self, testing the limits of the family boundaries as well as the boundaries of each existing individual in the nuclear family. Infants and children are the best researchers in the world. If a rule holds true in the kitchen at lunchtime, does it also hold true in the living room at bedtime and in the bathroom at bath time? Each child tests out not only the behavioral limits in the family but also the emotional limits. How many times is it possible to ignore mother's requests or commands before she gets angry? How far is it possible to push brother or sister before getting walloped? What is the best way to approach father to get something?

As the child tests the emotional waters in the family he detests those topics and issues that are connected with anxiety and avoids them. If mother gets anxious when her son approaches new situations and attempts to protect him, the son will become anxious about new situations and learn to look for protection. If a mother becomes anxious when her daughter makes decisions that differ from hers and subsequently imposes her own decisions, her daughter will learn to count on others to make decisions for her.

An individual's level of emotional differentiation is largely dependent on the degree of emotional differentiation of the parents. In general the more open and flexible the family system is, the more differentiated the individuals in the family will be. Conversely, the more closed and rigid the family system is, the less differentiated the individuals in the family will be. Criteria for evaluating the level of differentiation include decision making, the degree of personal responsibility, and the ability to discriminate between thoughts and feelings.

It is not uncommon to hear the words "I feel" when the speaker really intends to convey "I think" or "I believe." The statement "I feel that nurses are qualified health professionals" is inaccurate in that the intent of the statement is a thought or a belief. Feelings have to do with emotions: "I feel sad," "I feel happy," "I feel tired." Thoughts have to do with ideas or beliefs: "I think the sun will rise tomorrow," "I believe the world is round," "I think families operate on systems principles." Most people are able to discriminate between their thoughts and feelings when the difference is called to their attention, even though common usage is inaccurate. There are some people, however, who are unable to discriminate between thoughts and feelings and literally do not see the difference between the two. To the extent that people are able to discriminate they make decisions based either on principles of behavior or on what "feels right." Those who make decisions based on what feels right are people who are more concerned with maintaining personal comfort than they are with attaining planned goals. It requires a great deal of time and energy to maintain the status quo and to keep things comfortable. When people use considerable energy in maintaining comfort they do not have the time left either to make long-range plans or to take steps to implement their plans.

The idea of personal responsibility is not pervasive in our culture. What is far more usual is the casting of blame, fault finding, and scapegoating. When a problem occurs it is often attributed to sources outside the self instead of realistically evaluating the part one might play in the problem. This is a carryover from traditional cause and effect thinking: either the cause is seen outside the person with the problem or the person with the problem causes everyone else in the family to be upset. Individuals with a high level of differentiation tend to take a greater degree of personal responsibility for their feelings, thoughts, and behavior. They do not typically use such phrases as "he makes me angry" or "She makes me happy" but rather phrases such as "I get angry when he does that" or "I'm happy when I'm with her." The difference may seem subtle but even semantically it reflects the difference in taking credit for one's own feelings as opposed to attributing them to others.

In therapy one of the major emphases is placed on considering each person in the family as an individual and examining how each participates in, and perpetuates, the present problem. Given the operating principle that it takes at least two to have a problem the task then becomes one of assisting each family member to examine how he contributes to the problem. This is not a particularly easy task because in some families the problem does seem to reside clearly in one person: when dad drinks, son misbehaves and mother gets depressed; it is difficult to determine the source of the problem. However no matter where the problem seems to reside family members have defined some behavior in another as a problem for them and that is a convenient place to start. The discovery of how each family member perceives and reacts to the problem provides beginning clues to how each member of the family participates in keeping the problem going. It also provides data about what each might do to change his participation in the problem during the problem-solving process.

In many families there is a tendency to blame and to attack others while at the same time defending the self. If the family therapist focuses on how each individual is experiencing what is happening instead of listening to reports about how bad another person is he or she can short-circuit the blaming and attacking tendencies in the system. As family members relate how they are affected by whatever problem exists they also become aware of behaviors that may be ineffectual and inappropriate in dealing with their own reactions. They also be-

come aware that the only person anyone can do anything about is oneself. Although most people recognize intellectually that it is impossible to change another person, many people keep trying to do so. As a matter of fact some people make a career of trying to change others. It is no small task to focus on one's own reactions, thoughts, and behavior because the tug is so great to report about another person. The therapist must stay alert to when the emphasis shifts to another and maintain focus on the individual at hand. The desired outcome is for each family member to take responsibility for his own feelings, thoughts, and behavior and for each to define some kind of stand in relation to the problem as well as in relation to other family members.

In attempting to assist family members to discriminate between thoughts and feelings, to describe decision-making patterns, and to assess personal responsibility the family therapist assists each member to more clearly define a perception of self in the family system. When the members are able to appreciate how they influence, and in turn are influenced by, other family members the chances for continued blaming are diminished. This provides the basis for a more thoughtful examination of behavior the next time a problem appears or when the stress level in the family rises.

TRIANGLES

According to Bowen (1976), the basic stable unit of human interaction is the triangle. When tension increases in a two-person system, or dyad, a third person or issue is triangled in to relieve the tension. Since dyads are basically unstable, it is not long in any kind of interaction before a triangle exists. Triangles involve the irresistible urge to talk about another person. Characteristically, Bowen adds, an emotional triangle has two relatively calm sides and one relatively uncomfortable side. In times of low stress the preferred position is to be a member of the comfortable dyad; the outside position is to be avoided. In times of increased stress the outside position is the preferred one; the twosome position is uncomfortable.

An easily identifiable, culturally sanctioned triangle is one that includes a wife, a husband, and his mother, which is known as the mother-in-law syndrome. This triangle begins operation before marriage; the emotional intensity escalates after marriage and it is then that the discomfort becomes apparent to the parties involved. When two individuals engage in a relationship whose goal is marriage, at some point each will be introduced to the family of the other. This introduction can be either by way of information given about the family or by way of actual contact. In most relationships both types of introduction occur. During the time of engagement and courtship each individual experiences the need to impress or please the family of the other in order to be accepted by the family.

There are some common cultural patterns involved in the process of acceptance into the family of one's spouse. One pattern is for the wife to actually take on the husband's family by becoming increasingly responsible for doing such things as remembering birthdays and anniversaries and maintaining contact via letters and telephone calls. Since mothers are the emotional caretakers in most families, the son's wife may have frequent contact with her husband's mother. It is through this relationship that the facilitation of acceptance becomes most important. The wife soon finds that she is receiving all kinds of information about her husband from her mother-in-law. Since some of this information is positive and some is negative the wife begins to experience subtle pressure to do something about her husband, either to make him better or quit making him worse. She may also experience cues that if she were a better wife he would be a better husband and son. This then leads either to covert or overt conflict between the mother-in-law and daughter-in-law about the way in which the new

household should be run and how the new relationship should be handled.

Interestingly enough, often a husband seems oblivious to the developing struggle between his wife and mother. From the husband's standpoint his marriage is working well and his relationship with his mother is tolerable. If the conflict is brought to his attention he may disregard it, take sides with one or the other, or account for it by stating that women certainly have a hard time getting along with each other. What has in fact happened is that the wife has gotten triangled into the relationship between her husband and his mother in her attempt to be accepted into the family.

During periods of low stress the husband and wife are comfortable with one another and are able to discuss objectively his mother's "interference" in their relationship since the mother-in-law is in the outside position. During times of increased stress the husband ignores the conflict between his wife and mother and maintains the comfortable outside position. This pattern can go on uninterrupted for years. Some people believe that this is the way life is and that there are some things that just need to be tolerated. What people often fail to do is to look at the part each plays in maintaining the triangle. A series of steps can be undertaken to break up the triangle and to achieve a more satisfactory way of relating. One beginning step is for the wife to give the husband's mother back to the husband and to stay out of their ongoing emotional relationship. Although this is difficult to do because it involves going against cultural proscriptions, it is possible to accomplish.

When a husband and wife present themselves for family therapy with the stated problem of difficulties with the in-law system the therapist first assesses who is responsible for what in each family. The most common complaint is that the wife feels inadequate, overwhelmed, and angry about her relationship or lack of relationship with her husband's mother. The therapist's next step is to obtain a history of how that relationship evolved and on what it is based. It is not uncommon for a wife to feel that she has no support from her husband in dealing with her mother-in-law and she subsequently blames her husband for not controlling his mother's behavior. It often emerges that the wife is overinvolved in the husband's family and is assuming far more responsibility for dealing with them than the husband is. The family therapist proceeds to help the wife evaluate what is realistic responsibility to her husband's family and what is not realistic. The wife has a definite relationship with her husband's mother but the relationship revolves around a third person—either the husband or a child. As issues are identified between the husband and his mother the wife is encouraged to stay out of those issues and leave their resolution or nonresolution to her husband and his mother instead of jumping in and either protecting or defending her husband. It is fascinating how often a wife thinks she must protect her husband from his own family.

As a case in point, one couple stated that the husband's mother was disappointed and dissatisfied with the job her son had chosen for his career. She never discussed this with her son directly but would bring up the subject regularly with his wife in letters, telephone calls, and whenever the two were together on visits. The wife spent a great deal of time explaining how it was that her husband had chosen his job and defending his right to do so; as a result she consistently ended up being angry with her mother-in-law because she did not understand her son and was not supportive of what he was doing. When the wife reported these conversations to her husband he responded by shrugging his shoulders and commenting that his mother had always been a difficult person to deal with. He was not at all uncomfortable with the situation and only came to therapy to help his wife calm down since she seemed so upset about his mother.

The initial goal was to assist the wife to become less reactive to the mother-in-law's input and then to put the issue of the mother's dissatisfaction with her son back between mother and son where it belonged. One technique that has proven effective in many instances where defensiveness and frustration are issues is to encourage the defensive one to agree with statements that had previously been defended; that is, the next time the mother-in-law complains that her son's work was a poor choice the daughter-in-law is encouraged to agree rather than argue with her. She is counseled to list all of the material things the couple might have if indeed he did have a better job. She is further encouraged to describe that she has tried everything she can think of to get her husband to reconsider changing jobs but he remains adamant. She then is to appeal to her mother-in-law for help in talking to her son directly about what can be done. The purpose of this strategy is not to change the mother-in-law's behavior in any way, but to give the wife the option of not being caught up in the old pattern, which has in the past led predictably to anger, defensiveness, and dislike of the mother-in-law.

It is amazing what can happen when one individual changes a usual pattern of reaction in a triangle. One result is a fairly dramatic relief of anxiety; the other is that the rest of the system will respond by getting upset and trying to get the person who has made the change, even if the change is in a positive direction, to revert to predictable ways of behaving. This latter point must be emphasized regularly when working with families. Whenever one person changes the system reacts by attempting to force the changed individual back to the usual patterns of behavior. This illustrates the operating principle that things will get worse before they get better. It takes some measure of courage to maintain change when other people are saying that things are terrible, that the person who changed has either gone crazy or does not care anymore, or that he is bad or worthless.

However if the change is maintained in spite of system pressure the system will adapt to the change in one way or another. This, of course, involves a risk on the part of the person who is changing.

Family therapists can easily become involved in triangles. One of the most frequent ways is to see one member of a family who spends a lot of time reporting to the therapists about the other members of the family. If the therapist begins to see family members in the same way that the person reporting about them sees them, the therapist is caught in an emotional triangle. It is important to remember that every member of a family has distinct and individual impressions of every other family member and that perceptions are colored by the relationship each has with the other. If the therapist accepts reported perceptions as "true" without validating or checking out his own perceptions then triangling will occur. One useful way to avoid getting caught in an emotional triangle is by focusing on the person at hand and simultaneously attempting to discover what part he plays in the ongoing emotional system.

Since triangles are potentially dysfunctional (Fogarty, 1974), the goal of family therapy is to "detriangle" which means encouraging a person-to-person relationship between members of the family. Instead of spending time talking about the mother-in-law, the husband and wife are encouraged to spend time talking about their relationship. Also rather than talking about their husband and son the wife and mother-in-law are encouraged to talk about their own relationship. The husband and mother are discouraged from talking about the wife and the husband is encouraged to talk to his mother about their relationship. This not only provides a strategy for more open and direct communication in families but also diminishes distortions and prevents the perpetuation of triangles in the system.

Teaching clients about triangles and how they operate in systems has a preventive po-

tential. Individuals become increasingly aware of the part they play in keeping anxiety and tension operative in the system and how that tension is maintained and perpetuated. If individuals can achieve that perspective, particularly in periods of calm, they have a beginning knowledge base and experience on which to draw the next time tension arises in the family system. They are thus better prepared to consider their own behavior in dealing with future problems. Another preventive aspect is to offset the transmission of ongoing family issues to the next generation.

MULTIGENERATIONAL TRANSMISSION PROCESS

Bowen (1976) states that unresolved emotional issues in families are passed down from generation to generation and have the potential for evoking increasing intensity and dysfunction. This can be demonstrated by collecting at least a three-generational history and identifying recurring issues. It is not at all unusual to discover that there are issues apparent generationally that either are consistent or skip a generation. For instance alcohol ingestion is a pattern that can frequently be traced generationally. Great-grandparents may have had difficulty with alcohol; the grandparents were teetotalers; the parents had trouble with alcohol and the children won't touch a drop. The issue of alcohol is an ongoing one but it is handled differently in each generation. When such generational issues are identified it is possible to intervene by developing an awareness of the issues, by observing how the patterns affect the current generation, and by implementing strategies that may preclude the transaction of the same issue to future generations.

This theoretical concept has the most preventive potential for families in therapy but, as with any preventive measure, it is difficult to assess the outcome without longitudinal generational studies. Since family therapy as a way of thinking is still young, the results of longitudinal study are not as yet available. However, it is the responsibility of those invested in family therapy to design and undertake carefully constructed research protocols in an effort to test out hypotheses and to modify approaches based on the results of those hypotheses.

SUMMARY

Family therapy departs from the more traditional forms of therapy in that it considers problems in living as indications of difficulty in a system—the family—instead of problems in an individual. Systems concepts are not concerned with cause and effect but rather with interaction and with the interplay of emotional forces that evoke dysfunction in the family. The dysfunction may be exhibited by one particular family member and is considered a signal of distress in the family rather than dysfunction in that particular person. All people are a part of systems and influence, and are influenced by, those systems. The family is chosen as a focus since the most intense emotional relationships are found in the family and since the family system by virtue of its intensity has the most profound impact in shaping a person's life-style.

Family therapy is not only a treatment modality but also a vehicle for educating individuals about systems principles and concepts. The ultimate goal of any therapy is the prevention of dysfunction. Whether or not this actually occurs is yet to be determined through meticulous research and follow-up. In most instances people do the best they possibly can in any given situation. Through the use of family therapy and education, health care professionals can provide information to families that will enable them to have more specific and appropriate tools at their disposal for negotiating their way through this difficult business of living in a complex technological society. If in fact families are the building blocks of society then strengthening families will result in a strengthened society.

References

Bowen, M.: Theory in the practice of psychotherapy. In Guerin, P. J., Jr., ed.: Family therapy, New York, 1976, Gardner Press, Inc.

Fogarty, T.: Fusion in the family system. In Andres, F. D., and Lorio, J. P., eds.: Georgetown family symposia, Washington, D. C., 1974, Georgetown University Medical Center, vol. 1.

Peplau, H. E.: A working definition of anxiety. In Burd, S. F., and Marshall, M. A., eds.: Some clinical approaches to psychiatric nursing, New York, 1963, The Macmillan Co.

Sullivan, H. S.: The interpersonal theory of psychiatry, New York, 1953, W. W. Norton & Co., Inc.

CHAPTER 18

Therapeutic intervention with children through art

DONNA BLAIR BOOE

Art as a symbolic means of communication can be viewed both historically and evolutionarily. The history of art provides a visual index to prehistory and to civilizations through the ages in that art is found in every culture and gives testimony to the universal importance of man's use of the graphic elements in his "expressive" life. Whatever its purpose, it is a uniquely human experience. Art has been a part of man's history for thousands of years and can be traced to the earliest cave drawings of the late Ice Age with the discovery of beautiful rock paintings such as those found in the caves of Altamira, Spain, dated from 30,000 to 12,000 B.C. (Lommel, 1966). The fact that most of these 150 paintings were of bison and other animals is significant in the context of the environment. Early man's survival depended on the animals and this late Ice Age was the high point of the hunting culture. In considering the paintings of untutored prehistoric man one cannot escape concluding that art is an elemental activity.

Art forms are present in all cultures no matter how simple or complex; apparently an innate creative impulse exists in man. Similar beginnings in the development of children's art forms were demonstrated in a cross-cultural study done by Kellogg (1967). Drawings by children from each of the 30 different cultures in the study were so similar that the natural origin of the child could not be determined. It was only

after the child perceived his own particular culture and developed his own style that differences were noted.

Limited attention was given to the systematic study of children's art until Ballard's (1958) work in 1912, when he reported on the subject matter of approximately 20,000 children living in London. He found that interest in human figure drawings declined at about the age of 9, then rose slightly, and dropped again after the age of 12. The order of preference in subjects drawn was as follows:

Boys: Ships, miscellaneous objects, plant life, houses, human beings, vehicles, animals, weapons, and landscapes.
Girls: Plant life, houses, miscellaneous objects, human beings, vehicles, animals, weapons, and landscapes.

Considering the era when this study was done and the fact that England was a great naval power it is not surprising that the boys' preference for subject matter was ships. It appears that, again, as in the cave drawings of animals by Paleolithic man, the social environment influences the subject matter chosen for drawings.

PURPOSE OF ART

Artistic expression is symbolic and has meaning both for the artist and for others. Mumford (1952) writes that through the "detachable and durable form of symbols" man can abstract and

179

represent parts of himself, his experience, and his environment. Through these symbols man's essential experience of life can be recalled, perpetuated, and shared with others.

According to Read (1958), mental images are translated into a medium of communication in the form of speech and gestures. In addition, man elaborates various graphic symbols that become a medium of communication by agreement between two or more people. The symbols may be arbitrary, obscure, or abstract; children's first drawings may be quite abstract or nonfigurative and have no basis in immediate visual experience. These drawings are representations with imaginary associations rather than conscious attempts to imitate and translate images into graphic form. Children's drawings represent original self-expression; they represent how children perceive reality. Similarly Kris (1952) believes that pictures not only convey a thought or meaning but "catch reality of the man who is able to see them. Seeing contains both elements: that of recognizing what is known, the elements of thought, and that of actually holding reality."

Grozinger (1955) alludes to the emotional aspect of art rather than the visual by saying that children make statements about themselves rather than the objects and figures they draw. DiLeo (1970) thinks that children's drawings represent mental impressions "imbued with emotional and imaginative elements." In contrast to Freud's view, Jung and Fromm have pointed out that artistic symbols, like dreams, serve to reveal their referents, not veil them. Jung further notes that symbols are "pregnant with meaning" and "image and meaning are identical" (Arnheim, 1967a). Read (1958) claims that the child's graphic activity is a specialized medium of communication with its own characteristics; it is governed by inner subjective feelings and not determined by objective realism.

Artistic expression represents an attempt to communicate with the intention of affecting others. Further, artistic expression is not an ex-

perience for its own sake but rather an overture that demands a response from others.

Berlo (1960) describes the primary purpose of communication as that of altering the original relationship between self and the environment. More specifically it is "to affect with intent," the basic purpose being to reduce the probability of becoming a target of external forces and to increase the probability of becoming an influencing agent.

Hayakawa (1966), in his writing on communication with children, says that first there is the vast area of nonverbal communication that takes place through touching, holding, and caressing long before speech becomes a communicating vehicle. After speech is established there is always the constant problem of interpretations. Significantly he points out that one of the things we tend to overlook in our culture is the tremendous value of the acknowledgment that a message is being sent. Agreement or disagreement is not the issue but rather acknowledgement of the message, which says in effect, "I acknowledge you and your thoughts." Through the stimulus of art, messages can be communicated. These cues provide the nurse with an opportunity to acknowledge and reinforce personal worth.

Society's tendency to move toward complexity increases stress. In childhood there are unlimited stresses or anxiety-producing situations, which are compounded by the child's helplessness in controlling his environment. The way in which he interprets his experience is probably one of the most important factors that influences his adjustment to it. Awareness of the child's interpretation of a stressful situation and the meaning it has for him can be discovered through the media of art. This point was unexpectedly demonstrated to me one day in the playroom of a children's hospital:

A 9-year-old girl was admitted for diagnostic tests because of unexplained abdominal pains. Her mother was staying with her around the clock and from all overt behavior she appeared well adjusted and even happy during hospitalization. She came willingly to the playroom when it was announced that the nurse had come to take her there so she could play with others or draw. Immediately on arrival in the playroom she began to draw a house with windows, a door, a chimney, flying birds, a fence, a tree, and flowers. She became increasingly intent on her drawing; as time went on and the picture got closer to completion she said, "You know, I'm worried about something." The nurse answered, "You are? Do you know what it is?" Averting eye contact and methodically concentrating on drawing the rows of flowers outside the house she said, "Yesterday I heard my mother talking to the doctor in the hall, and he said I might not go home!" Her drawing and comments could not be discounted for they had purpose and required understanding. At this point the misunderstanding of the feared incomplete message was clarified. What actually was said was that unless the results of the tests were back from the laboratory she might not go home that next day. Fortunately, in drawing the house to which she so wanted to return she was able to express her fears, harbored and greatly elaborated on overnight. With this experience, the nurse's appreciation for art as a therapeutic modality and a means of intervention began to evolve.

INTERPRETATIONS OF ART

Art is described in a variety of ways. Art is diversionary, an escape from the real world, an expression, a representation, a release or catharsis, a therapy, a communication. However it is defined it is a mode of genuine experience and gives an indication of how reality is perceived. An art form is feeling conceptualized, organized, objectified, and expressed in significant symbolic form; it graphically states the emotional experience.

Read (1951) makes a penetrating analysis of the manner in which psychoanalysis has attempted to deal with the creative process in general and how the psychoanalyst is "concerned with the dynamics only of the esthetic experience and not with value judgments." He writes that psychoanalysis "has come to the aid of the philosophy of art in two ways. . . . the first stage was to show that art could have hidden symbolic significance and that the power of art in civilization was due to its expression of the deeper levels of personality." The second stage was more important for it showed that

"the process of symbolic transformation which is fundamental in the creative process of art is also biologically fundamental."

Creativity is not uncommon in children under stress: sublimation through drawings offers a defense of the child's ego. These creative expressions give glimpses of uncensored fantasies, provide insight, and serve a self-healing function by facilitating release. Further, new lines of communication are opened and the drawings provide a starting point for interpretation.

The value of children's art as a technique by which the child communicates about himself is becoming more and more recognized; during the last decade there has been increased interest and use of art as therapy both as a primary and as a supportive technique. Champernowne (1971), a Jungian analyst, speaks of the "uneasy partnership" of art and therapy and of the possibility that art may override the therapy. She states that with the right measure of consciousness (meaning nonexploitive) art can be healing and can be used as a means of creative change, growth and development, and transformation that is goal directed.

The usefulness and widespread applicability makes art an important therapeutic modality. Its success as a medium of communication and therapy has been demonstrated in studies of clients with psychopathology (Kramer, 1971), mental retardation (Wilson, 1977), drug abuse (Wittenberg, 1974), and various physical and physiological disorders with overlying emotional distress (Cohen, 1971; Silver, 1975). Art as an adjunctive or primary form of therapy can be practiced on an individual or group basis. The goals are similar to other forms of therapy in that resolution of conflicts, self-reliance, and growth are the desired outcomes. Approaches may vary with the therapist and depend on the needs of the client.

Interpretations of the use of art in the therapeutic process, include developmental, Gestalt, and psychoanalytical approaches. Williams and Wood (1977) approach art therapy within a developmental framework based on the work of Lowenfeld and Brittain (1970). They provide a useful resource for planning appropriate stage-related art experiences with therapeutic objectives based on four areas: behavior, communication, socialization, and preacademics. Multi-objectives are designed for five developmental stages to facilitate mastery of each level.

The Gestalt approach is taken by Rhyne (1973). Principles of Gestalt perception are used in the art experience. The active experiencing of art provides a "bridge between inner and outer reality" by which the client creates art forms and becomes the sender and receiver of self-messages. The correlation of visual perceptions with inner thoughts and feelings is made apparent through the medium of art. Selectivity of patterns seen within the total configuration become obvious and the discovery of the relationship of the parts that make up the whole has meaning for the artist. Through the perception of graphic productions, insight into the self is offered and personality integration and self-awareness are facilitated.

In a psychoanalytical interpretation of art the client's spontaneous art productions are accepted as communication in symbolic speech with interpretations of the art made by the client to the therapist (Naumburg, 1973). Art therapy can be the primary mode of treatment; however, it can also be adjunctive to any therapeutic method and need not be exclusively identified with any particular school. Kramer (1971) conceives of art therapy as essential in a therapeutic milieu that offers a mechanism to support the ego, promote maturation, and foster the development of a sense of identity.

Spontaneous drawings, according to Cohen (1971), are symbolic and serve as a canvas for revealing subconscious conflicts by tapping "primitive layers." Further, productions offer a glimpse of the client's "inner world," his traits, attitudes, behavior characteristics, personality strengths and weaknesses, and the de-

gree to which he is able to mobilize his inner resources for handling both interpersonal and intrapsychic conflicts.

Summarizing the value of spontaneous art from a psychoanalytical viewpoint, art productions are more than just a means of expression. They facilitate the conscious realization of conflicts, encourage abreaction of emotion, and promote catharsis. Rambert (1949) believes that drawings allow one access into the child's unconscious but qualifies this by saying that to understand the child's drawing it is necessary to be initiated into his logic and symbolism. She makes a most significant point: "We would never be able to understand a child's drawings if he did not explain them."

Understanding drawings and making valid interpretations of symbols in art forms is addressed by Arnheim (1967b). He notes the limitations of making one concrete symbol or object stand for another equally concrete object or representational fact by stating that this approach is arbitrary and cannot be proved. Arnheim, like Rambert, emphasizes that direct information is required to validate whether or not a particular association was or is in the conscious or unconscious mind of the artist or the interpreter.

In a study to determine if one group of health care workers could identify psychopathology from paintings, Ulman and Levy (1974) found that there were no differences in the ability to identify pathology among art therapists, other mental health professionals, and judges with no special experience in working with clients with psychiatric disorders. All three groups scored better than would occur by chance, but no one group scored better than the others. In a later study, Levy and Ulman (1974) also conclude that the ability to identify psychopathology from paintings can be improved with training.

In a study of spontaneous drawings and identification of fears in children hospitalized for orthopedic disorders, Booe (1972) demonstrates that the media of art when accompanied with dialogue can be used as a valid technique in uncovering feelings of fear. It is emphasized that the combination of the art work and the accompanying dialogue provides a more accurate picture for assessment.

ADVANTAGES OF ART AS A THERAPEUTIC TECHNIQUE

Many advantages exist in using art as a therapeutic technique with children. It can be employed effectively even with young children once they learn to scribble. Graphic communication is done physically and tactily; from birth, babies begin to express themselves in physical and tactile ways. With growth and experimentation they develop an expressive vocabulary at the preverbal level. Chocolate pudding smeared on the tray of the high chair may precede the manipulation of crayons or other media in learning to control movements and produce visual forms.

Even at the verbal level children do not have the vocabulary to express themselves or the capacity to make abstractions that adults usually possess. The difference between concrete drawings or paintings and abstract speech is obvious, and it is far more difficult to be evasive graphically than verbally. When a child draws he is usually specific about numerous details that would be left out of a strictly verbal account. Content such as expressions, clothes, body parts, omission or exaggeration of body parts, motion, and other input show up and can readily be explored.

Assessment is fundamental to the nursing practice and the actions taken by the nurse are based on assessment skills. These can be enhanced and broadened by using the media of art. The diagnostic value of projective drawing tests is well established and drawings are used to measure intelligence, emotions, and feelings as well as to screen for delays in physical and mental development.

Projective drawings obtained in intelligence and psychological test designs have a testing protocol and are prompted. Drawings and other art works used in art therapy are produced spontaneously.

In the discussion of diagnosing psychopathology from spontaneous paintings in art therapy, Levy and Ulman (1974) state that diagnostic ability can be improved with training. They recognize the limitations of making accurate diagnoses based on "talented hunches" and advocate assessment based on tested and reliable measures. Recognized psychological tests that use projective drawings could provide a means for bridging diagnosis and therapy.

The nurse is in a unique position to use spontaneous drawings and recognized psychological tests that are based on prompted drawings. These can be used singly or in combination and can help assess as well as provide cues for intervention.

Establishing a relationship is a primary factor in any therapeutic encounter and art is often the key in reaching a child who is frightened or withdrawn. Anxiety is lower during painting or drawing than in direct conversation because art, like play, is something most children naturally like to do and are enthusiastic about. Their own pleasure is reinforcing and stimulating and they feel a sense of accomplishment when another is interested in their work. Satisfaction, pleasure, and self-esteem can result from materializing a product in which the child is the master. In this omnipotent role the child can create a paper world on his own terms.

Associated with the establishment of a relationship is the facility and ease with which a diagnostic or therapeutic session can begin. Like play, art is an excellent means for assessing and interviewing because it begins immediately. Art immediately provides clues to physical and mental development as well as insight into the child's world. It is physiologically and neuromuscularly a more intense activity than verbal interaction. The child's complete involvement in a drawing usually decreases self-consciousness and allows an acceptable and productive outlet for release of tension or aggression.

One of the most significant advantages in using art is its facilitation of communication. The child usually draws things that have meaning for him. He then talks about features of the drawing that he considers to be meaningful. Involvement in drawing promotes the surfacing of feelings and enables a child to talk about things that are not easily verbalized. Safety is provided for perceived unacceptable feelings as they are readily and safely displaced onto the nonthreatening drawing.

The child may spontaneously talk about his drawing when his work is acknowledged with interest. Should spontaneous verbalization not occur, it can generally be encouraged after the drawing is completed. Interruptions are regarded as disruptions and the child needs complete freedom to create, including freedom from inquiries and prodding. Acceptance of a drawing, whether complete or incomplete, means acceptance of the child. The nurse can make a verbal overture using the drawing as the focal point. Open-ended statements that are not threatening usually will elicit willing responses from the child. Instead of saying "What is this?" or making a value judgment such as "This looks like a gun," a workable approach is to acknowledge the drawing in a positive way and say "Tell me about your picture." Dialogue is easily maintained following the child's lead. For example, when the response is a comment such as "That's the mother and she's all tied up in the spider web and being eaten," the dialogue can be continued by saying "Ooh, I wonder how it feels to be all tied up and be eaten by a spider?" Other productive leads could be "I wonder how that makes the mother feel," or the spider, or the daddy, or the children. Guided dialogue eliciting fantasies, feelings, and imagination can proceed until the child signals that it is time to terminate the discussion of that particular drawing.

Whether spontaneous speech occurs when a child draws is variable. The pleasure some children derive from their drawings is sufficient and they feel no further need to communicate. It appears that very young children who do not yet have the verbal skills to express themselves seldom vocalize during art activities but will do so when prompted (Williams and Wood, 1977). Also for some children so much psychic energy is expended in mobilizing their thoughts and executing the art work that the extra energy required to verbally communicate is just not available. Older children may say nothing or may discount their art as not worthy. Possible contributing factors include low self-esteem, inadequacy felt when comparing drawings with others in the peer group, or early socialization in an environment or school system in which discipline, structure, and order overrode the fostering of individual creative expression and actualization.

Establishing communication with children who are reticent or are unable to make contact or who are unable to draw requires innovative approaches. Attempts can be made to stimulate interest and to reduce the stress of producing a drawing or of being the center of attention. Games can be tied in with drawings and an effective technique is to suggest a game that uses art media. Taking the dominant role in playing a game while describing it takes the child off "center stage," and usually reduces his self-consciousness. He sees that the activity is progressing even if he is not initially engaging in it. Also his anxiety is lower because the interaction is displaced onto the inanimate paper.

Winnicott (1971) describes therapeutic consultations in which the "Squiggle Game" is used to get into contact with a child; this game or variations of it can be used to encourage communication. For example, initiating the encounter, the nurse says, "I've got an idea! Let's play a game of Squiggle," or Curly Q or some other word that might capture the child's interest and imagination. Then, taking a pencil or crayon, the nurse shuts his or her eyes and says, "I'm going to make a squiggle and you turn it into something. Then you get a turn to make one and I'll turn it into something." It is difficult for children to resist participating in this game, particularly if there are colored pencils and imaginative squiggles.

This back and forth interplay of making squiggly lines facilitates communication because it is both provocative and productive. The technique is flexible and can be used in a directive way when background material is known. Some games and art activities can be used in group work and have value; however, this one is consistently more effective on an individual basis.

Freedom of expression is a primary characteristic of art therapy and while exposure of psychic material is one by-product it also permits keeping selected conscious knowledge at bay. Kramer (1971) points out that because children are dependent and need their parent's love, they may find themselves in a double bind; they may be unable to express feelings that would disturb their tenuous sense of trust in the parent-child relationship. When verbal expression is unsafe, art provides a need-fulfilling experience that allows for safely symbolizing feelings that cannot and should not be put into words.

Another advantage in using art therapy is that it provides a graphic record. Serial productions become progress notes and provide a visual account of process. The collection of art works in a serial order over a period of time is a necessary requirement and while a single drawing may be deemed more significant than the others, there is danger in using an isolated drawing. The data base is more reliable and more complete if the series of drawings and accompanying dialogue is used in making interpretations. The nursing process includes evaluation and this systematic collection contributes a tangible and objective measure.

In the light of current psychiatric practice with the widespread use of psychotropic drugs, short-term hospitalization, and community mental health centers Williams (1976) demonstrates the effectiveness of art in crisis intervention and short-term therapy. She reports that while art therapy evolved mainly for long-term use positive effects of rapidly establishing rapport, facilitating communication, and providing a safe arena for expressing feelings are evident in short-term therapy.

Art is especially advantageous in preventive mental health, a priority for community health practitioners in today's society. Increased population and escalating rates of mental illness mandate attention. Accompanying trends are increased numbers of one-parent families and mothers working outside the home. There is a demand for placement facilities for infants and toddlers; kindergartens, nursery schools, and day care centers offer alternatives for early childhood care.

Schools have always been in a position to observe children and identify those who present problems that might range from excessive passivity or aggressiveness to a total inability to relate to authority figures or peers. In day care centers there is also an opportunity to observe children for potential problems such as separation anxiety and feelings of abandonment. The parent, too, may experience this anxiety, have guilt feelings, and be depressed over the separation.

Art work that children do as a matter of course in schools and preschools is generally thought of as educational and recreational. However, art can serve as a means for the early detection of potential problems and be included in planned prevention programs.

Salant (1975) writes on preventive art therapy with a preschool child and describes two phases of prevention: the first is immediate intervention, which occurs when the situation is problematic and not pathological; the second is intervention before dysfunctional behavior patterns become reinforced and established.

Preventive mental health in schools and pre-school settings is based primarily on two things: (1) initial and periodic conferences with the parent, parents, or parent surrogate; and (2) detection of the child's behavioral cues, verbal and nonverbal. Nurses, teachers, and child-care workers have a significant role to play in preventive mental health and this goal can be served by art. Since art activities are already an integral part of virtually all school programs and a part of the daily routine, recognition of clues that are present in the child's "symbolic speech" becomes a significant factor. Assessment and evaluation can be practiced on an ongoing basis; there are usually slight nuances or cues that might be detected before behavior problems or mental disorders become full-blown. An aware staff that not only looks at but sees and listens to what children say about their art work is in an influential position to intervene and actively foster mental health.

DEVELOPMENTAL SEQUENCES IN ART

Basic to any evaluation and assessment task is knowledge of developmental norms and sequences. The developmental approach is widely accepted in physical, cognitive, and psychoanalytical theory of personality development. Research demonstrates that stages of learning to draw are identifiable; DiLeo (1970) summarizes the American and European literature on the sequential and developmental aspects of drawings. He indicates that there is general agreement that at least two distinct stages of graphic activity can be identified: a kinesthetic, or scribbling, stage followed by a representational stage. Sequences are most apparent in the drawings of the human figure during the representational stage, although transitional phases are present in this continuum. He observes that the diagnostic use of projective drawing tests—used to determine intellect, perceptual and motor function, and emotional and social adjustment—gives credence to these beliefs.

A fundamental requirement in using drawings in assessment is that they "be viewed within the framework of chronological age." What is normal for a 4-year-old would be considered highly irregular for a 7-year-old. In chronological time individual variation occurs but the sequence is uniform "until variations in the environment are great enough to deviate the organism from its predetermined course" (DiLeo, 1970).

The extensive and significant work of Lowenfeld and Brittain (1970) offers understanding of children's art within a developmental context based on analyses of normal children's artwork. Through these developmental sequences parameters are established for making interpretations about the child's skill, his cognitive and conceptual development, and his emotional and affective processes. Using this framework one can predict expected modes of graphic and artistic expression at chronological stages. These developmental sequences are summarized in Table 2. Further expansion of these stages follows.

Random marks. Random marks are the first building blocks of graphic expression with "circular reaction" experimentation while holding and using objects or fingers and hands.

Disorderd scribbling. About the age of 18 months to 2 years of age the child begins his first graphic record called scribbling and this tends to follow a fairly predictable order. There is a continuous elaboration of kinesthetic experience, which is usually done in large sweeps. The child at this stage does not have the fine motor or visual control over his scribbling; some 20 basic scribble patterns have been identified by Kellogg (1967). There are sequences in the development of directionality in drawing; DiLeo (1970) reports that initially the scribble is a continuous, horizontal zigzag stroke; vertical and circular strokes appear more consistently in the third year.

Controlled scribbling. This stage may occur 6 months later and is important because the

TABLE 2

Summary of developmental sequences*

Age (approximate)	Stage	Description
18 months	Random marks	Images made by kinesthetic experimentation with hands; waving objects or fingers smearing food.
2-4 years	Scribbling	
18 months-2 years	Disordered scribbling	Continued and elaborated kinesthetic experimentation.
2-2½ years	Controlled scribbling	Beginning physical and visual control appears; marks are experimented with by repeating and varying them; lines begin to take on meaning.
3-3½ years	Naming of scribbles	Recognition of shapes.
4-7 years	Preschematic	Conscious attempt to make recognizable representations such as human figures; spatial relationships not established.
7-9 years	Schematic	Individual and definite concept of man and environment, which is often repeated (schema); awareness of spatial relationships evident through use of base line and sky line; creative and continued experimentation with space relationships.
9-12 years	Dawning realism	Peers influential; drawings express characteristics of sexual identity; attention given to detail and realistic color; transition from base line and sky line to perception of plane.
12-14 years	Pseudonaturalistic	Continued elaboration of perspective, detail, proportion, and color; drawings reflect interest in surroundings and sexual characteristics.
14-17 years	Decision	Conscious manipulation of media and forms; abstractions become designs; drawings reflect social and environmental themes.

*Data from Lowenfeld, V., and Brittain, W. L.: Creative and mental growth, ed. 5, New York, 1970, Macmillan Publishing Co., Inc. © 1970, Macmillan Publishing Co., Inc.

child now discovers visual control over the marks he is making. Variations and repetitions characterize this stage and the control exhibited in his drawings is reflected in the child's beginning control over other parts of his body and environment. As the child starts to control his scribbles he discovers shapes and forms and these take on meaning. Naming of scribbles has great significance for now the child's thinking is changing from kinesthetic to imaginative. This can be recognized usually in a child of 3 or 3½ years of age. Perhaps he does not have a plan when he starts his drawing but when it is finished he sees it as an entity and can say what it is.

Naming of scribbles. Only when the child reaches the naming of scribbles stage is there an attempt to use different colors for different meanings. He also must have reached the first stage of color perception and be able to distinguish between colors.

Generally speaking, scribbling begins at the age of 2 and continues until the age of 4 years old. If a child is still scribbling at 6 or 7 years of age one must consider that he is not functioning at the level normal for children of his age. Evaluation must be made if this is a transitory response to frustration or anger or if this is a consistent pattern.

Preschematic stage. There is a conscious creation of form usually spanning ages 4 through 7 years. The transition from a mainly kinesthetic activity to a representational one of visual objects gives the adult and the child clues to his thinking process and what is important to him. Drawing by children in this stage evolves from an undefined collection of lines into recognizable forms, and usually the first symbol achieved is from the mandala with two vertical lines. It resembles a tadpole and appears to represent a man with head and legs. Soon other lines, representing arms, and a "belly button" are added. Inclusion of the body follows. The child strives for balance and arranges the head, arms, and legs in appropriate places. Ears and often hair are added to achieve a balance. This is a common drawing for most 5-year-olds and it has been found that having them look at a person while they draw does not alter the way they draw a man.

Most writers believe that the child's early drawings are projections of his own body image and this view of egocentricity is commonly accepted. DiLeo (1970) thinks that these early renditions represent a parent and states that young children portray themselves when they draw their family.

It is interesting to note that, as with play, children of an earlier age draw alone and are uninterested in others' work. By the time they reach 5 they are more interested in others' drawings and begin to make judgments and comparisons.

During this stage there is little relationship between the color used and the object represented; however, this does not mean that the colors selected do not have significance. Color choice may be highly individualized such as a child who has long, red braids coloring the hair red.

Spatial relationships are not established at this period of egocentricity. Objects are often seen revolving around the child in space and the way they are peripherally placed is intricately tied in with the whole thinking process.

At this stage there is great flexibility; change in drawings indicate the rapid changes in the mode of thinking. At the age of 5, one can expect representational attempts; the more different they are, the more developed the cognitive processes are. By the time the child is 6 years old he has developed a fairly elaborate drawing of a man. Intelligence can be scored on the basis of the completeness of the drawing (Harris, 1963).

There is a growing development in perception of surrounding objects including not only the visual appearance but an awareness of all the senses such as the kinesthetic and auditory senses. The way things are represented is an indication of the type of experience the child has had with them and exaggerated sizes indicate the importance of the experience. Fig. 18-1 was created by a little boy 5½ years old. He graphically imparts his feeling about walking in the rain. Notice the long toes particularly. One can almost experience his "feel" for walking in the wet grass with his umbrella and yellow slicker.

Schematic stage. The schematic stage is the achievement of a form concept by a child of 7 to 9 years of age. Representational symbols of a man, house, and tree change after much experimentation and the child arrives at a definite concept of man and his environment. He establishes his "schema," which is a concept that is repeated over and over again unless there is an intentional experience that influences him to change. The difference between the use of repeated schema and stereotyped repetitions is that the schema is flexible and has many deviations, while the stereotyped repetitions are fixated. There is no specific time for the formation of a schema although most children reach this stage at about 7 years of age.

The milestone at this age level is finding a definite order in space relationships. A "base line" is established and appears as an indication of the child's realization of the relationship between himself and the environment. A counterpart to this base line is the "sky line" drawn across the top of the page giving further evidence of orientation in space.

Along with space, time representations are

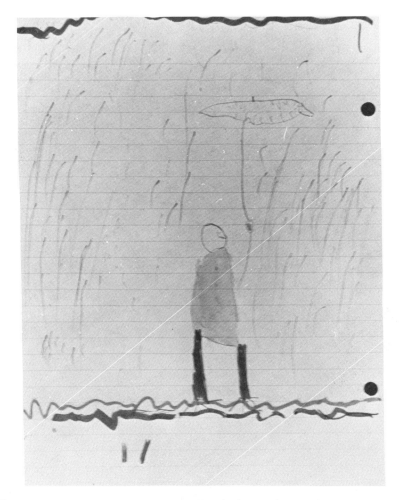

Fig. 18-1. Boy, 5½, consciously portrays kinesthetic experiences of preschematic stage.

presented; these are often done in comic book fashion where different time sequences or spatially distinct impressions are included in one drawing.

Color schema is an indication that the child has begun to make abstractions and to generalize from one situation to another; colors realistically portray the object.

With the emergence of the schema, sharing and understanding of others' feelings begin to develop and the child moves from a position of egocentricity to one of social interaction. Fig. 18-2 demonstrates this awareness of others' feelings. It was drawn by an 8-year-old girl who had allergies and was given injections by her mother, a nurse. The little girl draws herself crying and she says the handkerchief is in the mother's pocket "in case Mother starts to cry." The mother had said, "I could just cry every time I have to give her a shot."

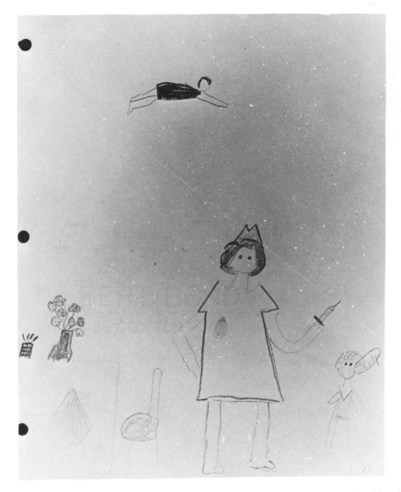

Fig. 18-2. Girl, 8, demonstrates growing awareness of other's feelings and size relationships that have emotional significance.

One can gain insight into the child's experience and feeling through variations or deviations in the normal schema. Three principal forms of deviation can be noticed in children's drawings: (1) exaggeration of important part or parts, (2) neglect or omission of suppressed parts, and (3) change in symbols for significant parts. In exaggerating parts children create size relationships that are "real" to them. The origin lies in the relative importance of specific

parts or in the emotional significance the particular part has for the child. In Fig. 18-2 the anxiety produced by the hypodermic syringe is apparent: it is longer than Molly's arms, the site of the "shot." She draws herself calling "Help," in comic book fashion and when asked about the figure over the mother's head she says with some optimism, "That's Superman coming to save me."

At this developmental stage when spatial

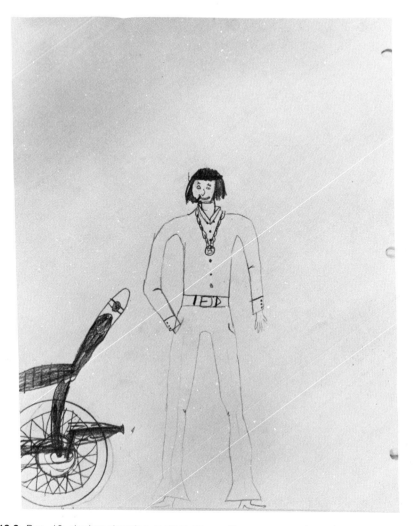

Fig. 18-3. Boy, 10, depicts dawning realism stage with awareness of gender, peer group, and increased attention to detail.

relationships are being established children often use another space representation called "folding over." This concept is best explained by visualizing the paper folded over so that two surfaces are represented simultaneously. In Fig. 18-2 Molly shows the design in the table cloth that is really under the vase of flowers and the container of shots.

Dawning realism. The dawning realism stage occurs during the "gang age" when the child is from 9 to 12 years old. A recurring pattern at this time is being or not being a part of the peer group. The importance of the opinions of authority figures about a child's artwork is replaced by the peers who freely give opinions. The child becomes very conscious of his actions

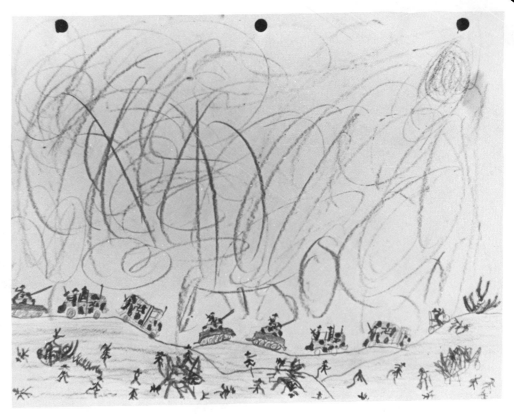

Fig. 18-4. Boy, 9, demonstrates cognitive shift from separated base and sky lines to spatial concept of plane.

and no longer has the uninhibited approach to drawing that characterized earlier stages. In artwork two factors that offer clues concerning whether or not the child identifies with his peer group are the content of the work and his willingness to participate in group work.

The drawings of children at this stage express characteristics of their sex and there is marked attention to accuracy of detail that has not been previously seen. Realistic interpretation becomes important with an increased awareness of hues and shades of color. This attention to detail is notable in Fig. 18-3, drawn by a 10-year-old boy in 1970. Long hair, head bands, and medallions characterized the mode of dress that were stereotypic of youth in the United States during the 1960s. The attention to detail is seen in the cuff buttons, belt buckle, creases in the pant legs and behind the knees, creases in the sleeves at the elbow, and in the spokes, "sissy bar," and muffler of the motorcycle. Boys at this age like to draw cars, plans, and motorcycles while girls like to draw figures of girls and choose another means of conveyance to draw—the horse.

Perceptual and cognitive development is recognized in changing spatial representations. During this stage there is a rapid transition from the use of the base line to the discovery of plane. Earth and sky are no longer separate

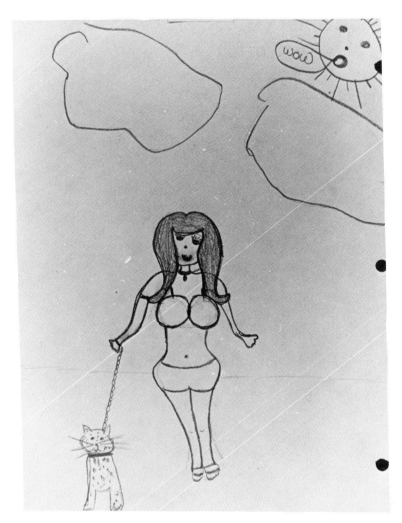

Fig. 18-5. Girl, 12, depicts feelings about sexual identity characteristic of pseudo-naturalistic stage.

entities divided by a void. They now touch. Fig. 18-4, drawn by a 9-year-old boy, demonstrates this concept. He says that the sky is full of smoke "from the explosions." Apparently the origin for the content of this picture is from televised World War II movies. He says that the Americans are winning the war and that the figures in the foreground are dead Germans. It is interesting that a boy on a bicycle is leading the tank battalion to victory.

Pseudonaturalistic stage. The pseudonaturalistic stage is a transitional step identified with young people from 12 to 14 years. It is an age of turmoil and excitement with the struggle for identity being the prime developmental task. In artwork greater interest is shown

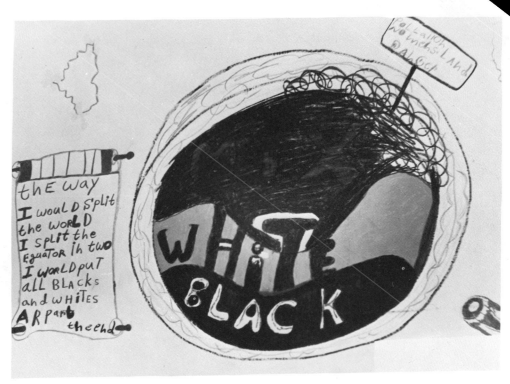

Fig. 18-6. Hospitalized boy, 15, demonstrates adolescent art of decision stage characterized by individual, societal, and cultural concerns.

in perspective, proportion, and detail. Generalizations about color cannot be made and reactions to color are highly individualized and subjective.

At this age level rapid biological changes and individual differences become obvious. The child is often critical of himself and his work and visual likenesses are taken seriously. Sexual characteristics receive attention and are often greatly exaggerated in drawings. The drawing of the self becomes a reflection that may be an idealistic representation or a fairly accurate appraisal. Fig. 18-5 was drawn by a 12-year-old girl who gave marked attention to hair style, eyes and mouth and other body parts, and jewelry. She made only a few erasures in

drawing the hips and the stance of the legs but made many in successively enlarging and emphasizing the breasts. She was apparently pleased and impressed with this idealistic representation, for she even drew the sun saying "wow" as she walked her tiger with all her blossoming womanhood and developing feminine identification.

Decision stage. The decision stage is the last of the developmental sequences and is a period of conscious adolescent art of youths from the ages of 14 to 17. Various types of media are used; an elaboration in the organization of spaces occurs with abstractions becoming designs. Aside from abstract designs and studied artwork spontaneous art productions at this age level reflect themes of environmental concern as well as those of relationships in society.

Fig. 18-6 is an example of these concerns, although it is different from the previous examples in that it was drawn by an "identified patient." The artist was a 15-year-old Puerto Rican boy hospitalized in a psychiatric unit in New York City. He and his mother had arrived in New York a year earlier speaking only Spanish and had moved in with relatives. The boy was learning English and his problems in dealing with the new culture in which he found himself was influential in his hospitalization; they were graphically portrayed in his drawings. In this particular one, he depicts a universe with separate spheres for blacks, whites, and "mix." He elaborated on, and scribbled over, the grey-colored "mix" sphere and posted a sign saying "Pollation—Nomehs Land—Danger." The scroll he drew tells how he would split the world. He omits the mix, denying them (him) a place in his proposed order of existence and there ia sense of finality with his closure, "The End." This drawing has been presented in a developmental context for its dramatically and explicitly depicts individual, societal, cultural, and universal concerns that characterize this age group.

Aside from this drawing's usefulness as an example of the final developmental sequence, there is an overlay of psychological content that cannot be ignored. This drawing and two others by the same adolescent boy demonstrate recurring themes in his art work and serve as symbolic speech. Primarily they concern aggression, identification, and sexual conflicts. The identification theme has been previously mentioned and the content and dialogue of Fig. 18-6 indicate his feelings about his place in the greater society as well as about his being from an ethnic minority.

He defines the projectile symbol in the lower corner of Fig. 18-6 as the destructive force that would "split the world." The same themes of aggression and sexual conflict are drawn in vivid black and red in Fig. 18-7. He pointedly bisected the lower figure and "X'd" out, cross-hatched, and shaded in the lower trunks of the other figures. The "X" syndrome and shading or cross-hatching the area below the waist is not an uncommon theme for adolescents preoccupied with attempts to control sexual impulses. Cross-hatching is related to obsessive thoughts and is a "controlled" indication of anxiety, preoccupation, or fixation of that part (Machover, 1971; Burns and Kaufman, 1970).

Other content deals with aggressive impulses. The violence expressed is unmistakable: one figure is yelling, "Kill"; another is stomping on a person whose visible head lies in a pool of blood. Notice the expression and the intensity of the eyes of the figure yelling, "Kill." Facial expressions are believed to be one of the more reliable signs revealing various emotions (Machover, 1971).

Fig. 18-8 reveals a commentary that literally elaborates on his symbolic speech. There is a representation of "toughness" in the figure drawn, with much detailed attention given to hairy arms and fingers, stubby whiskers and scars on the face, and an obviously broken nose. With all this expression of "hardness," the flower, with its innate features of softness and delicateness, presents a disconcerting effect. Notice the "crucified" bleeding wound in the hand that is holding the flower. It is impossible to say if the figure drawn is getting ready to sniff the flower or bite a petal. He did not comment on this. Machover (1971) claims that the depiction of teeth is associated with aggression.

The unresolved Oedipal conflict is made apparent in the armband saying "Mother" and the arrows drawn through the red hearts. Notice the accepted symbol for the wind. It is blowing the word "MOMmm." Added significance of this drawing was seen later in his hospitalization when he stated that, although his mother

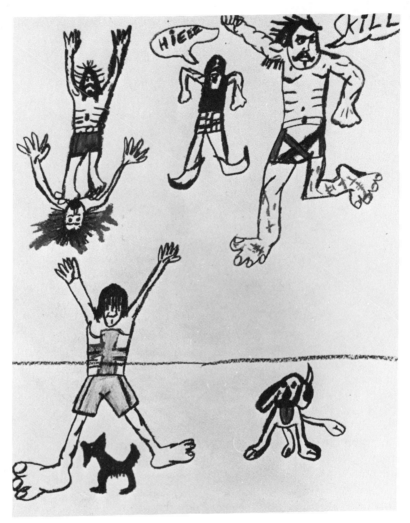

Fig. 18-7. Same boy who drew Fig. 18-6 portrays themes of aggression and sexual conflict.

was "in the business," he was going to support her when he got out.

These few drawings were selected for their clarity of expression and because they succinctly present the impact of visible symbolic speech. It is recognized that if one were to attempt to communicate with every client by using art there would be disappointments and possibly even added blocks to the therapeutic process. The way the art media are presented and the astute recognition of the client's cues about it are both influential in its use. With this particular adolescent the use of art was positive. Even if no one had ever seen or used his creations in assessment, in establishing a relationship, and in communicating, perhaps just pro-

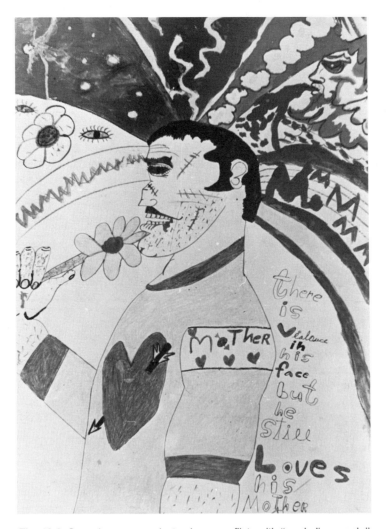

Fig. 18-8. Same boy communicates inner conflicts with "symbolic speech."

viding the media so that he could graphically express himself would have had a therapeutic effect.

CONCLUSION

The first half of the twentieth century witnessed the revolutionary view that mental disorders might be psychological rather than organic. Freud's psychoanalytical model dominated psychological thought and was the first systematic and developmental theory aimed at understanding psychological processes in human nature and behavior.

Hartmann (1950) recognized that the greatest practical importance for the mental health of children was in the field of prevention. Today, as at midcentury, the challenge still lies in prevention. It is a difficult task, however, since early recognizable diagnostic signs of mental disorders in children are not easily identified. Single approaches to prevention are unreliable; innate and environmental factors that contribute to the etiology add to the complexity of the problem.

Since 1950 the number of treatment modalities and available facilities for the treatment of mental disorders has shown a marked increase, and there has been a concerted effort directed toward understanding the mental health problems of children.

Epidemiologists distinguish three levels of preventive actions. Primary prevention is directed toward etiological factors and includes biological, psychosocial, and sociocultural measures designed to foster mental health. Secondary prevention aims at early detection and treatment of maladaptive behavior and tertiary prevention refers to preventing the "aftereffect" of chronic or permanent disability.

Contrary to popular opinion, the task of prevention is not to insulate the child from frustration, stress, or conflict. The ability to test reality requires exposure to stressful or anxiety-producing experiences that are essential for learning to make decisions and resolve conflicts. Achieving this fine balance is not easy and Anna Freud (1958) points out that there is "ample evidence that the date at which we take therapeutic action is of extreme importance." She advises beginning therapy "immediately after appearance of trouble."

The use of art may provide graphic signals of distress that might otherwise remain obscure and insidious. Art as a preventive measure and therapeutic modality finds its effectiveness in ready acceptance and easy accessibility because children like to draw and it is a common and natural activity for them. While it is undoubtedly true that the very best primary preventive methods cannot eradicate mental disorders—even if one knew what the very best methods were—carefully exploring and weighing all possible approaches provide health professionals with options and challenges in the prevention and treatment of mental disorders.

References

Arnheim, R.: Toward a psychology of art, Berkeley, 1967a, University of California Press.

Arnheim, R.: Art and visual perception, Berkeley, 1967b, University of California Press.

Ballard, P. B.: What London children like to draw. In Read, H.: Education through art, New York, 1958, Harcourt, Brace & World.

Berlo, D. K.: The process of communication, New York, 1960, Holt, Rinehart & Winston.

Booe, D. B.: Identification of children's fears through their drawings and dialogue (unpublished Masters thesis), Denton, 1971, Texas Woman's University.

Burns, R. C., and Kaufman, S. H.: Kinetic family drawings, New York, 1970, Brunner/Mazel.

Champernowne, H.: Art and therapy: an uneasy partnership, Am. J. Art Ther. **10:**131-142, April 1971.

Cohen, F. W.: Mark and the paint brush: how art therapy helped one little boy, Austin, 1971, University of Texas.

DiLeo, J.: Young children and their drawings, New York, 1970, Brunner/Mazel.

Freud, A.: Child observation and prediction of development, psychoanal. study child **13:**99, 1958.

Grozinger, W.: Scribbling, drawing, painting: the early forms of the child's pictorial creativeness, New York, 1955, Praeger Publishers, Inc.

Harris, D. B.: Children's drawing as measures of intellectual maturity, New York, 1963, Harcourt, Brace & World.

Hartmann, H.: Psychoanalysis and developmental psychology, Psychoanal. Study Child **5:**14-16, 1950.

Hayakawa, S.: On communication with children, etc.: Rev. Gen. Semantics **23:**175, 1966.

Kellogg, R., and O'Dell, S.: The psychology of children's art, San Diego, Calif., 1967, CMR-Random House.

Kramer, E.: Art as therapy with children, New York, 1971, Schocken Books, Inc.

Kris, E.: Psychoanalytic explorations in art, New York, 1952, International Universities Press.

Levy, B., and Ulman, E.: The effect of training in judging psychopathology from paintings, Am. J. Art Ther. **14:**24-25, Oct. 1974.

Lommel, A.: Prehistory and primitive man, New York, 1966, McGraw-Hill Book Co.

Lowenfeld, V., and Brittain, W. L.: Creative and mental health, London, 1970, Macmillan Publishing Co., Inc.

Machover, K.: Personality projection in the drawing of the human figure, Springfield, Ill., 1971, Charles C Thomas Publisher.

Mumford, L.: Art and techniques, New York, 1952, Columbia University Press.

Naumburg, M.: An introduction to art therapy, New York, 1973, Teachers College Press.

Rambert, M.: Children in conflict, New York, 1949, International Universities Press.

Read, H.: Psychoanalysis and the problem of esthetic value, Intl. J. Psychoanal **32:**75-82, 1951.

Read, H.: Education through art, London, 1958, Brace & World.

Rhyne, J.: The Gestalt approach to experience, art, and art therapy, Am. J. Art. Ther. **12:**237-248, July 1973.

Salant, E. G. Preventive art therapy with a preschool child, Am. J. Art Ther. **14:**67-74, April 1975.

Silver, R.: Children with communication disorders: cognitive and artistic development," Am. J. Art Ther. **14:**39-47, Jan. 1975.

Ulman, E., and Levy, B.: Art therapists as diagnosticians, Am. J. Art Ther. **13:**35-38, Oct. 1973.

Williams, G. H., and Wood, M. M.: Developmental art therapy, Baltimore, 1977, University Park Press.

Williams, S.: Short term art therapy, Am. J. Art Therapy **15:**35-41, Jan. 1976.

Wilson, L.: Theory and practice of art therapy with the mentally retarded, Am. J. Art Ther. **16:**87-97, 1977.

Winnicott, D. W.: Therapeutic consultations in child psychiatry, New York, 1971, Basic Books, Inc.

Wittenburg, D.: Art therapy for adolescent drug abusers, Am. J. Art Ther. **13:**141-149, Jan. 1974.

CHAPTER 19

Reality therapy: one approach to enhancing man's relationships

LINDA COLVIN

HISTORY OF REALITY THERAPY

Reality therapy was developed in the 1950s by William Glasser, a psychiatrist practicing on the West Coast (Strupp and Blackwood, 1975). Glasser's questioning of the fundamental beliefs of freudian-oriented psychoanalytical teachings began as he neared the end of his residency at the Neuropsychiatric Institute at the University of California, Los Angeles. When he expressed his feelings that even with all he had been taught something was lacking, most of his teachers and fellow residents considered him a radical. One teacher, G. L. Harrington, shared Glasser's concern. Harrington's own questioning had begun years earlier through supervision by his training analyst, H. Kaiser (Glasser and Zunin, 1973).

Glasser's (1969) ideas that there had to be more to mental disorders than he had been taught led to the search and eventual development of his own theories. He left his residency determined to try out his own ideas and did so in his small private practice and as a consultant for the Ventura School for Girls. His work at the school proved successful; the girls began to enjoy the program and express feelings of hope, and the staff became increasingly involved in the helping process. His approach was successful with patients and the staff responded favorably to his radical approach; thus reality therapy as a treatment modality evolved.

In 1964 Glasser first used the term "reality therapy." The following year saw the publication of Glasser's book, *Reality Therapy,* dedicated to Harrington. In 1969 Glasser formed the Institute for Reality Therapy, which continues to offer training courses for clergymen, judges, lawyers, nurses, physicians, police officers, probation officers, psychologists, social workers, and teachers. People are trained to work in the many helping agencies that serve as primary prevention resources throughout the community. Incorporating reality therapy in schools was a strong attempt to lower the number of new cases of mental disorders (Glasser, 1969).

THEORY OF PERSONALITY

Reality therapy holds that people develop an identity image by the age of 4 or 5 years and come to view themselves as either a failure or a success. This self-image may vary greatly from the image that society has of the person. The individual may see himself as a failure when society acknowledges him a success. People who have developed a failure identity are generally lonely people with difficulty facing the real world since they find it an uncomfortable place. They see the world either as frightening, depressing, or anxiety producing.

To develop a success identity each individual must have two basic psychological needs met: (1) knowing that at least one person loves him

200

and loving at least one person, and (2) viewing himself as worthwhile while simultaneously believing that at least one other person sees him as worthwhile. The person needs *both* love and a feeling of being worthwhile, not just one or the other (Glasser, 1965).

To have these basic needs met, man as a social being needs involvement with others. Involvement with others is also an integral part of an individual's motivation toward responsible behavior. By nature man has a desire to be content, to be involved, and to have a success identity. Inherently each seeks to demonstrate responsible behavior and to form satisfactory relationships with other people. So where do individuals stray from their basic nature for responsibility and involvement? Since a person develops a success or failure identity at an early age involvement with parents is important in the development of identity. Moreover identity is strongly influenced by peer relationships, school, and other aspects of the culture and environment (Glasser and Zunin, 1973).

A success or failure identity is not fixed for life; rather a person can change his identity as a result of involvement and responsible behavior from a failure identity to a success identity. To a great extent man is what he does; therefore if what a man does involves irresponsible behavior and he changes what he does to responsible behavior, he increases his feelings of self-worth.

THEORY OF MENTAL ILLNESS

People who have developed a failure identity feel uncomfortable in the real world and handle this discomfort either by denying reality or by ignoring it. What is referred to by other mental health professionals as mental illness is, according to Glasser, an individual's attempt to deny reality. The specific ways of denying reality are generally viewed by other mental health professionals as the symptoms of various diagnoses. Reality therapists do not use the standard diagnosis; they do not consider it helpful in

assisting a person to change. Further a client may even use the diagnosis as an excuse for current irresponsible behavior by describing his behavior as acceptable since he is "ill."

There are two major ways in which people deny reality: (1) they may change the real world in their minds to make themselves feel more comfortable, or (2) they may simply ignore reality. In the first instance the denial of reality by changing it in his mind protects the individual from facing feelings of worthlessness, meaningless, or insignificance in the world. An individual can believe himself to be not worthless Joe Blow but rather a president or any great hero. This alteration in reality may encourage a retreat into an entirely "made up" world. In the second group reality is not changed; it is simply ignored. These people are aware of the real world and make a decision to ignore it by consistently breaking the rules and laws of the world.

According to Glasser and Zunin (1973) both changing reality in the mind and ignoring it indicate a problem with responsibility. Thus the treatment follows a prescribed format (except in mental disturbances caused by biochemical disorders and brain damage). The first step is to help the client become aware of the self-defeating nature of his behavior and discover behavior that will help him meet his basic needs without causing harm to himself or others.

OVERVIEW OF REALITY THERAPY

In order for reality therapy to be effective each of a sequence of steps must be completed. The steps include (1) involvement, (2) examining current behavior, (3) making a value judgment of the behavior, (4) identifying a plan to change the behavior, (5) committing oneself to the plan, and (6) if the plan fails, accepting no excuses and altering the plan. Each step must be executed in sequence for reality therapy to be effective (Bassin et al., 1976). Attempts to examine behavior prior to the establishment of involvement or trying to make a plan before behavior has been studied and judged is unsatisfactory. It is recommended that no step be skipped or taken out of sequence; the value of reality therapy comes from the process whereby one step leads to the next.

The reality therapist is not interested in the client's past. If the past had provided adequate developmental support, the client would currently be able to act responsibly and would not be seeking therapy. Each person has the potential for being either responsible or irresponsible. His decisions, not the conditions of life, determine behavior. Thus the entire focus of treatment is on current behavior and the generation of future plans. Clients are helped to define and clarify life goals as well as to examine ways by which they prevent their own progress toward these goals. The counselor helps the individual to interact more productively with the environment by looking at alternatives, ways in which compromise can increase goal-directed behavior, planning, and modifications of behavior when indicated. The counselor teaches people to behave in a more productive way by assisting them to make specific plans as well as by helping them to make a commitment to follow through with the plans. Through reality therapy people learn ways of living and behaving that enable them to fulfill basic psychological needs.

Reality therapy can be considered an ecological approach to mental health because it strives to strengthen the man-environment interface. Intervention serves to help a client change his behavior to deal more effectively with life situations. Encouragement and guidance are provided so that clients can make plans and implement actions that help them as well as others around them. By helping others and doing the responsible thing they feel increased self-worth and thus are helped. Since reality therapy considers that man has two basic psychological needs—to love and be loved and to be worthwhile to self and others—it seems obvious that man's relationship with others is of

utmost importance in therapy. In the process man's relationship with self, others, and the universe can be affected positively through therapy.

Reality therapy sessions are verbally active. The client and counselor sit in comfortable chairs facing one another. Fees are discussed early and openly with the amount varying in different parts of the country. Generally sessions are held once a week for approximately 45 minutes.

PROCESS OF REALITY THERAPY

Six major steps comprise a guide for helping clients move toward more responsible behavior and better feelings about themselves.

Step 1

The first step is involvement. The therapist becomes involved responsibly with the person who has come for help. Involvement is an extremely important step since none of the other steps can be started until involvement has occurred. If involvement is not established, the therapist cannot help the client. Becoming involved may be the hardest part of therapy since the person seeking help often has difficulty establishing an emotional relationship. The therapist, realizing that involvement is fundamental in helping people learn to fulfill their needs, uses skill to interrupt the barriers people have built against involvement. Glasser (1965) indicates that the major skill in doing reality therapy is the therapist's ability to get involved. Involvement—the building of a relationship between two people—begins as the client gains confidence that the therapist can be trusted and will not desert him.

This caring relationship has clearly defined limits. The appropriate levels of involvement are honestly discussed and the client is never promised what cannot be given (Glasser, 1972). Basically involvement is confined to the office, although phone calls for achievements and/or emergencies are permissible and sometimes encouraged. By having the client call about a success the therapist indicates that he is interested in the positive experiences that the person has. It is important to focus on the client's strong points and accomplishments rather than on his failures.

The initial topics of discussion vary from one client to another in order to promote involvement and also to help the client become aware that there is more in life than dwelling on unhappiness or on symptoms of irresponsible behavior. Whatever is discussed is seen as valuable, since involvement between therapist and client is promoted and the client's involvement with his own misery is broken.

Counselor's role in achieving step 1. The counselor must be willing to become meaningfully and responsibly involved with the client. In order for involvement to happen the counselor must communicate that he cares. Aloofness and cool detachment are not acceptable. Transference is not encouraged; instead the counselor should attempt to present himself as a genuine, real, warm, understanding, concerned person who is interested in the person seeking help. This interest in the client is the cornerstone of therapy. The therapist consistently conveys the belief that the client has the potential to be happier and that he is capable of more responsible behavior. Throughout every interaction the therapist conveys acceptance of the client as a person. The therapist gets involved with the client and explains the therapeutic situation so that the client has a clear understanding of the relationship (Glasser, 1972).

Step 2

The second step is to focus on and discuss the client's present behavior. Clients must be helped to look at their behavior. Awareness of one's behavior precedes movement toward increased responsibility.

Regardless of past life experiences each person is accountable for his behavior. Past life events, no matter how traumatic, are not accepted as an excuse for irresponsible behavior; an individual is responsible for what he does. The task of therapy is to help the client to recognize the part that he plays in determining what happens to him.

Behavior is considered far more important in reality therapy than feelings or past experiences, since people can more easily control their behavior than their feelings. Emphasis is placed on what is happening in the client's life at the present time; the past has already happened and cannot be changed. By dealing with the present the client can look at his behavior to become aware of what changes are indicated for a more productive future. This is not to say that the importance of the past is being denied. The past has a great deal to do with how an individual behaves in the present; therefore he is assisted in relating his past experiences to present behavior. For example, when a client discusses a terribly traumatic event that occurred in his past, the therapist listens carefully and then responds by directing the client to examine how the impact of this event is affecting his present behavior.

Working with feelings per se, just as with working with the client's past, is not helpful in leading a person to a success identity. Actions and feelings occur in a cycle:

$$\text{Do bad} \rightarrow \text{Feel bad}$$
$$\text{Feel bad} \leftarrow \text{Do bad}$$

Feelings and their importance are not denied; however it is easier to break the cycle at the doing level. Therefore the therapist guides the client to focus on what he is doing rather than on what he is feeling (Glasser and Zunin, 1973). A person does not decide to change his behavior if he has never really looked at specific aspects of the behavior. Once the behavior is changed the cycle becomes:

$$\text{Do good} \rightarrow \text{Feel good}$$
$$\text{Feel good} \leftarrow \text{Do good}$$

Therapist's role in achieving step 2.
When a client discusses his feelings the therapist helps him relate those feelings to his current behavior. The therapist accepts the client's statements that he feels badly by responding with comments such as "Now that I understand how you feel, tell me exactly what you've been doing," or "Tell me what you did today that led to your feelings." Although statements of this sort initially surprise the client they may enable him to become aware that he is responsible for his own behavior and feelings. The goal is to help the client acknowledge that he feels uncomfortable because he has been behaving in an unsatisfactory way. The person is guided toward an awareness that anyone would feel badly if he were doing what the client has been doing.

The therapist constantly focuses on the behavior that can be changed as well as positive behavior. The therapist can bring out positive behavior by asking, "What are you doing that is keeping you from getting even more depressed?" As the client elaborates what he does to keep himself from feeling worse he is forced to look at his positive actions. As the client begins to describe ways that keep him from becoming more depressed he is focusing on his positive behavior and a beginning is made toward a success identity. The therapist first guides the client from the topic of his bad feelings, then tells him what he is doing, and then gets him to examine his positive characteristics.

Step 3

The third step is to guide the client to make a value judgment about his behavior. Once a client has examined a specific behavior, the behavior should be evaluated. Judging, or evaluating, behavior is important because the client is not going to move from an examination of behavior to automatically changing the behavior. He must at some point decide that the behavior needs changing, and in order to make a decision that the behavior needs changing the

client must see that the current behavior is not working to his advantage. By looking at the man-environment relationship, reality therapy applies ecological principles to the human condition by evaluating the whole person and how his actions affect the community. The question is posed: "Is the identified behavior good for you as well as for others?" If the person decides that the behavior or a part of the behavior is not good for him, then he is ready to plan ways to change the behavior.

Therapist's role in achieving step 3.
The therapist insists that the client look at his behavior and determine what he is doing that contributes to his failure. Considerable encouragement is required from the therapist to persuade the client to stop and evaluate his behavior. Making a value judgment of one's behavior is often painful. The therapist never tells someone else how to live life; instead the goal is to assist the client to find flaws in his behavior and move toward new behaviors that allow for a more productive interaction with others. The therapist guides the client in taking the responsibility for judging his own behavior without making the value judgment for him.

Step 4

The fourth step is to assist the client in making a plan to change his behavior. A plan with which the person can succeed will move him in the direction of a success identity. Both client and counselor carefully consider the client's motivations and abilities while devising the plan. The plan needs to have balance between elaborateness and simplicity. If it is too complicated the patient may not be able to carry it out, thus reinforcing a failure identity. An overly simplistic plan may make such an insignificant change in his behavior that the person cannot see any difference at all. The implementation of a balanced plan often leads to a feeling of success. Once the therapist and client decide on a mutually satisfying plan the plan becomes a written contract that is considered both official and important. The contract includes details of planning such as the day the activity is to take place, the time, and what the client is going to wear. In general the more specific the plan for change, the more efficiently it can be implemented.

Therapist's role in accomplishing step 4. The therapist serves as a teacher helping the client make responsible decisions and plans. The client should be helped to make a list of alternative behaviors without making any judgments of the alternatives. Some ideas will be absurd but the listing of as many alternatives as possible allows the client to see the unending number of options. Therapists should draw on their own satisfactory life experiences as they help list alternatives for clients who have less successful experiences. The client who is not in the habit of examining alternatives may have considerable difficulty listing his options. Once the client acknowledges that alternatives do exist, each should be weighed as to its value in order to guide him toward the most reasonable, responsible, and effective alternative. The next step consists of the therapist's turning the specific plan into a written contract for action.

Step 5

The fifth step involves asking the client to make a commitment to the plan. The best plan in the world, no matter how individualized it may be, is useless if the client does not make a commitment to carry it out. The client with a failure identity has difficulty making such a commitment. Commitments are generally between people, and the therapist becomes the person toward whom the client makes a commitment. Later the client is assisted toward making commitments to meaningful others and/or to himself. If the plan is well made and the client succeeds in it later commitments become easier.

Therapist's role in achieving step 5. The earlier established involvement helps the ther-

apist lead the client toward a commitment to the plan that they have defined. Each person needs support and encouragement to make a commitment to the therapist that he will carry out the plan. The therapist monitors the commitment to determine if it is realistic and suitable for implementation.

Step 6

The sixth step is to accept no excuses from the client for a plan that has failed. Even though considerable effort goes into making a good plan, some are unsuccessful. Not all commitments that a client makes are kept. The therapist does not spend time dwelling on the failed plan and making excuses for why it was found wanting. Rather the next step is either to make alterations or to design an entirely new plan. The combined energies of the client and therapist go into making a new plan, not into discussing what the old one lacked; such discussion reinforces failure. The goal in reality therapy is to move from failure to a success identity through a commitment to a new plan that has the potential to work.

Therapist's role in accomplishing step 6. The therapist avoids cross-examining the client about why he did not keep the commitment to the plan. Since it is important that the therapist not depreciate the client for failing, he or she spends no time blaming the client for the failure. The goal is to look at the present and determine if the client is going to fulfill the old commitment or make a new one. The client may want to dwell on the past and commiserate about why he did not fulfill the commitment; the therapist simply seeks to know if the client will now fulfill the commitment and if so, when. If not, work begins on a new plan.

No form of punishment is used; punishment reinforces a failure identity. There are times when natural consequences occur after irresponsible behavior, but this is not considered punishment. The person who is not punished when he fails assumes increased self-responsibility and is often motivated to make a new plan and carry it out successfully.

CASE HISTORY

The following case may help clarify the process of reality therapy:

Sue, aged 18, sought counseling from a nurse because of her increasing feelings of unhappiness. The first sessions in reality therapy dealt with establishing involvement between the nurse and client. The nurse used emphathetic listening and reflective statements to encourage elaboration about the client's current miserable situation. As Sue began to feel that she was being heard and understood, her trust and involvement began to grow.

Sue explained that a year before she had met and fallen in love with Mike. Although Mike planned to get married, he wanted her to move in with him for awhile before the wedding. Sue was hesitant about doing so, but Mike assured her that they would marry when the "timing" was better. Thinking that she had met the man of her dreams, who would soon marry her, Sue moved in with Mike. A virgin before meeting Mike, Sue remained sexually faithful to him throughout the year that she lived with him, although she felt guilty about the sexual relationship since they had not gotten married as planned. She feared that people would consider her promiscuous.

On moving in with Mike Sue gave up her friends and family ties and she missed her family a great deal. Mike did not want her to associate with them and to please him Sue remained aloof from her family. More than anything she could think of, she said, she wanted "for Mike to love me as he did when we first met and as I still love him; to be married, to have a small house, to have children, and to restore relations with my parents."

Basically Sue's goals were realistic, except for the part about Mike's loving and marrying her. Mike refused to discuss marriage, constantly criticized her, would not allow her to look for a job, and insisted that she call him each time she left the apartment for any reason. There was never any money available for recreation such as going to the movies or out to eat. Mike, who spent his days off watching TV in his underwear and drinking wine, expected Sue to stay in the apartment with him, which she did.

Sue was not able to correlate her behavior or activities with her current unhappiness. She could only see that Mike had to change back to the way he behaved when they first met and that he had to marry her. She somehow thought that the magical solution

was getting Mike to marry her. Sue sought counseling to help her get Mike to set a wedding date.

Some of Sue's pain originated from a lack of meaningful involvement. She had given up all of the important people in her life to keep Mike. Mike's involvement with her was lacking; indeed he did not seem to have the ability to engage in a mutually meaningful relationship.

Intervention included guiding Sue to recognize that she was in control of, and responsible for, her own actions and feelings. Once she recognized the scope of her responsibility, change could begin. The interaction between Sue and the external environment was tremendous. Her internal environment was deteriorating as she attempted to maintain homeostasis. Her old environment had been relatively comfortable, requiring only a slight effort to maintain a balance. Now, however, the environmental forces were great and her responses were inadequate and underdeveloped. Nevertheless once she realized that she must take control and be responsible some semblance of balance could be regained.

Sue was guided away from discussing her feelings of worthlessness and unhappiness in an attempt to focus on her action. The following conversation demonstrates the difficulty inherent in getting Sue to examine her behavior.

Nurse: "Sue, I hear your sadness." Pause. "Tell me what you did today before you came in."

Sue: "Well, I mostly stayed around the apartment. Mike didn't want me to go out."

Nurse: "Exactly what did you do? You got up . . . what, around 7 AM?"

Sue: "Yes I got up at 7 AM and made Mike's breakfast. He yelled at me as usual. This time the eggs were cooked too hard; yesterday he said they were cooked too soft. I try to get them perfect but it's no use. Before he never yelled and we had such fun together."

Nurse: "After you got up you fixed breakfast and then what?"

Sue: "Oh, I cried."

Nurse: "You cried for . . . what, 10, 20 minutes?"

Sue: Smiling. "Yes, I cried for a few minutes. You keep getting more picky about exactly how long and everything. . . . Oh, I cried about 30 or 40 minutes because things are so lousy between us and I can't see what I can do to make it back like it was. I just don't know how to convince Mike that we have to get married."

It was tempting at this point to try to help her see that marriage to Mike might not be so grand but the behavior needed to be examined. Alternatives would be explored in the planning stage.

Nurse: "You smiled just then when you said I was getting picky about what you did today." Smiling. "I really do want to look at what you're doing."

Sue: "Well, it sounds so silly telling you about every detail.

Anyway, I didn't do anything else until late afternoon when it was time to come in to see you. I just sat in my housecoat and drank coffee a couple of times. Mike sometimes calls but he didn't today. Today was just like yesterday and the day before that."

Nurse: "I think if I did that all day I'd be more depressed than you are." Big smile. "Really!"

Both laughed and the point was made. Her actions were not helping her or others. She was unable to get her basic psychological needs met sitting in an apartment all day. She needed to do some things that she was good at so that she could feel successful and worthwhile as well as become involved with others to decrease her loneliness and have her need for love met.

Nurse: "Okay, you've told me what you do; now tell me what you think about what you do."

Sue: "Mike's right. I'm just a lousy person who doesn't have sense to come in out of the rain."

Nurse: "Sue, what do you think about what you do each day? Is it behavior that's good for you?"

Sue: "No!" Begins to cry. "I've ruined my life. My days are so boring . . . and I'm sick of it all."

Sue finally looked at her current behavior and judged it. She had seen that her behavior was not helping her; yet she had not known what to do with the information. She had been overwhelmed with feelings of inadequacy as she listened to Mike's constant complaining and criticism. She felt that she was no longer good enough for him and since she had left everyone for him his opinion had become overly important. To have him she had made a decision to burn her bridges with her parents and old friends. She had given up a great deal to live with Mike and now he had no intention of marrying her. She was not looking at the situation clearly yet; she could see no alternative except getting Mike to marry her. She was afraid that if she did decide to change her behavior Mike might get mad and leave her. She insisted that she did not want this because she loved him too much to live without him. Life was terrible with him but she was sure that it would be worse without him. Almost as great as the fear of losing him was the realization that she had made her decision to go against the advice of family and friends when she moved in with him. She had assured them that she was doing the right thing and that she and Mike were getting married. She had fantasized that as soon as they were married the old spark of their initial relationship would return. To move away from Mike meant admitting that she had made a mistake. She feared that her family and friends might not take her back and that if they did they would constantly remind her of her mistake. Change involved considerable fear and Sue needed the relationship

with a supporting counselor to help her see potential solutions.

From the first time Sue came in she would say, "Don't tell me to move out. I'll never do that." Although her moving out had never been mentioned, she feared that it would be. She could see that leaving Mike was an alternative, although she would not list it as one. Once Sue decided that her behavior was not helpful to her adjustment she was able to look at new ways of relating to others. Since she desperately needed involvement, a positive change occurred when she called her mother. The following discussion took place after she was asked, "What do you do?"

Nurse: "Sue, what would you really like to do that will help you feel better and maybe help someone else feel better also? Let's make a list."

Sue: "I would love to talk to my mother and I think she would like for me to call. I heard that she is worried about me. I'd like to meet a girl that I see at the pool every afternoon. I'd like to start back swimming. I'm really good at swimming and used to be the best in high school. I'd like to make some new clothes."

Nurse: "Great, what a list! Let's look at each of these and make a plan for tomorrow."

Each alternative was weighed and listed according to priority rank. Since Sue needed meaningful involvement and an activity that she not only enjoyed but was good at, it was decided that she would call her mother and go to the pool.

Contract: I will get up tomorrow at 7 AM, fix Mike's breakfast, dress, and fix my face. 7:45 AM: See Mike off to work, straighten the house, and have a second cup of coffee. 9 AM: Call Mother. 10 AM to 12 noon: Mend last year's bathing suit and try it on. 12 noon to 1 PM: Fix and eat a light but nutritious lunch of boiled egg, sliced tomato, slice of bread, glass of milk, spinach salad, and two cookies. 1 PM: Put on a bathing suit and do some preswim stretch exercises. 1:15 to 2 PM: Rest and let lunch digest. 2 PM: Gather up towel, suntan lotion, magazine, sun glasses, sun hat, and slippers. 2:30 PM: Go out to the pool. 2:30 to 3 PM: Get settled at poolside table in the shade and look around to see if the girl I want to meet is there. 3 to 3:15 PM: Swim. 3:15 PM: Get out and sunbathe; watch for the girl to come to the pool, enjoy the sun, and think about how pretty I looked swimming. 4 PM: Go over and talk to the girl. (Mike would be home at 5 PM and the evening was not part of this plan.)

Signed: Sue
Witness: Linda

The plan and commitment were made. The plan was a success because Sue had a great day. Her mother was delighted to hear from her and invited her to meet her for lunch later in the week. The girl at the pool invited Sue in for a Coke, and Sue had so much fun that she was almost late getting home to greet Mike. Sue was doing things to get the involvement phase going and was reaching out beyond her limited world of Mike.

Subsequent plans turned out to be successful, which surprised Sue and increased her confidence. One new friend encouraged her to apply for a good secretarial job that had opened up in the office where the girl worked. Sue wanted the job badly but thought that Mike would never allow it.

All of these small successful plans helped prepare Sue for a traumatic confrontation with Mike. Sue learned that all the time she had been faithful to Mike, considering herself a wife and doing what he wanted, Mike had been seeing other women. The support gained from her outside involvement and increased self-worth were needed to help Sue make decisions and behave responsibly.

Her list of alternatives included shooting the woman, shooting Mike, and shooting herself. Other alternatives were listed between tears and outbursts of rage: stay with Mike and let him see other women; move out of his apartment into her own apartment; and move into her old room at her parents' house and look for a job. Because she had someone to turn to with whom she was involved, a realization of the impact of behavior on feelings, an evaluation of her prior behavior, and a new familiarity with making plans, Sue was able to select the best alternative. She decided to move in with her parents and start looking for a job. The plan was made and once again it was specific. Sue's feelings were strong and without proper planning she might not have stuck to the plan. Every detail from contacting her parents to putting her belongings in the car was planned.

Moving out was extremely painful for her and she needed to talk by phone with the nurse-counselor twice during the first day at her parents' home. During the first phone session she reported that she knew she was doing the right thing but felt ambivalent. She needed frequent encouragement and support to carry out the plan. She cried and told of her love for Mike and how much she missed him and wanted to call him. Then as she kept talking she said, "I can't go back to that. He isn't going to change. I'm not going to waste my life like that any more." After this statement it was necessary to look at the future positively and discuss the present plan. The nurse-counselor gave Sue an open invitation to call back if she had a good experience or if she felt the need for support.

The second call came about 5 hours later. Sue had stayed with the plan and she could not believe how much more content she felt. Her anxiety was greatly reduced when she was warmly welcomed back into her old circle of relationships and she saw that she could live without Mike for the first 24 hours. She could not believe how nice her first day had been. Also several subsequent good things had happened to her. She was able to add to the plan a phone call to the agency that had the job that she had wanted. The job was still open and they set up an interview.

When Sue obtained a job her attitude completely changed from that of the girl who had walked in for counseling and was so sad only 6 weeks before. Using the reality therapy approach, Sue moved from telling of her sad feelings to looking at, evaluating, and changing her behavior.

SUMMARY

Reality therapy is one way to help people find a more purposeful, successful, and fulfilled life. It can be used in conjunction with other modalities and certainly during the phase of involvement any number of therapeutic principles and techniques can be employed. There is no mystery about what the therapist is doing. The client is guided to look at his behavior, make a value judgment about the behavior and organize a plan to change that behavior. Attention thus focuses on the client's strengths, successes, and potential as he attempts to lead a responsible life.

References

Bassin, A., Bratter, E., and Rachin, R.: The reality therapy reader, New York, 1976, Harper & Row, Publishers.

Glasser, W.: Reality therapy, New York, 1965, Harper & Row, Publishers.

Glasser, W.: Schools without failure, New York, 1969, Harper & Row, Publishers.

Glasser, W.: The identity society, New York, 1972, Harper & Row, Publishers.

Glasser, W., and Zunin, L.: Reality therapy. In Corsini, R., ed.: Current psychotherapies, Itasca, Ill., 1973, F. E. Peacock Publishers, Inc.

Strupp, H., and Blackwood, G.: Comprehensive textbook of psychiatry, vol. 2, ed. 2, Baltimore, 1975, The Williams & Wilkins Co.

CHAPTER 20

Wholeness and integration: Gestalt theory and practice

LYNN W. BRALLIER

GESTALT THEORY AND HUMAN ECOLOGY

Gestalt theory represents an expansion and integration of several theories of psychotherapy. The result is an organized way of viewing human processes that is ecological in nature. Gestalt theory addresses the human experience in a comprehensive manner, paying attention to the dynamic quality of both the internal and the external environments. It both analyzes and synthesizes in that it insists on clear awareness of the parts of the personality or life experience before integrating these parts into a coherent whole.

The Gestalt concept of contact reflects an awareness of the internal and external environments as ecological universes. Contact can be defined as a sense of awareness and connection with these environments. Contact with oneself as an organism means being aware of bodily sensations, thoughts, feelings, and actions and claiming ownership of these aspects of the internal environment. When contact is made among various parts of oneself, experiences of being "centered," balanced, and sturdy are likely to occur. Contact with the external environment is also of concern to Gestalt theory. Emphasis is placed on the process of contact and withdrawal that goes on constantly as we interact with the "outside-our-skin" world.

Human ecology theory and Gestalt theory are related in another important way. Both recognize and appreciate all parts of the universe. As part of the human potential movement Gestalt theory promotes helping people reach into themselves and outside themselves to become all that they have potential for being. People are encouraged to make contact with and identify with all aspects of the universe available to them in order to expand and grow. Thus interaction between the internal and external environments is seen as holding possibilities for learning and changing.

GESTALT PERSONALITY THEORY

Gestalt theory of personality is a theory of the *processes* people utilize as they go from birth to death. It avoids static constructs such as states of personality development and types of personalities. It favors instead an existential-humanistic view that values the uniqueness of an individual's experience of the moment. The present moment's experience is acknowledged to have past experiences influencing it, but the important point is to deal with the wholeness experienced rather than analyzing why it is experienced the way it is.

Gestalt personality theory focuses on identifying the organismic processes used by people as they cope with life, grow, find meaning, and expand their potentials. The emphasis is on becoming whole and integrated. Psychopathology of the personality is treated as a departure from an individual's innate healthy processes.

Gestalt is a German word that has no precise English equivalent but generally translates to mean a cohesive pattern or whole. In Gestalt theory all of nature is thought of as a unified and organized whole. The healthy personality is also viewed in these terms. As with the holism exhibited in nature the personality is dynamic and contains many parts. When parts of the personality are differentiated, they can become polarized so that conflict between various opposing parts is active although perhaps outside of the awareness of the person. These splits in the personality must be healed for healthy integration or wholeness to become a reality.

To be healthy the person must also have a sense of being part of a natural order and process in the universe. Gestalt theory supports the belief that people have a built-in process for achieving wholeness just as other living beings demonstrate when their natural growth is uninterrupted.

The Gestalt concept of organismic self-regulation describes a universal, natural process of satisfying needs and relieving tension. According to this concept tension is caused by wanting something but not taking action to get it. This process operates smoothly when a person is healthy. The person satisfies needs by becoming aware of a need, taking action based on this perceived need, and fulfilling the perceived need. For that moment the person is in a balanced, or homeostatic, state. Soon, however, another need or want arises and the process replays. When there are blocks in this process needs go unmet and balance is lost. If a person has chronic blocks in the process of fulfilling needs the physical, mental, emotional, or spiritual well-being will be disturbed.

The concept of organismic self-regulation implies an ability to be aware of needs; it also implies that a person as an organism is an open system interacting with an environment that can supply inputs to satisfy needs. In Gestalt theory strong emphasis is placed on the process of awareness, which is viewed as the basic component of life experience and is thus basic to personality formation and maintenance.

What are we aware of and how do we become aware? We are aware of facets of our external and internal environments, which include values, feelings, thoughts, memories, fantasies, and wants. We are aware of aspects of these two environments mainly through the use of our physical senses—seeing, hearing, touching, tasting, and smelling. At times we are also aware of our environments through "paranormal" sensing, as in telepathic occurrences. These types of awareness experiences are also respected as a valid part of the individual's experience.

The process of becoming aware of only one perception at a time instead of being overwhelmed by thousands of sensory information bits perceived simultaneously has to do with the concept of figure and ground. All possible experiences are in the perceptual field, or ground. From this emerges, or becomes figural, a single perception. For instance, as I focus on writing these words I may become aware that my mouth is dry and decide to get a drink of water. For a short time my thirst becomes figural and my writing blends into the background.

As a sensory perception becomes figural from the background it is acted on—either to push it out of awareness if possible, let it go out of awareness, let it stay on the edge of awareness, or let it be fully impactful and motivate behavior.

Stratford and Brallier (1975) refer to awareness as being the first step in the need-satisfaction cycle. When a person is fully aware of a figural perception, energy and excitement are noticeable, action is taken that satisfies the excitement or need, and that piece of business is finished so that some other perception becomes figural. The more smoothly the process flows from allowing clear awarness to fulfilling a need, the more satisfied and balanced a person feels. Each time people go through this process they change in some way.

Gestalt theory is existential in respect to its emphasis on the fact that awareness is possible only in the present. Whatever exists for us exists only now. Thus it is more enlivening to be as fully aware of what is wanted now and to take action on that than to think about either past unmet needs or future needs.

Gestalt theory also emphasizes the concept of "aliveness" of the personality. Aliveness—the opposite of deadness and dullness—is a sense of wholeness and integration of a person's body, mind, spirit, and environment. Alive people are congruent and feel responsible for, and free to make, choices about their lives with input but not control from their environments. Aliveness is a quality everyone can develop further and its enhancement is seen as necessary in a healthy personality.

GESTALT THEORY OF PSYCHOTHERAPY

This section focuses on Gestalt theory as it applies to the process of assisting individuals to rid themselves of bothersome thoughts, feelings, and behaviors and/or expand their potential for finding satisfaction and enjoyment in life. A Gestalt therapist defines psychotherapy as an interactive experience in which the therapist assists the client to change and grow in an atmosphere of mutual respect and equality as opposed to arranging a "big healthy–little sick" therapist-client relationship. While the art of Gestalt therapy takes training, experience, and creativity on the part of the therapist it does not require that the therapist construct a position that is more interpersonally powerful than the client's position.

Self-responsibility

The Gestalt theoretical stand on the importance of self-responsibility supports the formation and maintenance of a person-to-person type of therapeutic relationship. The notion of self-responsibility reflects the belief that we have the freedom to choose who we are and what we do and that it is a waste of energy and time to blame others for our life experiences. When people are helped to be responsible for themselves they are likely not only to create more alternatives but also to make choices that lead toward satisfaction and joy. By promoting equality in therapeutic relationships the therapist avoids taking responsibility—or seeming to take responsibility—for clients' lives or for their well-being. Clients must then mobilize their own inner resources and be responsible for themselves. One of the major goals of Gestalt therapy is to enhance clients' abilities to be creatively self-responsible.

Self-awareness

Another aim of Gestalt therapy is to help clients become more self-aware individuals. Self-awareness means awareness of all possible aspects of experiencing oneself and one's external environment. Expanded awareness leads to a sense of wholeness and enables a wide range of possible choices aimed toward health. Awareness of many facets of oneself at any given moment also allows the identification of inappropriate or useless habits so that new behavior can be substituted immediately. Gestalt therapy is phenomenological. Attention is given to whatever can be observed about the client at the moment and brought to the client's awareness. Awareness is enhanced by inquiring as to *what* the client experiences and *how*. Intellectualizing about why the client is doing something is avoided since it robs the awareness process of its immediacy and aliveness.

At times the therapeutic task is to help a client remove blocks to awareness. Instead of making interpretations about the blocks the Gestalt therapist may make suggestions that help the client explore the block to awareness itself or experiment with new ways of being aware of the area that is being blocked. This method keeps the focus on the inner process and avoids much of the defensiveness that can be triggered by interpretive statements.

Learning the integrative process

When people can readily integrate prior life experiences with new experiences a unified personality is apparent, and it can operate efficiently and joyfully. Out of this observation emerges a third major goal of Gestalt therapy. This is to help clients learn the integration process so that they can gracefully integrate life experiences into their personalities.

In helping clients learn to integrate experiences both therapist and client focus on the client's intrapsychic processing as it happens. This can be in the form of asking a client to report a constant stream of awarenesses of both internal and external environments. Spontaneously reporting awarenesses usually leads to acknowledgment of memories, feelings, or actions that are being blocked from integration into the personality. Once these are experienced clearly work can proceed toward "owning" these "split-off" thoughts, feelings, or actions and thereby comfortably integrating them into the personality.

The concept of contact

As defined earlier, contact is a sense of awareness and connection with one's internal and external environments. Contact with others is viewed by Gestalt therapists as essential for protection against an overwhelming sense of aloneness and for a sense of support for growth of the personality. Attention is given in the psychotherapeutic situation to the nature and purpose of clients' processes of making contact with themselves and others.

Polster and Polster (1973) delineate two aspects of contact that are relevant to the practice of psychotherapy: (1) they define contact boundaries as the points at which one can experience the differentiation of self and nonself and (2) they describe the concept of contact functions as modes of making contact. Gestalt therapists also concern themselves with the balance of contact and withdrawal in a client's life.

Our bodies and value systems, our wishes to deal mainly with that which is familiar to us, and our selection processes about what parts of ourselves we make available to whom all serve as boundaries along which contact can be made or rejected. The characteristics and functioning of these boundaries in the personality interact to provide a sense of the entire boundary of the self. This sense is vital to contact between people because each must have a clear sense of separateness before healthy, gratifying contact can be achieved. Psychotherapeutic work to help clients become aware of the many facets of their boundaries is basic to the therapeutic process since the quality of contact between client and therapist depends on the clarity of each one's own boundaries. Naturally the more disorganized a client's personality is, the more important working on boundaries of the self becomes.

The senses of touching, seeing, hearing, tasting, and smelling as well as the ability to speak and move, are modes of making contact with others. These modes allow for testing and redefining of boundaries as well as for a sense of excitement and possibilities for growth. Shutting down the contact functions often leads to depression, boredom, and loneliness. Gestalt therapists pay considerable attention to helping clients become aware of how they use their modes of contact and what devitalizing blocks are operating to diminish the ability to make enjoyable contact.

The balance between contact and withdrawal is also of concern in Gestalt therapy. People become psychologically troubled when they either cannot maintain contact or cannot break it. As is typical of Gestalt therapy, work on the problem of being stuck at one end of the continuum of contact and withdrawal proceeds by paying attention to the client's process of flowing between these two extremes. Ideally clients are helped to become increasingly aware of their needs and wants at any given time to maintain contact with the inner or outer environment or to withdraw from it. Practicing this awareness is one way clients can discover their own balanced, rhythmic pattern of flowing from aloneness to togetherness and back again.

In addition to the concepts of contact boundaries, contact functions, and the balance of contact and withdrawal, Gestalt therapists use the notion of resistances to contact. Resistances are seen as attempts to avoid awareness of parts of the self as well as full contact with others. Some theorists of psychotherapy view resistances of the client as a negative factor in the therapeutic process, while Gestalt therapists respect clients' resistances as having arisen from a perceived need for protection or survival and welcome opportunities to work directly with the resistances as they manifest themselves.

The five most typical resistances are (1) confluence, (2) deflection, (3) introjection, (4) projection, and (5) retroflection. Each of these can provide both a positive and negative impact on the personality depending on the nature and extent of their use. For instance confluence—the sense of blending of boundaries with another so that a sense of separateness is lost—can be experienced as being in love if the feeling is mutual, pleasant, and temporally limited. Confluence with another, which involves a chronic submergence of one's own uniqueness, however, can become an empty attempt to be alike and in constant agreement. This precludes rewarding contact and leads instead to resentment. Release from the overuse of confluence as a resistance to nourishing contact comes from helping clients learn the process of defining their own boundaries, needs, or wants more clearly.

Deflection is used by people to dilute contact and make it less intense. At times this may be beneficial but if used in excess it prevents contact. Avoiding eye contact, talking too softly, or constantly interrupting the natural course of the contact are ways of deflecting. In Gestalt therapy clients who consistently use deflection

to break or avoid contact are helped to be aware of this pattern so that they can deliberately choose whether or not to use it.

Introjection is the process of bringing the environment inside one's boundaries. This can be done by swallowing it whole or by tasting, biting, and chewing carefully. Often clients have swallowed some beliefs whole and these become "shoulds," which act as blocks to authentic contact. For instance the belief that one should not raise one's voice precludes all sorts of interesting contact possibilities. In working with introjection problems the Gestalt therapist reacquaints clients with their choices of what to take in, how to do so, and how to rid the system of old perceptions that are no longer useful.

Projection is the ability to extend thoughts or feelings outward in time or onto people or objects in the external environment. This can be done creatively, as in conjuring fantasies of the future or in projecting our own experience accurately onto another so that empathy is the result. The use of projection in a destructive way is evident when clients have not claimed for themselves what is being projected but instead attempt to rid themselves of some trait, thought, or feeling by unloading it onto someone else.

Retroflection is an intent to expend energy in some form onto the environment but once started the action turns in on the self. Since the action that is retroflected may be a loving one, retroflection is not in itself seen as unhealthy. For instance, one could have an impulse to reach out and touch another person gently but block that impulse and stroke one's own body instead. Habitual retroflection can lead to an extensive loss of contact with others and a severe blocking of excitement so that tight areas in the musculature of the body and a depressed mood become evident. Retroflective behavior must be dealt with in a way that releases energy so that energy is available for work in psychotherapy sessions. Gestalt therapists usually help clients release the retroflected energy by having them pay attention to body movements that are retroflective in nature. As clients become more aware of their "holding-in" process they can experiment with letting go in order to follow through on their original impulse. In this way clients are able to restore their abilities to make contact.

THE PRACTICE OF GESTALT THERAPY

The theoretical framework for the practice of Gestalt therapy leaves room for a great deal of creativity in its application by the therapist. Dr. Frederick Perls (1970), the founder of Gestalt theory and therapy, demonstrated a highly creative and unique style of practice with clients. Generally speaking, Gestalt therapists highly value practicing from the point of awareness that contains an artful blend of theory and one's own sense of the moment. The following section illustrates my own approach to specific clients and may need to be modified to be useful in other therapeutic encounters.

Gestalt therapy is practiced with individuals, groups, and families. In group and family work the focus is likely to be on one person at any given time although some attention may be paid to the interaction process. Perls was well known for "hot seat" work in which he gathered a group together and members took turns on the "hot seat" of intensive, individual work while others watched and hopefully learned. Occasionally someone in a Gestalt group is helped to become fully aware of what he or she wants from other family or group members and can experiment with satisfying that want. At times group or family members participate in an individual's work by playing characters in dream or fantasy enactment.

Principles of Gestalt therapy are adaptable to a wide range of clients' goals and problems. They are used in crisis intervention, supportive therapy, and work on personality structure. A wide range of diagnostic and problem categories are amenable to intervention with Gestalt

therapy. Some of these are depression, anxiety, phobias, addictions, both borderline psychotic and acute or chronic psychoses, death and dying counseling, and management of pain. Modified Gestalt principles are also useful in helping a person with hysterical personality traits. Since hysteria can be viewed as an overly heightened awareness of feeling states, Gestalt work is best aimed at heightening awareness of thoughts rather than feelings, so that integration of the cognitive and affective systems can take place. Through this modified approach the client is helped to gain a balanced state of wholeness, which replaces the imbalanced overemphasis on feelings.

Whether Gestalt therapists are dealing with an individual, a group, or a family, some characteristic stances are taken. Honesty, openness, and the ability to be warm and supportive are valued and acted on to the best ability of the therapists. Respect is given for the client's ability to be a more self-responsible person. Therapists act as coaches, or guides, helping the therapy become a process by which the clients learn more about themselves through experiencing themselves in a new way. The therapists' central task is to maintain a clear awareness of themselves, the clients, and the environment. It is out of their own awareness base that Gestalt therapists can formulate their interventions.

Classical Gestalt methods

The remainder of this section on practice will illustrate some of the classical Gestalt methods as they are actually used with clients.

Experimentation. Underlying many Gestalt psychotherapeutic interventions is an attitude of experimentation—an encouragement to clients to experiment with their behavior as a way of broadening personal boundaries and claiming the wholeness of their personalities. The concept of experiment as a tool in therapy sessions leads the therapist to be aware of clients' inhibited, incomplete, or interrupted behaviors, verbal or nonverbal, and to ask the client to follow through into what may be new behavior.

A client, Alice, sits with her arms crossed during a session but occasionally makes slight lateral hand and forearm movements as she speaks of her devotion to her son's well-being. When she is asked to be aware of her arm movement and move it to completion several times she finds that she makes strong sweeping motions and becomes suddenly aware of wanting to sweep him out of her life. At this point the therapist might ask her to experiment with saying some sentences as though speaking to her son as she continues to make the complete sweeping motion. Awareness and integration of this new part of herself now gives Alice an opportunity to make clear, conscious choices about her relationship to her son.

Many people are uncomfortable with experimenting with new behavior during a therapy session, so the therapist is careful to help lower the clients' resistance by grading the experiment for comfort level. If clients are too uncomfortable to actually try new behaviors at some point in a session, the therapist may ask them to sit quietly and fantasize the new behavior. The next step might be to fantasize it and then report it to the therapist.

Unfinished business. Another concept used in the practice of Gestalt therapy is that of unfinished business. The therapist is alert to signs that indicate that a client is holding on to emotions that were not discharged in past situations. Signs of unfinished business are legion and include experiences within the awareness of clients by which they know they have "never gotten over" some event. When the unfinished business is not within clients' awareness, they cast people into roles that reflect an earlier unresolved situation rather than seeing how these people are currently behaving. Clients may also manifest useless or destructive behavior as a result of unfinished business.

The process of resolving unfinished business

through the use of Gestalt therapy entails helping clients bring into awareness of the original unresolved events and work on them as if they were happening in the present. An attempt is made to portray the experience vividly. From this impact-in-the-present type of work clients can have the opportunity to experience new closures to old life events. Because of the powerful way the event and its new resolution are felt, they now take precedence as a base from which to react to similar future situations.

Enactment. The process of enactment is another classical aspect of Gestalt clinical practice. Enactment is the dramatization of parts of a client's life experience. Often during a session when therapist and client are designing an experiment to help the client expand personal boundaries, enactment is a tool through which the client becomes aware of new parts of the self.

Enactment may be used as part of an experiment in which a client is helped to become more aware of the feelings behind a particular behavior. For instance a new client, Joann, habitually tightens her facial muscles as she walks into the therapist's office. The therapist asks her to dramatize this behavior by exaggerating the tightness of the muscles and then releasing the tension as completely as possible. The fourth time Joann releases the tension from the exaggerated state of usual tension she bursts into tears as she becomes aware of repressed sadness regarding the way in which she terminated with her former therapist 2 years earlier.

Enactment is also utilized to help clients claim disowned parts of themselves. For example, Terry complains that his younger brother is obnoxious when he openly displays his anger. Since Terry is a passive, intellectual young man the therapist asks him to enact delivering a speech on the virtues of being "out front" with anger. After the speech the therapist asks Terry to boast about his own (imagined) great capabilities to express anger clearly and openly and to illustrate his points by giving (imagined) examples. Through this strenuous work, Terry becomes more personally aware of a rationale for being open with anger and experiences a shift in his self-concept that allows that behavior to occur. In the next session the therapist suggests that Terry enact his brother being angry as a way to further expand Terry's experiential boundaries of his own expression of anger.

Dialogue. Dialogue is another common form of enactment used by Gestalt therapists to help clients sharpen their awarenesses of little known facets of themselves. One specific way that it is helpful is to provide clients with a way of being empathic with another's experience while broadening their own boundaries. Clients who complain that they had an upsetting argument with someone else may be asked to enact themselves and the other person alternately, speaking back and forth from each of the body positions and locations in the room that represents the self and other.

The concept of polarities or splits within the wholeness of the personality was mentioned earlier. When splits are present ambivalence and confusion become evident. This internal conflict is viewed by Gestalt therapists as a war being waged between two opposing parts of the self. Enactment of these polarities allows the parts of the self to carry on a dialogue and eventually make peace or show some appreciation or need for each other. When the polarized parts come to terms with each other the split is healed and the personality moves further along toward integration.

The best known of polarities in Perls' (1970) "topdog-underdog" split. The topdog is the master, the controlling and often highly critical part of the person that dictates to the underdog. The underdog part is the slave that makes passive and ineffective attempts to obey the master, thus constantly defeating the master. The possibilities for polarity conflicts within the individual are limitless. Other examples include struggles between the ambitious and lazy, the grandiose and self-effacing, the kind and cruel,

and the generous and selfish parts of oneself.

Often the polarities are worked less at an intellectual level and more at a feeling level through the use of metaphors. Instead of enacting part one and part two of oneself the client may work through a conflict by choosing to enact two objects or living things that represent opposing parts. Conflict can be creatively expressed, for instance, when a client plays the parts of an ant versus a sloth, Queen Victoria versus a flower child, or an orchid versus a dandelion.

Enactment of polarities is illustrated by discussing a session with Doris, who is stuck in a perfectionistic, critical part of herself. She complains that she asked her husband to dig a hole for a bush and told him exactly where she wanted it dug. When she returned she found that he had dug the hole a few inches to one side of the appointed spot, which annoyed her greatly. The therapist first asks Doris to enact herself and her husband, dialoguing in present tense the entire bush-planting scenario. By enacting her husband's part of the interaction she becomes aware of feeling angry at having such explicit demands made. She begins to get a feeling for what one part of herself does to other parts of herself, that is, constantly scolding and criticising her performance as a wife, mother, and lawyer.

The next step in helping Doris claim both of these parts of herself and getting them in contact with each other is to have her enact what she chooses to call "superdog" and "sneaky dog." As she enacts these characters, she is able to be less defensive about the superdog part of herself and creatively plays out a humorous dialogue. She delights in playing sneaky dog, who responds to superdog's demands to clean and shine their living area immediately by hanging superdog's rug out to air on the window ledge (where it is bound to be soiled by the local pigeon droppings). Thus superdog is easily defeated and the pigeons can be blamed.

From this enactment of her polarities, Doris

recognizes how tempting it is for both her and her husband to try to defeat in a passive and irresponsible way her rigid and demanding "superdog." She also gains a new sense of the choices available between the extremes she has just dialogued.

The next step in work on this polarity struggle is to have her enact in more metaphorical ways the battle between the perfectionistic and the "I'll try" parts of herself. As she tires from enacting the battles they give way to curiosity and finally to compromise with even a touch of admiration between parts. Resolution and integration then become possible in her daily life.

Part of the process of enacting polarity struggles is a point Perls calls the impasse. This point is usually experienced as a feeling of loss of energy, stuckness, or deadness, as if the opposing parts were locked in a battle that cannot be resolved. Clients may or may not need the therapist's assistance in getting through the impasse. Once they are through, their energy is restored and they often report a sense of rebirth or new awareness of strength.

Fantasy. Fantasy work is another classical tool of Gestalt therapy. As illustrated in some previous examples, fantasy is at times the only route to making contact with some people and with past events or possible future events. Fantasy can be very helpful in creatively exploring new approaches to old problems. It is also another powerful tool for expanding personal boundaries and shifting the nature of the personality.

An example of fantasy work directed toward change of the personality is work with Marcia, who is depressed and highly anxious and suffers multiple psychophysiological symptoms. At the outset of a session the therapist asks her to breathe deeply and abdominally, letting go of tension as she exhales. The therapist then asks Marcia to fantasize the words she is exhaling. The word "hate" comes clearly to her awareness and she reports feeling a heavy tenseness in her upper abdominal area, which she identi-

fies as the place she stores her hate. The therapist then asks her to fantasize what the hate looks like. Marcia reports that she visualizes it as a heavy purple sphere with a rough surface and that it is about the size of a bowling ball. As she continues with her fantasy she imagines removing the ball from her abdomen and holding it in her hands. She now reports that she feels much lighter and that most of the tension is gone from the stomach. Marcia is willing to imagine letting the therapist hold the "hate" ball while she fantasizes more about her abdominal area. She is quiet and then reports a picture in her mind of fragile but pleasant-feeling filaments growing in the empty place. Marcia stays with this fantasy until she is breathing more easily and feels confident that the filaments are part of her. Feeling much less tense and anxious and more free she imagines taking the old, heavy, rough hate ball from the therapist and crushing it into tiny pieces of dust, which she blows away. At the beginning of the following session Marcia reports that some of the buoyant feelings are still with her and that her abdomen has been only slightly tense. She also has decided that she wants to work on letting go of a specific hatred that she is now aware of having held on to from a broken romantic involvement 8 years before.

Body-mind integration. Working with body-mind intergration is another classical aspect of Gestalt practice. This may begin in a fantasy form or by focusing on body movement and awareness. If parts of a client's body appear to be ignored, avoided, emphasized, or immobilized a Gestalt therapist might encourage a client to become aware of that part of the body. Depending on the circumstances the therapist may ask clients to do such things as exaggerate something about a part of their bodies, fantasize a story about that part, or have a dialogue with the part. Another way the body is included in the therapy is by asking clients to express emotions—usually anger—in physical form. For example, if the anger is blocked a Gestalt therapist might arrange the environment so that a safe pile of pillows is available. The therapist may ask a client to begin by tapping the pillow, slapping it while exhaling, making a sound on the exhale, and then rhythmically pounding the stack of pillows. Often this procedure helps clients become suddenly aware of what the blocked anger is about and in the process discharge it.

Dreamwork. Another important part of Gestalt therapy is dreamwork. Gestalt therapists treat a dream as a reflection of various parts of the client's personality. The therapeutic task of dreamwork is for the client to become more fully aware of these split-off parts of the personality, claim them, resolve conflicts among the parts, and integrate them.

Rather than discussing a dream in an abstract, intellectualized manner the therapist and client approach a dream as if it were happening in the present. The therapist first asks the client to tell the dream in the present tense. The therapist may then repeat a summary of the dream for the client or feed back information about which part of the dream the client seemed most reactive.

A character or object in the dream is identified as impactful if the client has strong positive or negative feelings about it or tries to ignore its existence. The therapist usually asks the client at this point to enact that character or object. In this way the client has the opportunity to become vividly aware of the aspect of the self represented by the dream character. For instance, Jim reports a dream about his father's funeral several months after the actual funeral. When he is asked to "be" the casket he replies, "I am strong and solid and I enclose this man and hold him in a loving way." At this point Jim begins to cry, recalling forgotten times when he had actually been supportive and loving with his father. As he continues to recall these instances the guilt he had been feeling for not having done enough for his father great-

ly diminishes and he spontaneously allows himself a full sigh of relief and a comfortable smile.

Often two characters in a dream are in conflict. In that case the therapist asks the client to enact these characters in a dialogue of their conflict. The same principles apply as just described in the section on working with polarities. If the dreamwork is being done in a group and there are many characters in the dream, the therapist may ask group members to help enact the dream to make it an enlivening experience for everyone. Often the participants add new elements that help expand the dreamers' awarenesses of themselves.

SUMMARY

From the description of Gestalt theory and practice in this chapter the reader can see that emphasis is placed on people as unified beings. This holistic approach is the hallmark of Gestalt therapy. A sense of integrated wholeness, which includes tapping into every possible human potential of the client, is valued by the Gestalt therapist. The therapist's office is transformed during each session into a microcosm of the clients' lives. Into it they bring as vividly as possible their internal and external environments for the purpose of exploration, expansion, and integration.

References

Brallier, L. W., and Hoffman, B. S.: Assisting a psychotic patient with the integration process, Psychotherapy **8:** 304-306, 1971.

Latner, J.: The Gestalt therapy book, New York, 1973, Julian Press, Inc.

Perls, F. S.: Four lectures. In Fagen, J., and Shepherd, I. L.: Gestalt therapy now, Palo Alto, 1970, Science & Behavior Books, Inc.

Polster, E., and Polster, M.: Gestalt therapy integrated, New York, 1973, Brunner/Mazel, Inc.

Stevens, J. O.: Gestalt is, Moab, Utah, 1975, Real People Press.

Stratford, C. D., and Brallier, L. W.: Gestalt therapy with profoundly disturbed persons, unpublished paper, 1975.

CHAPTER 21

Holistic health practice: expanding the role of the psychiatric–mental health nurse

LYNN W. BRALLIER

HOLISTIC HEALTH PHILOSOPHY AND HUMAN ECOLOGY

Although the technological approach to health care is currently flourishing a divergent concept has been reborn and is attracting renewed interest. Both ancient and revolutionary, this concept is holistic health care. It is rapidly emerging as a companion to the medical model of health care delivery in the United States and in many respects is also a viable alternative to it.

In reference to this contemporary approach the word ''holistic'' (also spelled ''wholistic'' by many practitioners) is defined as an integrated state of wellness—specifically the integration of body, mind, spirit, and environment of a client. Rather than practicing a fragmentary approach to health care practitioners of holistic health seek to help liven and integrate the body, mind, spirit, and environment of each client. When these aspects of living are dynamically balanced and integrated clients are whole and fully well. They are far beyond an absence of symptoms and illness. They are physically fit, filled with vital energy, and relaxed; they find meaning in life and are busy creatively developing their own human potentials.

The holistic philosophy of health care and the human ecological perspective on health care are congruent in many respects. Both concepts acknowledge that the total human being, including the spiritual aspects of that person, relates to the total environment. Aware of the interrelatedness of all things, practitioners of these approaches are especially interested in the interaction of the individual's internal and external environments.

Historically holistic health care began with shamans, who were the healers of individuals and communities in ancient cultures. Shamans viewed healing as restoring the balance of the spiritual and bodily aspects of ill people as well as rebalancing their relationship to their community. Other early philosophers and religious leaders were aware of the wholeness of people as well as of the impact of the spirit, or soul, upon both mental and physical well-being. The Greeks knew that the body could be in a diseased state because of disharmony of the mind; curing the body in a lasting sense meant healing the spirit. Szasz (1978) reports that modern psychotherapy evolved directly from Socrates' concern that the welfare of the soul was the most important aspect of living.

Today, by way of Gestalt theory and family systems theory, the ancient concept of holism has become familiar to many modern psychotherapists. The term ''gestalt'' is used in one sense to indicate the experience of feeling complete and in harmony with oneself. Thoughts, feelings, bodily sensations, and actions all feel

219

balanced and a sense of well-being prevails. Another holistic concept, family systems theory, allows that the family is more than the sum of its parts and that change in one part of the system will change the character of the whole family.

One other example of holistic philosophy influencing health care delivery is the general practice or family practice model. Often people who were born prior to 1945 can recall visits to ''the'' doctor who knew their physical and family history; educational, mental, and emotional status; social interaction patterns; and religious persuasions. In the current practice of medicine superspecialists and computers are more numerous than family practitioners. Many people have learned a mechanistic and fragmented concept of themselves as a result of having to decide which part of themselves to take to what specialist. Too often these people assume that understanding and influencing the state of their health is so complicated an issue that they have shifted personal responsibility for their health to professionals and their technology.

In light of the present level of health of our general population, outcomes reflective of full and positive wellness may seem outrageously idealistic. Although modern medicine performs seeming miracles occasionally in the treatment of emergencies and serious illnesses, it has earned a failure mark in the promotion of excellence of well-being. This point is made clear by epidemiological research that indicates that only 6% of our population comes near to full wellness (Belloc, 1971).

Believing that wellness is a possibility for everyone, holistic health practitioners also hold that each person expresses wellness in a unique way. Since holistic health professionals are health ecologists they maintain a wide-angle view of a client's eco-system including the client's external environment. Clients are encouraged to be highly aware of the impact of their environments and to arrange them to sup-

port wellness as much as is possible. Once the environment is clean, free of noise, and beautiful it is safe to become harmonious with it and allow it to add to a sense of wholeness. Clients are also encouraged to live within the laws of nature by carefully monitoring and coping with stressors, eating food that is fresh and uncontaminated, and using mild natural medicines whenever possible.

Attending to a client's body, mind, spirit, and environment is more than practicing comprehensive health care. Checking fully the many aspects of a client's life is only a means with which to begin the serious work of moving toward a positive state of wellness. Holistic health philosophy and practice extend beyond comprehensive health care by emphasizing clients' spiritual values, the integration of all aspects of a client's life, and the belief that clients are responsible for their own health.

BASIC TENENTS OF HOLISTIC HEALTH PHILOSOPHY

A belief upon which much of the practice of holistic health is based is that human beings are naturally inclined to be vitally alive and in perfect health or wholeness. In spite of the fact that only 6% of the U.S. population demonstrates this soundness the potential for this state of well-being is within each person. The philosophical stance that wholeness is an important goal as a state of being is in sharp contrast to the mechanistic philosophy underlying much of modern medical practice in which attention is given to one organ or section of the body at a time as a focus for treatment. In psychosomatic medicine's attempt to connect mind and body some progress has been made but only in describing psychological causes for bodily ills, not in helping people use their minds to prevent illness and promote high-level wellness. With the addition of spiritual influences on health holistic health philosophy addresses the issue of the mind healing the body.

As mentioned earlier holistic health theory

describes a human being as more than the sum of the parts of the self—the body, intellect, emotions, spirit, and interaction with the social and nonsocial environments. Dynamic balance among these intimately connected parts is a state of wellness. Divisions or imbalances within this human gestalt result in tension and dis-ease. In evaluating a client's dis-ease, or departure from wholeness, the holistic health practitioner looks for parts of the self that are not in harmony either with each other or with the whole. Examples of disharmony can be manifested in an unlimited number of ways, ranging from the person who is generally healthy but suffers severe indigestion when faced with highly competitive situations to the person who ordinarily rates himself as very successful but occasionally has brief, severe depressive episodes and feels that life has no meaning. The first person illustrated a mind-body disharmony in which a mind in some state of upheaval disrupts bodily functioning. In holistic health terms the second example illustrates a spiritual problem in which the person is not in sufficient contact with the spiritual part of the self.

Since inclusion of spiritual matters is not usually associated with health care, a brief discussion of spiritual concepts may be useful at this point. The word "spiritual" is not to be confused with religious doctrines and practices. As defined in holistic health philosophy spirit is the life force that provides energy for all parts of the self to be in harmony with nature. It is the essence of humanness—the energy of being, or consciousness. Spirit is also a personal and vital connection to an inspiring force or forces greater than oneself, such as God, art, or a sense of fitting into history or nature. This commitment to something more expansive and powerful than the self can provide a basis for purpose, meaning, and style of life.

When people are not in contact with the spiritual dimensions within themselves they may complain of feelings of hopelessness, help-lessness, grief, and a sense of isolation and anomie. A cogent philosophy is missing—that of life and death from which the individuals can act in conducting their lives.

In contrast, people who are spiritually healthy are purposeful, committed, and have a sense of uniqueness and energy to actualize their ideals. Having the sense of contact with and dedication to a force beyond themselves allows people to develop and exhibit altruistic feelings and value systems, which holistic health practitioners believe are present naturally in all people. These value systems manifest themselves in acts of love, compassion, hope, courage, creativity, and wisdom. Thus when spiritual energy is high individuals are likely to behave in ways that result in receiving positive feedback from others. As every clinician knows positive intrapsychic and interpersonal experiences are beneficial both in preventing illness and in recovering from illness. The saying, "Your faith has made you whole," is adopted by holistic health practitioners as, "Your commitment to health can help make you well and keep you well." Another basic tenet of holistic health philosophy is the belief that people can take responsibility for their own health.

The conventional medical model often encourages a collusion between doctor and patient in believing that the doctor is responsible for and director of the patient's health care and that the patient should only cooperate. In contrast, the holistic health model defines the client's role as one of partner since clients are respected as being able, as was the health professional, to learn about health and illness. Further clients are seen as senior partners who take the ultimate responsibility for their own wellness. By now the reader has probably noticed the use of the word "client" to indicate a partnership role rather than "patient," which is easily experienced as a subservient role.

In carrying out the philosophical notion of client self-responsibility holistic health practitioners often function as teachers and coaches with clients. Principles of sound nutrition, exercise, and stress management are easily taught. The following practical suggestions and specific programs are offered by practitioners to help their clients:

1. Choose an exercise program that is appropriate.
2. Eat regular, wholesome meals.
3. Manage stress so that tension levels are not dangerous during waking hours and plan for restful sleep at night.
4. Manage unhealthy habits such as overeating, smoking, and excessive drinking.

Although holistic approaches emphasize prevention of illness and growth toward total wellness, other educational offerings such as classwork are made available to clients who are ill. Whether holistic health practice is used exclusively or as an adjunct to medical treatment of the illness the emphasis in these classes is on self-regulation and self-healing. An example of this approach is instructing clients in specific meditative methods that may help control hypertension.

A third fundamental philosophical concept of holistic health care is the theory that people are able to learn to control stress. This control may be exhibited by clients' learning to eliminate selectively stressors from their lives, reduce the intensity of the stressors, or cope with existing stressors more effectively by changing their responses to the stressors. Since prevention is the focus, educational approaches are quite useful. Often examination of clients' basic value systems and philosophies of life and death can be of crucial importance as to how clients manage stress. Discussion of these issues encourages clients' reformulation of values and revision of life-styles. A striking reduction in the number of stressors, particularly the number of stressful thought patterns, may then be experienced by clients, which may result in a higher level of wellness.

A fourth important tenet of holistic philosophy is that clients can combine both traditional and unconventional approaches to prevent illnesses and to heal themselves if they do become ill. By its very nature holism must respect or at least recognize the potential of healing methods that span time and cultures. Ancient remedies may be suggested to accompany modern ones as long as the two do not cause difficulties when combined. For instance, certain herbal teas and extracts as well as specific meditations may be recommended to help a client accelerate the healing process after surgery. Another ancient method of healing—currently being researched in the laboratory, clinically tested, and utilized as an adjunct to other forms of treatment—is healing by the laying-on of hands. Dolores Krieger of New York University teaches a course in what she calls the "therapeutic touch" to students in the graduate nursing school. She has also joined many physicists, psychologists, and others who are conducting research that has demonstrated remarkable results in healing human beings, animals, and plants by the laying-on of hands. It is possible that electromagnetic fields of energy are involved in this type of healing; whether or not this is so, the act of touching can certainly communicate a calming, comforting, caring, and loving influence that helps to heal a person by relieving his pain, anxiety, depression, and loneliness.

HOLISTIC HEALTH CENTERS AND PRACTICES

During the 1960s we witnessed the birth of community mental health centers across the country. In the 1970s holistic health clinics and practices began to take form. Perhaps the 1980s will be remembered as the decade of the health revolution in the United States.

One of the oldest holistic health clinics in the United States is in Springfield, Ohio. Developed by a clergyman, Dr. Granger Westberg, it was sponsored by three churches (Tubesing, 1976). Classroom space in one of the churches was converted on weekdays into clinic offices and a staff of both professionals and volunteers was collected. In the mid-1970s, Westberg and Tubesing, a pastoral counselor, started two other holistic health centers in Illinois. Sponsored by the Kellogg Foundation, the centers provided for a physician, a counselor, a nurse, a secretary, and volunteers from the community. The word ''wholistic'' is used by this group to indicate both the philosophical and pragmatic focus on wholeness of body, mind, and spirit. As practiced by the Westberg groups the process of engagement, evaluation, and treatment illustrates the delivery of services generally by holistic centers (Peterson et al., 1976).

The initial appointment is usually made by telephone. At this first meeting any urgent health needs are attended to but the main concern is the client's overall health status. The client fills out a personal health inventory prior to the appointment and it is reviewed by the entire staff at the initial meeting. By discussing life stressors, goals, and spiritual beliefs present health status and areas for growth are outlined jointly. Referrals are then arranged to whatever services the client and health team agree are appropriate. Frequently these referrals are for such services as a complete physical examination, a course in stress management and nutritional management, biofeedback, or perhaps a form of counseling. Many referrals are for the general purpose of prevention of illness and enhancement of wellness. Often the format is a group educational approach so that costs to the client are kept at a minimum and social support is maximized to help reinforce new health care behaviors.

Since long-term, comprehensive attention to health is the intended service to the client at the health center, many chronic problems are addressed early and followed closely. To encourage progress toward wellness for clients with chronic problems highly creative approaches are sometimes called for. In California and now in some other areas many holistic

health centers offer a wide range of services including various special diets and herbal treatments, therapeutic massage, acupressure, reflexology, and various forms of meditation, self-healing, and spiritual development.

Clients at a holistic health center tend to be college educated and employed as professionals or white-collar workers. An experimental center in Washington, D.C., however, serves an impoverished area of the city. This center, the Community of Hope Health Services, was founded, and is directed by Lois and Roy Smith, community mental health nursing specialist and clinical psychologist respectively, and a physician, Janelle Goetcheus. Following the Westberg model its services include helping people cope with the financial and legal stressors on their health caused by their environment.

Many private practitioners around the country are attempting to expand their roles to include the skills necessary to practice holistic health. My own practice is an example of this. As a clinical specialist in psychiatric–mental health nursing, over the years I have added biofeedback skills, knowledge of various meditative and spiritual practices, some expertise in therapeutic massage and acupressure, and a continuing teaching process regarding exercise, nutrition, and physical assessment. I teach a course in stress management and meditation to clients and other lay and professional groups. In light of the knowledge and wide areas of expertise required however a one-person holistic clinic is not practical. Most of us therefore must settle for constantly acquiring as much new knowledge and as many skills as possible, meanwhile referring clients to other holistic pracitioners. The independent practitioners of holistic health offer clients the same philosophy of health care and similar procedures as the clinics do.

In addition to various centers and practices around the country, an organization called the Association for Holistic Health in San Diego is becoming a national education and information center for the field. This association also publishes the *Journal of Holistic Health* and a newsletter called *Holistic Health Focus*.

CLINICAL ASPECTS OF HOLISTIC HEALTH PRACTICE

The number of "new" therapeutic approaches that are being included by their designers under the rubric of holistic health grows daily. While many of these approaches reflect holistic philosophy others do not. As yet the field is too young to have produced wise and seasoned teachers who can claim the authority to define resolutely what clinical methods do or do not belong in the practice of holistic health. In presenting clinical approaches then I hope to describe adequately some of my own clinical work as well as suggest other holistic methods that also have been beneficial. Because the spectrum of possibilities for helping clients toward wellness is very broad, this presentation highlights but a few of them.

Being both psychotherapists and nurses, psychiatric nurses who hold master's degrees are ideal candidates for practicing within the holistic health model since they deal with the mind-body aspects of practice with relative ease. To have a sturdy, well-rounded base from which to practice holistic health, the psychiatric nurse-therapist may also need refresher courses in physiology or medical nursing and nutrition as well as in spiritual and religious philosophies and practices. Estimates from various medical textbooks indicate that 50% to 80% of visits made to physicians are for illnesses best classified as psychophysiological. For this reason stress management is a major part of any holistic approach. Since psychiatric nurse-therapists are already knowledgeable about stress management, they may only need to update their knowledge and skills in this area.

Because stress management is one of the core concepts within the holistic health model we should look at how the clinician helps clients deal with stress. First stress must be defined. Selye (1974) notes that factors that cause stress are stressors and that stress is a nonspecific bodily response to a stressor. During stress the person's physiological homeostasis has been disrupted and the body is in distress while attempting to return to its balanced state. Stress responses are learned and patterning of stress responses becomes chronic. Usually one or two sites of the body such as the stomach or neck muscles are involved. If exposure to stressors is too intense or prolonged and if coping mechanisms are unable to reduce the stress responses, common illnesses such as headaches of various types, arthritis, respiratory and cardiovascular disorders, and many types of pain, lethargic states, and infections may result. Even some forms of cancer are now thought to be the result of stress interfering with the effectiveness of the immune system so that aberrant cells are not noticed and therefore are not destroyed. Although our frantic life-styles and polluted environment expose us constantly to stressors, we probably experience stress most by how and what we think. Part of any course in stress management given by a holistic health practitioner includes helping people focus on how their perceptions, beliefs, and thought patterns influence their level of stress. For instance, a person may discover that he believes he is never quite "as good as" other people are and that he consistently produces thoughts that reflect this belief. These self-denigrating thoughts trigger feelings of sadness, anger, and perhaps other emotions in varying intensities. Physiologically the body is now out of a calm, homeostatic state and is being controlled by the sympathetic nervous system. It will go through distress in trying to recover its balance. When this person becomes aware of his negative beliefs and consequent negative thought patterns about himself he can reevaluate them and perhaps will discard many that were causing unnecessary stress to his body. Many other principles of stress management can be taught in class to help clients learn to cope effectively with the stress of living.

In clinical practice some stress management principles are taught, as are many forms of psychotherapy and self-regulatory therapies such as biofeedback, meditation, and visual imagery. Although nearly any form of psychotherapy can be considered helpful in managing stress, the forms I have found to be most useful are both individual therapy and family therapy that are derived from theoretical vantage points of communication theory, systems theory, Gestalt therapy, behavior therapy, cognitive behavior modification, Gesalt body-mind awareness work, and guided imagery focused on both relief and prevention of further stress symptoms.

In keeping with the philosophy of client as partner, many of the methods used in a holistic health practice are of a self-regulatory or self-healing nature. For instance, biofeedback is a therapy in which delicate physiological monitoring instruments serve as teaching tools and allow clients to learn to control consciously many physiological variables previously thought to be automatic. Receiving audio and/or visual feedback from an electromyograph instrument on how tense or relaxed the muscles are in the forehead, jaws, back, or arm can help clients learn to release the tension. A general relaxation response is learned from practice with the electromyograph during office visits. This biofeedback work is supplemented by home practice in which clients strengthen a relaxation response by listening to relaxation tapes and practicing various forms of relaxation such as specific breathing methods, meditative methods, autohypnosis, and visual imagery work. As the relaxation of parasympathetic response is strengthened, it is integrated into clients' lives and is at first consciously and later automatically substituted for a stress response. For the purpose of relieving stress symptoms and preventing other symptoms from developing, a variety of biofeedback instruments and auxiliary relaxation methods can be used to help clients achieve the ability to control their own psychophysiology. A wealth of psychological benefits are possible from the regular practice of relaxation and meditation. Among those most frequently reported by clients are an increase in confidence in themselves to manage their own lives, a deepened sense of knowledge and acceptance of themselves; an ability to care and love and yet to remain detached enough from other people, thereby avoiding unproductive emotional struggles, and a decreased dependency on external factors such as alcohol, tobacco, and food as well as other people.

No matter what the specific stress illness may be, many methods of psychotherapy and self-regulatory therapies have a broad and basic usefulness with clients. Considering the range of psychophysiological illnesses possible, this is fortunate. In my own holistic practice, I see clients with problems typically brought to a psychotherapist such as depression, anxiety, phobias, psychosis, substance addiction, interrupted grieving, and problems in marital relationships and families. I use stress management principles with these clients and even more intensely with those who are coping with such illnesses as asthma, chronic pain, migraine and tension headaches, skin diseases, insomnia, colitis, stomach ulcers, aortic stenosis, hypertension, and cancer.

To illustrate a holistic approach with a client it would be helpful to present a case history of Ann, who actually represents a composite of several persons with whom I have worked to gain control over seemingly intractable migraine and tension headaches.

Ann is 38 years old. She says she has had headaches for as long as she can remember and has spent approximately 3 days in bed every 2 weeks with a migraine headache. She complains of mild to moderate tension headaches in between the acute migraines. Her neurologist is very concerned that continuing the high, constant dose of Cafergot will be harmful to her and has referred her for self-regulatory therapies.

A detailed assessment is made of Ann's body, mind, spirit, and environment. Information is collected about her health history generally—her major past and present life changes and her current nutritional and exercise habits. How she copes with stressors in her environment is given a great deal of attention. Her spiritual beliefs, life goals, and attitudes toward herself and others are discussed. It is made clear to Ann that she will be taking the basic responsibility for her health and she feels some fear but also welcomes the challenge. A biofeedback diagnostic evaluation is done, which indicates that Ann has high muscle tension in her forehead and neck and low hand temperature. Both of these readings are typical of people who have a combination of migraine and tenson-type headaches. At the end of the evaluation conference a preliminary wellness program is initiated. Ann agrees that the priorities should be to begin a biofeedback program for learning to control her headaches and to change some aspects of her general health habits.

In subsequent sessions Ann learns with aid from a biofeedback instrument how to warm her hands at will. She is able to do this at the earliest sign of the onset of a vascular headache and has had some success in aborting an acute migraine process. She is enthused about her successful experiences and reports many side benefits of the relaxation she has learned from biofeedback work. She has practiced a 20-minute "suggestions for general relaxation" tape two to three times each day as part of the biofeedback approach to helping her gain control of her vascular system and its response to stress. Ann has watched her diet more carefully and has managed to eat less junk food and more raw fruits and vegetables. She also takes a vitamin and mineral supplement each day and claims to have more energy as a result of her new relaxation and nutrition program. There was celebration when Ann managed to give up smoking and she is experimenting with how she feels when her alcohol consumption is curtailed drastically, saying that the meditations she does now make her feel both "high" and calm and that they seem to replace her need for alcohol and for those purposes.

Two new exercise programs have been instituted. Ann begins each day with some Feldenkrais (1977) body awareness movements and has begun to take long walks in preparation for a running program that is reasonable for her.

Over the next 5 months Ann returns twice each week for psychotherapy, biofeedback, and general health counseling. In psychotherapy Ann does some Gestalt work on her tendency to be a perfectionist and to be nonassertive and fearful of becoming fully well and "normal." This work leads to eight conjoint sessions with her husband and with her whole family. As the family system begins to change, allowing her to take a more assertive adult role, Ann experiences satisfaction in having a greater impact on others and is able to begin giving up using her headaches to manipulate others or to withdraw from conflict in the family. During one of the conjoint sessions with her husband he learns to do some of the massage and acupressure techniques that are used during each of her office visits to relieve tension and pain. Both Ann and her husband learn some reflexology points to massage in the hope that this method will also be helpful for pain relief.

Many types of imagery work are done with Ann. As part of the biofeedback goals of gaining more control over her hand temperature and muscle tension, suggestions that she visualize her hands as large and red and see her muscles as loose rubber bands or pieces of spaghetti are found to be helpful. For the purpose of integrating her new self-regulatory skills into her life Ann is encouraged to develop her own relaxation and self-regulatory images to "flash to" during the day. Images of herself as absolutely well are placed on custom-made self-regulatory cassette tapes that are given to Ann as needed.

Imagery is also a vital part of the psychotherapy done with Ann. At one point she is asked to imagine her heart being able to talk to her; she feels angry with her heart for beating too fast at times and starting a headache. This leads to more imagery work in which Ann in a very relaxed state is helped to imagine being able to go into a room and find the person (part of herself) who is responsible for causing the heart to beat too rapidly. Ann in imagery meets an old man who claims he must cause her headaches or she will become wild and immoral. This leads to several discussions of Ann's spiritual values and the conflict diminishes greatly.

After 8 months of therapy Ann feels in control of her symptoms and her life generally to a degree great enough to terminate her twice-weekly contract. She will stay in touch for regular health checkups and knows help is available should she need any further consultation for stress management.

Approximately half of the clients in my own holistic practice have cancer. Many of these clients have been given a terminal diagnosis but the focus of the therapeutic contract is on the highest level of wellness possible. After a thorough evaluation similar to that done with Ann priorities for therapeutic work are jointly set. The range of possible approaches is very broad. For instance following the holistic body-mind-spirit-environment framework various forms of psychotherapy may be employed to help the client reduce anxiety and depression and add a sense of hope and even intermittent joy. Both psychotherapy and biofeedback may be used to help clients experience a stronger sense of control over the course of their illness. Biofeedback and imagery may help clients control pain, alleviate the side effects of chemotherapy and/or radiation therapy, and master the ability to relax generally and to sleep well. Clients are asked to talk about their environments to see if their surroundings are conducive to energy conservation, minimal distress, and maximum comfort. Considerable attention is also given to discussing spiritual beliefs and philosophy of life and of death. If clients wish they are assisted in various ways to get in touch with their own reserve supplies of such qualities as courage, love, and wisdom.

Much of the work just outlined helps relieve damaging stress effects on an already severely stressed body. Close attention to other aspects of stress management may help relieve physical distress enough to allow the body to function more normally. The more clients' bodies stay in a homeostatic state, the greater the chances will be that the immune system will be more efficient in combatting the proliferating cancer cells. Simonton and Simonton, a radiologist and counselor team in Texas, have applied this information clinically in a holistic approach to stress, which includes having clients with cancer use methods of visual imagery to influence their immune systems (Simonton et al., 1978). Over the years they have collected clinical data that support this approach as a viable method by which some clients have apparently become cancer free and have maintained that

status for 5 years or longer. Many holistic health practitioners around the country are using the Simonton method with clients who have cancer and other severe chronic illnesses.

THE PSYCHIATRIC NURSE AS HOLISTIC HEALTH PRACTITIONER

Reorienting one's practice from medical model to holistic health model entails many changes in philosophical assumptions about attitudes toward those who seek assistance with their state of health.

Meanwhile the general public is becoming increasingly interested and knowledgeable about holistic health and self-care as can be noted by perusing the popular paperbacks such as "How to . . ."—relax, eat sensibly, exercise, stop smoking, and so on. A shift of philosophy and power is underway. Both professionals and the public may need help with this shift however since some professionals seem able only to relate well to sick people and some people "prefer" to be sick. For those who have unclear preferences new reinforcers might be helpful. These new reinforcers could be provided by the insurance industry in the form of refunds on insurance premiums if clients document attendance at classes on nutrition, exercise, stress management, and control of harmful habits or seek clinical assistance for the purpose of preventing illness and enhancing wellness. If holistic health nurse practitioners and much of the public are dedicated to the philosophy of holistic health such reinforcers may become a reality.

In closing, perhaps a review of some basic requirements and attitudes would be useful. First is the personal commitment to practicing holistic principles in one's own life. The holistic health practitioner must love being healthy. For the psychiatric nurse, learning medical nursing skills as well is important. Giving serious thought and study to refine one's own philosophy of life, attitudes toward death, and spiritual beliefs is also essential. An openness to both orthodox and unusual methods of healing is useful. Competence as a teacher and consultant is also necessary to carry out effectively the client-as-partner relationship. The role of holistic health nurse practitioner is obviously not for everyone. Since the areas for new learning are particularly varied and numerous, it is perhaps best suited to those who enjoy constant growth and change in their professional practice.

References

Belloc, N., Breslow, L., and Hochstim, J.: Measurement of physical health in a general population survey, Am. J. Epidemiol. **93:**328-336, 1971.

Bloomfield, H.: The holistic way to health and happiness, New York, 1978, Simon & Schuster, Inc.

Carlson, R.: The end of medicine, New York, 1975, John Wiley & Sons, Inc.

Feldenkrais, M.: Awareness through movement, New York, 1977, Harper & Row, Publishers.

Peterson, W., Tubesing, D., and Tubesing, N.: The process of engagement, Hinsdale, Ill., 1976, Society for Wholistic Medicine.

Selye, H.: Stress without distress, New York, 1974, New American Library.

Simonton, O., Simonton, S., and Creighton, J.: Getting well again, New York, 1978, St. Martin's Press, Inc.

Szasz, T.: The myth of psychotherapy, New York, 1978, Anchor Press, Doubleday Publishing Co.

Tubesing, D.: An idea in evolution, Hinsdale, Ill., 1976, Society for Wholistic Medicine.

CHAPTER 22

Transactional analysis: dealing with the man-environment relationship

PAT KURTZ

Transactional Analysis (TA) was developed
as a social-psychiatric theory recognizing humankind's needs and propensity for social
interaction. As a theory it attempts to explain
not only how the personality and unique behaviors of the individual develop but also how
the individual influences and is influenced by
the environment and people in that environment.

Before discussion continues about the specific concepts and theoretical formulations of
TA some general introductory background
information will be helpful. Like most "new"
theories TA has a basis in and many commonalities with earlier theories of personality and
behavior. TA's foundation includes the developmental theories, psychoanalytical theory,
ego psychology, and some of the learning
theories.

What is different about TA is its focus on
the social components of behavior, which includes providing an understanding of the how's
and why's of social interaction as well as an
understanding of the problems and remedies
for them. Additionally TA theory explains concepts and relationships on the basis of readily
observable behaviors and from a commonsense
point of view rather than from inferred constructs. Like most theories TA theory is not
considered a finished product. As behaviors

and human problems are tested in the light
of the theory, old concepts are elaborated, refined, or discarded and new concepts are developed.

VALUE ASSUMPTIONS

There are several assumptions basic to TA
theory. It is believed that in the natural course
of events every person is meant to grow physically and emotionally to a maximum potential
and that each person will do so unless blocked.
TA therapy is concerned with identifying and
removing those blocks. People have the capacity, the right, and the responsibility to participate in their own block removals; therefore the
concepts of the theory are identified in such a
way as to be meaningful to ordinary people.
Therapy is a contractual arrangement in which
client and therapist have mutual rights and responsibilities. It is also believed that people
have the right to get their needs met and that
they can be met in a way that is fun and does
not hurt other people. Children are considered
valuable and should be nurtured as should the
Child (ego state) in each adult.

Because of the belief that the concepts should
be made understandable and that it is permissible to have fun while figuring things out and
getting cured, the language of TA includes
many colorful and colloquial terms that keep

229

their everyday meanings. The terms and concepts will be introduced and explained as the theory is described.

Analysis of the individual and his relationship to the world is done on four levels: (1) structural analysis is based on the structure of the individual personality; (2) transactional analysis analyzes communication; (3) game analysis describes a series or cluster of transactions within a larger social context; and (4) script analysis is concerned with the individual's lifetime relationship to this world. Understanding and meaningful change is possible at all levels.

STRUCTURAL ANALYSIS—EGO STATES

In TA the personality of the individual is conceptualized as a system with three subsystems described as ego states. These three ego states—Parent, Adult, and Child—are unique developmental phenomena and describe how individuals relate to their environment in different ways. For this discussion the names of the ego states will be capitalized; when an individual person is referred to the term will not be capitalized. Each ego state is a set of related and consistent behaviors, feelings, and attitudes. In a healthy personality all three ego states are available for use and any given ego state is energized according to the needs of the situation.

Child ego state

The Child ego state is the first to develop. It is the ego state of birth and until the other ego states have developed it is the only ego state; therefore it is usually the ego state that we experience as the self. The Child is composed of those sets of feelings, attitudes, and behaviors that we experienced as children. The Child is the source of our feelings, curiosity, spontaneity, wishes, and intuition. The language of the Child ego state is that of ourselves as children and includes phrases such as ''Wow,''

''I want,'' ''Can't make me,'' ''I love you,'' and ''I hate you.'' The posture and activity of the Child is open, free, active, and relaxed. Smiles and hugs as well as temper tantrums and frowns come from the Child part of the personality.

Parent ego state

The Parent ego state includes a set of feelings, attitudes, and behavior patterns similar to those of an individual's parents. The parents in this instance may not be the biological parents but include those people who held that significant place in the individual's life. These early caretakers include parents, older siblings, grandparents, or other persons who may have had responsibility for the individual as a child such as maids or housekeepers. Although each person has a unique Parent ego state, Parents have many common characteristics. The language of the Parent ego state includes ''must,'' ''should,'' ''everyone,'' ''you,'' ''never,'' ''always,'' and a collection of mottos to cover all occasions such as ''Every cloud has a silver lining.'' The body posture of the Parent may be stiff and people who spend a lot of time in that ego state are likely to experience frequent neck stiffness and headaches. The pointing, accusing finger and the soothing pat are both behavioral characteristics of the Parent.

Parent words and responses are usually stereotyped and are passed down from parent to parent for generations. Characteristic of Parent communications is the fact that they are reproduced from the assimilated responses of other people and have not been subjected to analysis or reality testing by the individual. For this reason these responses are automatic in nature and can be thought of as tape recordings stored in the brain that play whenever the right button is pushed. These automatic verbal responses and other behaviors are referred to as Parent tapes. The content of the Parent tapes is related to moral values and represent the expected be's and do's of behavior. Button pushing to stimulate a particular tape comes from the environment in the form of particular situations, physical surroundings, or behavioral stimuli from other people such as childlike behavior.

Although automatic on the part of an individual, Parent tapes may well be astute observations or very practical problem solutions from a parent or grandparent. Part of the process of parenting involves passing on knowledge, moral values. and ready-made opinions, and the process is valuable because children then have the benefit of the experiences of earlier generations. Difficulties arise when those opinions or values interfere with healthy growth or are no longer of value in the current situation. The person who relies on Parent tapes for direction may not know what to do on occasions for which there are none or they are irrelevant.

The Parent ego state is a later development and becomes an autonomous structure somewhere between age 9 years and adolescence. There is some theoretical disagreement about whether or not the behaviors that appear to be Parent in early childhood are part of a separate ego state or whether they are incorporated in the Child ego state as pseudo-Parent and identified in second-order structural analysis.

Adding tapes to the Parent tape library does not stop after a certain age. Later tapes are acquired from bosses, teachers. and other authority figures who have importance in our lives. Nurses, for example, have tapes about how nurses behave and how patients are supposed to be treated. The strongest and loudest tapes are likely to be those that were repeated the most often over time and were related to issues of reward, punishment, and survival for the child at an early age.

Adult ego state

The Adult ego state is the least well defined of the three ego states but is nonetheless important. The major characteristics of the Adult are autonomy and adaptation to present reality.

The Adult ego state may be most easily conceptualized as a computer whose function is taking in, storing, and analyzing information; making predictions; and developing programs.

Developmentally the Adult makes its initial appearance around the age of 2 or 3 years, coinciding with parental demands that children meet some external standards for which they are not motivated and coinciding with the neurological development that makes this possible. Accomplishing the tasks required by the parents causes the child to develop the capacity for objective thinking (Schiff, 1975). Adult development is completed by about age 12 years.

The behavioral characteristics of the Adult ego state are those of erect posture, level head position, alertness of senses, even voice tone, and phrases such as ''I think,'' ''It is my opinion,'' ''The facts show that,'' and ''Under certain circumstances.''

The process of structural analysis

The most simple and basic analysis in the course of therapeutic intervention from a TA point of view is that of structural analysis, which means simply the process of identifying the content of each ego state of a given person and that person's learning to identify or diagnose which ego state is operating at a given time. Essentially this means being able to tell the difference between facts (Adult), feelings (Child), and opinions (Parent). Young children can easily learn these distinctions; however, many people are confused about these differences and need some time and practice making these differentiations. On a more complex level structural analysis means identifying individual Parent tapes, the circumstances of their recording, the Child feelings and development, and the Child responses to the parent tapes. Being able to identify ego states allows an individual to cathect other ego states at will and provides the person with more options for problem solving and for interacting with the environment.

The analysis of second-order structure, re-

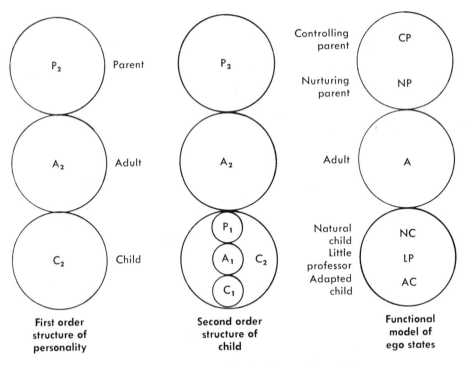

Fig. 22-1. Structural and functional ego state models.

ferred to earlier, is of a more theoretical nature and presupposes that before the Adult and Parent structures develop the young child has correlates of these structures (A_1 and P_1) within the Child ego structure (C_2) and that there is an early or infant (C_1) structure. The neuroses are thought to be problems of second-order analysis in the Child and some have suggested that psychosis is a problem of a proposed third-order structure, which is at a very early developmental level (Schiff, 1975). Fig. 22-1 shows a model of the person from the standpoint of first-order structure, second-order structure, and function.

For purposes of this discussion first-order analysis will be sufficient, together with an understanding of what is known as "functional analysis." Berne (1961) believed that these ego states were personality manifestations of actual structures in the brain and that later research would show that there was a relationship between structural areas in the brain and the organized sets of behaviors that make up the three ego states. For purposes of understanding and treatment, looking at ego states in terms of their function is easier than using the structure.

Functional analysis

In functional analysis the Adult ego state is considered essentially as it is from a structural viewpoint. The Parent ego state is divided into two parts according to the functions of Nurturing and Controlling Parent. Both functions of the Parent—nurturing and control—are meant to be in the service of the Child, promoting his safety, health, and adaptation to the world. The two major divisions of the Parent serve to support or develop different aspects of the

Child ego state. Neither function of the Parent ego state is inherently good or inherent bad. What is important for the Child's well-being is the particular Parent ego state that promotes or inhibits growth and well-being. Although generally it is good for the Child to be nurtured and comforted, if there are never any criticisms, demands, or proscriptions on behavior the person will have a more difficult time adjusting to parts of the environment that are not nurturing and protective. On the other hand, of course, if the child is subjected only to criticism and inhibition of action and feeling, the result is low self-esteem and lack of certain necessary behaviors that promote his own well-being and that enable him to properly parent his own biological child and behave in a nurturing way toward other people when this is appropriate and required.

The Child has three functional parts: the Natural Child, the Adult in the Child, and the Adapted Child. It is the Natural Child, sometimes called the Free Child, that is spontaneous, natural, and energetic. This is the part that reacts on the basis of instincts, feelings, and needs.

The Adult in the Child, or Little Professor, is functionally thought of as being similar to the A_1 structure. What is recognized with this functional part is the innate although poorly developed intellectual aspects of the young child. This part of the personality makes decisions of some sort at a very early age but on the basis of internally developed categories, meanings, and logic. Much of the basis for decision making at this level cannot be identified at a rational level and has been described as intuition.

The Adapted Child is essentially the Natural Child adapted to the environment, especially to the parents or parent figures. It is the function of the parents to help the child adapt to the world. The early adaptation is to the immediate environment, which is the mother first and then the expanded family. Later, of course,

adaptation is to the larger environment such as the neighborhood and school. The personality of a person is based on his genetic endowment and how he reacts and develops to his surroundings from that aspect. To a large extent it is also the adaptation the child makes to his parents. Not all children adapt the same way; nor does a child adapt the same way to everyone or everything. Generally, however, a person learns a standard adaptation pattern, which takes one of two forms: (1) complying, and most children do comply to the demands and expectations of their parents; or (2) rebelling, which can also be thought of as a particular form of compliance.

One way to conceptualize the adaptation process is to think of the child's needing certain nurturing and life-sustaining things from the parents. To get these things the child is expected to behave (adapt) in certain way. The child does whatever is needed to "make mother smile." It sometimes happens that rebellious behavior is "what makes mother (or father) smile" regardless of what they may actually say. Parents are commonly pleased (and smile) at children's noncompliant behavior.

An important facet of understanding adaptation is that most adaptation requires a modification of the spontaneous and instinctual responses of the Free Child. In some instances in order for the child to adapt to the parents' demands certain feelings, needs, or wants must be inhibited. Pleasing some parents may even require self-destructive behavior.

The Natural Child can also be rebellious when what is required is not what the child wants to do. There is a difference between the resistance and rebelliousness of the Natural Child and that of the Adapted Child. The Natural Child will rebel against things perceived to be against its best interests or instinctual needs or wants. The Adapted Child will rebel because it has learned this behavior as a response to Parent demands, and the response is as automatic as the compliant response is for others. The rebellious Adapted Child says "no" simply because an authority figure has said "yes." Unfortunately for the Rebellious Child not everyone in the larger environment will smile at the rebelliousness the way Mom and Dad did.

It is believed that there is a complementary relationship between the dominance of the Nurturing or Controlling Parent and the Natural or Adapted Child. The more of the Nurturing Parent the child has experienced, the more likely that he will be free to respond naturally and to get his needs met; conversely, the more of the Controlling Parent there has been, the more likely that the person will respond from an Adapted position in terms of automatic behaviors designed to please others.

The ideal seems to be some happy medium in which the Natural Child is nurtured and supported with enough control to make him civilized and able to get along in the world. However, one additional component is required besides the right balance of Parent—the Adult. It is considered far more healthy and productive for the individual to learn to use facts and logic in the service of getting needs met than to develop automatic adapted behaviors that may be appropriate as a child and for that particular family but not appropriate as a grownup with other people. Some of the healthiest Parent messages are those that include the instructions to think and to solve problems.

Functionally a person has five ego states available to use at any given time. Both theoretically and practically certain of the ego states are more appropriate than others at any specific time. Inappropriate use of ego states is one cause of interpersonal difficulties.

In summary, the individual personality is composed of three ego states. The Child ego state is the major part of the personality, responding to both internal needs and external environment. especially the parents. The Adult ego state provides the information and predictions that the Child needs to make rational decisions and is a later development of the personality. The Parent ego state is the storehouse

of parental, family, and cultural prescriptions and prohibitions.

As a result of the growing-up experiences the child has, the kinds of parenting, the kinds of Parent tapes that have been introjected, and his reasoning capacity at the time of the experiences every person by age 10 years or less has developed an existential view of the world having to do with how he sees himself and how he sees others. These views range on a continuum from every positive (OK) to every negative (not OK).

PSYCHOLOGICAL HUNGERS
Stroke hunger

Before further discussion of the analysis of transactions, games, and scripts it would be useful to identify several other concepts central to the TA theory—concepts that influence the motivation and kind of interactions the individual has with his environment. In his early work Berne (1961), using other works to support his conclusions, identified the concept of stimulus hunger, which he defined in terms of a need for sensory stimuli and intolerance for long periods of boredom or isolation. He believed that the hunger was particularly for the stimuli that are obtained through physical intimacy. Based on the belief that actual physical stroking of the skin is essential for the physical and emotional health of the infant, he later identified "stroking" as essential for grownups as well (Berne, 1964). To varying degrees people learn to substitute psychological strokes for physical strokes. A stroke is defined as "a unit of recognition" and this term is used to include any form of recognition from a loving kiss to the ritual "Hello" to an acquaintance to a scolding from a parent or teacher. As a rule the units of recognition that are perceived as positive are called "strokes" and those that are perceived as negative are called "kicks," although both serve the function of providing a recognition stimulus and sensory input. Positive strokes, known colloquially as "warm fuzzies," are preferable to kicks but kicks are better than no strokes at all and may be eagerly sought after by someone who is deprived of strokes. The absolute importance of stroking, both in infancy when it is considered a survival issue and later when it promotes our emotional survival, makes it a medium of exchange in the day-to-day and long-term transactions in our interpersonal environment.

There are many cultural and individual family rules that proscribe the kind, amount, and source of strokes that a person may ask for, take, or refuse. Much of the parental control comes from the parents' ability to give or withhold strokes.

Structure hunger

In addition to the stimulus and recognition hungers there is a third hunger called "structure hunger." This refers to needs that individuals have to structure their groups as well as their time. Six levels of time structuring have been identified; they have to do with the quality and amount of stroking that are taking place. At one level is "withdrawal," a state in which the individual is not involved with other people but is self-stroking or stimulating by fantasy, by reading or watching television, or by physical stroking with attention to body needs.

Next in intensity of stroking is the level called "rituals," which are stereotyped, programmed ways of getting strokes. The most common ritual stroking is that of our greeting and leave-taking behaviors in which the recognition units are clearly culturally defined and predictable. Influences in the amount and intensity of stroking at this level depends on the relationship to the other individual and the length of time between stroking episodes. For example, there are differences prescribed for intimates as compared with subordinate employees and differences between first encounters of the day and the sixth meeting by the end of the day.

A simple "Hi, how's it going?" will suffice for an acquaintance but not for a close friend who has been on vacation. At all times adherence to the prescribed ritual stroking is necessary to maintain a relationship at a given level. Any initiation of increased or decreased stroking intensity in terms of amount or quality is the signal for a possible change in the relationship. It may, however, only reflect the individual's own stroke level in his reservoir. It is difficult to give out strokes if no strokes or only kicks are coming in.

The third level is that of "activities," which is most commonly a work situation. Work is thought to require more time in the Adult ego state and getting the job done is more important than recognition. Of course, some jobs require more Adult time than others do and some people spend more time exchanging strokes on the job.

The next level is called "pastimes" and accounts for a large share of the time spent interacting with others. Much pastiming is socially programmed and predictable but has more variation and spontaneity for stroking than rituals or work. In the pastiming situation people talk about topics of general interest and social acceptability. Topics include who makes the best car or where you can find the best martini, the best bargain, the best food; how to cook something, sew something, fix something; inflation; the weather; and raising children, vegetables, and eyebrows. One of the functions of pastiming is for the Child to find someone who will be compatible at the next levels of time structuring—games and intimacy. Both games and intimacy have intense stroke value. The difference is that games are played for particular outcomes that reinforce the life position, produce bad feelings, or justify certain decisions.

Games are a series of interactions (transactions) that proceed in a predictable manner; on the surface they seem ordinary enough, but they have ulterior motivation. Intimacy is a game-free, caring, sharing relationship. Both will be discussed later in more detail. Characteristically persons who have a psychiatric diagnosis are more likely to structure their time at the levels that have little stroke value. Deliberate altering of the level of time structuring is an appropriate therapeutic action.

TRANSACTIONAL ANALYSIS

The basic unit of behavior in TA is the transaction, a unit of communication between ego states. The transaction can be a communication between two ego states of the same person or from an ego state of one person to an ego state of another. For example, the internal dialogue that we all carry on with ourselves is between two of our ego states, usually between the Parent and the Child, in which we may be applauding, criticizing, explaining, justifying, or bragging to ourselves. There is a certain amount of stroke value in our self-communications; for some people they are positive strokes; for others, kicks and guilt trips. Making this internal dialogue explicit has therapeutic value in that verbalization takes it out of the automatic realm and makes it accessible to the Adult state, which is usually bypassed in the internal exchange. For example, the person may then hear himself call himself ''stupid'' and understand why and from whence came the bad feelings, the way it was when he was a child.

A model has been developed showing the ego states involved and the direction of the communication vector in different types of transactions. There are two possible relationships for the vectors in a transaction. The first relationship is that of a parallel position, which occurs when the messages are exchanged between like ego states or a complementary Parent-Child. When the vectors are parallel communication is occurring and will continue indefinitely. The second relationship is that of a crossing of the vectors when the response to a communication stimulus comes from a noncomplementary ego state. In functional terms the controlling Parent, Nurturing Parent, Adapted Child, and Natural Child are different ego states. The Controlling Parent and Adapted Child are complementary to each other and the Nurturing Parent and Natural Child are complementary.

Other combinations are generally noncomplementary. When vectors are crossed communication stops and can be resumed only if one or another of the persons switches ego states so that they are again complementary.

When there is a single set of vectors between ego states the communication is a simple transaction. There are two types of complex, or ulterior, transactions—the angular and the duplex. In the angular transaction there are three ego states involved, with one person sending a message, usually from the Adult of the one person to two ego states of another person, usually the Adult and the Child. The duplex transaction involves four ego states—two from each person. At one level is the social, or overt, transaction, with a psychological, covert message at another level. The well-known double-bind communication is an example of the angular transaction. Examples of all four types of transactions are presented in Fig. 22-2.

When there are psychological messages these take priority over the social message. To further complicate the communication issue people tend to hear messages in terms of their existential position and may often hear an ulterior message when none is there. The overt message is translated into a different message by means of the internal dialogue between the Parent and the Child. By this means people are able to turn kicks into strokes and more commonly strokes into kicks.

GAME ANALYSIS
Rackets and trading stamps

Most everyone likes to get something for free, which is why some commercial concerns offer trading stamps. In the course of an ordinary business transaction, in addition to the merchandise that has been paid for, there is a bonus of free stamps. If enough of the right color stamps have been acquired the collector is entitled to a ''free gift.'' A similar psychological system of collecting bonuses from ordinary transactions that can be traded in for something free operates in interpersonal transactions.

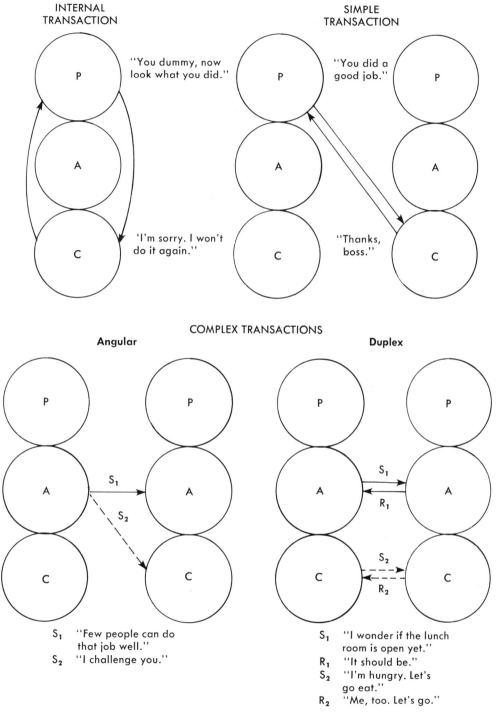

INTERNAL TRANSACTION

"You dummy, now look what you did."

'I'm sorry. I won't do it again."

SIMPLE TRANSACTION

"You did a good job."

"Thanks, boss."

COMPLEX TRANSACTIONS

Angular

S_1 "Few people can do that job well."
S_2 "I challenge you."

Duplex

S_1 "I wonder if the lunch room is open yet."
R_1 "It should be."
S_2 "I'm hungry. Let's go eat."
R_2 "Me, too. Let's go."

Fig. 22-2. Types of transactions.

If a transaction can be initiated or if a response can be reinterpreted so as to elicit or promote particular feelings, these feelings can be used as stamps and collected for a later trade-in for something free—''guilt free'' in this instance. For example, over a period of time a person may collect ''unappreciation'' from his boss at work. The events about which he feels unappreciated may be the actual transactions of his job (which he may set up in some way) or may be his later translations of those transactions through internal dialogue. He may trade in his collection of unappreciation stamps after only one book for a free ''call in sick'' or he may save several books for a big prize and get a free ''quit his job.''

Similarly a person may collect a few anger stamps for a free ''slam the door'' or several books for a free ''homicide.'' Or a person may collect enough nobody-loves-me depression stamps for a free ''drunk,'' a ''shopping spree,'' or ''suicide.'' The point is that the prizes are guilt free. The person has collected enough of whatever kind of feelings are necessary to justify the action. In many instances the person has to justify even seemingly simple and ordinary actions like taking a day off because the Parent in his head will not permit it without strong justification.

In the normal course of living children experience a wide variety of feelings and, initially at least, act on these feelings even before there is a conscious awareness that a ''feeling'' exists or before it is categorized. Parents teach children the names of their feelings whether or not they may legitimately act on them (''Yes, I know that you're mad at your brother, but you may not hit him'') and whether or not the feelings themselves are approved or allowed in that family (''Don't ever say that you hate anyone''). Feelings that are approved may vary from family to family or according to age or sex roles. For example, in some families the way to be heard is to shout; in others raising the voice is unheard of. Boys may be encouraged to feel anger but never to be afraid and girls may be allowed to be afraid but never angry.

The result of these reinforcements and prohibitions is that feelings that are supported and responded to become automatic responses or initiators in transactions rather than specific to a real here and now situation. Another consequence is that certain feelings that otherwise would be spontaneous responses are blocked from awareness. In that instance the child must substitute a more acceptable response such as feeling depressed rather than angry. Generally each person adopts a favorite response that becomes automatic and is the ''racket.'' A racket, then, is a substitute for feeling or it is the feeling known to get strokes and reinforcement. Rackets are not conscious substitutes. The adoption of a particular racket is integrated as part of the Adapted Child. The person may be aware that something is missing or feels wrong but has not learned to feel the prohibited feeling or knows no other way to elicit the needed nurturing or stroking. Identifying and experiencing the missing feelings is an appropriate therapeutic goal. The racket feeling is the feeling used for psychological trading stamps.

Games

The earlier discussion of time structuring indicated that game playing and intimacy had high stroke value. Intimacy is a relationship that is game free with straight transactions and a mutual sharing and caring. Being intimate requires that a person be able to reveal oneself, including the bad parts, to take responsibility for one's own behavior and to allow others to do the same. Few people are able to achieve intimacy and resort to game playing for most of their intense strokes and the reinforcement of their life position. It is believed that everyone plays some games. What is important for health is that the games are at a low level and generally do not interfere with achieving some intimacy and with being a winner in life.

By definition a game is a series of ulterior transactions with a predictable payoff in bad feelings. By "bad" feelings it is meant that they are the racket feelings, or trading stamp feelings, which are then used for some purpose—either to reinforce an existential position ("See, I knew you couldn't trust men") or to further the life plan, or script, which is a decision about how life will be. That may mean, for example, collecting enough rejection stamps to finally commit suicide or enough anger stamps to get a divorce, withdraw from people, and live out a lonely life.

There are five basic elements necessary to diagnose a game. The first element is the con and the gimmick. The person who initiates the game presents a stimulus that hooks some need into the other person. That need is called the gimmick. The presence of both of these factors leads to the response. If it were not a game the transactions would proceed in a complementary way to a conclusion. In a game, however, the initiator pulls a switch; that is, he changes ego states and causes confusion in the other person who is trying to figure out what happened. The final element is the payoff for both of them, which is the racket feeling or stamp collection. In addition to the elements named, in order for the transactions to be a game the ulterior aspects must be transacted out of the players' awareness. If the ulterior transaction and the switch are done deliberately it is not a game but a maneuver performed for some overt gain.

A common example of a game is the one called "Why Don't You—Yes, But" (WDYB). The opening move in this game (the con) is a presentation of a problem and an invitation for others to help solve this problem. In this instance that which is hooked is the respondents' needs to be wise and helpful, and they respond by offering suggestions. The switch in this game is that all suggestions are rejected as not workable for some reason and the end result is a silence in which the helpers feel inadequate to help and the helpee reinforces the belief that no one else is any smarter than he is and the wise helpers (Parents) do not win.

If this were not a game a request for help would be made, suggestions offered, and good suggestions accepted with a thank you. Even if a con is offered a person can refuse to play by letting the other person have the responsibility for his problem and crediting him with being able to think of solutions.

Karpman (1968) has pointed out that the moves in a game involve a switch from one of three positions—rescuer, victim, and persecutor. In the above game the initiator starts in the apparent position of victim and the other players come out to rescue. The switch in the game occurs when the victim becomes a persecutor in the sense that the continual rejection of suggestions is an implied criticism of the inadequacy of the would-be helpers, who then become the victims.

Games are numerous and include those designed for two to five players. Everyone has favorite games and can usually play more than one position. For example, the initiator of a WDYB can just as easily take the part of Wise Parent if someone else initiates the game. Each game also has its degrees of depth depending on the severity of the consequence: first-degree games involve psychological damage—bad feelings. Second-degree games involve social damage—disruptions of relationships or jobs such as divorce or being fired. Third-degree games result in tissue damage—liver deterioration in the game "Alcoholic" or death in a third-degree "Rapo" game, and so forth.

SCRIPT ANALYSIS

The concept of scripts includes all of the elements previously discussed. According to TA theory, by the age of 9 or 10 years every child has made some basic decisions about the Parent messages he has perceived or misperceived and has a general plan, or script, for his life based on these decisions. Three basic script outcomes have been identified: (1) "winner," (2) "non-winner,'' and banal, and (3) ''loser'' or harm-artic'' (tragic and dramatic).

The script includes the kinds of relationships, their outcomes, and the roles, games, and feelings that are needed to further the script; unless redecisions are made along the way the play is carried out to its end. A few people have identified themselves as winners. Most people have ordinary garden-variety scripts and live out lives of ''making it,'' but they may not be particularly happy or may not end up where they would really like to be. The losers are those who wind up in the hospital, the morgue, the courtroom, or the prison. Psychiatric illness is thought to be a script or script ending in which the person has decided that he will always be helpless, miserable, confused, scared, crazy, depressed, and/or mistrustful and behaves in such a way so that he will be labeled sick.

One part of the script is the counterinjunction. These are the ''be'' and ''do'' messages from parents that are incorporated into the Parent ego state and offer the general behavioral objectives that the culture and the family prescribe. These are generally positive messages that are consistent within the family and the culture.

A second part of the script includes the messages that come from the Child ego state of the parents rather than the Adult or Parent and are incorporated by the Parent-in-the-Child, or P_1. These are the secret and not so secret messages, which may be in direct conflict to the Parent messages, and reflect the fears, ambitions, disappointments, needs, and other feelings of that mother or father. When these messages are happy and consistent so that the child is nurtured to grow and be healthy there is no problem. However often these messages may be damaging to the child. They may be incorporated because of the child's survival and love needs, as previously discussed in terms of ''what makes mother smile.'' When these messages are the type that inhibits health and normal growth they are called injunctions.

Goulding and Goulding (1976) have identified twelve common injunctions with variations: (1) ''Don't be,'' or ''Don't exist,'' (2) ''Don't be you,'' (3) ''Don't be a child,'' (4) ''Don't grow,'' (5) ''Don't make it,'' (6) Don't,'' (7) ''Don't be important,'' (8) ''Don't belong,'' (9) ''Don't be close,'' (10) ''Don't be well (sane),'' (11) ''Don't think,'' and (12) ''Don't feel.'' Each of these injunctions has variations and degrees.

Simply because an injunction is given by a parent does not mean that the child will automatically obey it. What the child decides to do will depend on his age, his experiences, his ability to figure out other options, and whether other important people are sending countering messages. This decision is the third element in the script.

A fourth part of the script is the program, or how to carry out the injunctions. Often the ''how to'' is taught by the parents who may be operating with the same injunctions themselves. For example, the way not to be close is to fight. The way not to feel sexy is to work all the time. The way not to think is to drink. The child may pattern his chosen script after a fairy tale or a story that seems to fit and important script information can be obtained by asking about and identifying the elements of that favorite story.

Other parts of the script include the life position, which is a result of the decision; the games needed to set up the payoff rackets; and the complementary roles taken by other people. A script analysis includes identification of all these parts. The purpose of the analysis is to identify the decisions made by the child in the context of the environment so that the individual can make another decision about his script and script ending and decide to be a winner instead of a loser (Steiner, 1974).

THERAPY

TA therapy is done on a contractual basis and, depending on what the client wants to be ''cured of,'' the therapy relates to any or all of the concepts that have been described. On a basic level structural analysis in which the client learns that he has three distinct ego states and how they function may make life easier. If the person is having interpersonal difficulties, understanding transactions, learning to be straight as well as to use different ego states and to diagnose other's ego states can clear up a lot of transactional difficulties.

Many difficulties require a script analysis because it is on the basis of decisions made about injunctions that a person organizes his games, uses his ego states in transactions, runs his rackets, or blocks out one or another ego state. It is helpful if the therapist knows his or her own script and has made redecisions as necessary since these rackets or injunctions may interfere with being aware of those of the client.

The analysis is not "done" by the therapist. Rather it is a joint effort by therapist and client in which the therapist uses all three of his or her ego states to listen intuitively, to provide professional training and ethical committment, to provide Adult information when needed, and to nurture and protect when the client is unable to do it for himself because of the unavailability of part of his personality, lack of information, or lack of appropriate internal parenting. The most important functions of the TA therapist are to provide protection to the client's Child by providing information and available support, to give permission to the Child to disobey the injunctions, and to support the redecisions to be a winner; the therapist should use everything that he or she knows how to do well and safely, getting help if needed. Once a redecision is made it is necessary to give the client a period of

support in which he can try out the new behaviors, learn to use his Adult instead of his Controlling Parent and Adapted Child, process his Parent tapes through his Adult for updating, and change his relationships so that the people around him support his new decisions rather than invite him into his rackets and destructive games.

Because TA is a social theory and therapy, it works particularly well in groups where people get involved with each other, play their games, and demonstrate their script decisions. The group then provides the matrix for trying out the new behaviors. The presence of other people adds to the likelihood that there will be people who do not play particular games and can call them or who may have good parenting skills or good Adult information when it is needed. For example, a group member may have an effective Nurturing Parent and can demonstrate what it means and how to use it to nurture oneself as well as others. At all times the group members can practice giving and receiving good strokes with each other.

References

Berne, E.: Transactional analysis in psychotherapy, New York, 1961, Grove Press, Inc.

Berne, E.: Games people play, New York, 1964, Grove Press, Inc.

Goulding, R., and Goulding, M.: Injunctions, decisions, and redecisions, Trans. An. J. **6**(1):41-48, 1976.

Karpman, S.: Fairy tales and script drama analysis, Trans. An. Bull. **7**(26):39-43, 1968.

Schiff, J.: Cathexis reader, New York, 1975, Harper & Row, Publishers.

Steiner, C.: Scripts people live, New York, 1974, Grove Press, Inc.

Part five

CLIENT–HEALTH CARE SYSTEM INTERFACES

■ The chapters in Parts two through four have dealt with nurse-client interactions designed to enable the client to learn more effective ways of responding to his multiple internal and external environments. In contrast, this last section looks at the broader perspective in community mental health; this section examines and summarizes crucial factors that affect both the client and the nurse in the community mental health setting.

Chapter 23 describes a business approach for looking at the community. Specifically the community is assessed in relation to mental health needs through the eyes of a marketer. Critics contend that too often health care programs are developed to meet the needs and satisfy the whims of the provider rather than in response to a community need. In contrast, few business enterprises can be sustained if they do not meet a community need. The community must support and desire the product of any business if it is to realize a profit and thereby justify its existence.

The marketing approach described, while by no means new, is novel to the health care industry whose product is largely service. This approach describes how a community can be assessed in a systematic fashion by attempting to determine the specific health care needs of the community rather than by providing for needs that members of the health care team believe the community ''ought'' to have. This approach is truly consumer oriented rather than merely providing lip service to the concept of meeting the client's needs as the client defines them.

Chapter 24 ties together each of the threads in the text as it succinctly relates community mental health nursing to human ecology. The chapter highlights how an ecological approach demands a responsiveness to the community as well as to the client as a unique individual. Table 3 details the procedures required for the performance of community mental health nursing roles and provides a noteworthy summary for the text.

CHAPTER 23

The application of marketing concepts to community mental health nursing

WADE LANCASTER

As the eighth decade of the twentieth century begins it is becoming apparent that man's progress may have been purchased at a price far greater than the costs recorded in his accounting ledgers. Many of these additional, unexpected costs are now being illuminated in the form of a severely damaged environment. Less visible but equally distressing is the disintegration of many social institutions; unable to keep pace with man's rapidly changing needs these institutions are crumbling under the onslaught of "future shock."

Man's sojourn from the forest to the precipice has been an amazingly short trip, and now the moment has arrived for man to take account not only of where he has been but also of where he is going. Many social scientists as well as ecologists have noted the grim problems awaiting man in the future. These new problems are both complex and pervasive; they affect everyone, with total disregard for social levels, classes, cultures, and so on.

For the most part man's attempts to solve new problems with old solutions have fallen short of their goal; whether or not he solves these new problems will be determined not alone by what he tries to do about them but by the very ways in which he thinks about them and about himself. As man continues to search for new solutions to these problems, he must learn from the past. However, as he learns from the past and moves into the future, he must avoid employing

obsolete dogmas. The issue is not whether knowledge and know-how are transferable; instead the issue is one of applicability.

Currently many American social institutions are undergoing a period of sedition. All of the hallowed institutions are feeling varying degrees of pressure for reorientation: there is a clamoring for an increasing amount of responsiveness, openness, and humaneness. On the surface this assessment and self-evaluation might be unsettling; however, it very well may be regarded as a healthy prelude to change. In a dynamic environment society is both ruthless and benevolent—ruthless in eliminating inappropriate social institutions, benevolent in rewarding institutions that change to meet new conditions.

One of the many American social institutions presently feeling the pressure for change is the health care industry. Professionals and consumers alike have become increasingly aware of, and concerned with, the nature and distribution of health resources and the patterns of medical practice as well as the problems of medical economics. The American health care industry has been characterized by some experts as having "uniformed consumers, a lack of management skills, small and fragmented delivery units; noncompetitive cost-plus pricing features, and inefficient incentives for both the buyers and sellers of health services" (Ellwood and Herbert, 1973).

The pressure for more responsive, open,

245

humane health care is being felt in all areas of the industry. Indeed even the treatment, care, and prevention of mental health problems have not been exempt from the pressures of societal change. The community mental health movement, which started in the early 1960s, has been severely criticized for not having achieved the goals and mandates originally established. According to the critics the problems stem from poor planning and implementation of services, inadequate funding, too few mental health centers, a lack of collaboration between providers, and a reluctance toward viewing the community as the client as well as a lack of responsiveness to the needs of the individual community.

Although many criticisms have been directed toward community mental health its advocates have acknowledged the benefits such as increased utilization by new clients, changes in the type of clientele, the treatment of more children and adolescents, and the elimination of bias toward the consumers of mental health services. The acknowledged benefits of community mental health unfortunately have not been sufficient to offset its criticisms and shortcomings. Consequently a call for a "bold new approach" is being sounded. This new approach is to be based on a thorough assessment of community needs, comprehensive planning, and a subsequent emphasis on the community as the client.

MARKETING AND ITS IDENTITY CRISIS

The theme of this chapter was selected with the full knowledge that it entailed some risks, just as all decisions do. But as one rational decision maker long ago pointed out all of man's existence entails a quest for certainty in an increasingly uncertain world. Clearly the health problems we will be facing in the future are uncertain ones. Those of us charged with the responsibility for suggesting some alternative solutions to these problems must attempt to deal

with some problems dimly illuminated by only a zodiacal light.

The suggestion that marketing be applied to community mental health nursing may seem a crass and inappropriate application of a discipline usually associated with hucksterism and products we do not want or even need. Much of the bad press associated with the marketing field comes from the tendency to view marketing only in terms of advertising and selling. Marketing often raises images of attractively packaged goods of marginal quality, offensive and misleading advertising, and deceptive selling tactics. Given the negative images held by many people outside the marketing field one might ask why should community mental health nurses get immersed in such a tawdry area?

The truth is that modern marketing suffers from an identity crisis. The layman who thinks about marketing often associates it with only one of the major components involved in the total marketing process. Consequently in the popular mind marketing is viewed as the task of influencing and persuading people to buy goods and services. Since most people resent these persuasive attempts, many individuals develop a negative image of marketing. Unfortunately the public forgets, overlooks, or does not understand the remaining components of the marketing process (Kotler, 1972).

The purpose of this chapter is to present the positive sides of marketing by briefly exploring the nature and scope of modern marketing, by explaining what is meant by the contemporary philosophy of marketing known as a consumer/client orientation, and to outline a planning framework that centers on a consumer/client orientation for a community mental health program.

NATURE AND SCOPE OF MODERN MARKETING

The process of marketing is as old as man, having been in existence since barter, trade, or exchange began among primitive people. In contrast, the formal study of marketing as a discipline is relatively new. Most marketing scholars agree that the beginning of marketing thought occurred around 1900 when the word marketing was first used as a noun (Bartels, 1962).

Evolution of marketing thought, 1900-1950

Since its inception the marketing discipline has been in a constant state of transition; the concept of marketing has undergone a number of conceptual as well as perceptual changes. The introduction of new ideas as to what marketing is and what it ought to do has stimulated continual reconceptualization. Simultaneously an endless search for new realms for the application of marketing has provided for perceptual changes (Bartels, 1974).

Early in its development marketing thought was primarily concerned with the distribution of products. This emphasis stemmed from the notion that the economic process was divided into two components: production and distribution. Marketing was viewed as a technical process, that began on the completion of production; consequently the concept of marketing early in this century was limited to the macro aspects of the distributive process (Bartels, 1974).

By the early 1920s the concept of marketing included the functions and problems of institutions responsible for distribution. Although broadened to a degree, marketing was still limited to the distribution of products and remained associated with the discipline of economics as a macroeconomic activity (Barels, 1974).

Marketing advances in the 1950s

In rather sharp contrast to the earlier study of marketing grounded in institutional economics, the 1950s witnessed a dramatic change for marketing with the emergence of new approaches to and concepts of marketing. One

development of extreme importance was the increased emphasis on the marketing management approach, that is, the management of products, price, promotion, and channels of distribution. This advance moved the concept of marketing a step further from the macroscopic to the microscopic level and from the general to the specific, as well as enlarging the marketing manager's role within the internal organizational structure (Bartels, 1974).

In the late 1950s traditional approaches to the study of marketing were supplemented by focusing attention on managerial decision making, the societal aspects of marketing, and quantitative marketing analysis. New concepts in marketing were borrowed from the field of management as well as from other social sciences. This increased interest in the social sciences imbued marketing scholars with a greater appreciation for the humanistic aspects of marketing, which in turn lead to an awareness of the consumer and subsequently to the study of consumer behavior (Bartels, 1974).

BROADENED CONCEPT OF MARKETING

Although vigorous debate concerning the basic notion of marketing has alternately waxed and waned since the early 1900s, marketing has traditionally been associated with the sale of physical products and consumer services. The formal study of marketing dealt primarily with how transactions are created, stimulated, facilitated, and valued between profit-seeking business firms and want-gratifying consumers. For the most part marketing scholars focused their attention on the managerial problems of large consumer goods producers who cater to the needs of the mass market. In contrast, relatively little attention was devoted to the marketing of services in the private sector, while even less attention was given to the marketing of public services.

During the late 1960s and 1970s not only was the traditional view of marketing challenged but the possibility of expanding the scope of marketing was also vigorously debated. After raging throughout most of the 1970s, the controversy has since waned. However, while the controversy appears to be over, the broadened concept of marketing is not without its critics. Unfortunately, because of space limitations, only the essential issues of the broadened scope of marketing will be discussed.

In 1969 Kotler and Levy published their now classic article, "Broadening the Concept of Marketing," in which they criticized the then prevailing view of marketing as "a function peculiar to business firms." They suggested that marketing is a more pervasive societal activity performed by different organizations in a wide variety of contexts. They observed that nonbusiness organizations have products and services as well as customers and use marketing tools; however, it is the business organization that has developed and used the science of effective marketing. Therefore Kotler and Levy (1969) argued that since all organizations perform marketing or at least marketing-like activities "the choice facing those who manage nonbusiness organizations is not whether to market or not to market, for no organization can avoid marketing. The choice is whether to do it well or poorly, and on this necessity the case for organizational marketing is basically founded" (Kotler & Levy, 1969). The authors concluded that marketing tools developed "in the most forwardlooking business organizations" should be adopted by nonbusiness organizations as they recognize their marketing role and make the choice to do it well.

The Kotler and Levy (1969) article was intended to be provocative. And indeed it stimulated a debate that continued for several years. As a result of these debates nonbusiness marketing became integrated into the mainstream of both marketing thought and practice in the 1970s. The movement to expand the concept of marketing probably became irreversible when the *Journal of Marketing* dedicated the entire July 1971 issue to marketing's changing social and environmental role. That issue included applications of marketing technology to fund-raising, population problems, solid waste recycling, health services, and other aspects in social marketing. In fact it was in this issue that Kotler and Zaltman (1971) coined the term "social marketing," which they defined as "the design, implementation, and control of programs calculated to influence the acceptability of social ideas and involving considerations in product planning, pricing, communication, distribution, and marketing research" (Kotler & Zaltman, 1971).

Shortly thereafter Kotler (1972) reevaluated his earlier positions concerning broadening the concept of marketing and articulated a "generic" concept of marketing. He proposed that marketing is concerned with "how transactions are created, stimulated, facilitated, and valued." The focus is on transaction, which is "the exchange of values between two parties." Thus marketing takes place whenever (1) there are two social units, (2) one is seeking a specific response from another, (3) the response probability is not fixed, and (4) one attempts to produce the desired response by creating and offering values to the market. When a functional view of marketing is adopted the generic concept does not limit marketing to specific institutions, specific responses, or specific response units.

In summary the work of Kotler, Zaltman, Levy, and others has pressed toward emphasis on the fundamental character of marketing in business as well as other contexts, identifying its root character in the nature of exchange. All human interactions are then potentially susceptible to a marketing analysis so that, in addition to the transactions included in traditional business marketing, there is the possibility of other types of marketing such as social marketing, and the marketing of organizations, persons, and places. From mass marketing phenomena to what may be termed intimate marketing in private dyadic relations, elements basic to giving and receiving are at work.

The broadened concept of marketing has

attracted widespread comment and response, and the literature is now both substantial and diverse. Recognition and increasing acceptance have led to a growing interest in applying marketing concepts and tools to both quasi-business and nonbusiness situations. Zaltman and Jacobs (1977) suggest several reasons for the rapid acceptance of the broadened concept of marketing:

1. An increased recognition that the practice of marketing is simply the practice of applied social science and thus applicable to practical problems in action-oriented social science settings.
2. An increase in the perceived seriousness of social problems.
3. The realization by managers in nonbusiness, social change settings that conventional social change tactics are of limited effectiveness and that marketing techniques provide a new perspective and a new arsenal of tools.
4. The increased role and importance of the non business sector and public sector as a provider of goods and services (p. 399).

Marketing is simply a set of planning concepts previously used mostly in business. The possibility of its use in the health care field has been investigated and promoted by others, so the idea is not new. The health care field has traditionally avoided marketing, and some aspects of the process are undoubtedly difficult to accept in regard to health care delivery: advertising, competitive pricing, and so forth. By avoiding the whole of the marketing process, a health care organization too often falls into another trap: namely, it is responsive to market realities and changes. To date an implicit philosophy in health care organizations has been to provide the ''best possible services'' that the agency can provide. Historically health care organizations have decided those services that they want to provide with minimal attention to what the public wants, needs, or is willing to purchase.

The marketing philosophy is dramatically different in that it holds that the organization has an obligation to determine what the public perceives as its needs, to establish a plan of action, and to implement the program in an expedient and cost-effective fashion that can ultimately be evaluated and modified as needed.

Hence marketing provides an approach for examining, predicting, planning, managing, and evaluating the exchange process between provider and consumer. In order that marketing might be useful in health care delivery a slight reordering of thinking is imperative. The recipients of health services have long been considered patients, which denotes passivity in the exchange process. The marketing approach addresses the recipient of services as client or consumer thereby denoting an increasingly active involvement in the exchange process. The application of marketing concepts to community mental health addresses the notion of consumer as recipient of services as well as acknowledges the necessity for thorough assessment of community needs prior to program development.

CONSUMER-ORIENTED MARKETING: FOUNDATION OF MODERN MARKETING

A consumer orientation toward the marketing of services acknowledges that the marketing process must commence prior to the initiation of production. Such an orientation necessitates a reordering of thinking whereby the steps in the planning process begin with an assessment of consumer needs, desires, and wants. In a commercial market profitable entrepreneurs determine the need for their product before goods are produced. Likewise the successful marketer packages, offers, and distributes his goods in ways that attract the attention of consumers and stimulate the need to obtain the product.

The implementation of a consumer orientation directs the attention of the organization to a specific segment of the total population. The process of community assessment and market segmentation is essential to delineating a market that is the appropriate size, that is in reasonable geographic proximity to the service program, and whose members believe they will benefit from consuming the product (service).

In order to utilize marketing concepts in community mental health nursing an appreciation of ecology's value would prove useful. Ecology refers to the way in which organisms or social systems adapt to the environment. With its holistic perspective ecology focuses on the "capacity of an organized behavior system to sustain itself by drawing upon the resources of its environment" (Dawson, 1969). Survival and adaptation are key ecological concepts. Similarly consumer-oriented marketing seeks to provide services that allow clients to make the best possible adaptation to their environmental insults and constraints. Programs are planned based on identified client needs and on those services that provide maximal opportunities for mental health growth. There are a number of steps that lead to effective assessment of consumer needs. These steps are delineated in the next section and are followed by some suggestions for program planning.

MARKETING: A PLANNING FRAMEWORK FOR COMMUNITY MENTAL HEALTH PROGRAMS

Consistent with the concepts introduced in the previous section the following is suggested as an approach that applies marketing concepts to planning community mental health programs. Such an application is recommended as one answer to society's criticism that community mental health has never achieved its maximum potential largely because programs are planned and implemented without due consideration for the needs of the consumers. In an era in which cost effectiveness is a requirement that mandates the viability of a program, marketing strategies seem particularly relevant.

If providers of community mental health services are going to be responsive to the needs of the public they serve, an orientation toward community as client is imperative. A public health orientation facilitates the overall assessment of the mental health needs of the community. In general program planners need to know about the environment in which the service is to be provided; the characteristics, lifestyle, and degree and type of mental health morbidity of the consumers; and the consumer's perceived need for mental health services as well as the types and quality of mental health services that are currently being provided in the community. Thus a systematic process for program planning is described that begins with a recognition of the need after completion of a comprehensive community assessment. A carefully planned assessment yields specific data as to what is "right" as well as which areas of the mental health system need further development.

Community mental health nurses should possess considerable information about the communities in which they work: the nature of community mental health nursing necessitates interfaces with individual clients and families as well as with groups and organizations both within and outside of the community.

Community assessment

Regester (1974) has identified several groups from whom problem awareness within a community might originate. The groups include the community at large, health care providers, politicians, recipients of services, and institutions such as hospitals, clinics, and penitentiaries as well as special interest or power groups.

Specifically three major sources of information constitute input for assessment of the community in regard to the need for specific types of mental health services. Each of these (community attitudes, assessment of resources, and identification of the target market) requires a two-way flow of communication between the providers and each of the constituent groups. The first input is an assessment both of the community's attitudes toward mental health services and the currently available mental health facilities. Specific attitudinal information should be gathered from the professional community including private practitioners, public and private hospital administrators and staff, social workers, and other professionals from institutions and organizations that provide community mental health services. In addition, attitudinal information should be gathered from special interest groups including parents of emotionally disturbed or mentally retarded children, families of patients in psychiatric hospitals, and power groups such as black political groups, neighborhood associations, and women's groups. Also, attitudinal information should be gathered from the community-at-large, for example, from the total populace within a specifically designated geographic region (Regester, 1974). The establishment of health care boards or panels have proved valuable as one way to become responsive to mental health needs as perceived by the community. These groups, generally consumers as well as providers, establish ongoing communication networks between the community and the program developers (Echeveste and Schlacter, 1974).

The second major input for a community analysis is an assessment of the community's resources and constraints. Information should be gathered to determine the availability of professionals who have training in the traditional mental health disciplines such as psychiatrists, clinical psychologists, social workers, and psychiatric nurses. In addition, the availability of professionals outside the traditional mental health disciplines should be considered. Included in this group would be general practitioners and medical specialists other than psychiatrists, clergymen, school teachers, and counselors (Beigel, 1971). A determination should be made of the availability of existing mental health facilities and services such as hospitals, halfway houses, and nursing homes. In many communities existing services are fragmented and a mentally disturbed person may

receive services from several agencies, none of which is aware of the work being done by any of the other agencies (George and Barrett, 1974).

While a community may have adequate professional and physical resources available it may still suffer from a serious deficiency resulting from a lack of coordination among the various resources; a subsequent fragmentation of efforts may occur that would deter the provision of beneficial services. Treatment and rehabilitation services tend to become segmented, indirect, and inefficient when they are not coordinated. Clearly there is good reason for seeking alternatives to present methods of treating the mentally ill. A broad range of integrated services is needed to cope with the problem of the delivery of mental health services. The barriers to developing these alternatives may be formidable in both cost and complexity; however, the price of not developing them may be even costlier (George and Barrett, 1974).

Identifying the target market is the third major source of data for a community assessment. In order to determine the target market general parameters such as geographic area, population size, and problem delineation are established. The more precise aspects of market targeting are determined by a subsequent process known as market segmentation.

In identifying the target market the following information is procured at the outset of the project:

1. The geographic area of the community is defined thereby limiting the target market to those individuals who reside in a certain geographically limited area.
2. Determination of the size of the target market should be based on the greatest number of people currently and potentially requiring treatment; consideration should be given as well to the location of the target market within the community or perhaps even more appropriately the

heterogeneous market should be divided into homogeneous subtarget markets.

3. Critical to the assessment is a concern for determining the problems, needs, attitudes and perceptions of the target market.

Market segmentation

Market segmentation allows for a finer delineation of the needs of the target population for whom community mental health services can be planned. The task of market segmentation often seems overwhelming at the outset since such a wide array of variables could be used as criteria for the segmentation process. Three conditions are used to define the parameters for market segmentation:

1. Segment measurability. Unless information exists or can be obtained regarding a specific characteristic or consumer, segmentation is impossible. This condition often rules out segmentation according to determinants such as values, beliefs, or attitudes that are difficult to measure.

2. Segment accessibility. The data about each characteristic must be available to the community mental health nurse.

3. Segment substantiality. Substantiality refers to the necessity for segments to be sufficiently large to be subdivided and measured.

On meeting the conditions of measurability, accessibility, and substantiality the program planner must decide how the market will be divided into segments. Since there is no unique or ''best'' way in which to segment a market, a variety of approaches are identified.

One approach would be to segment according to age, thereby examining the mental health needs of each age group, and then to plan a program that would meet the identified needs. The population might also be segmented according to demographic factors other than age including education, income, occupation, race, religion, or sex. It is important to realize that demographic variables in isolation are not sufficient for a thorough segmentation; rather demographic variables generally constitute the foundation for more detailed segmentation processes.

Additional possibilities include segmentation according to a variety of socioeconomic variables, stages in family development, diagnostic category, and consumer-expressed desire for a specific service. Still another possibility is to segment a population according to levels of prevention—primary, secondary, or tertiary. For example, one way to segment a community while maintaining an orientation toward prevention is to determine the at-risk groups and organize programs or strategies to reinforce coping ability and thereby intervene in mental health description. Families under stress from death of a member, divorce, birth of a defective child, return to the home of a discharged psychiatric patient, or victims of human abuse or aggression constitute readily identifiable target markets for preventive psychiatry.

In segmenting a market it is essential to maintain an awareness of cultural differences within the population. Variations exist among cultural groups as to incidence of selected diseases; for example, blacks are high risks for sickle cell anemia whereas Jews are especially susceptible to Tay-Sachs disease. Moreover, different cultural groups hold specific opinions and beliefs regarding health values and theories of disease causation as well as preferences for mode of treatment.

Perhaps the key issue in market segmentation is determining what the consumer believes he needs and what he wants to do to alter his health status. In some instances consumers change their health beliefs subsequent to health education whereas with other groups beliefs and attitudes are tenaciously held. Prior to any attempt at program planning the community mental health nurse must assess the target population's wants, needs, beliefs, opinions, value systems, and receptivity to new ideas.

Planning for a community mental health program

Once the market has been segmented and a specific group identified or targeted to become involved in a community mental health program, the planning phase begins. The decision to plan a community mental health program requires a systematic and comprehensive approach to the planning process itself. Since the resulting program must operate within a society that is composed of many subsocieties, this process is bound to be complex. Therefore, a piecemeal planning approach will not suffice (George and Barrett, 1974).

There are five major elements to be considered for effective community mental health planning.

1. Recognition of the limitation of uncoordinated planning on an agency-by-agency basis, thereby duplicating services in some areas and omitting services in other areas.
2. Emphasis on the need for community sanction of planning.
3. Consideration of the need to define the spectrum of essential community mental health services.
4. Combining the skills of mental health professionals and members of the broader community.
5. Recognition of the benefits of a system approach to planning.

The systems approach views the community as a vast service network composed of interrelated components that serve a unitary purpose, namely the restoration of those individuals who come in contact with the system at any point to optimize personal and social functioning (Lindenberg, 1968). The systems approach to planning is excellent for a community starting a community mental health program from scratch. Most communities start with a hodgepodge involving many agencies; a systems approach to planning offers a method by which existing programs and new services are linked in an effective mental health network. The basic criterion for any service program, new or old, then is how it fits into the overall constellation of services (Lindenberg, 1968).

The result of the planning effort should be a definition of goals, specification of physical facilities, and funding requirements. The importance of local, state, and federal funding and regulatory bodies cannot be discounted. Consequently the publics to whom most community mental health programs are accountable are numerous.

It is crucial at the beginning of the planning phase to make a sound estimate of the needs of the target market to establish performance criteria for evaluating existing and future services. The community assessment phase culminates in the delineation of a specific set of program objectives. A specific time plan is set forth and the establishment of a marketing mix occurs. Developing the marketing mix includes four planning variables: product, price, promotion, and physical distribution policies. According to Kotler, there are six different types of products including physical goods, services, organization, persons, places, and ideas (Kotler, 1972). In community mental health programs the product—service—is defined as primary, secondary, or tertiary prevention.

In order for the product or service to be used by consumers it must be promoted so that it becomes familiar, acceptable, and desirable by individuals in the target market. The development of a promotional program involves complex issues in community mental health. The program planner has to determine the size of the advertising budget (if the funds are available). He must select the form of appeal to be used, develop or select forms of media, schedule advertising plans, and evaluate the results. Moreover, each person employed in the program must realize that he is advertising his service in each contact with the community.

In the social marketing context, place or channel of distribution calls for providing adequate distribution and response facilities. Specifically this aspect of planning includes selecting or developing outlets for the service and deciding on their number, size, and location (Kotler and Zaltman, 1971).

The last variable in the marketing mix is cost, or the price that the consumer must pay to obtain the product. Four different but interrelated costs must be considered—money, opportunity, energy, and emotional costs. In planning a program one should be aware that the cost to the consumer generally excees the actual monetary outlay for the service: additional costs may include medication, transportation, loss of wages, and charge for baby sitting as well as emotional drain from fear or apprehension.

Once the program has been planned, promoted, and implemented, consideration must focus on evaluation. Crucial to determining whether or not a program is efficient and effective in delivering mental health services to the community is an analysis of the program's impact on the identified target market. A determination of the occurrence of specific forms of mental health disruption within a population for whom primary preventive efforts were developed would constitute one form of evaluation.

Measuring the effectiveness of a program could be accomplished by establishing reporting systems, developing performance criteria, measuring program results, and then taking corrective actions. Community mental health programs have been evaluated in a variety of ways including work load data, number of hours spent in service, number of active patients, referrals, change in incidence of suicide, and specific diagnostic entities. Lombello et al. (1973) consider these measures too gross to be useful; they recommend evaluation based on treatment outcome, which although difficult to accomplish yields valuable data about the effectiveness of the program. In this mode of evaluation the mental health provider and client set treatment goals and negotiate a contract.

At the completion of the treatment contract the patient and a follow-up worker review the contract and evaluate its effectiveness.

SUMMARY

Historically marketing has moved from a focus on advertising and selling to a discipline well grounded in concepts both from the traditional business area of management and the more recently included behavior science emphasis. The application of marketing concepts to community mental health nursing, especially in relation to program planning, demands a reorientation of thinking for providers. Recipients of mental health services must be viewed as active participants in program planning in order to demonstrate effectiveness of provider activities. In community mental health nursing a captive audience of program recipients is unavailable. Individuals who seek community mental health services generally do so voluntarily; hence program consumption depends on a substantial cadre of consumers who perceive themselves desirous of or in need of the service. Thus mental health offerings must be such that clients believe their functioning will be enhanced and that they will obtain relief from stress or learn new and more effective coping techniques.

References

Bartels, R.: The development of marketing thought, Homewood, Ill., 1962, Richard D. Irwin, Inc.

Bartels, R.: The identity crisis in marketing, J. Marketing **38:**73-76, October 1974.

Beigel, A.: Communicating with the catchment area, Hosp. Community Psychiatry **22:**87-90, March 1971.

Dawson, L. M.: The human concept: a new philosophy for business, Business Horizons **12:**29-38, December 1969.

Echeveste, D. and Schlacter, J.: Marketing: a strategic framework for health care, Nurs. Outlook **22:**377-381, June 1974.

Ellwood, P. M., Jr., and Herbert, M. E.: Health care: should industry buy it or sell it? Harvard Business Rev. **51:**99-107, July/August 1973.

George, J. A., and Barrett, J.: Systems planning for treatment and rehabilitation programs, Res. Outlook **6:**29-33, 1974.

Kotler, P.: A generic concept of marketing, J. Marketing **36:**46-54, April 1972.

Kotler, P. and Levy, Sidney.: Broadening the concept of marketing, J. Marketing **33:**10-15, January 1969.

Kotler, P. and Zaltman, G.: Social marketing: an approach to planned social change, J. Marketing **35:**3-12, July 1971.

Lindenberg, R.: One community's approach to integrated mental health planning: challenge, accomplishments, problems, Am. J. Public Health **58:**1173-1180, July 1968.

Lombello, J., Keresuk, T., and Sherman, R.: Evaluating a community mental health program contract fulfillment analysis, Hosp. Community Psychiatry **24:**760-762, November 1973.

Regester, D.: Community mental health: for whose community? Am. J. Public Health **64:**886-893, September 1974.

Zaltman, G., and Jacobs, P.: Social marketing and a consumer-based theory of marketing. In Woodside, A.G., Sheth, J. N., and Bennett, P. D., eds.: Consumer and industrial buying behavior, New York, 1977, Elsevier North Holland, Inc.

CHAPTER 24

An ecological approach to the practice of community mental health nursing

JOHN G. BRUHN and F. DAVID CORDOVA

A new approach to the treatment of the mentally ill was undertaken throughout the United States in the early 1960s. Community mental health centers were established to care for patients in their locales. Yet 15 years later large numbers of mental patients are worse off than they were before. The problems stem from poor planning at all levels of government, lack of funds, an inadequate number of mental health centers, and lack of welcome in the attitudes of communities. As a consequence many mental patients are poorly housed and fed, unemployed and socially isolated, and receiving no medical treatment. Many have disappeared between the cracks of society.

According to Drs. Ellen L. Bassuk and Samuel Gerson of Harvard University, the 603 existing community mental health centers are short of the need—1,500 centers—and can serve only 40% of the population (The New Snake Pits, 1978). Each patient in a state institution costs an average of $11,250 a year and, since state budgets are limited for mental health care, patients have been discharged as a means of saving money. As a result patients are dumped precipitately into communities that are not ready to receive them. These patients are susceptible to exploitation by landlords of substandard, unsafe hotels, rooming houses, and nursing homes and by private agencies that often make great profits without providing adequate care.

To complicate these problems federal programs such as Medicaid pay little for care at mental health centers and the Supplemental Security Income (SSI) program often will not support former mental patients living in halfway houses or other residential centers. Mental illness still carries a stigma at all levels in our society.

One reason for the ineffectiveness of the innovative community mental health centers has been the lack of coordination between the agencies that are responsible for health care. In Detroit, for example, three separate agencies are supposed to monitor a program funded by four different sources and carried out by 40 nonprofit organizations. The result of this is chaotic: a hospital may provide a patient with an adequate plan to follow on discharge but fail to alert a clinic; then when the patient fails to show up the clinic does not realize it and the patient is lost because no one has any overall responsibility (The New Snake Pits, 1978).

The need to recognize the support systems that exist within the community and to strengthen the linkages between these support systems and the formal mental health services systems was emphasized in the *Final Report of the President's Commission on Mental Health* (1978). It is our premise that these linkages between systems exist and that interfaces between clients and professional helpers occur whether or not they are planned. If the linkages between agencies and institutions are planned, well-established, and widely known, the interfaces between clients and helpers will be more likely to be beneficial. This is the premise that underlies an ecological approach to community mental health.

The purpose of the present chapter is to explain what is meant by an ecological approach to community mental health; to examine the nature of the various types of interactions between nurse, client, and community as they relate to mental health; and to outline the procedures for using an ecological approach in community mental health nursing.

It is important at the outset that we do not believe that mental health is a separate concept distinguishable from physical health. Indeed the work of *health* professionals should be the *health* of their clients. Our emphasis on mental health in this chapter is mandated by the nature of this textbook, which focuses on special issues to be studied in depth by nurses who are specializing in mental health services. The ecological approach discussed here is applicable to other subspecialties of health as well as to the broad concept of health and the delivery of services to promote, maintain, or restore it.

WHAT IS AN ECOLOGICAL APPROACH?

An ecological approach is founded in flexibility and adaptation. For example, depending on the needs of a particular situation, it might be helpful for the health professional to obtain more information than a patient can, or will, tell. It might be necessary to talk with the family, to visit the home and the patient's employer, and to obtain information about the community in which he lives. The extent to which the health professional will want to pursue such further information will depend on the purposes this information will serve. Perspective may be limited or broadened to fulfill specific needs. Whereas more data might

help professionals to understand and treat the patient, too much data or irrelevant data will merely waste time and add nothing of value in understanding the client.

Similarly an ecological approach can be used by a health professional who works for a community agency or institution. When the agency decides, for example, to suggest, or initiate, changes in referral policies or admission procedures that will affect others in the community, it might be helpful, or even essential, to learn something about the attitudes of individuals who will be the sources of support or resistance. The health professional might gather details about specific groups or organizations or individuals within them to assist in implementing policy changes.

Thus an ecological approach is taken by the health professional who recognizes that, no matter how thorough his investigation or understanding is, there are always other forces that affect the client directly or indirectly, whether the client is a community, agency, family, or individual. An ecological approach involves recognition of both the interdependence and the uniqueness of people, whatever their level of social organization, and the cumulative effects that a single change will have on a family, group, or community. An ecological approach implies that an effort will be made to obtain information at all levels of a social organization so that it can be used to plan and coordinate activities that will have a maximum effective impact on the client. Finally an ecological approach takes into account the fact that clients and helpers themselves are continually changing as a consequence of forces in their own worlds as well as a consequence of their interaction. Thus the health professional must continually update his or her knowledge about the client.

Past implementations of the community mental health center concept have not involved planning, coordination, or careful analysis of the impact that establishing the centers would have on mental institutions. As a result what was thought to be an innovation in the care of the mentally ill has usually created chaos in the health care delivery system, engendered negative attitudes among the public, and actually promoted mental illness by removing ill people from sources of professional help and discharging them to fend for themselves.

AN APPROACH, NOT A MODEL

We have stressed the phrase "an ecological approach" because it is only one of many approaches that can be used by health professionals. The term "approach" implies approximation, tendency, or nearness. Furthermore, we have avoided the term "model" because models have a way of becoming theories that are perpetuated but never tested. The so-called medical model with a focus on cure is such an example. Indeed the advent of the community mental health center concept was a reaction to the limitations of the curative model.

Since precise etiologies and cures for mental diseases have not been found, as they have for many physical illnesses, mental health professionals have begun to emphasize prevention and education and maintaining patients in the community. Glidewell (1974) notes that the specialized skills and training of mental health professionals may conflict with meeting real community needs. Therefore there are limitations to the helping dyad of psychiatrist and patient and a need for greater public responsibility of mental health professionals in meeting community needs. Chu and Trotter (1974) were more explicit in stating that psychiatry has persistently thought primarily of cure and that it has preferred to ignore those whom psychiatry has been unable to cure. Jones (1968) elaborated on this theme in discussing the lack of early intervention in community psychiatry. He stated that the established role of the psychiatrist is one of the major stumbling blocks to early involvement: "The usual medical model in consultation is about as far from prevention as one can get."

An ecological approach, by contrast, is a nonmedical approach that is broad enough to view human behavior along the entire health continuum from illness to wellness. In addition, the ecological approach does not require only experts in its practice. Professional territoriality and models have helped to perpetuate separatism and to limit the perspective of clients and what can be done for them. Jones (1968) claimed that one of the major limits to progress in community psychiatry has been that each discipline thinks of the total situation in terms of its own needs. Auerswald (1969) stressed that solutions for mental and social problems cannot be solved within the framework of any single discipline.

The terms "team" and "interdisciplinary" have been in use for a long time (Bowen, et al., 1965; Pepper, 1976). A precise definition of a team process has not been developed but it is clear that if people from different disciplines work together on the same problem they are likely to perceive the problem better and develop a greater variety of approaches to a solution than if each were to tackle the problem alone. Teams and interdisciplinary groups do work, although at times painfully (Wise et al., 1974).

The ecological approach requires some degree of teamwork and interdisciplinary interaction, since it involves processing physical, biological, and social sciences and humanities. The ecological approach is a systems approach: it facilitates thinking about things and people in terms of interdependence and interrelationships, and with this perspective it provides a rough framework for learning how things and people work. The ecological way of thinking is to obtain as complete and unified a picture as possible, which requires collecting information on all the elements that impinge on the issue. The art of the ecological approach is to piece these elements together and examine the interfaces between them to obtain as complete a picture as possible. No one can do this alone; it requires teamwork. If teamwork and interdisciplinary interaction were brought to bear more often on health issues, we could guide our actions and regulate their consequences rather than make blind choices with insufficient data.

ELEMENTS OF AN ECOLOGICAL APPROACH

Kelly (1966) observed that the concept of ecology is particularly useful in defining a community mental health program. An ecological analysis of mental health services can be applied in three areas. One analysis can be done of social or organizational systems. The assumption to be made is that any change in the operation of one service will affect all other services. A change in the number of admissions to one local mental health facility will affect not only the operation of all other health facilities and resources but also the social structure of the community, for example, through changes in the size and nature of the labor force and in the economy.

A second area that lends itself to ecological analysis is the relationship between the physical environment and individual behavior. The assumption is made that factors such as population density, public housing, urban renewal, environmental design, and migration, affect social behavior.

A third area for analysis is the relationship of individuals to their immediate social environment such as family, work place, and school. The assumption is that social structure and social behavior are reciprocal. In 1966 Kelly suggested that these three areas be subjected to analysis in planning community mental health center activities. He predicted that otherwise these community centers might perpetuate outmoded treatment methods rather than initiate a new concept of psychological service.

Rapaport (1977) identified four sources for intervention in an ecological approach to mental health services: (1) the individual, (2) the small group, (3) organizations, and (4) social institutions and communities. Since mental health problems are often a result of the inability of an individual or group—or even an entire community—to fit into society, the values that underlie each component need to be identified before the individual (or group) can be assisted in adjusting to society. He suggested that an analysis of the values and goals of each component would help mental health professionals in determining the level at which the problem lies as well as in prescribing intervention suitable to that level. Furthermore, he believes that mental health problems require intervention at several levels; thus strategies must be planned for each level.

Some common elements are found in the opinions of both Kelly (1966) and Rapaport (1977) on how to view mental health services: they both stress that (1) the various levels of social organization interact and are interdependent and that social structure and physical environment affect the biological well-being of a person, family, organization, or community; (2) a health professional acquires inadequate knowledge if he or she focuses only on one level and indeed the intervention may even be ineffective; and (3) ecological information is not esoteric but has practical value in planning and problem solving in mental health.

Health professionals must have their own role clearly in mind before they can be effective in helping to define a community mental health program. The client (an individual, family, or community) may differ in his expectations of the health professional and if health professionals are not clear about their role, they may complicate the existing problem merely by their presence as outsiders.

Health professionals can assume various roles in providing community mental health services, for example, as change agents, sources of support, and coordinators. The way in which health professionals will become involved in the process of providing services will depend on the role assumed. Indeed the individual, family, or community may not want health professionals involved in defining their problem or formulating strategies but only in the provision of services. On the other hand the individual, family, or community may see health professionals as rescuers and gladly turn over the entire problem to them.

PATTERNS OF INTERACTION

A common image of a health professioal in interaction with a client or patient is that of a helping relationship in which the health professional is the dominant person giving advice to, or doing something to, a sick patient. The image also tends to emphasize the one-to-one interaction between health professional and client. This pattern of interaction is only one of several types that can exist between health professionals and patients. Indeed in community mental health nursing the client is likely to include the patient's family and community agencies in addition to the patient. This has been referred to as a "social network," which is composed of all the interactions that are impor-

tant to the health of the client (Garrison et al., 1977). An examination of some of the types of relationships that can exist for the community mental health nurse will allow the possible roles to be more clearly defined and better understood by all participants in the interactions that might occur.

Four patterns of interaction between nurse, client, and community are illustrated in Fig. 24-1. The emphasis in each pattern is the overlapping (shaded area) of the circle, which represents interaction and interface. The interface includes that which each person brings to the situation (culture) as well as the nature of the situation (physical environment, purpose for meeting) and the attitudes and behavior of each person as they interact. The emphasis is on reciprocity between client and community, nurse and client, nurse and community, and finally nurse, client, and community. It is when all three circles interface that a social network is formed. Indeed it is our view that no inter-

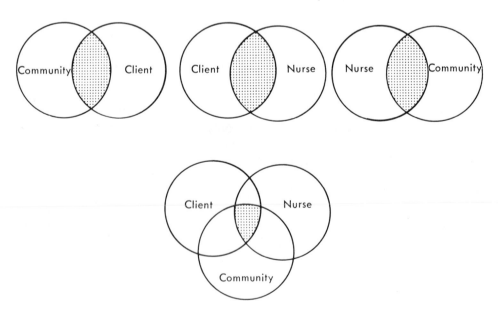

Fig. 24-1. Patterns of interaction between nurse, client, and community.

action between a health professional and client can be fully understood without a consideration of "the community" each brings to the interaction.

Each of the four patterns of interaction as they relate to community mental health nursing is discussed below.

Client-community interaction

Each of us, whether labeled client, consumer, or patient, is a product of a culture, that is, a melding of genes, social experiences, values, and expectations that make us unique. We carry our uniqueness with us to all of the situations that we encounter throughout life, and through experience learn how we feel most comfortable behaving, both when we are sick and when we are well. We also have incorporated other people's reactions toward us into our uniqueness, which tends to reinforce patterns of behavior that are rewarding to us.

Some of the behavior that is unique and individual is overt and some is covert. Oftentimes we need to look beyond that which a person can tell us to understand him more fully as a person. This might require observing the way he speaks, what he does not discuss or tell, and the bodily gestures or movements that reinforce or contradict what he says. Each client, patient, consumer, and health professional therefore brings to any interaction a myriad of complex experiences; these experiences all influence that interaction on conscious and unconscious as well as on overt and covert levels. Since mental illness does not occur suddenly out of the blue but is a process involving an individual's social network, it is important for the community mental health nurse to be aware of both their own and their client's uniqueness.

Nurse-community interaction

The interaction between the nurse and the community can take place through any combination of a number of roles that the nurse might choose to play. The selection of a role for interacting with a community is important in gaining entry to it. The role that is chosen may determine whether or not the nurse is permitted access to the community and if the access is to the total community or only to specific groups.

The nurse's role is dependent partially on how the community defines its need for a community mental health nurse. The community's assessment of its need will place limits on what the nurse can and cannot do in the community and will also dictate the criteria for evaluating the success of the nurse's interactions. For this reason it is important for the nurse and community to agree on their expectations before the nurse's formal entry into the community. Roles and expectations do change and, when they are clarified at the outset, later confrontations and disappointments can be minimized.

Without clear goals both community and nurse can unwillingly subvert one another's purposes. Communities can subtly co-opt health professionals into altering their role to coincide with changes in community attitude and opinion. Similarly, because community health professionals work in a community, they often see other roles for themselves and slip into undertaking too many projects, which results in confusing the community about what they were originally intended to do. Although the nurses' personal backgrounds will influence how they see and interact with communities in a professional role, they must remain aware of their personal biases and minimize them as they perform professionally.

Nurse-client interaction

The professional relationship of nurse-client is often seen as one in which a client comes for therapy or help and the nurse provides it in the form of advice, clinical intervention, or social support. In community mental health nursing, however, the client is more likely to include the family and the community agencies and resources that have influenced the client's total life. Although the focus here is on the mental health nurse in the community we recognize that much of what we have to say will apply to the mental health nurse in inpatient settings as well.

The most common nurse-client interaction is one in which the nurse plays several roles simultaneously, for example, arranging school transportation for the children and homemaker services for a family while the mother is hospitalized or providing social support to a mother and obtaining prenatal care for her pregnant teenage daughter who is unmarried and living at home. To be effective in each of these roles and to arrange all activities so that they work together for the benefit of the patient the nurse must know those community resources that are available and how to mobilize them. A nurse whose roles are clearly understood should experience little difficulty in performing them.

With the passage of time and with greater community acceptance the community may permit the nurse to take on new roles. Increased credibility also offers the opportunity for innovation and suggestions for social change. One guideline that should be suggested for any nurse-client interaction, however, is to begin with a specific role and then to expand to take on new roles as success allows. Health professionals may be tempted to respond to a situation in which they are obviously needed by assuming too many roles too soon before they fully understand the total situation and the needs of all parties. Indeed attempting to be too helpful may not only overwhelm the client but the actual helpfulness may be the wrong therapy. A too-helpful health professional may be easily co-opted into being a rescuer by a client (individual, family, or community).

The community mental health nurse also has to be aware of subtle or even obvious changes in a client's behavior caused by illness, recovery, or reassessment that may affect the equilibrium of their interaction. For example, an indi-

vidual, family, or community may present itself as increasingly helpless and ask for more and more guidance and direct involvement from the nurse. If the nurse is not aware of this behavior, it soon will be impossible to be unbiased and free from alignments in the client's world. The consequence can be a dangerous game and the outcome will be an unprofessional situation of winners and losers. Health professionals must realize that they cannot help everyone in all situations. The relationship between clients and health professionals should be terminated if it becomes apparent to either party that their interaction is not professional or is not meeting the client's needs.

Nurse-client-community interaction

The processes that bring about change occur at the points where nurse, client, and community interact. The multiple roles of health professionals, the interrelating roles of a person or of family members, and the power, communication, and interest groups in a community all connect in various ways. Changes at these connections take place among living systems (which are all open systems) in contact with their environment, with input and output across system boundaries (Chin, 1969). When two open systems connect with one another, they can be said to interact. It is the area of interface that is of major concern to mental health nurses.

Interfaces are the lines of communication in a work group or the mutual role expectations of nurse and client or the affective ties between family members. Interfaces can be functional or dysfunctional. The community mental health nurse's role is to assist open systems to function effectively through methods that can be described as preventive, corrective, or rehabilitative. *Preventive* measures involve the anticipation of sources of dysfunction in a system and intervention to maintain or enhance equilibrium. *Corrective* measures are those that treat or counteract or otherwise intervene to correct disequilibrium or dysfunction in a system. *Rehabilitative* measures provide continuity of care and create an environment that is favorable to a steady or improved state of functioning.

Another way of viewing these three activities is to consider them as levels of intervention. Primary intervention involves the early detection and diagnosis of mental illness, public education about signs of mental illness, and public education about ways of coping and relaxing to prevent the accumulation of unsolved interpersonal and personal problems. Secondary intervention involves the provision of treatment in the patient's own environment, preferably in the family, so that all who have contact with him can participate in restoring a positive environment. Tertiary intervention involves rehabilitation, the efforts to keep the client functional in the environment that will help restore his identity and confidence. Arranging the necessary social support and continuity of health care to habilitate the client is an essential part of this level of intervention (Banchevska, 1976). Bolman (1968) has described primary intervention as those activities that are aimed at reducing the incidence of mental illness through prevention, secondary intervention as those that are aimed at reducing the prevalence of mental illness through treatment, and tertiary intervention as those that reduce the extent of the disability.

Intervention in community mental health nursing is seldom focused exclusively on preventive, corrective, or rehabilitative activities. All three activities are usually involved because a mental health problem is not limited to a specific behavior or to a single individual and because any behavior of an individual, who is an open system, has effects and implications for the family and community as well. Intervention to correct a dysfunction in a system therefore must include efforts to help restore the system to a steady state as well as efforts to prevent the recurrence of future dysfunction in the system.

Several major skills must be mastered before intervention in open systems. One skill is to observe the growth and development (life cycle) of communities, families or groups, and individuals. Another is to be able to assess community, family or group, and individual needs and how needs change as a function of time and state of health. Still another is the identification of sources of stress and indications of mental illness. The final skill is the ability to identify and use support systems that mitigate or prevent dysfunction and enhance a steady state in a system and between systems (Skrovan et al., 1974).

COMMUNITY MENTAL HEALTH NURSE AND HEALTH CARE TEAM

The majority of health professionals and laymen acknowledge the interrelationship between physical and mental health, yet the health care system is bifurcated, directing the mentally ill down a different path from that of the physically ill. Each system has its own specially trained personnel, its own care facilities, and separate community agencies and resources. A person with a mental and physical problem has to unravel the complexities of two health care systems that seldom meet. Indeed the public has been educated to separate mental from physical ills. The mass media conveys the message that mental ills can be alleviated through self-medication or self-taught techniques to relax or find oneself, whereas physical health must be monitored by periodic checkups by a licensed physician. It is not surprising therefore that we do not find mental health professionals included in the term ''primary health care team.''

Primary health care is defined as front line, first contact, readily accessible care that is provided by a team of professionals responsible for a patient's total health care in the context of his environment. Even so, primary health care clinics often exclude mental health practitioners. Indeed an unspoken attitude prevails among the physical care practitioners that their patients might not be willing to come to a clinic or facility that also includes mental patients. Fundamental to the success of a health team, however, is its ability to work together as a coordinated unit. Perhaps the first step toward a health care team that is truly oriented toward caring for the whole person is attitudinal and behavioral changes among health professionals that will unify the two health care systems. Changes in patient attitudes and behavior will no doubt follow.

One of the continuing difficulties that a community mental health nurse will encounter is how to interface with the system of health care for physical health. These difficulties arise when a patient has both a mental and a physical problem and decisions need to be made about who the primary physician (health provider) is or when a patient needs to be referred across systems. The team concept, even within each of the two health care systems, evokes many highly charged issues of professionalism, leadership, control, authority, responsibility, and legal liability (Pluckhan, 1972). Ironically the problems of interfacing between the individual, family, and community that are encountered by the mental health nurse will be encountered within the microcosm of the health care team, because the team is an intimate group whose success depends on cooperation. It is essential therefore that the community mental health nurse obtain and continually sharpen skills in leadership, small-group dynamics, and social organization as well as in the understanding and practice of social change.

PUTTING THE ECOLOGICAL APPROACH INTO PRACTICE

The importance of the ecological approach to community nursing is based on the premise that the causes and treatment of health problems extend beyond the individual client—that the nurse should be concerned not only with the care of individuals but also with the health of families and communities. Furthermore, nursing intervention should be directed not only to-ward correcting a problem but also toward enhancing the health status of individuals and groups, becoming an advocate for total community health efforts, and assisting individuals, groups, and communities in health planning.

Many community health nurses still define a community in terms of a resident case load. This is a limited view because case load implies a grouping of people who are different or sick or who need to be taken care of. In addition, community health nurses sometimes limit themselves to the identified needs of individuals and families who are the target population of one agency's specific program. Community health nursing involves a greater commitment and responsibility than just being in the community or taking care of the sick in their homes.

Recently the community nurse practitioner has emerged as a new role in nursing. One graduate program trains nurses to focus on the health of the total community and become involved in community self-help (Skrovan, 1974). Also community nursing electives are available in some nursing schools where students can apply the nursing process in the community by becoming directly involved in real community problems and issues (Knight, 1974).

PERFORMING COMMUNITY MENTAL HEALTH NURSING ROLES

Among the numerous possible roles for the community mental health nurse (Fig. 24-1) we have selected one role as an example (being an effective team member) and have outlined the procedure for performing it (Table 3). In this case the task is to integrate data from experience, knowledge, and skills. To be an effective team member requires not only knowledge, experience, and skills but also an ability to integrate them. The terminal objective for the role of being an effective team member is to analyze the impact of intervention on the client: did team intervention have an effect on the client and, if so, why did it succeed or fail?

Several specific objectives must be met be-

TABLE 3

A procedure for performing community mental health nursing roles

Role and function ↓	Being an effective team member		
Task identification ↓	Integrate data from experience, knowledge, and skills		
Terminal objective ↓	Analyze impact of intervention on client		
Specific objectives	**Concepts**	**Strategies**	**Resources**
1. Establish structure, organization, and goals of team	Health care team organization, management, job descriptions, communications flow, goal priorities, role clarification Team building	Role playing Simulated experiences Group discussion	Videotapes on team building Book by H. Wise et al. (1974) Institute for Health Team Development (Montefiore Hospital, New York)
2. Define client problem	Human ecology Social systems analysis Community health	Interviews Surveys Observation Group discussion and decision-making workshops	Books by D. M. Connor (1968, 1969a, b) and A. T. Brown (1978) Community organization consultant Department of Health, Education, and Welfare
3. Initiate collaborative activities for clients' benefit	Comprehensive health care Continuity of health care Client needs	Team conferences	Community agencies and organizations Book by J. G. Dugger (1975)
4. Determine timing of interventions in client situation	Social change Preventive intervention	Case conferences Planning conferences Interviews with family Crisis intervention techniques	Family and community agencies Book by G. M. Gazda et al. (1977)

fore the terminal objective can be reached. Naming specific objectives helps to clarify the steps that must be taken as well as the order in which to tackle them in the process of reaching the terminal objective. We have identified four specific objectives along the path toward becoming an effective team member (Table 3), and under each specific objective, examples of concepts, strategies, and resources that will help to accomplish the objectives. The procedure shown in Table 3 should make it possible for a community nurse to define and carry out any specified role (Cohen, 1973; Davis and Underwood, 1976; Harris and Soloman, 1977; Wooster Development Project, 1977).

In addition to a procedure for carrying out a role the community nurse must have a plan for intervening in a health problem. An example of such a plan is shown in Table 4, in which a high rate of venereal disease among teenagers is used as an example of a community problem. The major components in developing a plan to intervene are (1) specifying the types of data needed and their possible sources, (2) drawing inferences for nursing intervention in the problem, (3) identifying ways of implementing the plan, and (4) evaluating the effectiveness of the plan.

Every plan should involve community, family, and individual levels of analysis (Table 4). Seldom does an individual have a health problem that does not affect others, and it is sim-

TABLE 4
Plan for intervention in community problem: a high VD rate among teenagers

Data needed	Data sources	Inferences for nursing intervention	Implementation	Evaluation of implementation
Community level				
1. Characteristics of population at risk (age, race, education, culture)	City-county health department	Is VD viewed as a community problem or seen as a problem only by health professionals?	Increase community awareness if needed	Decrease in VD rate Use of VD clinic Establishment of sex education classes in schools
2. Attitudes of community (is VD seen as a problem? by whom?)	Records in neighborhood clinics	Will community support a VD clinic and sex education classes?	Involve parents in planning	
3. Is sex education taught in schools?	Census data		Establish VD clinic in community or neighborhoods to provide care	
4. Is VD a problem in neighboring communities?	Survey of community attitudes		Teach sex education in schools	
5. Prevalence of social problems in community (alcoholism, drug use, crime, unemployment)	Interviews with community groups (PTA, church leaders, teachers, etc.)			
6. Leisure and recreational habits of community and at risk group				
7. Motivation to solve problem				
8. Services offered				
Family level				
1. Characteristics of families (size, one or two parents, income levels, religious affiliation, divorce rate, degree of cohesiveness, etc.)	Interviews with community agencies (Family Service, Visiting Nurses' Assoc., Mental Health Assoc., etc.)	Lack of information about family attitudes toward sex and VD	Seek to involve parents and children in sex education classes	Participation in classes and groups on sex education
2. Attitudes toward sex and contraception				
3. Does VD cluster in families or neighborhoods?				
4. Degree of family cohesiveness and responsibility for family members				
Individual level				
1. Attitudes and knowledge about sex, knowledge and use of contraceptive devices	Personal interviews with teenagers	Agencies don't know enough about teenager attitudes and habits to initiate intervention program	Use peers for personal contact with resistant persons	Increase in knowledge of sex Use of contraceptive devices
2. Attitudes and practices of peers				
3. Working, going to school, how time is spent, source of income				
4. Need for information and willingness to obtain it				

ilarly rare that a family is ill by itself. Since communities are made up of individuals and families, so the health and functioning of one part of this ecological system in some way affects other parts. Caplan (1974) has discussed the ecological system model and its implications for nursing in detail.

MAKING A COMMUNITY ANALYSIS

A key step in the plan for intervention in a community problem is to make a community analysis. This step follows the collection of information and data about the community and what it sees as the problem. An analysis must be made before inferences can be drawn about why and how a community nurse should be involved. We should emphasize that a community analysis differs from a community diagnosis. Diagnosis involves a deductive process and often results in a label. The label in turn calls to mind a set of procedures that were used successfully in the past to treat a similar problem. A tentative diagnosis often causes a health professional to limit data collection to the suspected diagnostic category. Certainly no one is free of bias. Bias is not perforce bad, but the risk is that often we are not aware of our biases, or worse, that we deny them.

Several guides and sources of information are available that provide techniques to analyze communities.* Such an analysis is important because the visible surface of the community is only a small part of the total. Although these techniques for learning about communities are useful, no model can be applied to all of them. The community mental health nurse will need to add to, and subtract from, the various strategies available in conducting a community analysis. A thorough community analysis will enhance the probability that the choice and timing of an intervention will be appropriate

and that it will have beneficial effects on the client.

PRIMARY PREVENTION AND HEALTH PROMOTION IN MENTAL HEALTH

Perhaps one of the most important roles for the community mental health nurse, and yet a role that has remained undeveloped, is that of a health promoter. So much of mental health is crisis oriented, mainly because individuals, families, and communities do not know what they can do to prevent crises or how to take steps to enhance their total well-being. Others have the knowledge but do not assume the responsibility for prevention or for health promotion.

As health professionals we do have some knowledge of the behavior that helps to regain health or promote it. We give such advice to individuals and families following a heart attack or stroke. Advice is given to communities about the quality of air, water, and recreational facilities. A logical extension of these roles lies in recommendations to individuals or programs for communities that will contribute to, and foster, mental health.

An argument can be offered that it is difficult to promote health in a society that values its ability to solve crises with technology and that promotes illness behavior through the mass media. However, community health nurses who understand and value the concept of health promotion and who want to put into practice the concept of holistic health and teamwork are in a prime position to assume leadership in this area. Community health nurses could provide the linkages between the now separate (physical) health and mental health systems in applying an ecological approach to the practice of community nursing.

References

American Medical Association: Guidelines for community health programs, Chicago, American Medical Association (no date).
American Public Health Association: Guide to a community

---

*See the following references: Blum (1969), Conner (1968, 1969), American Public Health Association (1961), Littrell (No date), Roen and Burnes (1968), and Ross (1967).

health study, ed. 2, Washington, D.C., 1961, American Public Health Association.

Auerswald, E. H.: Interdisciplinary versus ecological approach. In Gray, W., Duhl, F. J., and Rizzo, N. D., eds.: General systems theory and psychiatry, Boston, 1969, Little, Brown & Co.

Banchevska, R.: The role of the community mental health centre in prevention, Ment. Health Soc. **3:**329-335, 1976.

Blum, H. L. et al.: Health planning, 1969, San Francisco, 1969, Western Regional Office of American Public Health Association.

Bolman, W. M.: Preventive psychiatry for the family: theory, approaches and programs, Am. J. Psychiatry **125:**458-472, 1968.

Bowen, W. T., Marler, D. C., and Androes, L.: The psychiatric team: myth and mystique, Am. J. Psychiatry **122:**687-690, 1965.

Brownlee, A. T.: Community, culture, and care: a cross-cultural guide for health workers, St. Louis, 1978, The C. V. Mosby Co.

Caplan, G.: Support systems and community mental health, New York, 1974, Behavioral Publications, Inc.

Chin, R.: The utility of system models and developmental models for practitioners. In Bennis, W. G., Benne, K. D., and Chin, R., eds.: The planning of change: readings in the applied behavioral sciences, ed 2, New York, 1969, Holt, Rinehart & Winston.

Chu, F. D., and Trotter, S.: The madness establishment, New York, 1974, Grossman Publishers, Inc.

Cohen, R. E.: The collaborative coprofessional: developing a new mental health role, Hosp. Community Psychiatry **24:**242-246, 1973.

Connor, D. M.: Strategies for development, Ottawa, 1968, Development Press.

Connor, D. M.: Diagnosing community problems, Ottawa, 1969a, Development Press.

Connor, D. M.: Understanding your community, ed. 2, Ottawa, 1969b, Development Press.

Davis, A. J., and Underwood, P.: Role, function, and decision making in community mental health, Nurs. Res. **25:**256-258, 1976.

Dugger, J. G.: The new professional: introduction for the human services mental health worker, Monterey, Calif., 1975, Brooks/Cole Publishing Co.

Garrison, J., Kulp, C., and Rosen, S.: Community mental health nursing: a social network approach, J. Psychiatric Nurs. **15:**32-36, 1977.

Gazda, G. M., Asbury, F. R., Belzer, F. J., Childer, W. C., and Walters, R. P.: Human relations development: a manual for educators, ed. 2, Boston, 1977, Allyn & Bacon, Inc.

Glidewell, J. C.: A nonmedical model for community mental health. In Bellak, L. ed.: A concise handbook of community psychiatry and community mental health, New York, 1974, Grune & Stratton, Inc.

Harris, M., and Soloman, K.: Roles of the community mental health nurse, J. Psychiatric Nurs. **15:**35-39, Feb. 1977.

Jones, M.: Beyond the therapeutic community: social learning and social psychiatry, New Haven, 1968, Yale University Press.

Kelly, J. G.: Ecological constraints on mental health services, Am. Psychol. **21:**535-539, 1966.

Knight, J. H.: Applying nursing process in the community, Nurs. Outlook **22:**708-711, 1974.

Littrell, D. W.: The theory and practice of community development: a guide for practitioners, Columbia, Mo., University of Missouri (no date).

The new snake pits, Newsweek, May 15, 1978, pp. 93-93C.

Pepper, B.: The team: a means of achieving continuity of care. In Dean, A., Kraft, A. M., and Pepper, B. eds.: The social setting of mental health, New York, 1976, Basic Books, Inc.

Pluckhan, M. L.: Professional territoriality: a problem affecting the delivery of health care, Nurs. Forum **11:**301-310, 1972.

The President's Commission on Mental Health: The President's Commission on Mental Health, Washington, D.C., 1978, U.S. Government Printing Offiice, vol. 1.

Rapaport, J.: Community psychology: values, research and action, New York, 1977, Holt, Rinehart & Winston, Inc.

Roen, S. R., and Burnes, A. J.: Community adaptation schedule: manual, New York, 1968, Behavioral Publications, Inc.

Ross, M. G.: Community organization: theory, principles, and practice, ed. 2, New York, 1967, Harper & Row, Publishers.

Santopietro, M. C., and Rozendal, N. A.: Teaching primary prevention in mental health, Nurs. Outlook **23:**774-777, 1975.

Skrovan, C., Anderson, E. T., and Gottschalk, J.: Community nurse practitioner: an emerging role, Am. J. Public Health **64:**847-853, 1974.

Wise, H., Beckhard, R., Rubin, J., and Kyte, A. L.: Making health teams work: an organizational development approach to team building, Cambridge, Mass., 1974, Ballinger Publishing Co.

The Worcester development project: planning and coordination, Nurs. Times **73:**1064-1066, 1977.

Index

A

Abused husbands, 107
Abusive parents, 115-117
  characteristics of, 117
  treatment of, 117
Acceptance, 45
Activity group therapy, 163-169
  benefits of group experience, 166
  case illustration, 168-169
  definition, 163
Adaptation, 11-12, 17-19, 40, 51-53, 155, 250, 257
  in aging, 51-53
  in continuity of care program, 155
  ecological principle of, 52-53, 257
Adaptive mechanisms, 53
Adaptors, 51, 54
Addiction, 88, 91
Ageism, 66
Agent, 41, 51, 123, 129, 132
Aggression, 106, 185, 195
  art therapy for, 185-195
  in spouse abuse, 106
Aging, 50, 54-57, 71-73
Ainsworth, M., 116, 118
Alcohol, 90-92, 127, 171, 177
  addiction to, 92
  cost of use, 92
  and rape, 127
  usage in families, 171, 177
Alienation, 107, 124, 167
Altered state of consciousness, 88, 95
Amphetamines, 90
Amputation, 141-142
Anger, 95, 104-105, 112, 135-138
  in abusive situations, 105, 112
  in drug abusers, 95
  in rape victims, 135-138
  verbal expression of, 112
Anticipatory guidance, 53, 69, 155
  in aging, 53, 69
  with chronically ill psychiatric patients, 155
Antisocial personality disorder, 126
Anxiety, 143, 171-172, 183
  in families, 171

Anxiety—cont'd
  levels of, 171
  and nonterminal loss, 143
  reduction through art, 183
  responses to, 171
Apathy in child abuse, 117
Art
  in activity therapy groups, 167-168
  advantages of, 183-184
  developmental sequences in, 186-197
    controlled scribbling, 186
    disordered scribbling, 186
    naming of scribbles, 186
    preschematic stage, 187
    random marks, 186
  form, 181
  as graphic record, 185
  interpretations of, 181
  as preventive therapy, 185
  purposes of, 179-187
Art therapy, 167, 168, 179-198
Association for Holistic Health, 223
Atkenson, P., 112
Attachment, 115-117
Auerswald, E. H., 258

B

Ballard, P. B., 179
Barbiturates, 90
Basic human needs, 104
Behavior
  changes in, 204
  evaluating one's own, 204
  in reality therapy, 203-204
Behavior modification to reverse gender dysphoria, 81
Behavior setting, 19
Berlo, D. K., 180
Berne, E., 234
Bernstein, A., 89
Bessell, H., 42
Blacher, R. S., 144
Blum, R., 94
Body image, 140-150
  alterations in, 141

Body image—cont'd
  alterations in—cont'd
    effects of, 141
      coping with, 141-147
    and self-esteem, 140
Bolman, W. M., 263
Bonding behaviors, 116
Bowen, M., 172, 174, 177
Bowlby, J., 115-116
Branden, N., 165
Burgess, A., 125, 135, 137
Burn trauma, 143-144
Burnside, I., 56

C

Caffeine, 90, 92, 99
Caplan, G., 36, 42
Carlson, S., 59
Carter, J., 6
Cautela, J., 57
Child abuse and neglect, 115-122
  legal aspects, 117-118
  reporting of, 117
  as symptom of family distress, 117
  treatment, 117-122
Child advocacy, 117
Childbirth, 33, 38
Chu, F. D., 258
Clark, A. L., 37
Class, E., 117
Cohen, F., 182
Cohort, 59-62, 67
Colostomy, 141
Combs, A., 165
Comfort, A., 56
Communication, 45, 170-178, 180, 183-184
  through art, 179-180
  with children, 180
  in families, 170-180
  graphic, 183
  in human development program, 45
  nonverbal, 180
Community, 7, 13, 15, 18, 50, 152, 155, 250-252, 257,
    267
  analysis of, 267
  assessment of, 250-251
    attitudinal information, 250
    constraints on change, 251
    identifying target market for, 251
    resources for, 251
  diagnosis, 156
  responsiveness to mental health planning, 152
Community mental health, 4, 13, 19, 40, 152, 154, 156-
    160, 246, 257

Community mental health—cont'd
  criticism of, 152, 156-160, 246
  ecological approach to, 257
  program planning phases, 156-160
    decision making, 156
    diagnosis and assessment, 156
    evaluation, 156
    idea generation, 156
Community Mental Health Centers Act, 151-152
Community Mental Health Centers Amendments of 1975,
    6
Community mental health consultation, 135
Community mental health nursing, 1-3, 7, 51-52, 62, 69,
    124, 134, 155, 246, 260-267
  in continuity of care program, 155
  in gerontology, 51-52, 69
  interfaces with clients and community, 260-263
  for rape victim, 124, 134
  role, 260-265
  systems level intervention, 263-267
  use of marketing approach, 245-254
Confluence, 213
Consumer, 90-91, 96, 246-250
  marketing orientation toward, 249-250
  orientation in health care, 246-250
  self-help groups, 96
Consumer Reports, 91
Consumer Union Report, 91, 99
Contact, 210-212
Continuity of care with discharged psychiatric patients,
    151-160
  client advocacy, 158
  community acceptance, 157-158
  decision making, 156-157
  evaluation, 156-157
  group supervision, 159
  individual supervision, 158
  patient education, 158-159
  planning, 155
Cooley, C. H., 165
Crisis, 31, 36, 42, 54, 69, 107, 112, 124, 134-139, 185,
    197, 214
  developmental, 31, 36
  intervention, 42, 124, 134-139
    with aging person, 54
    and art use, 185
    counseling principles for, 138-139
    Gestalt therapy for, 214
    in rape, 124, 134, 137
  maturational, 69
  situational, 31, 112, 137, 197
    during pregnancy, 107
    of rape, 137
    during unemployment, 107

Cross-dressing, 83
  anxiety caused by, 83
  transitional need for, 83
Culture, 12, 17-18
Cumming, E., 64
Custodial care, 4
Cycling of resources; *see* Ecological principles

D

Dawning realization in art therapy, 191
Decision stage in art therapy, 193
Deflection, 213
Dehumanizing support institutions and spouse abuse, 103-
    105
Deinstitutionalization, 150, 152, 157
  legislative mandates, 153
  program for continuity of care, 150, 157
Denial, 145-146
  of disability, 145
  expression of, 145-146
    inward, 145
    outward, 145
DeRios, M., 93
Developmental sequences in art; *see* Art, developmental
    sequences in
Differentiation of self, 172-174
  criteria for measuring level of, 173
  emotional, 173
DiLeo, J., 180, 186, 188
Discharged psychiatric patients, 152-160
  community acceptance of, 157-158
  fear of, 157
Discipline, 116
  in child abuse, 116
  as expression of parental anger, 116
Disengagement, 64
  differential, 64
  process of, 64
Dix, D., 4
Drawings, 167-168, 182-197
  in activity therapy groups, 167-168
  by children, 182-197
  projective, 183
  for promoting communication, 184
  spontaneous, 182
Drug abuse, 88-99, 104
  and altered states of consciousness, 93
  consequences of, 90
  cross-cultural study of, 93-94
  definition, 92
  education about, 98-99
  in fulfilling the need for personal control, 93
  motives for usage, 94
  nursing implications, 95-99

Drug abuse—cont'd
  overdose, 99
  personality characteristics of abusers, 93
Drugs, 89-90
  amphetamines, 90
  barbiturates, 90
  psychoactive, 89
Dyads in family systems, 174
Dysphoria, gender, 79-81
  adolescent, 81-82
  treatment of, 81

E

Eaton, M. T., 124
Ecology, 10, 13, 16-18, 22-23, 154, 250, 259
Ecological analysis of mental health services, 259
Ecological approach; *see* Ecological perspective
Ecological concepts, 50
Ecological niche, 61
Ecological panorama, 22
Ecological perspective, 2, 8-10, 13, 22, 26, 50, 54, 123,
    154, 219, 257
  for community mental health, 257
  in continuity of care program for discharged psychiatric
      patients, 154
  in gerontology, 50, 54
  and holistic health care, 219
  in rape, 123
Ecological principles, 52-53, 154-155
  adaptation, 52-53, 155
  cycling of resources, 52
  interdependence, 52, 154-155
  succession, 52, 155
Ecosystem, 10-11, 17, 23, 50, 52-54, 67, 155, 220
  gerontological, 50-52
  intervention, 67
Ego states, 230-236
  adult, 230-234
  child, 230-234
  parent, 230-234
Emotional maturity, 172
Energy in systems, 171
Engel, G., 142
Environment, 1, 7, 13, 16-19, 22, 26-29, 33, 38, 40-41,
    51, 57-59, 125-126, 128-131, 155, 209-210, 212,
    220
  biological, 41
  in continuity of care program, 155
  definition of, 155
  external, 40, 212
  of fetus, 33
  in Gestalt theory, 209-210
  and holistic health, 220
  internal, 40, 212

Environment—cont'd
  internal—cont'd
    of rape victim, 126
    of rapist, 125
  physical, 41
  in pregnancy, 38
  prosthetic, in aging, 57-58
  psychosocial, 33
  in rape, 128-131
  sociocultural, 41
  stimulation of, for geriatric patient, 58-59
Epidemics, 104
Epidemiological process in studying rape, 123
Epidemiological triad, 41, 123, 129
Epidemiology, 128-133
  descriptive, 129
  of rape, 128-133
Equifinality, 12
Equilibrium, 12, 38
Erikson, E., 115
Evaluation
  of psychiatric programs, 159
  purpose of, 156-159

F

Family, 34, 41, 106
  changing character of, 41
  communal, 41
  historical perspective of, 34
  nuclear, 34
  role of anxiety, 171-172
  in spouse abuse, 106
  violence within, 106
Family history, 172
  collecting, 172
  three-generational, 172
Family issues, 171, 177
Family secrets, 171
Family therapy, 170-178, 219
  differentiation of self, 172-174
  goal of, 175-177
  and holism, 219
  multigenerational transmission process, 177-178
  responsibility for self, 173-174
  taking family history, 172
  triangles, 174-177
  use of anxiety, 171
Fantasy, 217
Fatherliness, 116
Fear, 135, 138, 157
  of discharged psychiatric patients, 157
  in rape victims, 136, 138
Feedback, 11
Feelings, 46, 173, 203, 210, 230

Feelings—cont'd
  awareness of, 210
  in family therapy, 173
  focusing on, 46
  in reality therapy, 203
  in Transactional Analysis, 230
Fetus, 33, 36-39
Figure and ground concept, 210
Foster care for abused children, 118
French, J. R., 72
Functional analysis, 232-234
  adult ego state, 232
  child ego state, 232-234
    adapted child, 232-234
    child in adult, 232-234
    natural child, 232-234
  parent ego state, 232
    controlling parent, 232
    nurturing parent, 232

G

Galdston, R., 117
Game, 126, 235
  definition of, 126
  as described in Transactional Analysis, 126
Game analysis, 230, 236, 238-239
  definition, 239
  elements, 239
  games, 238
  rackets, 238
  trading stamps, 238-239
Gender dysphoria, 79-80, 84
Gender role, 81
General systems theory, 1, 8, 23, 155, 225
Gestalt approach, 182, 214-218
  in art therapy, 182
  methods used with clients, 214-218
    body-mind interaction, 217-218
    dialogue, 216-217
    dreamwork, 218
    enactment, 215-216
    experimentation, 214-215
    fantasy, 217
    integration, 215
    unfinished business, 215
Gestalt concepts, 209-210
  contact, 209
  figure and ground, 210
  organismic self-regulation, 210
  resistance, 213
Gestalt theory, 209-218, 219, 225
  and "aliveness" of personality, 212
  contact, 212
  and holistic health, 219

Gestalt theory—cont'd
  and human ecology, 209
  integrative process, 212
  as personality theory, 209
  and process of awareness, 210
  self-awareness in, 211
  self-responsibility in, 211
Glidewell, J., 258
Gordon, T., 44
Goulding, R., 240
Grief, 145-149, 221
  education for professionals dealing with grieving person,
    147-148
  process for dealing with, 145
  related to body loss, 145
  societal reactions to, 148-149
Groth, A. N., 126
Grozinger, W., 180
Guided dialogue, 184
Guilt, 135-138
  feelings of, in rape victims, 135, 138
  nursing interventions to deal with, 135-138

H

Hallucinogens, 93
Harrington, G. L., 200
Harrison Narcotic Act of 1914, 91
Hartmann, H., 197
Hayakawa, S., 180
Healing, mental, 3
Health, 13-14, 19, 27, 51
Health promotion, 267
Helfer, R., 115
Helplessness, 221
Heroin, 90-91
Hierarchy of needs, 51
  belongingness, 51
  physiological, 51
  safety, 51
  self-actualization, 51
  self-esteem, 51
High-risk groups, 118, 128-129, 134, 152
  discharged psychiatric patients as, 152
  for child abuse, 118
  for mental illness, 134
  for rape, 128-129
Holism, 1, 95, 210, 219
  in Gestalt theory, 210
  as philosophy, 219
Holistic health care, 219-228
  basic tenets, 220
  with cancer patients, 226
  case illustration, 225
  clinical aspects, 224-228

Hostilic health care—cont'd
  definition, 219
  history of, 219
  and human ecology, 219
  role of client in, 221
  self-healing, 222
  spiritual aspects of, 221, 227
Hollender, M. H., 143
Homeostasis, 9, 16, 155, 210, 224
Homosexuality, 79, 82, 125
Hopelessness, 107, 221
Hormone therapy, 83
  androgen, 83
  estrogen, 83
  for transsexuals, 83
Horney, K., 42
Host, 41, 123, 128-130
Hostility, 140-150
  and nonterminal loss, 140-150
  and grief, 146
"Hot seat," 214
Human development program, 42-46
  curriculum, 43
  theoretical base, 44-46
    awareness, 44
    mastery, 44
    social interaction, 44-46
Human ecology, 1, 10, 12, 16-20, 24, 28, 154,
    219

I

Ileostomy, 141, 143
  adjustment after surgery, 143
  postoperative reaction, 143
Illness as result of unfavorable ecological factors, 51
Institutionalization, 152, 163-164
Interaction, 260-263
  client/community, 260-261
  client/nurse, 260-261
  nurse/client/community, 262-263
  nurse/community, 261
  patterns of, 260-263
Interdependence; see Ecological principles
Interdisciplinary interaction, 258, 263-264
Interface, 22, 24, 28, 236, 258, 262
Introjection, 213
Involvement, 202

J

Jealousy, 105
Johnson, Judge Frank, 153
Joint Commission on Mental Illness and Health,
    6
Jones, M., 5, 258

K

Kaiser, H., 200
Karpman, S., 239
Kellogg, R., 179, 186
Kelly, J. G., 259
Kempe, C., 115
Kennedy, J. F., 6
Knorr, N. J., 143
Kolb, L. C., 141-142
Kotler, P., 248
Kramer, E., 185, 192
Kreiger, D., 222
Kris, E., 180
Kuypers, J. A., 67

L

Languor, 146-147
Legislation, 6, 90-91, 96, 153
  for drug abuse, 90, 96
  mental health, 6
  for psychiatric patients, 153
Levy, B., 182-183
Levy, S., 248
Life review, 54, 70
Life space, 19
Lindsley, O. R., 57, 65
Loneliness, 95, 166-169
  of drug abusers, 95
  in schizophrenia, 167
  ways to counteract, 166-169
"Looking-glass" self, 165
Lowenfeld, V., 182, 186
Lynch, A., 117

M

Magic Circle, 42-43, 46-49
  guidelines for, 43
  implementation of, 46
    active listening, 46
    involving everyone, 46
    paraphrasing, 46
    providing recognition, 46
    review, 46
    transferring leadership, 47
  leader in, 43
  obstacles to progress of, 47
    copying, 47
    gaining good feelings from unacceptable behavior, 48
    ignored members, 48
    nonlistening, 47
    rambling, 47
Marcel, G., 165
Marijuana, 90-91
Marital violence, 106

Market segmentation, 251-252
Marketing, 246-254
  broadened concept of, 247-249
  consumer orientation, 246-249
  evolution of, 247
  and health care, 249
  identity crisis in, 246
  nature and scope of, 246-247
  philosophy of, 249
  as planning framework, 250-254
Masculinity, 105
Maslow, A., 51
Mastectomy, 140-142
McClannahan, L. E., 57
Mead, G. H., 165
Mechanic, D., 153
Medicaid, 256
Medicalization of human condition, 89
Meditation, 223, 225
Mental health, 51, 155
  gerontological, 51
  systems theory approach to, 155
Mental Health Study Act, 6
Mental illness, 153, 201
  chronic, 153
  theory of, according to reality therapy, 201
Mental images, 180
Mental incompetence, 153
Mental Retardation Facilities and Community Mental Health Centers Construction Act of 1963, 6
Meyer, A., 4-5
Mimicry, 35
Model, 1, 8, 24, 26-29
Mothering process, 116
Motherliness, 116
Mumford, L., 179
Myocardial infarction, 144

N

Nason vs. Superintendent of Bridgewater State Hospital, 153
National Institute of Mental Health, 5, 151
National Mental Health Act, 5
Niche, 12
Nicotine, 90-92
  addiction to, 91
  cancer and, 92
  incidence of usage, 91-92
Nonterminal grief, coping measures, 145-147
  anticipation, 147
  anxiety, 146
  depression, 146
  emotional release, 145
  hostility, 146

Nonterminal grief, coping measures—cont'd
  languor, 146-147
  physiological symptoms, 146
  shock and denial, 145
Nonterminal loss, 140-150
  coping with, 140-150
  denial stage, 145-146
  due to surgery, 143
  reactions of professionals to, 148

O

Object loss, 140-144
  by amputation, 141-142
  and body image, 140
  due to burns, 143
  myocardial infarction and, 144
  surgical, 141-143
    colostomy, 141
    ileostomy, 141
    splenectomy, 144
    urostomy, 141
O'Connor vs. Donaldson, 153
Opiates, 91
Ounsted, C., 117

P

Palmore, E., 52
Palomares, U., 42
Panic, 146
Paradigm for evaluating bonding, 118-122
  differences between abused and nonabused children, 119-120
  discriminating variables, 119
Parent discussion groups, 112
Parenthood, 33
Patient advocacy, 153, 157
Payoff in psychological game, 126
Pelvic exenteration, 143
Peplau, H., 171
Perls, F., 214, 216
Personality, 210
Phantom limb, 141-142
Phobic reaction, in rape victims, 137
Physical-environmental subsystem of aging, 57
Physiological changes of aging, 54-57
  cardiorespiratory, 55
  decreased sensory acuity, 54-55
  genitourinary, 56
  neurological, 55-56
  nursing implications, 56-57
  physical appearance, 54
Pinel, P., 3
Planning for community mental health programs, 253-254
Poetry, in activity therapy groups, 167-168

Polarities, in Gestalt therapy, 216
Polster, E., 212
Powerlessness, 107
Pregnancy, 33-38
  physiological aspects, 35
  psychological aspects, 36
  tasks of, 36-38
Preschematic stage in art, 187-188
President's Commission on Mental Health, Report of, 6-7, 152, 256
Prevention, 6, 13, 31, 40-42, 50, 62, 72, 123-124, 134, 200, 222, 263
  and holistic health practices, 222
  of mental illness, 6, 222
  primary, 13, 40-42, 50, 62, 72, 110, 123-124, 134, 263
    with children, 40-42
    community level, 263
    in elderly persons, 50, 62, 72
    in rape victims, 123, 128
    with reality therapy, 200
    in spouse abuse, 110, 112-113
  secondary, 13, 15, 41, 103, 123-124, 163, 263
    with children, 41
    in community, 263
    in spouse abuse, 103
  tertiary, 13, 15, 41, 103, 124, 163, 263
    activity groups as, 163
    with children, 41
    on community level, 263
    in rape victims, 124
Preventive mental health, and art therapy, 185-186
Preventive psychiatry, 13
Primary gain, in rape, 125
Primary health care, 263
Primary prevention; see Prevention, primary
Projection, 213
Proximity-maintaining behaviors in children, 120
Proximity-seeking behaviors in children, 120
Pseudonaturalistic stage in art, 193
Psychoactive drugs, 89
Psychoanalysis and creative process, 181
Psychological hunger, 234-236
  stroke hunger, 234
  structure hunger, 235-236
Psychological subsystem of aging, 65-70
  assessment of self-esteem, 70-71
  social-breakdown syndrome, 67
  social competence, 67-70
    creative adaptation, 68-69
    effective social-role performance, 67-68
Psychotherapy, 170-180, 200-241
  family, 170-180
  Gestalt, 209-218
  holistic, 219-228

Psychotherapy—cont'd
  reality, 200-208
  Transactional Analysis, 229-241
Public education, 97-99, 128-129, 134, 157
  for communities receiving discharged psychiatric patients, 157
  for persons working with rape victims, 134
  for rape prevention, 128-129
  in substance abuse, 97-99

R

Rambert, M., 182
Random marks in children's art, 186
Rapaport, J., 259
Rape, 123-137.
  anger as motivator, 125, 135
  as crisis, 124, 134
  definition of, 123, 135
  as denial of homosexuality, 125
  ecological perspective of, 123
  emergency treatment for, 124, 134-135
  frequency by epidemiological factors, 130-133
    age of victim, 130
    location in city, 131
    number of rapes by month, 130
    time of day, 131
  legal system and, 134
  as motivated by need for sexual gratification, 125
  myths related to, 135
  nursing intervention for, 134-137
  physical examination after, 136-137
  profile of, 132, 135
  reaction of victim, 136
    acute phase, 136
    emotional reactions, 136
    reorganization phase, 136
  societal attitudes, 135
Rapist, 123-126
  antisocial personality, 126
  displaced anger, 125
  feelings of incompetence, 125
  sadistic needs, 125-126
Rapo, 126-127
Read, H., 180-181
Reading in activity therapy groups, 167-168
Reality therapist, 202-208
  case illustration, 206-208
  role of, 203-205
Reality therapy, 200-208
  as ecological approach, 202-204
  personality theory of, 200
  process of, 202-204
  steps, 202
  theory of mental illness, 200

Reality therapy—cont'd
  as treatment approach, 200
Regester, D., 250
Resistance, in Gestalt therapy, 213
  confluence, 213
  deflection, 213
  introjection, 213
  projection, 213
  retroflection, 213
Reticular activating system, 57
Retirement, 54, 62-64, 69
  phases of, 64
  as "roleless role," 63
Retroflection, 213
Reusch, J., 144
Rhyne, J., 182
Rituals, 235
Rogers, C., 165
Role, 62-63, 68, 170, 259, 263-265
  alternatives in aging, 62
    association member, 63
    citizen, 62-63
    of community mental health nurse, 263-265
    family, 62, 170
    friend, 62
    retiree, 62
    user of leisure, 63
  insufficiency of, 68
Rouse vs. Cameron, 153
Rubin, R., 35-37
Rush, B., 4

S

Sadistic rapist, 125-126
Sadness, 95, 112
Salant, E. G., 185
Schematic stage in art, 188-197
  deviations from normal, 189-197
  repeated symbols, 188
  representational symbols, 188
    color, 189
    space, 191
    time, 188
  stereotyped repetitions, 188
Schilder, P., 140-142
Schizophrenia, 163-169
  described as, 169
  self-concept of, 163
  and use of activity group therapy, 166
Schoenberg, B., 142
Script analysis, 230, 239-240
Secondary prevention; *see* Prevention, secondary
Sedatives, 99
Self-actualization, 51, 72

Self-actualization—cont'd
  self-development, 72
  self-utilization, 72
Self-concept, 43, 65-66, 140-144, 163-166
  of aging persons, 65-66
  attitudinal component, 164
  and body image, 140-141
  conceptual component, 165
  definition, 165
  and description of normal self, 164
  development of, 164
  existential view, 165
  need for positive, 165
  perceptual component, 164
  personal self, 66
  physical self, 66
  of schizophrenic person, 163-164
  stability of, 165
  and surgery, 144
Self-esteem, 45, 66-67, 140, 167, 183-184
  in aging, 66
  and art therapy, 183-184
  as related to body loss, 140
  in schizophrenia, 167
  socially influenced, 66-67
  task specific, 66
Self-image, 200
  failure identity, 200
  success identity, 200
Selkin, J., 123, 127
Selye, H., 224
Sensitivity training, 99
Sensory training, 58-59
Separation anxiety, 116
Sex reassignment, 79, 82-84
  presurgical treatment, 82
  psychotherapy for, 82
  transition phase, 83-84
Sexual deviation, 124
Sexual functioning, 56
Simonton, C., 227
Social change, 105
Social isolation, 111, 116, 144
  in child abuse, 116
  in spouse abuse, 111
  following surgery with body loss, 144
Social Security Act, 5
Sociocultural subsystem, 59-63
  age stratification, 59-60
  role alternatives, 62
  status, 60-62
    implications for older client, 62
    involvement dimension, 61-62
    status dimension, 60-61
Sociocultural subsystem—cont'd
  status—cont'd
    value dimension, 61
Spiritual/philosophical subsystem, in aging, 71
  religion and, 71-72
  self-actualization, 72-73
Spouse abuse, 103-113
  case history, 108-110
  community support, 103, 112-113
  cultural factors, 106
  definition, 103
  dynamics of, 110
  environmental factors, 106
  etiology, 103
  multidimensional approach to, 103
  nursing intervention, 110-113
  prevention, 105
  societal myths, 106
Stark, R., 107
Steinmetz, S., 107
Stern, L., 116
Stimulation, 58-59
  environmental, 58
  sensory, 58-59
Stratford, C. D., 210
Stress, 13, 92, 116, 140, 180, 222-224
  in childhood, 180
  definition, 224
  due to body loss, 140
  environmental, in child abuse, 116
  management of, 222-224
  response of, 224
Stressors, 51, 54, 155, 224-228
  environmental, 155
  management of, 224-228
  response to, 224
Stroke, 234
  definition, 234
  positive, 234
  psychological, 234
Structural analysis; *see* Ego states
Substance abuse; *see* Drug abuse
Succession; *see* Ecological principles
Sullivan, H. S., 42, 65, 115, 164-165
Supplemental Security Income, 256
Symbols in communication, 180
Systems, 1, 8, 11, 23, 155, 170-172, 210, 225, 258
  closed, 11
  dysfunction, 170-172
  as ecological approach, 258
  energy in, 171
  family, 170
  levels of, 170
  living, 11

Systems—cont'd
  open, 11, 210
  principles of, 170
  theory, 1, 8, 23, 155, 225
Szasz, T., 90-91, 93, 219

T

Tasks, 36-38
  developmental, 37
  maternal, 37
  of pregnancy, 36-38
Team process, 258, 263-264
Terr, C., 117
Territoriality, 25
Tertiary prevention; *see* Prevention, tertiary
Test, M., 158
Theory, 23-24
Therapeutic milieu, 5
Therapeutic touch, 222
Tobacco, 90-91
"Topdog," 216
Transaction, 236, 248
  angular, 236
  complementary, 236
  crossed, 236
  duplex, 236
  marketing, 248
  parallel, 236
  social, 236
Transactional Analysis, 229-241
  assumptions, 229
  ego states, 229-236
Transcendental meditation, 99
Transsexual, 79-86
  counseling, 85
  family of, 84-85
  surgery for, 84
Transvestism, 79
Trauma, 124, 134-139, 143
  burn, 143-144
  rape, 124, 134-139
Triangles, in family systems, 174-177
Trickett, E. J., 52
Tuke, W., 3

U

Ulman, E., 182-183
"Underdog," 216

Unification, 23
Urostomy, 141

V

Values clarification, 112
Ventura School for Girls, 200
Victim of rape, 123-125, 128-129, 134-139
  emotional reactions, 136-138
  follow-up counseling for, 137-139
  internal environmental dynamics of, 126
    naïveté, 127
    "rapo," 126-127
    vulnerability, 127
  long-term reaction, 137
  needs of, 135
  nursing intervention for, 134-138
  physical examination, 136-137
  testing by rapist, 127
Violence, 106-107
  family, 106
  marital, 106
Visual imagery, 225, 227
Vulnerable old, 60, 67

W

Weil, A., 94-95
Wellness, 220, 223
Westberg, G., 222-223
Wholeness, 209, 214
Widowhood, 62
Williams, G. H., 182, 185
Winnicott, D. W., 184
Withdrawal, 212
Women's liberation movement, 105
Wyatt vs. Stickney, 153
Wylie, R., 165

Y

Yoga, 99

Z

Zaltman, G., 248
Zen Buddhism, 99
Zusman, J., 152

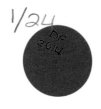

Monika Habermann
Leana R. Uys
(eds.)

Violence in Nursing

International Perspectives

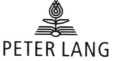

PETER LANG

Frankfurt am Main · Berlin · Bern · Bruxelles · New York · Oxford · Wien

Bibliographic Information published by Die Deutsche Bibliothek
Die Deutsche Bibliothek lists this publication in the Deutsche Nationalbibliografie; detailed bibliographic data is available in the internet at <http://dnb.ddb.de>.

ISBN 3-631-50180-3
US-ISBN 0-8204-6047-8

© Peter Lang GmbH
Europäischer Verlag der Wissenschaften
Frankfurt am Main 2003
All rights reserved.

Printed in Germany 1 2 3 4   6 7

www.peterlang.de

Acknowledgements

We would like to express our thanks to the following people or institutions:
The contributors, for their contributions, and the way in which they worked
with us to see this book published.
The translators of different chapters from original languages:

o Birte Mangouras,
o Dr Bärbel von Braun and Margret Lampe (chapter 1, 5, 6) Julia Leonhardt,
  (chapter 1)

Collaborators on different chapters:

o Dr Chika Ugochukwu, who did the data collection for chapter four in Nigeria.

Assistance with preparing the manuscript:

o Mrs Ruth Brinkmeier
o Mr Andreas Stutzig

Financial assistance of the Hochschule Bremen

Bremen Juli 2002   Monika Habermann and Leana R. Uys

5

Preface

As we enter the 21st century, the movement to democratic societies has become a global phenomenon. Changes in Central and Eastern Europe, large parts of Latin America and South Africa provide inspiring examples of this recent trend. With these changes we have also witnessed a shift in the humanitarian and human rights thinking and action. Part of the thinking is how new societies can respond to the demands of political and social change and how to deal with the legacies of the past. These changes have also had an impact on established democracies. Health workers, and nurses in particular, form a large part of society and as such make a significant impact on whether or not these societies respond humanely to the social and development needs in a new or established democratic order. Despite this important contribution to society, nurses are at risk of violence and abuse and are in some instances perpetrators of violence.

According to recent research in the United States the majority of nurses remain unfamiliar with the knowledge that health workers, especially nurses, are assaulted more frequently in the workplace than any other working group or that the actual incidence of violence exists in their profession. The World Health Organisation (WHO)[1] defines violence as the "intentional use of physical force or power, threatened or actual, against oneself, another person, or against a group or community, that either results, or has a high likelihood of resulting in injury, death, psychological harm, maldevelopment, or deprivation." This book is an important contribution to our understanding of the significance of this global health issue. It focuses not only on the problem but seeks to understand the causes, manifestations of the various forms of violence and points to solutions to this "international human resource issue." The work draws from empirical research as well as the stories of those who have been affected by violence. The significance of the issue of violence in the workplace is well documented in the literature and substantiated by this work. Violence in the health care is not diminishing in importance or frequency. It is imperative to provide health care to all, but there are circumstances and situations in care settings that predispose this environment to incidents of workplace violence. In hospitals there is unrestricted movement of

---

1   World Health Organisation (n.D.) Document CRC 28/WHO 1, available: www.crin. org/docs/resources/treaties/crc.28/WHO1.pdf.

people, patients, families and other visitors from one area to another. There is an increase in use of the hospitals and health facilities by substance abusers, gang members, alcohol-dependant persons, and individuals with a history of violence or criminal records. Emergency units are open day and night and during the weekends. Patients or family members may have been traumatised by an event that decreases their ability to cope and leads them to violence. As more and more people use emergency departments for health care, waiting times are increased causing impatience and tempers can flare. Societal factors too lead to health care violence, including increased access to weapons, prevalence of drug use, and changes in family and community support.

Many nurses work in extremely volatile and politically dangerous situations as members of multi national care and humanitarian aid organisations. Hundreds of nurses work in remote rural villages with scant resources and security and are exposed daily to war and its consequences. Often nurses are targeted as victims because of religious belief or ethnicity and cannot provide adequate services because they are seen as agent of unwelcome change. Poor or inappropriate training may lead nurses to feel ill prepared for their work causing them to perpetrate violence against vulnerable patients such as the young, very ill or the elderly. These issues are dealt with in this book.

This important publication comes at a time when many nurses are grappling with new challenges related to both the theory and practice of nursing. New insights regarding care in ever increasing cross-cultural settings confront the nurse with the need to understand diversity and to seek new ways to facilitate conflict resolution and mediation. The importance thus to understand and critically reflect is underscored by the inclusion of chapters on theoretical analysis and empirical research that deals with nurse-directed and patient-directed violence.

In so far as this publication brings together philosophical discourse analysis of workplace violence in the literature, the different faces of violence in various settings, elder abuse, preventions strategies and guidelines for management of workplace violence, it provides an impetus for increased international awareness of the seriousness of the problem yet the possibility of the creation of a concerted joint effort to the establishment of a humane work environment free of intimidation, abuse and injury. The variety and richness of the experiences of the contributors will certainly be a useful guide not only to students and researchers in nursing, but to all in the health sector and in popular efforts to reorganise society.

The collection, editing and organisation of the best material on the subject of workplace violence in nursing is an important contribution to the field facilitating comparative analysis of issues that many nurses have felt are unique to their own experience.

I hope that this publication raises the profile of scholarship on violence in the health setting; it is extraordinarily important that we restore trust between the communities and the profession and work in partnership to create better humane societies.

Glenda Wildschut, South Africa

Contents

Acknowledgements   5

Preface
Glenda Wildschuth   7

Chapter One: Introductory Remarks: Violence in Nursing – International
Perspectives
Monika Habermann   13

Chapter Two: Workplace Violence in U.S. Nursing Literature – A
Discourse Analysis
Penny Powers   29

Chapter Three: Violence in Health Care: A Finnish Nursing Perspective
Maritta Välimäki, Johanna Taipale and Anneli Pitkänen   55

Chapter Four: Violence in Nursing in two African Countries
Leana R Uys and Rhosta S Gcaba   81

Chapter Five: Violence in Psychiatric Care: German Experiences
Dirk Richter   99

Chapter Six: Violence against Elderly People and its Prevention in Nursing
Care Institutions in Germany
Rolf D. Hirsch   113

Chapter Seven: Physical Restraint in Gerontology in Ireland
Róisín Gallinagh   141

Chapter Eight: Violence against Caregivers in Nursing Homes in the USA
Donna M. Gates   157

11

Chapter Nine: Identifying and Reducing Nurse-Nurse Horizontal Violence and Bullying through Reflective Practice and Action Research in an Australien Hospital
Bev Taylor _____ 177

Chapter Ten: The Content and Development of Management of Violence Policies in Inpatient Psychiatric Settings
James Noak and Steve Wright _____ 199

Chapter Eleven: Education for Violence Prevention – A Danish Example
Vibeke Sjøgreen; Anne Jensen, and Pia Kielberg _____ 217

Editors and Authors _____ 237

Chapter One: Introductory Remarks: Violence in Nursing – International Perspectives

Monika Habermann

Violence in Nursing

Care, support and affection – these terms characterise the self-image of professional nursing since its origins in the last century. Violence in nursing – the subject does not seem to fit into this notion. But ordinary and specific forms of violence in society are also manifest in nursing. Thus, several phenomena, which are classified as violence in a sociological context, may become effective within nursing relationships and the environment in which they develop.

Even if the extent of the problem cannot easily be identified, the World Health Organisation (WHO, 1996) decided that the subject of violence in the health care setting should be treated as one of the main topics of health care and nursing. This was followed by alarming reports also from the International Labour Organisation (ILO) which brought the issue world-wide to the public's attention (WHO, 2000; ILO,1998; Chappell and di Martino, 2000) The debate of the WHO focuses mainly on violence that health care-workers encounter as well as on the growing need for treatment of victims of violence by health care-workers. Apart from supporting research with the objective to identify forms and magnitude of violence in the health care sector (WHO, 2002) the WHO is also engaged in prevention programmes for vulnerable groups like the primary health care workers and the numerous women working as nurses in the health care field (WHO, 2000).

The International Council of Nursing (ICN) has also repeatedly tackled the problem through its press releases, guidelines and statements (ICN, 1999, 2000, 2001). The latest statement was summing up the results of a common investigation by the WHO, ILO, ICN and PSI (Public Services International). Violence within the health care-sector is described as epidemic with considerable consequences for the world's largest professional group in each health sector, that is to say those working in nursing (ICN, 2002). This group is not only likely to be effected by the probability of personal experiences with violence, due to the fact that they are the group highest in numbers in the health sector, but also because professional nursing is still mainly a female profession. According to the ICN 95% of professional nursing staff world-wide are women (ICN, 1999). Women are at risk of becoming victims of violence due to their position in society because violence of all sorts is being channelled and finds its targets primarily among those who appear powerless (Elwert, 1999). Apart from children, elderly people or other apparent outsiders of society, women are therefore especially vulnerable. The ICN (1999) therefore developed guidelines for dealing with violence at the workplace and initiated a zero-tolerance campaign.

Even if the previously-mentioned investigations and findings of international organisations focus primarily on the victims within health care-professions, it also becomes clear that the realities of violence are complex. Victims of violence in its different forms may also appear as the ones committing the crime. Five dimensions of violence in nursing have been found to be addressed in the literature which has been examined prior to the conception of this volume: nurses as perpetrators of violence; nurses as victims of violence; nursing in a violent environment; preventive measures for the control of violence and nursing care for people who either have already become victims of violence, or are empirically proven to be vulnerable groups, a fact which needs to be included in the concepts of nursing for this group.

The subject of violence in nursing presently receives intense attention – in the international specialised literature as well as with the general public – in the first four mentioned dimensions. Under the headings of "Workplace violence and its prevention" and "Violence towards those in need of care and its prevention" the importance of these dimensions for the discussion of violence, within the health care sector is documented through the contributions in this volume, which are exclusively dedicated to the different forms of these phenomena.

This limitation seemed necessary. The analysis of concepts of nursing for people who have become victims of violence is covered primarily in North American literature. Under the term of "domestic violence" for instance, the fragmentation of society and its consequences for the field of nursing are frequently discussed (Davidzhar et al., 2002; Varcoe, 2001; Merrell, 2001; Davis, R.E. et al., 2001). Contrary to the neo-conservative ideologies, that identify families as nucleus of societal development, the family seems to be an arena for conflicts and violence (Englander, 1997). Even if the growing sensitivity regarding this field of nursing, is impressively proven through the counselling of victims of violence within the family or other vulnerable groups, shown by many contributions which have been published in the last years, we refrained from including this subject matter in our publication. The necessity of describing and comparing concepts of nursing which apply to victims of violence, i.e. to battered children and wives, to young and old people who have suffered through war and expulsion and to people who have been subjected to everyday violence produced by modern society, as well as the discussion of desirable characteristics of such nursing concepts has to be reserved for a future compilation.

Violence in Nursing-Relationships and Workplace Violence

Whenever nurses use violence, this represents a reversal of their professional and social mission which creates fear and defensiveness and calls for more adequate professional and social control. Even though it was already conceived in the seventies for the specific field of psychiatric in-patients care, and even though it was staged in a dramatic way, the well-known portrayal of the nurse in the movie "One flew over the cuckoo's nest" still today conveys the reservations and fears of the public. In this movie, a display of power, striving for dominance and cool reserve determine the image of nursing. An image which – as shown also in the picture- can easily be shaken with a lasting effect. It thus becomes clear which forms of violence needs to be considered in a discussion of not only psychiatric care, but also a range of other health care and nursing settings. Apart from the immediate physical violence towards those in need of care, their conditioning and adaptation to everyday life in an institution can be part of the reality of violence. Experiences with violence of those in need of care have so many different facets. Apart from the institutional restriction there is namely neglect, verbal humiliation, physical irritation, damage or constraint, in extreme cases even the killing of patients. In the past few years such killings have repeatedly become the subject of legal, public and also scientific disputes, in a number of countries (Beine 1997, 1998; Payne, 2000; Hall, 1996). As an ultimate reversal of the professional mission of care, the analysis of these events discloses structural and cultural conditions of nursing over and above from individual pathologies of perpetrators.

When the direction of violence is reversed- i.e. where nurses become the target of attacks – similar forms of violence can be named: patients and their relatives offend and insult nursing staff, they threaten them and put them under psychological pressure or even attack them physically (Squire, 2001; Kingma, 2001; Duncan, 2001; ANA, 2001; Morgan, 2001; Rippon, 2000). As a primarily female profession, sexual harassment is also a form of violence which is experienced by nurses also in the work with patients and relatives (Madison, 1997; Madison et al, 2000), even so sexual harassments seems to be committed in general more by co-workers (Kinard, 2002; Duncan, 2001; Robinson, 1993). Furthermore, risks arise in many regions for nurses working in health care institutions in areas which are particularly dangerous or where home-based care take place in such areas.

Finally, under the term of "workplace violence" attention has to be paid to horizontal forms of violence. This is a phenomenon which can be considered as an extreme form of failed co-operation among staff within institutions which can only negatively influence the care given. Nurses who feel intimidated, attacked and humiliated by colleagues – these are only a few of the typical forms of horizontal workplace violence that can be classified as "bullying" – will only be able

15

to care and support in a limited manner, due to their own problems in the workplace (Bray, 2001; Vartia, 2001; Cusack, 2000; Kivimaki, 2000; Quine, 1999; Alderman, 1997).

It is rather difficult to quantify the importance of the phenomenon of violence in nursing even in the regional or national context. It becomes more difficult with regard to the international situation or when a comparison of countries is intended. Even the limitation of the exploration to only these cases when nurses and those in need of care are involved is not helpful. The difficulty of describing the phenomenon sufficiently are closely connected to the strong taboo attached to the subject: Violence which is, for example, carried out in a nursing relationship by nurses, contradicts in an elementary way – as indicated already earlier on – the self-image of nurses. In the first place, distinct methods are therefore required to address violence in nursing (Schiffhorst et al, 1999). In most countries nurses as perpetrators are dealt with through legal procedures, nursing associations and/or employers. A fact, which in turn may be obstructive to a disclosure for the purpose of scientific research. Even those cases where nurses become victims of violence within a nursing relationship, may be subject to taboos. This is especially true in cases where the experience of violence by a patient is regarded as a failure of the personal, professional nursing activity. This is assumed, for example, where experiences with violence within psychiatric care are concerned (Sauter and Richter, 1998). Due to these taboos regarding violence within an immediate nursing relationship where nursing staff either commit violence or become victims, a large number of unreported cases world-wide is assumed as far as this form of violence is concerned (ICN, 2001; WHO, 2000).

The difficulty in recording violence in an adequate way and the resulting problems in international comparative context, also result from the fact, that the definition of the phenomenon of "Violence in nursing" and its description and interpretation are ambiguous. There may be doubts as to whether the chosen structure of the subject, which has been drawn up initially through the above-mentioned dimensions in this volume, is a useful one. Are we not opening a discussion which – by pretending to be extensive – causes a levelling out and an easing of extreme cases of violence in nursing? Should the description and analysis of "violence in nursing" not be limited to those phenomena, where physical attacks as well as psychological attacks with proven serious effects for the victims are concerned? And, thus, should all further considerations, like, for example, the quoted misguided nursing concepts and institutional conditions, be left out? These questions include problems which determine the discourse of violence within the field of sociology in general. A brief reflection on this debate may therefore be useful, in order to categorise the present dimension of the subject of "violence in nursing" and to further examine it.

16

What is Violence? – The Discourse of Violence Portrayed through Sociological Reflection

Different connotations are connected to the term of "violence" within different languages through which a wide field of meanings is created. Thus, Webster distinguishes between up to seven definitions of violence which stretch from physical injury, to the deprivation of individual rights and liberty. Within the usage of the French and English language it is possible to further distinguish between the negative notion of the German term "Gewalt" (violence) and the positive force and state authority ("la force" resp. "power"). The German language does not know such differences. State authority and forms of violence in social life are classified here under the same term. One thing that the quoted language traditions have in common, is the fact that the discourse about violence always is a morally tainted discourse. This is even the case when the sceptical question arises, if and under which circumstances fragile human relationships and communities may develop, as well as if and how violence may be avoided or kept to a minimum in this process. The question of guilt and making up for it is also asked when violence is discussed. Similar to the terms of "poverty", "disablement" or "illness", sociological terms and theories regarding violence are thus determined by a contradictory approach, in which their embedment in socio-cultural experiences and political interests can be perceived (Thiersch, 1994). Thus, the spectrum of the discussion is determined by the opposite positions, the contours of which are specified here in a simplified manner:

on the one hand, the description and analysis of violence towards human beings is supposed to be limited to physical violence due to the "*Verletzungsmaechtigkeit* = the power of using violence" of the human being (Popitz,1992). This is classified as archetypical, universal language (Thiersch, 1994) and thus regarded as the essential characteristic of violence, the limitation on attacks which cause physical harm or humiliation: "We kick, beat, slap, choke, tie up (...) Violence is a physical means, a physical injury and physical pain – this is the indispensable point of reference for any kind of analysis of violence" (von Trotta 1997, p. 26). Works marked by Anglo-Saxon influences which compare cultures have traditionally looked at violence from this point of departure.

On the other hand, the specification of violence has experienced an extension which also includes terms like structural and cultural violence further to the physical and psychological effects on the victims, their physical and verbal situation of blackmail, constraint, isolation and humiliation. The indirectly effected forms of "structural violence" describe restrictions of people regarding their physical, psychological and mental potential (compare for example: Galtung, 1975, Faulseit et al., 2001, p.21), which document their powerless social position. "Cultural violence" manifests itself through the predominance of symbols, through which structural violence is experienced and handed down in the social process (Galtung in Kinkelbuhr, 2000, p. 26 f.). With this characterisation of the term of violence – according to its protagonists – the consequences of the systematic discrimination of social fringe groups or discrimination within the relationship of the sexes could be shown (Böhnisch, 1994).

If the critical analysis accuses the first quoted notion of violence for being restrictive for the purposes of commissioned stately research (Albrecht et al., 1990), the extension of the phenomenon to the mentioned non-physical forms of violence is also considered by others as being an unproductive generalisation, as a "catch-all concept", which leads to a "moral overheating" of the stated conflicts and thus impedes the development of strategies for a solution (Neidhardt, 1986). Furthermore, an extension of the term to new phenomena of suffered damages might cause a levelling of the power of description and analysis of the term: "Where everything is described as violence, nothing can be considered violence anymore" (Ahlers in Faulseit et al., 2001 p.15).

Whether an extended notion of violence or a limitation to the physical is valid – the answer cannot easily be found also in anthropological or socio-historical analyses. Still, there are some essential theoretical points of reference: a restricted definition of violence follows a social model of development which – as shown by Elias (1969) – connected the "process of civilisation" with the gradual transfer of the monopoly of violence to public authorities. This created the modern individual who has renunciated force on an individual level. The process is still effective today since the regulating force of the state keeps penetrating areas that were formerly declared private; nowadays, it sanctions, for example, the corporal punishment of children or rape within marriage which would have been unthinkable only a few decades ago. Other approaches also connect the emancipation of the individual from the formerly religiously sanction against violence to an increasingly rationally founded renunciation of violence. This is not an unbroken belief in progress, but endangered through the "dialectics of Enlightenment" (Adorno, Horkheimer). Violence is interpreted as a relapse by these progressive development models, as a reflection of a barbaric origin. It is connected to a decay of culture and its most important values. Prevention of violence – according to the conservative discourse within politics and society of this approach – thus requires forced protection, which may also be based on violence, of traditional values and its institutions.

Other results, however, led to a subdivision of violence into increasingly subtle forms, which characterise modern life. Foucault (1982), for example, described the subtle forms of influencing individuals through the control of their self-perception and –conception as "micro-physics of power". The disciplinary society and its "modes of objectivations which transform human beings into subjects" (ibidem 1982, p. 777) takes the place of a non-violent society as expected by those who believe in progress. A radical renunciation of power and violence is therefore impossible since individuals, as such are the products of disciplinary measures. Still, it can be shown how power and violence subtly take effect and this is what Foucault demonstrates impressively in his numerous analyses (e.g. Foucault 1977, 1988).

By way of transferring these aspects of sociological discourse to nursing, the following considerations are not to be neglected: if one adopts Foucault's above-mentioned point of view, violence in a nursing relationship is not only documented through manifest forms of physical detriment. These could only be interpreted as an impressive expression of the failure of more subtle attempts in the exercise of power. In this case, violence would be also part of the professional established relationship, e.g. the scientific discourse and its effect on practical use as to what "good" and "correct" nursing really implies. Let us use an example by way of explanation: while striving for professional recognition, nursing worldwide adheres to structural characteristics, e.g. through schemes of classification and the orientation on nursing processes within certain nursing models. The person in need of care is thus subjected to an adaptation to the growing power of experts in nursing, depending on the relevant model and philosophy of nursing. In view of the growing necessity to render nursing transparent, verifiable in terms of costs and quality and in view of the necessity to indicate epidemiologically which kind of nursing is required by the population, the resistance of some nursing theorists to the said structural approaches seems problematic. Still, if, for example, Parse (1987, 1990) attests to the traditional nursing theories a "totalitarian paradigm" which provides for a "holistic understanding" of someone in need of care, sets people thinking: Can the limitation and adaptation of the patients' situation to a diagnosis and narrow criteria for assessment not be considered as subtle violence?

Structural and cultural forms of violence as explained in the above definitions by Galtung may be less disputed regarding the interpretation of violence in nursing. The forced subjection of patients within the daily routine of a nursing institution and its symbolic staging was already pointed out by Goffmann (1961) in the sixties. The terms of 'focusing on patients' as well as 'customer service', which apply to those countries where private elements of nursing are significant, therefore describe now new standards for the adaptation of processes in nursing institutions to those they are meant to serve. Structural violence is also discernible where its counter-strategies start to take effect. The call for a larger representation of patients and their rights, which is becoming increasingly effective in many countries, can be regarded as such a kind of counter-strategy. Finally, reflections

19

on structural violence in nursing cannot be separated from certain aspects regarding women in particular: the lack of recognition or even disregard for the female profession of nursing, combined with a lack of adequate payment in many countries and an enormous workload and responsibility, have to be considered as being potential causes for subtle and open violence towards those in need of care. People who do not receive enough good care themselves, will only be able to pass on care in a very limited manner.

The quoted debate in social sciences as well as in the public health sector and nursing seems to recommend to pursue an open and detailed notion of violence. The process of development of violence becomes the focus and the connections and transitions between different forms of violence become clear. It thus becomes possible to also pursue a morally inspired casuistry (Thiersch, 1994). The distinction and the identification of the phenomena which are actually discussed, i.e. the immediate, physically violent act, the verbal humiliation or structural and cultural forms of violence, will make it possible to create precise individual investigation, despite the large range of perspectives.

Violence in Nursing – the Contributions

The present book is a collection of country-specific studies. The analysis of violence in nursing, therefore, takes into consideration various spheres of action in the nursing and health care system. Most contributions to this book can be summarised under the term of "workplace violence" The term, however, is defined somewhat vaguely in the international debate: The most recent press release of the International Council of Nursing (2002) defines workplace violence as violence directed against nurses in the workplace. Powers, however, shows in her contribution (chapter 2), how the term has evolved in the United States since the 1980s. And how the original concept of violence as a physical experience of violence directed against care givers has been defined and redefined to the more general term of workplace violence. Therefore, violence against the recipients of care might also be subsumed under this definition. This would then be an approach explaining the dynamics of the origin and development of violence: Because the consequence of violence against nurses can result in the passing on of violence to the recipients of care, as Hirsch (chapter 6) illustrates in his "triangle of violence" model. As is well-known from non-nursing social settings, victims can more easily turn into perpetrators than persons without the experience of violence. To do justice to the above-mentioned definitions employed by international organisations we have made the subject of violence against nurses a separate section besides the narrower definition of "workplace violence" which will

20

be dicsussed in four chapters (Powers, chapter 2; Taylor, chapter 9; Välimäki et al., chapter 3). The analysis of violence against patients especially refers to the sensitive areas of nursing care where the power and powerlessness of the affected persons create difficult relationships as e.g. in the field of psychiatry (Gallinagh, chapter 7; Richter, chapter 5) and nursing care for the elderly (Hirsch, chapter 6; Gates, chapter 8). Most contributions discuss approaches to prevent violence. The last three chapters of the book, however, predominantly focus on its prevention (Taylor, chapter 9; Noak et al., chapter 10; Sjøgreen et al., chapter 11).

The authors employed their own definition of violence in their research. Correspondingly, the articles reflect various meanings of the concept of violence, although the researchers regarded the physical and mental suffering of the victims an essential part of their definitions. An expanded concept that also includes social and cultural factors is used especially by Hirsch (chapter 6) and implicitly by Noack and Wright (chapter 10), Sjøgreen et al. (chapter 11) and by Powers (chapter 2) who integrates structural and (organisation-oriented) cultural forms of violence in nursing care. Taylor (chapter 9), Uys and Gcaba (chapter 4), Richter (chapter 5) and Välimäki et al. (chapter 3) use a field- and research-oriented qualification of violence.

In the USA, where the academic debate on violence in nursing care is most extensive, a multitude of papers on this subject has been written during the last four years. Lacking comparable country-specific surveys it is difficult to determine if these papers reflect a higher incidence of violent actions resulting in higher sensitivity to the issue or if there are simply more academic resources available. Powers refers in her analysis of workplace violence to the dominant discourse of medicine/epidemiology in nursing care. She argues that by using descriptive statistics that illustrate an "epidemic" in workplace violence, victims – mostly female– are created. A scientific approach following a dominant discourse of medicine/epidemiology produces new experts, channels the flow of money and neutralises the social issues in the process of medicalisation of everyday life. Powers indicates that current research ignores the individual narratives of perpetrators and victims. "Truth" is produced on the basis of quantitative evidence. Her critical comments call for not ignoring the discourse of violence in nursing care. She rather asks to define and reflect on the "speaking positions" for victims and perpetrators, that are recognisable in this discourse, and to make e.g. a conscious choice concerning methodologies in research.

Contrary to the USA, in most European countries both the individual voices having experienced violence in the health care system and knowledge of violence and its consequences are in general fragmentary, as Valimäki et al. (chapter 3) show. Assessing the existence of violence in the Finish health care system they included an illustration of important societal changes that took place during the last years. These changes are also relevant to understand the increase in violence in other countries: shortage of resources in the health care system, enforced changes in the world of employment, enforced mobility resulting in the loss of regional and social relationships. Although some studies conducted in the health care system identify the experience of violence in the workplace as a growing problem, the outlines of this problem, especially considering the violence against the recipients of care, are obviously defined very insufficiently.

The lack of empirical data in Africa was the reason for Uys and Gcaba (chapter 4) to conduct surveys in Nigeria and in South Africa in order to collect data on the forms and the extent of violence in nursing care. Both countries are characterised by considerable societal changes which are met by means of violence, especially in South Africa. As the data show, violence has considerable effect on the provision of nursing care, since e.g. ambulatory care had to be abolished or significantly reduced due to existing dangers. It can be assumed, however, from the results of the interviews that the experience of violence is only marginally more pronounced compared to other countries. However, the authors write that there obviously is a problem, that cannot be solved in the foreseeable future due to lack of resources and other urgent problems.

Richter (chapter 5) presents in his article the violence as experienced by care givers in the psychiatric clinics and its consequences. His surveys in Germany support the results of international studies that indicate a special potential for danger in this area. The daily danger is taken for granted by care givers and management and consistent preventive measures are missing. Assaults inflicted by patients, their triggers and their courses are often not recorded by the nurses, which shows a lack of self image and understanding of their duties on the part of the care givers. Therefore, preventive techniques, de-escalation measures, forms of communication with patients, successful and unsuccessful coping strategies of the care givers cannot be analysed systematically. Correspondingly, research on violence in psychiatric care is not available in Germany apart from a few selective studies.

Hirsch (chapter 6) discusses surveys on violence against the elderly in Germany against the backdrop of a comprehensive model dealing with the emergence and dynamics of violence and including relevant data on the situation in German nursing homes and possibilities to improve the situation. The fact is obvious that an appropriate professional care in nursing homes cannot be guarantied despite an improved financial security of the care recipients granted by the nursing care insurance established in Germany in 1995. There are serious quality problems. The social acceptance of neglecting the elderly, however, is not only in Germany a grave problem but also in other post-industrialised countries. According to Hirsch it is the result of our society collectively warding off old age, physical and mental decline and death.

Gallinaigh (chapter 7) confirms and expands on Hirsch's analysis by investigating a special form of violence in Irish nursing care, namely the practice of restraining the elderly and the consequences thereof. Her research indicates that it is often lack of staff and time that lead to employing restraints but also ignorance on the part of the care givers who regard restraints as a precaution against falling. The care givers do not take into consideration the contrasting evidence that the habitual restraining of patients increases falls. The nurses also document insufficiently and justify the grave measure of restraining which is a further indication that these techniques are used with great self-assurance in daily practice.

Gates (chapter 8) explores the depressing findings gained in gerontological and geriatric nursing, as discussed by Hirsch and Gallinagh, from the point of view of the nurse assistants who present the highest share of nursing staff in the USA and other countries. Nurse Assistants frequently suffer from aggressive and violent acts inflicted by the recipients of care. The reasons for the violence can be found in the daily work realities that Gates integrates into a model describing the genesis and promotion of violence: A growing share of very old persons increasingly afflicted with mental deterioration, insufficient training and social recognition of staff, especially of the nurse assistants, as well as non-existent management-related solutions of the problems result in violence on part of the recipients of care.

The final section of the volume provides a review of preventive measures and solutions to difficult workplace realities. Taylor (chapter 9) evaluates the possibilities to intervene against horizontal forms of violence among the personal in health and nursing care institutions such as bullying or mobbing. Taylor assumes, that shortage of resources and time as well as lacking communication expertise encourage social tensions in the workplace that can put individuals or groups under considerable pressure. The author presents an interaction strategy based on action research enabling the care givers to deal with such problems and to solve them.

Noak and Wright (chapter 10) highlight the strategies coping with violence on the management level, their desired content and their translation into the workplace. Interrupting the circle of violence in health care institutions demands the perception and recognition of the problems on the part of the management as well as the policies to solve such problems. Although their research and conclusions refer to the field of psychiatry, their approach is of general significance: Not only the care givers, but also those responsible for the institutions such as the management have to come to terms with the phenomenon of violence in nursing care and accept their responsibility for the prevention of violence.

In the last chapter Sjøgreen et al. (chapter 11) present as an example the training of staff in psychiatric care institutions to highlight the translation of preventive techniques into the workplace. Originally, this volume was supposed to include case studies from Asia, Latin America and Oceania. The editors did not succeed in their efforts to integrate them in spite of their international contacts. Although it can rightly be assumed, that violence in nursing care plays a role in these regions, the scientific discussion on violence in nursing care, with a focus on country reports, as displayed in this volume, unfortunately remains incomplete.

References

Albrecht, P.-A. and Backe, O. (1990) *Verdeckte Gewalt.* Frankfurt a.M. Suhrkamp.

Alderman, C. (1997) Bullying in the workplace. A survey. *Nursing Standard,* 11(35), 22-24.

American Nurses Association (ANA) (2001) ANA demands stricter violence protection. *Home Health Care Nurse,* 19 (7)449.

Beine, K.-H. (1997) Leben oder Tod. Einstellung zur aktiven Sterbehilfe bei Altenpflegepersonal. *Altenpflegeforum,* 5, 3, 2-9.

Beine, K.-H. (1998) Sehen, Hören, Schweigen. Patiententötungen und aktive Sterbehilfe. Freiburg im Breisgau, Lambertus.

Böhnisch, Lothar (1994) Ist Gewalt männlich? *In:* Thiersch, H., Wertheimer, J. and Grunwald, Kl. (Ed) *"...Überall in den Köpfen und Fäusten." Auf der Suche nach Ursachen und Konsequenzen von Gewalt.* Darmstadt, WBG S.103-113.

Bray, C. (2001) Bullying nurses at work: Theorizing a gendered perspective. *Contempory Nurse,* 10(1-2), 21-29.

Chappell, D. and di Martino, V. (2000) *Violence at work.* (second edition. Genf, International Labour Organisation.

Cusack, S. (2000) Workplace bullying: Icebergs in sight, soundings needed. *Lancet,* 356(9248),2118.

Davidzhar, R. and Giger, J.N. (2002) Domestic violence. *Journal Practical Nursing,* 52(1), 18-22

Davis, R.E. (2001) Confronting barriers to unviersal screening for domestic violence. *Journal of Professional Nursing,* 17(6)313-320

Duncan, S.M., Hyndman, K., Estabrooks, C.A. et al. (2001) Nurses' experience of violence in Alberta and British Columbia Hospitals. *Canadian Jorurnal of Nursing Research,* 32(4),57-78.

Elias, N. (1969) *Über den Prozess der Zivilisation.* Köln

Elwert, G., Feuchtwang, S., Neubert, D. (ed) The Dynamics of Collective Violence – an Introduction. In: Sociologicus, Supplement 1: *Dynamics of Violence.*

Faulseit, A., Müller, K., Ohms, C. & Soine, S. (2001) Anregungen zur Entwicklung eines lesbisch-feministischen Gewaltbegriffs als Grundlage für politisches Handeln. *Sozialwissenschaftliche Forschung und Praxis für Frauen e.V.*, 56/57, 13-30.

Foucault, M. (1977) *Discipline and punsih: The birth of the prison.* Berkely. Random House

Foucualt, M. (1988) *Die Geburt der Klinik. Eine Archäologie des ärztlichen Blickes.* Frankfurt, Suhrkamp.

Foucault, M. (1982) The subject and the power. *Critical inquiry,* 8, 777-795.

Galtung, J. (1975) *Strukturelle Gewalt.* Rohwolt, Reinbek.

Goffman, E. (1961): *Asylums: Essays on the Social Situations of Mental Patients and Other Inmates.* Anchor, Garden City, N.Y.

Hall, P. (1996) Alleged role of medical personnel in genocide in Rwanda. *Lancet,* North America Ed., 347(9010), 1265.

International Council of Nursing (ICN) (1999) Violence a world-wide epidemic. Available: http://www.icn.ch/matters_violence.htm.

International Council of Nursing (ICN) (2001) Increasing violence in the workplace is a thread to nursing and the delivery of health care. Press release. Available: http://www.icn.ch/prviolence_99.htm.

International Council of Nursing (ICN) (2000) Position Statement. Abuse and violence against nursing personnel. Available: http://www.icn.chpsviolence 00.htm.

International Council of Nursing (ICN) (2002) New research shows workplace violence threatens health services worldwide. Press release, Geneve. Available: http://www.icn.ch/pr10_02.htm.

International Labour organisation (1999) Violence against women in the world of work (Gender and Work Series, No. 1). Geneva.

Englander, E.(1997) *Understanding Violence.* Lawrence Erlbaum Associates, Baltimore.

Kinard, J. and Little, B. (2002) Sexual harrassment in the health care industry: a follow-up inquiry. *Health Care Management,* 20(4), 46-52.

Kingma, M. (2001) Workplace violence in the health sector: a problem of epidemic proportion. *International Nursing Review,* 48(3), 129-130

Kinkelbuhr, W. (2000) Sozialformen der Gewalt. In: Mader, G., Eberwein, W.-D. and Vogt, W.R. (eds): Konflikt und Gewalt. Münster, Agenda Verlag.

Madison, J. (1997) Australien registered nurses describe the health care workplace and its responsiveness to sexual harrassment: An empirical study. *Australien Health Review*, 20(2),102-115.

Madison, J. and Minichiello V. 2000 Recognizing and labeling sex-based and sexual harrassment in the health care workplace. *Journal of Nursing Scholarship*, 32 (4), 405-410.

Merrell, J. (2001) Social support for victims of domestic violence. *Journal of Psychosocial Nursing and Mental Health Services*,39(11), 46-47.

Morgan, S. (2001) The problems of aggression and violence for health care staff. *Professional Nurse*, 17(2), 107-108, 110.

Neidhardt, F. (1986) *Gewalt. Soziale Bedeutung und sozialwissenschaftliche Bestimmung des Begriffes.* Bundeskriminalamt, Bd.1 Wiesbaden.

Parse, R.R. (1987) *Nursing Science: Major paradigms, theories and critiques.* Philadelphia, Saunders.

Parse, R.R. (1990) Human becoming: Parses's theory of nursing. *Nursing Science Quaterly*, 5, 136-140.

Payne, D. (2000) Accountability. Psychotic nurse went on to kill. *Nursing times*, 96(29), 8.

Popitz, H. (1992) second edition *Phänomene der Macht.* Tübingen, J.C.B. Mohr.

Quine, L. (1999) Workplace bullying in NHS community trust: staff questionnaire survey. BMJ, 23,318 (7178): 228-232.

Rippon, T. (2000) Aggression and violence in health care professions. *Journal of Advanced Nursing*, 31(2), 452-460.

Robinson, R.K. (1993) Sexual harrassment at work: issues and answers for health and care administrators. Hospital Health Service 38(2), 167-180.

Sauter, D. and Richter, D. (eds.) (1998) *Gewalt in der psychiatrischen Pflege.* Huber, Bern.

Schiffhorst, G. and Hirsch R.D. (1999) Zur Meßbarkeit von "Gewalt". In: Hirsch, R.D., Kranzhoff, E.U. and Schiffhorst, G. (eds) *Untersuchungen zur Gewalt gegen alte Menschen.* Bonner Schriftenreihe "Gewalt im Alter", Vol 2.

Squire, V. (2001) What about our rights?...Violence sparks calls for action. *Australien Nursing Journal*, 9(4),3.

Thiersch, Hans Gewalt (1994) Bemerkungen zur gegenwärtigen Diskussion. *In:* Thiersch, H., Wertheimer, J. and Grunwald, Kl. (ed) *"...Überall in den Köpfen und Fäusten." Auf der Suche nach Ursachen und Konsequenzen von Gewalt.* Darmstadt: WBG, S.1-22.

Trotha von, T. (1997) Zur Soziologie der Gewalt. *In:* Trotha, von T. (ed) *Soziologie und Gewalt.* Sonderheft 37 Kölner Zeitschrift für Soziologie und Sozialpsychologie, 9-59.

26

Varcoe, C. (2001) Abuse obscured: an ethnographic account of emergency nursing in relation to violence against women. *Canadian Journal of Nursing Research*, 32(4), 95-115.

Vartia, M.A. (2001) Consquences of workplace bullying with respect to the well-being of its targets and the observers of bullying. *Scandinavian Journal of Work Environment and Health*, 27(1), 63-69.

World Health Organisation (1996) Prevention of Violence. Resolution of the 49th World Health Assembly (WHA49.25) Genf.

World Health Organisation (2000) Violence and Health. Proceedings of a WHO global symposium in Kobe, Japan. WHO Genf.

World Health Organsiation (2002) Report on global reserach. In preparation. Available:http://www5.who.int/violence_injury_prevention/main.cfm?p=0000 000585.

Chapter Two: Workplace Violence in U.S. Nursing Literature – A Discourse Analysis

Penny Powers

Introduction

This chapter is an analysis of the written discourse of workplace violence in nursing literature in the United States. Discourse analysis is a philosophical approach to the analysis of situated text in the tradition of critical social theory and post-modern feminism (Gavey, 1997; Gray, 1999; Hinshaw et al., 1999; McNay, 1992). Discourse is defined as a systematic integrated body of knowledge that can include one or more of the following: text, images, social structures, spoken language and behaviour. A discourse may be very large and widely known, such as the text of speeches at the United Nations. On the other hand, a discourse may be small, specialised, and clearly circumscribed, such as the discourse on pseudo-scalar mesons in physics. There is no single unity to a discourse. Instead, discourses (also called discursive fields) can be shown to demonstrate the influence of competing discourses, each with its own history, context and power relations. These discourses, in turn, could also be analysed as discursive fields composed of co-existing and competing discourses.

For example, in an analysis of the discourse on AIDS in sub-Saharan Africa, Seidel (1993) identified six discourses that have contrasting accounts, different histories, different paradigms, different power relations, differential access to public policy and funding, and different outcomes (p. 176). Seidel argued that oppression is created as an unintended consequence of two of these discourses, the medical and the medico-moral. It is the task of the discourse analyst to produce well-supported claims regarding the existence of dominant and resistance discourses and the power relations that they support, reproduce and resist.

Discourses are products of the time and the context in which they are situated (Cheek, 1997). In fact, it has been argued that statements about experiences should not be regarded merely as objective accounts, or even subjective reports, but as performances in a rhetorical context that reproduce situated power relationships (Allen, 1999). A discourse analysis seeks to describe a specific situated discourse and the power relations in context.

Discourse analysis produces interpretive claims that are based on a description of the power relations in a situated discourse. Discourse analysis shares with post-modern feminism the critique of post-positivist epistemologies, seeking to produce transformations in everyday life with regard to conditions of oppression. In the post-colonial world, where repeating diasporas have created hyphenated identities in the U.S. (Hispanic-American, Japanese-American) and complex power relations, the project of discourse analysis also shares with interpretive ethnography the notion of a gendered moral politics of action (Denzin, 1997, p. xv).

Discourse analysis differs from other traditions of content or narrative analysis such as semiotics and ethno-methodology in that discourse analysis emphasises the power inherent in situated social relations (Lupton, 1992). There are, at present, different versions of the method of discourse analysis because the application to diverse disciplines has so far prevented a coherent perspective (Cheek and Rudge, 1994). This discourse analysis follows the method described by Powers (1999). As a method of inquiry, discourse analysis has much to offer to nursing (Cheek and Rudge, 1994).

Nursing, being a genderised discourse (and, according to Valentine (1996) therefore "ghetto-ised") contains many discourses suitable for analysis because the target of dominant patriarchal discourses such as medicine is often the female body (McNay, 1992; Ussher, 2000). A discourse analysis provides situated evidence for actual or potential oppression of groups of people (Powers, 1999). No claim is made for generalisable truth and it is acknowledged that other, competing claims may be equally useful in provoking the transformation of oppressive conditions. Discourse analysis draws from the post-modern emphasis on language in the reproduction of power relations (Fairclough, 1995). "Those who have the power to regulate what counts as truth are able to maintain their access to material advantages and power." (Gavey, 1997, p. 52).

The evidence for the claims of a discourse analysis is organised into the following categories: a) the history of the discourse is documented in a genealogy, b) the system of knowledge is described in a structural analysis, and c) the power relations are analysed in a power analytic (Powers, 1999). The discourse in this case, the target of this analysis, is the discourse of workplace violence in the U.S. nursing literature.

In 1999, a survey by the Colorado Nurses Association of nurses in seven states found that 32% of the respondents said they had been victims of workplace violence (Carroll, 1999). "The risk for patient violence against nurses is still vastly underestimated." (Nield-Anderson et al., 1999). Under reporting is also a problem in England. A 1999 Nursing Times survey of 1,000 nurses in England found that 50% had been physically assaulted in the past year and 85% has been verbally abused (Downer, 1999).

For this analysis, the entire discourse on workplace violence in the U.S. nursing literature was analysed. No interviews were conducted and no visits were made.

Genealogy

The first of the three parts of a discourse analysis, the genealogy, presents the historical context of the construction of the discourse, including how the discourse came to be produced, whose interests were furthered by the development of the discourse, whose interests were ignored, what power struggles occurred during the development of the discourse, and what words in the discourse have a significant social history.

Nurses and others, such as police officers, have always lived with violence and aggression in their daily work. Violence from co-workers, psychotic patients, febrile patients, demented patients, visitors, physicians, etc., has always been present in the work of nursing. The act of one or more persons harming one or more other persons has historically been dealt with by the criminal justice system. The crime of assault has a long history in any country. The discursive origin of the need for another legal term to refer to assault that occurs in the workplace is not entirely clear. What is clear is that the social definition of assault has changed over the years.

Historically, assault was not reported or prosecuted as a crime when it happened to women and children where the perpetrator was a husband or father. The idea of women and children as personal property instead of human beings with rights equal to men had to change before an assault on a woman was regarded as anything other than discipline properly being administered by a man. In certain countries in the world today, for example, a woman who has been raped can expect to be killed by a male member of her family because of the disgrace. This act is not considered homicide. The recognition of assault against nurses as something other than an expected part of daily work did not occur until U.S. attitudes with regard to assault against women in general had changed.

Nursing in general is a genderised discourse and therefore the discourse of workplace violence against nurses became co-mingled with the discourse of assault against women. The genealogy of the discourse of workplace violence in nursing is difficult to untangle from the genealogy of the discourse on gender-motivated violence. Because of the power relations inherent in this discourse, workplace violence in nursing is a good candidate for a discourse analysis.

Statistics regarding homicides are routinely studied by the disciplines of occupational health, occupational medicine, public health and industrial medicine.

31

Before the term workplace violence was used, the terms occupational homicide, occupational violent crime, murder at work and fatal occupational injuries were used. The term occupational violence is still used in the occupational health literature (Findorff-Dennis et al., 1999).

The term, "workplace violence" is a relatively new phrase that came from the discipline of law and from mass media into government and the business world. The earliest reference to workplace violence was found in an editorial in the law journal *Trial* in 1988, where it was reported that "workplace violence" was increasing (Workplace violence a growing problem, 1988). An article in the journal *Security Management* in 1991 referred to workplace violence as a problem for security managers (Franklin, 1991).

OSHA provided an interpretation of the Occupational Safety and Health Act of 1970 in May 1992, stating that an employer could be cited under the general duty clause for failing to adequately protect its workers from acts of violence in the workplace (OSHA, 1992). Under this interpretation, OSHA compliance officers could penalise employers who allow assaults or opportunities for violence to persist. In 1994, the insurance firm of Cigna offered a rider for the Accidental Death and Dismemberment policies offered to corporations that included workplace violence (Koco, 1994).

Incidents reported in the mass media in 1994 were described as "workplace violence" (Gest, Wilkin, Hetter and Wright, 1994; Toufexis, 1994). Mantel and Albrecht (1994) quote a Pinkerton Security Service survey regarding the top concerns of business. In 1992, workplace violence was not mentioned as a concern by those surveyed. In 1994, however, workplace violence was in sixth place among the list of top ten concerns (p. 2).

The definition of workplace violence has changed over its short career. In 1993, the National Institute for Occupational Safety and Health (NIOSH) issued an alarm regarding the rising incidence of what was called "homicide in the workplace" which was also reported as "workplace-murder" among commentators (Castelli, 1993). Later, in 1996, NIOSH expanded its definition of workplace violence to include non-fatal injuries. In the 1996 report, NIOSH used a working definition of workplace violence as "physical assaults and threats of assaults, directed toward people at work or on duty" (NIOSH, 1996).

Before the 1996 NIOSH report, separate statistics for "fatal occupational injuries" and "non-fatal assaults" were kept by the Bureau of Justice and by the Bureau of Labour respectively (NIOSH, 1996). The NIOSH report of 1996 compiled both of these sets of statistics and reported them both under the name of workplace violence. In July 1998, the Department of Justice released a special report called "Workplace Violence, 1992-96" based on a redesign of the survey which had been used up until 1992 (U.S. Department of Justice, 1998). This special report took into account both fatal and non-fatal injuries.

In 1994, an article in the Wall Street Journal called workplace violence a "false crisis" (Larson, 1994) stating that the numbers of incidents were so infrequent as to be negligible. Various authors have discussed the expansion of the definition from murder in the workplace perpetrated by a co-worker to any kind of crime, perpetrated by any kind of person, from co-worker to stranger, during a robbery, during work hours, on the way to and from, or related to work in any way. Podolak (2000) argues that these expanded definitions of workplace violence have been caused by mass media coverage and have been used by others to advance their own treatment, prevention, legal, and insurance corporate ventures. Certainly the absence of a consistent definition over time complicates the comparison of figures from year to year without careful scrutiny of definitions (Myers, 1996). Definition and redefinition are discursive acts and therefore, moves of power. In this case, careers are being fostered by defining and redefining workplace violence. Redefinition has thereby created a discourse, a realm of power/knowledge, that has been addressed by many different disciplines including nursing.

In December 1994, the American Journal of Nursing published a news item to report that emergency room nurses were calling on state legislatures to pass laws to stop the rising violence against emergency room nurses (American Journal of Nursing, 1994). A bill introduced into the California State Legislature by the California Emergency Nurses Association was passed into law and took effect in January 1995. This law initiates mandatory reporting of acts of violence against health care professionals. In 1999, the State of Washington passed a bill requiring all health care facilities to report all incidents of workplace violence and to develop and implement a plan to protect employees (Washington Nurse, 1999).

In the context of the development of the discourse of workplace violence in nursing, it is important to note that in 1994 the U.S. Congress enacted the Violence Against Women Act regarding the crimes of domestic violence, sexual assault, and stalking. These crimes were named, described and penalties were prescribed. Since this law was enacted, the Department of Justice has awarded more than $ 800,000,000 through grant programs established under this Act to support efforts involving community-based social services, prosecutors, judges, victims, health care professionals, educators, religious groups and police departments.

The Violence Against Women Act created new federal criminal offences for violent acts against women and strengthened the penalties for existing crimes. It provided for civil remedies for the victims of gender-motivated violence, enabling them to bring a civil suit for damages against their attackers in either state or federal court. This legislation established a national advisory council to im-

33

plement the new law and create an awareness of the crimes of sexual assault and domestic violence. The National Advisory Council on Violence Against Women was created in 1995 and was chaired by Secretary of Health and Human Services Donna E. Shalala and Attorney General Janet Reno. In addition, the council included more than forty experts in the fields of domestic violence and sexual assault appointed by the President, including health care professionals, survivors, and representatives from religious groups, education, sports, the corporate world, media, and research. In the year 2000, the Council was expected to release an Agenda for the Nation on Violence Against Women to present specific strategies for ending gender-based acts of violence.

In the year 2000, however, the U.S. Supreme Court declared the Violence Against Women Act unconstitutional in Brzonkala v. Morrison (Dolan, 2000). It is not yet clear what effect this ruling will have on legal cases that attempt to hold the employer responsible for gender-motivated violence against women in the workplace, including nurses. It seems that the courts are moving away from defining crimes against women as something different from crimes against men. The social discourse on gender-motivated violence continues, however.

In the development of the discourse in nursing, workplace violence has been defined in the expanded sense, including non-fatal injuries as well as homicides. In the 1980's workplace violence in nursing was called assault, violent behaviour, the violent patient, aggression, crime, disruptive behaviour, homicides, verbal abuse, threats and occupational hazards. It has been defined as verbal abuse (including verbal threats), sexual assaults, harassment and physical violence (Carroll and Goldsmith, 1999) and as a range of behaviors from offensive language to homicide (Summers, 1999). Workplace violence has been defined to include violence from co-workers, patients, and outsiders, such as attacks on abortion clinics (Hampshire, 1999). The terms "workplace violence" and "workplace abuse" have been used interchangeably in the nursing literature (Carroll and Goldsmith, 1999). The International Council of Nurses defines workplace violence in the most expanded manner possible, "Being destructive towards another person." (ICN, 1993).

It is significant that no single definition of workplace violence in the U.S. nursing literature was found that defined workplace violence against nurses as gender-motivated violence. Motivation is a difficult concept to measure. This analysis argues that a strong resistance discourse in the U.S. nursing literature on workplace violence is a feminist view of workplace violence as gender-motivated violence against women.

In the previously mentioned 1998 report of the U.S. Department of Justice (1998), 24.8 per 1,000 nurses were reported as being victims of workplace violence. The report also noted that male victims were more likely to report the crime to the police than were female victims. The report did not give any explanation for this notation.

In 1999, the Joint Commission on Accreditation of Healthcare Organisations released the fifth product in the Commission's Computer-based Competency Training Series, on Security and Workplace Violence. Also in 1999, the American Nurses' Association (ANA) House of Delegates (June 17-20, in Washington, D.C.) called for legislation and regulations to ensure safer working conditions for nurses. The ANA has two statements with regard to workplace violence. The ANA states that nurses have the right to reject assignments that put themselves or patients in "serious or immediate jeopardy" (ANA, 1994) (The ANA also recognises that nurses have the right to weigh the risk of personal harm against the ethical obligation of care in their practice and to take action to protect themselves (ANA,1995).

This genealogy has described the developmental context of the discourse of workplace violence. It is clear that the interests of certain groups have benefited by the development of this discourse. Lawyers benefit from being able to prosecute and defend new infractions. Mass media has a new category of story to report. Consultants and institutes have benefited by being able to provide consultation regarding workplace violence prevention programs, debriefing services, and security measures (see: http://noworkviolence.com/). Academics have benefited by the description of a new field of power/ knowledge in which to perform research and pronounce truth. Certainly not least of all, the description of workplace violence has provided victims a speaking position, a way of discussing the incident that people can understand as a specific incidence of a category of events that happen at work. It is socially acceptable to speak about workplace violence in nursing.

The only power struggles involved in the development of the discourse of workplace violence seem to have been the disagreement over the definition of the phenomenon and the extent of the problem. The expanded definition that includes both fatal and non-fatal injuries has prevailed in business, government, and nursing. The question of whether or not victims of the violence have benefited by the discourse will be addressed in the power analytic.

It is not clear whether the interests of perpetrators are furthered. The voice of the perpetrator is represented only in interviews and case studies where it is used to determine a typical case that can be viewed as representative. The purpose of studying perpetrators is to be able to predict further events and therefore prevent them. The purpose is of studying perpetrators is not meant to benefit them individually through treatment, but to prevent other possible perpetrators (who are assumed to be similar in some way to the ones being studied) from committing the same acts.

Structural Analysis

The second of the three parts of a discourse analysis is the structural analysis. In this section, claims are made regarding how the discourse presently functions. The claims are grouped in the following three categories: 1) the axis of knowledge, 2) the axis of authority, and 3) the axis of value or justification.

The Axis of Knowledge

The axis of knowledge addresses the objects, subjects and processes of the discourse; the rules of evidence, the rules for the application of the discourse and the order that governs the appearance, disappearance, multiplicity, diversity, and styles of statements, theoretical strategies and concepts in the discourse.

The objects of the discourse of workplace violence in nursing are incidents that can and do happen to nurses while on duty. The objects are assumed to have a pre-interpreted reality in an objectively real world. The discourse produces its subjects from the objects by naming and defining these incidents as cases of workplace violence. The discourse of workplace violence in nursing defines these incidents in order to control the incidents within the discursive field of nursing in the same way that the discourse of workplace violence in business defines the incidents in order to control them within the discursive field of business. Defining a new category of events creates a body of knowledge that serves to enhance the power and influence of some groups over others. This is to say that new "turf" is created for some discipline to study, publish, control, and claim expertise sufficient to pronounce truth based on amassing agreed-upon types of evidence. This kind of totalising narrative focuses attention on the generalised perpetrator-as-example and nurse-as-victim, and not on social conditions surrounding the event or the discursive action used to study the event(s).

In this case, nursing has chosen to adopt the same discursive language used by business and government used to call the incidents workplace violence. Significantly, nursing has chosen not to follow the discourse of law and crime to determine the processes used by the discourse to manipulate the subjects. Business and government, including human relations, security and insurance interests, have chosen to use the discourse of law and crime to determine the strategies and styles of statements in their body of knowledge.

Nursing has chosen the dominant discourse of medicine/epidemiology to determine the rules of evidence, the styles of statements and the theoretical strategies of the discourse. This means that the discourse describes these incidents not in terms of criminal activity to be prosecuted in a legal manner, but in terms of an epidemic that needs to be researched and controlled in a scientific manner by eliminating the causes of workplace violence, treating the victims, and preventing further incidents. The goal of the discourse of workplace violence in nursing and in business is to reduce the number of incidents because of the loss of productivity among employees and the financial cost of these incidents to the institution.

The words in the nursing discourse follow the model (the dominant discourse) being used to describe and define what is happening. The significant words therefore include risk factors, causes, incidence, prevalence, spread, epidemic, public health problem, victims, sequelae, and prevention. For example, a news item in the journal *Safety and Health* in 1994 was titled, "On-the-job violence becomes 'epidemic'" (On-the-job violence becomes 'epidemic', 1994). It is important to emphasise that discourses are not "chosen" in a deliberate sense to structure a discursive field. The dominant discourse may emerge from many possible ways to think about, discuss, and otherwise perform or reproduce the discursive event in context. An unconscious consensus, probably reached through repetitive efforts of many people or groups, results in one or more dominant discourses accompanied by one or more resistance discourses.

The rules of evidence in the discourse of workplace violence in nursing follow the dominant discourse of medicine/epidemiology. Scientifically gathered knowledge with regard to the causes, incidence, prevalence, risk factors, etc. of the incidents is analysed to produce prevention and treatment strategies. The goal is phrased in the scientific language of prediction, control and prevention.

Theoretical strategies and styles of statements are also modelled on the discourse of medicine/epidemiology. Whereas the discourse of law focuses on punishment after the incident, the discourse of medicine/epidemiology focuses on prediction and prevention before the incident. The trade-off for society can be stated using the language of research. One disadvantage of focusing on prosecuting offenders is the risk of Type II error. That is, the risk is of not being able to identify offenders even when evidence to that effect exists before the crime happens. The disadvantage of prediction and prevention strategies is misidentifying people as possible perpetrators before the act, when they really are not – Type I error. The literature is clear that there is no definitive "profile" of a possible perpetrator in an incident of workplace violence.

The Axis of Authority

The axis of authority addresses the rules for who is and is not allowed to speak, what they can say and cannot say, and the systems for education, association and advancement. In the discourse of workplace violence in nursing, there is no for-

37

mal organisation that requires dues or membership, and no degree or certificate program in workplace violence. There are researchers who choose to publish on workplace violence in nursing (such as Caroll, Carmel, Cox, Hunter, Lanza, Morrison, Ryan, and Simonowitz) and there is the "Workplace Violence Prevention Reporter" journal published by James Publishing in Santa Ana, California . No one would publish about workplace violence in nursing without consulting the work of these authors, so there are some experts in the field whose voices are strong.

There are policy statements by ANA, ICN and various state, national and provincial nursing organisations. There are institutes devoted to the investigation of issues in workplace violence and counsellors who specialise in treating victims of workplace violence and other employees. There are consultants who charge fees to businesses and corporations to help them put security measures into place. Business insurance companies and lawyers can specialize in workplace violence issues.

There are other voices outside of the academic publications, institutes and policy statements. There are websites specifically devoted to workplace violence in nursing in the U.S. and in other countries. The main site in the U.S. (www.nurseadvocate.org) is maintained by Carrie Lybecker and has an extensive bibliography, links to national and international sites; links to books and articles; and contains an excellent list of definitions of workplace violence from many sources. The site contains the stories of individual nurses and posts news items from all over the world. This site lists books on workplace violence in general, workplace violence in nursing, and also violence against women in general.

In this website we can see the association made between workplace violence against nurses and violence against women. The resistance discourse of feminism is strong here and the implication is clear that violence against a nurse is a case of violence against women in general and implies that we should think and act with that understanding.

In the discourse on workplace violence in nursing, speakers include researchers, managers, institutional representatives such as human relations directors, and victims. The voice of the perpetrator is present only in case studies.

The Axis of Value or Justification

The axis of value or justification addresses how the discourse justifies its power, knowledge and technologies. The discourse of workplace violence in nursing justifies its power to define and pronounce truth by using the dominant discourse of medicine/epidemiology. This makes it appropriate to cite descriptive statistics that demonstrate the "epidemic" of workplace in violence in nursing and that the number of incidents is increasing. This creates "victims" that need "treatment" and organisations that need policies, insurance and in-services.

The discourse justifies its power/knowledge by using the processes called the medicalisation and clinicalisation of everyday life. Social and moral "issues" become defined as medical "problems" so that a scientific model can be used to describe and control the outcomes. In 1996, NIOSH clearly advocated this position, saying "We must also change the way we think about workplace violence by shifting the emphasis from reactionary approaches to prevention, and by embracing workplace violence as an occupational safety and health issue." (NIOSH, 1996, p. 1) The discourse can then expand its influence, receives money to perform the function and the general public can feel assured that the problems are being dealt with in clinical research settings using scientific methods. Subsequently, those employees determined to be outside the normal range of behaviour can be identified and targeted with normalising strategies designed to uphold the status quo of power relations and prevent incidents of workplace violence from happening. Public discussions of moral issues and social context are thus avoided.

Power Analysis

The third part of the discourse analysis, the power analytic, identifies the dominant and resistance discourses and their effects on groups of people. The power analytic focuses on the following questions: whose interests are furthered by the continuation of the discourse? What dominations are established, perpetuated or eliminated and is there evidence for the co-optation of other discourses?

Dominant Discourse

The dominant discourse is medical/epidemiology and not legal. Words like "incidence", "prevalence", "widespread", "victims", "public health problem," "risk factors" and "high risk occupations" are used to describe workplace violence in nursing (Findorff-Dennis et al, 1999). The word "victim" is used in both the legal discourse (as in "victim of a crime") and in medicine/epidemiology (as in "victim of a disease"). Health care workers are spoken of as among the occupations at "high risk" for workplace violence. Retail sales people have the highest risk, followed by police officers and security guards, taxi drivers, prison guards, bartenders, and mental health professionals. Nurses are not in the top 16 occupations unless they are in mental health (OSHA, 1999). Most of the research on workplace violence in nursing has been performed in psychiatric facilities, and secondly in the emergency room.

The dominant discourse of medicine/epidemiology is also demonstrated by the choice of using post-traumatic stress disorder (PTSD) to describe the "sequelae" of workplace violence. These sequelae include depression, chronic pain, behaviour changes, job loss, increased chemical use and sleep disturbances (Findorff-Dennis, et al, 1999). Researchers investigate post-traumatic stress syndrome and other "sequelae" of the event in some cases in order to be able to quantify the monetary damages and result in the justification of higher claims for the victims. The discourse does not emphasise prosecution of offenders or describe the events in terms of crime.

The purpose of focusing on how much money these incidents cost the facilities (Mitiguy, 1999) and how to reduce such expenditures is to generate interest in prevention. Events that cost facilities in terms of lost productivity; sales, etc. are possible revenue sources for individuals and groups who contract to reduce such losses. Hospitals implement systems to help prevent workplace violence, including special security systems (Freeman, 1999).

The dominant discourse of medicine/epidemiology is also demonstrated by research regarding characteristics of nurses that are associated with workplace violence. These include adoption of authoritarian attitudes, failing to involve the medical staff in an incident, poor communication skills, incompetence, job dissatisfaction and less than ten years' experience (Nolan et al., 1999). Other predictors of violence in perpetrators include: people with a history of violence, a stressful environment, male gender, drugs, youth, head trauma, low socioeconomic status, and cognitive impairment (Durkin and Wilson, 1999). Other researchers, however, argue that there are no pre-disposing factors among perpetrators and no consistent profile for a violent patient (Whittington and Wykes, 1994; Nield-Anderson et al., 1999).

Resistance Discourses

Discourses are multiple and offer competing ways of constructing knowledge, sometimes called subject positions, for people to identify with and use (consciously or unconsciously) as a way of enacting or embodying or performing meaning in a situation (Gavey, 1997, p. 54). Dominant discourses and resistance discourses co-exist and serve to constitute each other. In a shifting web of influence over time and in context, dominance may be consolidated by various means or may lose influence as more people choose to enact another subject position for various reasons.

In the case of the discourse of workplace violence in nursing, there seem to be two resistance discourses. The first resistance discourse is the feminist discourse of power and oppression. Instead of describing workplace violence as an epidemic with certain criteria, profiles, risk factors, associated characteristics of the victims, etc., this discourse describes workplace violence in terms of continuing male violence against women.

The resistance discourse of feminism is less strong in the academic publications where the discourse of medicine/epidemiology is strongest. The resistance discourse is stronger in the more informal writings and on websites, and stronger among victims than among researchers. In this resistance discourse, the events of workplace violence are spoken of as examples of gender-motivated violence against women. The voice of male nurses is absent in this resistance discourse.

In the dominant discourse of medicine/epidemiology, nurses are blamed for causing or provoking the assault by research that identifies characteristics of nurses involved in a violent incident. Nurses are warned that condescending attitudes and "rude or bossy" behavior "provokes" patient violence (McHale, 1999). The resistance discourse of feminism responds to some of these identified risk factors for workplace violence among nurses. So-called "domineering" behaviour of (female) nurses is claimed to contribute to triggering the violence. The speaking position of feminism points out that the wording of such claims is similar to the wording that is used to blame women for the crime of rape because they wore "provocative clothing" or behaved in a "sexually provocative manner". Another similarity between the discourse on workplace violence in nursing and the discourse on rape, is that nurses who experience workplace violence often blame themselves for the assault. Lanza (1999) uses catastrophe theory to explain why nurses blame themselves in mild assault cases and why female victims are blamed for the attack more than male victims.

In the feminist discourse of resistance, the statistics regarding under-reporting are highlighted. The discourse seeks to de-bunk myths such as "It would not occur to me" "There's nothing I can do." "Once a violent episode begins, I'm sunk." and "Take cover during a violent incident." (Stewart-Amidei, 1999). The purpose is to provide empowering strategies for women through the provision of a speaking position that defines these events as examples of oppression.

To the extent that the discourse of feminism encourages speaking up, and not blaming self, the strategy supports women. Home health nurses are reminded not to stay in a house when violence is occurring or when a patient will not put a gun away (Durkin and Wilson, 1999). Self defence classes for home health nurses have also been recommended (Durkin and Wilson, 1999).

41

To the extent that the feminist discourse creates a victim mentality among nurses, however, it supports a view of "otherness" that separates a woman's experience of workplace violence from a man's experience. This discourse also discourages thinking about the incident as assault or homicide. Instead, the incident is described as an example of women's oppression. The response to an incident thus described is social action and legal action.

The second resistance discourse is that of law. Violence against anyone is a crime, but nurses often "excuse" workplace violence when the patient is mentally ill, or delirious, or in pain or otherwise out of control. Some nurses want to exclude these types of assault from the definition of workplace violence. It has been argued that nurses have learned to produce documentation that causes nurses and the work of nursing to disappear into the text, thereby becoming invisible (Heartfield, 1996). The resistance discourse of law is very limited in the discourse of workplace violence in U.S. nursing and confined mainly to discussion of laws to be used to prevent incidents of workplace violence and laws mandating the reporting of incidents of workplace violence.

Whose interests are supported by the continuation of this discourse? Researchers can continue to study the subject, health care facilities can use the results to educated employees on methods to prevent violence, and victims can continue to receive support from people who specialise in treatment of the ongoing after-effects of the incidents.

Other people who benefit from the continuation and expansion of this discourse are people who create consulting corporations with regard to the prevention, treatment, insurance, and legal aspects of workplace violence. Recommendations in research studies include strong leadership, documentation and system requirements, support groups, de-briefing sessions, task forces, staff training, mandatory reporting and changes in individual nurses. Follow-up after violent events is always cited as crucial to the well-being of the organisation. The interests of perpetrators are ignored except as sources of clues for the creation of prevention strategies.

The domination of research discourse over personal experience discourse is perpetuated by the dominance of the discourse of medicine/epidemiology. Research deals with abstraction and generalisable statements. The resistance discourse of feminism deals with personal experience as evidence for oppression of women.

The discourse of workplace violence has co-opted other discourses by combining the study of statistics from several sources under one concept. This redefinition of workplace violence combined fatal and non-fatal injuries at work with incidents of assault and verbal abuse and degradation.

Conclusions

It is the claim of this analysis that the discourse of workplace violence in U.S. nursing literature provides two speaking positions for nurses. The dominant discourse is that of medicine/epidemiology. This discourse uses research language and methods to create categories of experience and generate strategies of control by prevention and treatment. There is evidence that the discourse of medicine/epidemiology perpetuates the oppression of female nurses by naming their own behaviour as a risk factor and producing self-blame. The dominant discourse ignores the experience of individual nurses in favour of totalising general narratives. The interests of researchers and entrepreneurs benefit from this discourse in that they are able to regulate what counts as truth. There is no input of voices from individual nurses or perpetrators except as self-confessing research subjects.

There are two resistance discourses. The strongest is that of feminism. In this discourse, nurses are given a way to talk about personal oppression in the workplace that includes verbal and physical abuse as well as assault and homicide. The discourse of feminism supports a victim mentality with regard to the incidents that encourages an "other" speaking position for nurses. This speaking position shifts the definition of the incident from the crime of assault or homicide to a case of gender-motivated violence that further enfeebles the position of the nurse as an oppressed female. The voice of the male nurse is absent in this discourse.

Implications

Understanding the power relations in a discourse enables participants and observers to choose to reproduce or resist the discourse. As a tool for empowerment, discourse analysis encourages discussion regarding the advantages and disadvantages of the selection of speaking positions. Other analyses are welcomed and discussion should be stimulated. Further analyses on related discourses would expand our understanding of the power relations in nursing and the potential for empowerment and oppression.

References and Bibliography

Alspach, G. (1993) Nurses as victims of violence. *Critical Care Nurse*, 13 (5), 13-17.

American Journal of Nursing (1994) ED nurses enlisting legislatures against rising workplace violence. Newsline, *American Journal of Nursing*, 94(12), 61, 65.

Anderson, L. N. and Clarke, J. T. (1996) De-escalating verbal aggression in primary caresettings. *Nurse Practitioner*, 21(10), 95, 98, 101-2.

American Nurses Association (ANA) (1994) *Position Statement: Risk vs. Responsibility in Providing Nursing Care*. [Online] Available: http://www.nursingworld.org/readroom/position/ethics/etrisk.htm (accessed June 6, 2002).

American Nurses Association (1995) Position Statement: *The Right to Accept or Reject an Assignment*. [Online] Available: http://www.nursingworld.org/readroom/position/workplac/wkassign.htm (accessed June 6, 2002).

Bensley L., Nelson N., Kaufman J., Silverstein B., Kalat J. (1993) *Study of assaults on staff in Washington State psychiatric hospitals*. Olympia, WA: State of Washington Department of Labor and Industries.

Blair, T. and New, S.A. (1991) Assault behaviour. *Journal of Psychosocial Nursing*, 29(11), 25-29.

Brayley, J., Lange, R., Baggoley, C., Bond, M., Harvey, P. (1994) The violence management team: An approach to aggressive behaviour in a general hospital. *Medical Journal of Australia* 161, 254-58.

Bruser, S. (1998) Workplace violence: Getting hospitals focused on prevention. *American Nurse*, 30(3), 11.

Bureau of Justice (1998) Special Report: *National crime victimization survey, workplace violence*, 1992-96. Publication NCJ 168634. Washington, D.C.: U.S. Department of Justice.

Butchart, A., Burrows, S., Griffin, S. (1999) Wounding the healers. *Reflections*, 25 (3) 19-21.

Caldwell, M.E. (1992) The incidence of PTSD among staff victims of patient violence. *Hospital and Community Psychiatry*, 43 (1), 838-839.

Carmel, H. and Hunter, M. (1989) Staff injuries from inpatient violence. *Hospital and Community Psychiatry*, 40 (1), 41-46.

Carmel, H. and Hunter, M. (1990) Compliance with training in managing assaultive behaviour and injuries from in-patient violence. *Hospital and Community Psychiatry*, 41(5), 558-560.

Carroll, V. (1999). Workplace violence. *American Journal of Nursing* 99 (3)60.

Carroll, V. and Goldsmith, J. (1999) One-third of nurses are abused in the workplace. *Reflections*, 25 (3), 24-27.

Castelli, J. (1993) NIOSH condemns workplace-murder epidemic. *Safety & Health*, 147 (3), 77.

Chambers, N. (1998) 'We have to put up with it – don't we?' The experience of being the registered nurse on duty, managing a violent incident involving an elderly patient: a phenomenological study. *Journal of Advanced Nursing*, 27, 429-436.

Cheek, J. and Rudge, T. (1994) "Inquiry into nursing as textually mediated discourse." In: P. Chinn, Ed., *Advances in Methods of Inquiry for Nursing*, 59-67. Gaithersburg, MD: Aspen Publications.

Chen, M. B. (1999) Day shift is most violent time. *Reflections*, 25(3), 28.

Chou, K. (1996) Assaultive behaviour in geriatric patients. *Journal of Gerontological Nursing*, 22 (11), 30-38.

Cooper, A., Saxe-Braithwaite, M., Anthony, R. (1996) Verbal abuse of hospital staff. *The Canadian Nurse*, 92(6), 31-34.

Cox, H. C. (1988) Verbal abuse in nursing practice. *Nursing Management*, 19 (11), 58-63.

Cox, H. C. (1994) Excising verbal abuse. *Today's OR Nurse*, 38-40.

Cox, H. C., Kerfoot, K. M. (1990) Changing verbal abuse into a syntonic interactive mode: The nurse manager's challenge. *Nursing Economics*, 8 (6), 416-417.

Craig, T. (1982) An epidemiological study of problems associated with violence among psychiatric inpatients. *American Journal of Psychiatry*, 139 (10), 1262-1266.

Croker, K. and Cummings, A.L. (1995) Nurses' reactions to physical assault by their patients. *Canadian Journal of Nursing Research*, 27 (2), 81-93.

Davidson, P. and Jackson, C. (1985) The nurse as a survivor: delayed posttraumatic stress reaction and cumulative trauma in nursing. *International Journal of Nursing Studies*, 22 (1), 1-13.

Dawson, J.; Johnson, M.; Kehiayan, N., Kyanko, S., Martinez, R. (1988) Response to patient assault: A peer support program for nurses. *Journal of Psychosocial Nursing*, 26, 8-15.

Denzin, N. (1997) *Interpretive Ethnography: Ethnographic Practices for the 21st Century*. Thousand Oaks, CA: Sage.

Diaz, A. L. and McMillin, D. J. (1991) A definition and description of nurse abuse. Western *Journal of Nursing Research*, 13 (1), 97-109.

DiBenedetto, D.V. (1992) Occupational hazards of the healthcare industry: Protecting healthcare workers. *American Association of Occupational Health Journal*, 43 (3), 131-137.

Dolan, J. B. (2000) Workplace violence: the universe of legal issues. *Defense Counsel Journal*, 67 (3), 332.

Downer, K. (1999) Operation Zero Tolerance of violence towards nurses. *Nursing Times*, 95 (9), 16.

Dublin, W. and Lion, J. (1992) *Clinician Safety*. Report of the APA Task Force, Report 33. Washington, D.C.: American Psychiatric Association.

Durkin, N. and Wilson, C. (1998) The value and impact of violence prevention training in a home healthcare setting. *Home Healthcare Nurse Manager*, 2 (6), 22-28.

Durkin, N. and Wilson, C. (1999) Simple steps to keep yourself safe. *Home Healthcare Nurse*, 17 (7), 430-436.

Edelman, S. (1978) Managing the violent patient in a community mental health center. *Hospital and Community Psychiatry*, 29 (7), 460-462.

Edwards, R. (1999) Prevention of workplace violence. *Aspen's Advisor for Nurse Executives*, 14 (8), 8-12.

Emergency Nurses Association. (1987) Verbal abuse in nursing. *Nursing Management*, 18 (9).

Emergency Nurses Association. (1995) *Fact Sheet: The 1994 Emergency Nurse Association Survey on Prevalence of Violence in U.S. Emergency Departments*. Park Ridge, Ill: Author.

Engle, F. and Marsh, S. (1986) Helping the employee victim of violence in hospitals. Hospital and Community Psychiatry, 37 (2), 159-162.

Fairclough, N. (1995) Critical Discourse Analysis: *The Critical Study of Language*. London: Longman.

Findorff-Dennis, M.J., McGovern, P.M., Bull, M., Hung, J. (1999) Work related assaults. *American Association of Occupational Health Nurses*, 47 (10), 456-465.

Fineberg, N., James, D.,and Shah, A. (1988) *Agency nurses and violence in a psychiatric ward*. Lancet, 1, 474.

Fisher, J., Bradshaw, J., Currie, B.A., Klotz, J., Robins, P., Searl, K. R., Smith, J. (1996) Violence and remote area nursing. *Australian Journal of Rural Health*, 4, 190-199.

Franklin, F.P. (1991) Over the edge: managing violent episodes. *Security Management*, 35 (9), 138-142.

Freeman, S. (1999) Saint Vincent tackles workplace violence. *Aspen's Advisor for Nurse Executives*, 15 (1), 6-9.

Gates, D.M. (1995) Workplace violence. *AAOHN Journal*, 43 (10), 536-543.

Gavey, N. (1997) Feminist poststructuralism and discourse analysis. In:M. Gergen,S. N. Davis (Eds.) *Toward A New Psychology of Gender*. 49-63. New York: Routledge.

Geis, A. (1986) *Community health nurses' perceptions of safety in the field: A descriptive study*, Unpublished Report, University of Illinois, Graduate College of Psychiatric Nursing.

Gest, T., Hetter, W.K., Wright, A. (1994 January 17) *Violence in America.* US. News and World Report 22-32.

Goodman R.A., Jenkins E.L., Mercy J.A. (1994) Workplace-related homicide among health care workers in the United States, 1980 through 1990. *JAMA,* 272 (21),1686–1688.

Gosnolk, D. K. (1978) The violence patient in the accident and emergency department. *Royal Society of Health Journal,* 98 (4), 289-190.

Gray, P. (1999) *Feminist Methodology.* Preconference Workbook: Tenth Annual Critical and Feminist Inquiry in Nursing Conference, October, 1999, Williamsburg, Virginia.

Graydon, J., Kasta, W., Khan, P. (1994) Verbal and physical abuse of nurses. Canadian *Journal of Nursing Administration,* 7 (4), 70-89.

Hampshire, M. (1999). Scarred for life. *Nursing Times,* 95 (25), 12-13.

Heartfield, M. (1996). Nursing documentation and nursing practice: a discourse analysis. *Journal of Advanced Nursing,* 24, 98-103.

Hinshaw, A.S., Feetham, S.L., Shaver, J. L.F., Eds. (1999) *Handbook of Clinical Nursing Research.* Thousand Oaks, CA: Sage.

Hodgkinson, P., Hillis, T.,Russell, D. (1984) Assault on staff in psychiatric hospitals. *Nursing Times,* 80, 44-46.

Hunter, M., Carmel, H. (1992) The cost of staff injuries from inpatient violence. *Hospital and Community Psychiatry,* 43, 586-588.

Hunter, E. (1997) Violence prevention in the home health setting. *Home Health Nurse,* 15 (6), 403-409.

Huston, H.R.; Anglin, D.,Mallon, W. (1992) Minimizing gang violence in the emergency department. *Annals of Emergency Medicine,* 21 (10), 1291-1293.

Infantino, A. J. and Musingo, S. (1983) Assaults and injuries among staff with and without training in aggression control techniques. *Hospital and Community Psychiatry,* 36, 1312-1314.

International Council of Nurses (1993) *Abuse or violence against nursing personnel.* Policy statement (available at: http:www.icn.ch) ICN: Geneva, Switzerland.

International Council of Nurses. (1994) *Guidelines on coping with violence in the workplace.* (Brochure). Geneva, Switzerland..

International Council of Nurses. (1999, May 05) *Escalating violence in the healthcare workplace.* Socio-Economic News (January-March). Available: http://icn.ch/newsletters.htm

Irish Nurses Organization. (1999, Feb/Mar) *News-Zero tolerance on attacks against nurses urged.* World of Irish Nursing. Available: http://www.ino.ie/NEWS/April1999/News9.html

Jones, M. K. (1985) Patient violence report of 200 incidents. *Journal of Psychosocial Nursing and Mental Health Services*, 23 (6), 12-17.

Keep, N. and Gilbert, P., (1992) California emergency nurses association's informal survey of violence in California emergency departments. *Journal of Emergency Nursing*, 18 (5), 443-442.

Kinkle, S.L. (1993) Violence in the emergency department: How to stop it before it starts. *American Journal of Nursing*, 93 (7), 22-24.

Koco, L. (1994, Sept. 26) Cigna adds violent crime rider to AD&D insurance policy. *National Underwriter Property & Casualty – Risk & Benefits Management*, number 39, 35-36.

Kurlowitcz, L. (1990) Violence in the emergency department. *American Journal of Nursing*, 90 (9), 34-37.

Lam, L. T., Ross, F. I., Cass, D. T., Quine, S., Lazarus, R. (1999) The impact of work related trauma on the psychological health of nursing staff: A cross sectional study. *Australian Journal of Advanced Nursing*, 16 (3), 14-20.

Lanza, M. L. (1983).The reactions of nursing staff to physical assault by a patient. *Hospital and Community Psychiatry*, 34 (1), 44-47.

Lanza, M. L. (1984a) Factors affecting blame placement for patient assault upon nurses. *Issues in Mental Health Nursing*, 6 (1-2), 143-161.

Lanza, M. L. (1984b) A follow-up study of nurses' reactions to physical assault. *Hospital and Community Psychiatry*, 35 (5), 492-494.

Lanza, M. L. (1984c) Victim assault support team for staff. *Hospital & Community Psychiatry*, 35 (5), 414-417.

Lanza, M. L. (1985a) Counselling services for staff victims of patient assault. *Administration in Mental Health*, 12 (3).

Lanza, M. L. (1985b) How nurses react to patient assault. *Journal of Psychosocial Nursing*, 23 (6), 6-11.

Lanza, M.L. (1996) Violence against nurses in hospitals. In: G.R. VandenBos& E.Q. Bulatao (Eds.), *Violence on the job: Identifying risks and developing solutions*,pp. 189-198. Washington, D.C.: American Psychological Association.

Lanza, M.L. (1992) Nurses as patient assault victims: an update, synthesis, and recommendations. *Archives of Psychiatric Nursing*, 6 (3),163-171.

Lanza, M. L. and Carifio, J. (1991) Blaming the victim: complex (non-linear) patterns of causal attribution by nurses in response to vignettes of a patient assaulting a nurse. *Journal of Emergency Nursing*, 17 (5), 299-309.

Lanza, M.L., Kayne, H.L., Hicks, C., & Milner, J. (1991) Nursing staff characteristics related to patient assaults. *Issues in Mental Health Nursing*, 12(3), 253-265.

Lanza, M. L. and Milner, J. (1989) The dollar cost of patient assaults. *Hospital and Community Psychiatry*, 40 (12), 1227-1229.

Lanza, M.L. (1999) Catastrophe theory: application of non-linear dynamics to assault victim responses. *Journal of the American Psychiatric Nurses Association*, 5 (4),117-121.

Larson, E. (1994, October 13) Trigger happy: A false crisis: How workplace violence became a hot issue. New York: *Wall Street Journal*.

Lavoie, F., Carter, G. L., Denzel, D. F., Berg, R. L. (1988) Emergency department violence in United States teaching hospitals. *Annals of Emergency Medicine*, 17 (11), 1227-1233.

Levin, P. F., Hewitt, J. B. and Misner, S. T. (1999) Violence against emergency room nurses: Effects and solutions. *Workplace Violence Prevention Reporter*, 5 (7/8), 12.

Levy, P. and Hartocollis, P. (1976) Nursing aides and patient violence. *American Journal of Psychiatry*, 133 (4), 429-431.

Lewis, M. L. and Dehn, D. S. (1999) Violence against nurses in outpatient mental health settings. *Journal of Psychosocial Nursing*, 37 (6), 28-33.

Lion, J. R. and Reid, W. H. (Eds) (1983) *Assaults within Psychiatric Facilities*. Orlando, FL: Grune & Stratton, Inc.

Lion, J.; Snyder, W., Merrill, G. (1981) Under- reporting of assaults on staff in a state hospital. *Hospital and Community Psychiatry*, 32 (7), 497-498.

Lipscomb, J. A. and Love, C. (1992) Violence toward health care workers. The Journal of the *American Association of Occupational Health Nurses*, 40 (5), 219-228.

Liss, G.M. and McCaskell, L. (1994) Injuries due to violence: Worker's compensation claims among nurses in Ontario. *AAOHN Journal*, 42 (8), 384-390.

Lusk, S. L. (1992) Violence experienced by nurses' aides in nursing homes. *The Journal of the American Association of Occupational Health Nurses*, 40 (5), 237-241.

Lybecker, C. J. (1998) Violence against nurses – a silent epidemic. *Workplace Violence Prevention Reporter*, 4 (6), 12.

Mahoney, B.S. (1991) The Extent, Nature and Response to Victimization of Emergency Nurses in Pennsylvania. *Journal of Emergency Nursing*, 17 (5), 282-94.

Manderino, M. A. and Berkey, N. (1997) Verbal abuse of staff nurses by physicians. *Journal of Professional Nursing*, 13 (1), 48-55.

Mantell, M. and Albrecht, S. (1995) *Ticking Bombs: Defusing Violence in the Workplace*. New York: Irwin.

McHale, S. (1999) From insult to injury. *Nursing Times*, 95 (49), 30.

McNay, L. (1992) *Foucault and Feminism*. Boston: Northeastern University Press.

Metropolitan Chicago Healthcare Council. (1995) *Guidelines for Dealing with Violence in Health Care.* Chicago: Author.

Mitiguy, J.S. (1999) Facing up to the problem of workplace violence. *Nursing Spectrum* (New York/New Jersey ed.), 11A (14), 8-9.

Morgan, L. (1999) In harm's way: Nurses face increasing abuse in workplace. *NurseWeek* (August 23), 12 (17), 13.

Morrison, E. F. and Herzog, E. A. (1992) What therapeutic and protective measures, as well as legal actions, can staff take when they are attacked by patients. *Journal of Psychosocial Nursing,* 30 (7), 41-44.

Morrison, E.F. (1993) Toward a better understanding of violence in psychiatric settings: debunking the myths. *Archives of Psychiatric Nursing,* 7 (6),328-335.

Morrison, E.F. (1994) Evolution of a concept of aggression and violence in psychiatric settings. *Archives of Psychiatric Nursing,* 7 (4), 245-253.

Mrkwicka, L. (1999) Violence and stress in nursing. *Reflections,* 25 (3), 22-23.

Myers, D.W. (1996) The mythical world of workplace violence – or it it? *Business Horizons,* 39 (4), 31-7.

National Health Service. (1999, December 18) *Managers' guide: Stopping violence against staff working in the NHS.* London: NHS Executive. Available: http://www.doh.gov.uk/zero.htm

National Institute of Occupational Safety and Health. (1996) *Violence in the workplace.* Available: http://www.cdc.gov/niosh/violpurp.html

Navis, E. S. (1987) Controlling violent patients before they control you. *Nursing,* 87 (17), 52-54.

Nield-Anderson, L. and Doubrava, J. (1993) Defusing verbal abuse: A program for emergency department triage nurses. *Journal of Emergency Nursing,* 19 (5), 441-445.

Nield-Anderson, L., Minarik, P.A., Dilworth, J.M., Jones, J., Nash, P.K., O'Donnell, K.L., Steinmiller, E.A. (1999) Responding to 'difficult patients' manipulation, sexual provocation, aggression, how you can manage such behaviour. *American Journal of Nursing,* 99 (12), 26-34.

NIOSH (1996) Current Intelligence Bulletin 57: *Violence in the Workplace*: Risk Factors and Prevention Strategies. Publication No. 96–100, available from the National Institute for Occupational Safety and Health, Cincinnati, OH.

Nolan, P., Dallender, J., Soares, J., Thomsen, S., Arnetz, B. (1999) Violence in mental health care: the experiences of mental health nurses and psychiatrists. *Journal of Advanced Nursing,* 30 (4) 934-941.

Occupational Safety and Health Administration (1992) OSHA Standards Interpretation and Compliance Letters 05/13/1992 – *Criminal Violence in the Workplace.* Available at: http://www.osha-slc.gov/OshDoc/Interp_data/ I19920513C.html.

Occupational Safety and Health Administration. (1996) *Guidelines for preventing workplace violence for health care and social service workers* (OSHA 3148): U. S. Department of Labor. Available: http://www.osha-slc.gov/Osh Doc/Additional.

Occupational Safety and Health Administration. (1999) *Workplace Violence.* Available at: http://www.osha.gov/oshinfo/priorities/violence.html.

Olson, N. (1994) Workplace violence: Theories of causation and prevention strategies. *Journal of the American Association of Occupational Health Nursing*, 4 (2), 477-482.

On-the-job violence becomes 'epidemic'. (1994) *Safety and Health*, 149 (2), 85.

Palmer, J. (1999) Emergency room nurses look at violence. *Reflections*, 25 (3), 28.

Patterson, B. and McCmomish, S. (1998) The physical management of violent behaviour. *Psychiatric Care*, 5 (6), 228-231.

Phelan, L. A., Mills, M. J., Ryan, J. A. (1985) Prosecuting psychiatric patients for assaults. *Hospital and Community Psychiatry*, 36 (6), 581-582.

Podolak, A. (2000) Is workplace violence in need of refocusing? *Security Management*, 44 (6), 152.

Poster, E. C. and Ryan, J. A. (1989) Nurses' attitudes toward physical assaults by patients. *Archives of Psychiatric Nursing*, 3 (6), 315-322.

Powers, P. (1999) *Der Diskurs der Pflegediagnosen.* Bern: Verlag Hans Huber.

Queensland Nurses' Union. (1998, May 26) *Workplace bullying.* Queensland Nurses' Union. Available: http://www.qnu.org/bullying.htm

Quine, L. (1999) Workplace bullying in NHS community trust: Staff questionnaire survey. *British Medical Journal.* Available: http://www.bmj.com/cgi/content/full/318/7178/228

Richardson, T. (1997, January) *Nurse abuse workplace violence: UNA examines nurse abuse*, Part II, News Bulletin. Available:http://www.ccinet.ab.ca.una/Publications/Newsbulletin/jan97nb.html Rossi, A. M.,

Jacobs, M., Monteleone, M., Olson, R., Surber, R. W., Winkler, E., Wommack, A. (1985) Violent or fear-inducing behaviour associated with hospital admission. *Hospital & Community Psychiatry*, 36 (6), 643-647.

Ryan, J. A. and Poster, E. C. (1989a) The assaulted nurse: Short-term and long-term responses. *Archives of Psychiatric Nursing*, 3 (6), 323-331.

Ryan, J. A. and Poster, E. C. (1989b) Supporting your staff after a patient assault. *Nursing*, 89 (12), 32k, 32n, 32p.

Ryan, J. A. and Poster, E. C. (1991) When a patient hits you. *Canadian Nurse*, 87 (8), 23-25.

Sanchez-Gallegos, D. and Viens, D.C. (1995) When the client is armed or dangerous: management of violent and difficult clients in primary care. *Nurse Practitioner*, 20 (6), 26-32.

Schwartz, C., and Greenfield, G. (1978) Charging a patient with assault of a nurse on a psychiatric unit. *Canadian Psychiatric Association Journal*, 23 (4), 197-200.

Seidel, G. (1993) The competing discourses of HIV/AIDS in sub-Saharan Africa: Discourses of rights and empowerment vs. discourses of control and exclusion. *Social Sciences and Medicine*, 36 (3), 175-194.

Shepherd E. (Ed.) (1994) *Violence in Health Care: a Practical Guide to Coping with Violence and Caring for victims*. New York: Oxford University Press.

Simonowitz, J.A. (1994) Violence in the workplace: You're entitled to protection. *RN*, 57 (11), 61-64.

Simonowitz, J.A. (1995) Violence in health care: A strategic approach. *Nurse Practitioner Forum*, 6 (2), 120-129.

Simonowitz, J.A., Rigdon, J.E., Mannings, J. (1997) Workplace violence: Prevention efforts by the occupational health nurse. *AAOHN Journal*, 45 (6), 305-316.

Snyder, W., III. (1994) Hospital downsizing and increased frequency of assaults on staff. *Hospital and Community Psychiatry*, 45, pp. 378-379.

Smith-Pittman, M.H. and McKoy, Y.D. (1999) Workplace Violence in Healthcare Environments. *Nursing Forum* 34,(3), 5-13.

Sommargren, C.E. (1994) Violence as an occupational hazard in the acute care setting. *Critical Care Nursing* 5, 516-522.

Stearley, H. (1998) To kill a nurse. Revolution: *The Journal of Nurse Empowerment*, 8(3/4), 64-74.

Stewart-Amidei, C. (1999) Violence in the workplace: Debunking the myths. *Journal of Neuroscience Nursing*, 31 (4), 199.

Sullivan, C. and Carl, M.S. Workplace assaults on minority health and mental health care workers in Los Angeles. *American Journal of Public Health*, 85 (7), 1011-1014.

Sullivan, E. J. (1999) Nurses take issue with workplace violence. *Reflections*, 25 (3), 4.

Summers, B.J., (1999) Violence in the workplace: Are you safe? *Tennessee Nurse*, 62 (2),13-14.

Tardiff, K. and Sweillam, A. (1980) Assault, suicide and mental illness. *Archives of General Psychiatry*, 37 (2), 164-169.

Tardiff, K. and Sweillam, A. (1982) Assaultive behaviour among chronic inpatients. *American Journal of Psychiatry*, 139 (2), 212-215.

Tardiff, K. and Koenigsberg, H. (1985) Assaultive behaviour among psychiatric outpatients. *American Journal of Psychiatry*, 14 (8), 960-963.

Toufexis, A. (1994, April 15) Workers who fight firing with fire. *Time*, 34-37.

U.S. Department of Justice. (1998) *Workplace violence 1992-1996.* Available at: http://www.ojp.usdoj.gov/bjs/abstract/wv96.htm.

Ussher, J. (2000) "Women's madness: A material-discursive-intrapsychic approach." In: Fee, W., Ed., *Pathology and the Postmodern*, 207-230. London: Sage.

Valentine, P.E.B. (1996) "Nursing: a ghettoized profession relegated to women's sphere." *International Journal of Nursing Studies*, 33(1), 98-106.

Vandergaer, F. and Sud, S. (1997) Your thoughts: Decrease violence – increase safety. *Home Health Focus 3.*

Washington Nurse (1999) Workplace violence – SB 5312. *Washington Nurse*, 29 (3) 16-18.

Wasserberger, J., Ordog, G. J., Kolodny, M., Allen, K. (1989) Violence in a community emergency room. *Archives of Emergency Medicine*, 6, 266-269.

Whittington, R. and Wykes, T. (1994) Violence in psychiatric hospitals: Are certain staff prone to being assaulted? *Journal of Advanced Nursing*, 19, 219-115.

Williams, M.F. (1996) Violence and sexual harassment: Impact on registered nurses in the workplace. *AAOHN Journal*, 44 (2), 73-77. Workplace violence a growing problem. (1988) *Trial*, 24 (8), 14. Washington, D.C.

Chapter Three: Violence in Health Care: A Finnish Nursing Perspective

Maritta Välimäki, Johanna Taipale and Anneli Pitkänen

Introduction

Violence in societies is a very topical issue in general (Keeler, 2001) and specifically in relation to workplaces. The need to pay attention to occupational safety and health has increased in the European countries (e.g. Chappel and Di Martino, 1998; European Agency for Safety and Health at Work, 1999, 2000 a,b,c; Wynne, 2000).

The purpose of this chapter is to provide a Finnish perspective on violence especially in Finnish health care and the nursing setting. The chapter first portrays Finland and the societal changes affecting the Finnish health care system. This will hopefully help readers perceive the context in which violence in health care will be approached. Next, the definitions of violence in Finland will be addressed, followed by an account of the prevalence and types of violence encountered in the services sector, especially within health care, and by a description of the violence or threat of violence. Lastly, we will conclude by introducing guidelines for dealing with violence and the means to improve the management and prevention of violence.

The forms of workplace violence are manifold, workplace bullying being one of them (Jankola, 1991). Workplace bullying within the health care and social field has attracted attention in the 1990s especially in Europe (Quine, 1999; European Agency for Safety and Health at Work, 2000a,b,c,) and in the Nordic countries (e.g. Leymann, 1992). A number of Finnish studies have addressed workplace bullying in recent years (e.g. Sutela and Lehto 1998; Kivimäki et al, 2000). The present review focuses primarily on physical violence, although it is obvious that various work-related uncertainties as well as competition and pressure at work are associated with conflicts at workplaces. These factors are also associated with workplace bullying (Lehto and Sutela, 1999). Emotional abuse and workplace bullying deserve separate investigation and are therefore not the primary focus of this analysis.

Some Facts about Finland

Finland is sparsely populated with around 5.2 million people; our average population density is no more than 17 inhabitants per square kilometre. Maybe because of its historical background, Finland was a quite isolated country until it joined the EU in 1995. Our population is culturally homogenous: 92,4% speak Finnish, which differs greatly from other languages, and 85.1% belong to the Lutheran Church (Statistics Finland, 2001).

Although the overall health and wellbeing of the Finnish population have improved, great health disparities remain among various population groups. Protection for the wellbeing and financial safety of individuals and families has traditionally been provided by the government through social programmes and services (e.g. social insurance, unemployment benefits, maternity policies). However, economic downturn and changes in support services changed in the early 1990s. The number of unemployed people tripled in a short time and decreased the level of individual citizens' wellbeing. The first group to be affected by employment was 15- to 24-year olds, whose number nearly quadrupled (Viitanen, 1998). At the end of July 2001, there were 317,600 unemployed job seekers registered at the employment offices (Ministry of Labour, 2001).

Because of missing work opportunities, people migrated from rural areas to urban centres. These societal changes have given rise to new health problems. Rates of suicides, mental problems of children and adolescents as well as violence and drug problems have increased dramatically. AIDS is an emerging health problem in Finland. The number of HIV cases has increased during the last five years, but is still quite low compared with other European countries. By August 8, 2001 Finland had 1307 registered HIV cases (National Public Health Institute, 2001).

Mental problems remain among the most serious health problems in today's Finland. For instance, in 1999 the use of antidepressants increased by 16% (National Agency for Medicines and Social Insurance Institute, 2000). Mood disturbances and neurotic and schizophrenic disturbances are the leading causes of retirement due to mental health disorders, and the leading cause of retirement among young people has been schizophrenia (Social Insurance Institute, 2001). As in the other Western countries, the population in Finland is getting older. About 14% of the population are over 65 years of age, and 5.9% are over 75 years old. The number of people over 85 years of age is expected to increase by one-third by the year 2010 (Statistics Finland, 2001).

Because of the economic burden placed on health services, health care and social services financing changed at the beginning of the 1990s. Due to economical and ideological reasons, the structure of mental health services has changed dramatically during the last two decades. The number of psychiatric beds has dropped from 20,036 in 1980 to 6,400 in 1995, and the average length of stay has been reduced between 1980 and 1999 from 166.8 days to 45.7 days. Despite these structural changes, total health expenditure still increased from FIM 44,842 million in 1996 to 49,198 million FIM in 1999 (Statistics Finland, 2001).

Finnish legislation obligates the municipalities to take responsibility for organising social and health services for the resident population. However, the law does not regulate the content, extent or organisation of the services in detail, and therefore big differences in the structure of health and mental services can be found in different parts of Finland. Furthermore, specialised health care services have generally shifted from conservative to intensified treatment modalities, leading to shorter hospitalisation periods and linked non-institutional care (Laine and Wickström, 2000).

The public sector, which is responsible for providing social welfare and health care services, is Finland's largest employer. The vast majority of the employees are women. The level of education among health care personnel has traditionally been high, and the introduction of the polytechnic system means that it will continue to rise (Wickström et al, 2000). Perhaps this is the reason why the work climate in the 1990s was increasingly marked by envy and competition between employees and by inadequate staffing compared with workload. On the other hand, work patterns have changed with the introduction of teamwork, which is supposed to foster mutual support, trust and appreciation among colleagues (Lehto and Sutela, 1999). The age structure of health care personnel has changed with the rise in the proportion of ageing workers. Within the next decade, the Finnish health care system will face a serious labour shortage as baby-boomers start to retire.

What is Violence from a Finnish Perspective? Violence from the Perspective of Criminal Law

Finnish legislation does not provide a definition of the concepts of threat and violence. Violence is usually seen as taking two forms. Violence 'vis absoluta' refers to a situation which completely excludes any exercise of will by the victim. Tying up the victim or shutting the victim in a room are supposed to involve such violence. The second form 'vis compulsiva', is defined as violence caused through the "bending" of the will of the victim. The effect of this kind of violence, that is, of psychological coercion, is indirect (Lakanen, 1999).

Violence may be unintentional or intentional. Intentional violence does not, however, necessarily fall under the Penal Code of Finland and is not always a criminal offence under the Penal Code. In practice, the difference between the two is not very clear (Aromaa and Heiskanen, 2000).

If health care professionals are exposed to physical violence or threats in their workplaces, they should naturally be entitled to similar legal protection as other crime victims. Crimes resulting in legal action in Finland include, among others, the following (Kokko, 2000):

- assaults: simple assault, assault, aggravated assault
- illegal threats (threatening with a gun or verbal threat; Penal Code 25, § 7)
- extortion and robbery
- breach of the peace in a public office (Penal Code 24, § 1)
- mischief (e.g. noise offence, disturbance of the peace in a public office, harassing telephone calls; Penal Code 17, § 13)
- vandalism (intentional damage to property; Penal Code, 35)

The mildest forms of hospital violence involve pushing and shoving, where the violence is relatively minimal. Tearing at clothes or beating the air does not usually meet the characteristics of a simple assault. Punching in the face resulting in an injury is the commonest form of assault. Kicking is also a common form of violence. By contrast, brutal kicking of a defenceless victim resulting in severe injures is to be interpreted as an aggravated assault. Hospital violence in Finland has rarely been serious enough to meet the characteristics of aggravated assault. The most typical form of aggravated assault is stabbing (Kokko, 2000).

In Finland, violence or threat of violence against public officials is liable to more severe punishment than if the violence were directed, for instance, at elderly people. Special legal protection of public officials has traditionally been justified by the fact that violent resistance against a public official is not only directed at the particular official but at the power of the state represented by that official. Of public officials, law enforcement officers are most often exposed to violence or threat of violence. The deaths of two Finnish policemen in Autumn 1997 ignited public debate about the violence and threat of violence against public officials as a larger societal phenomenon (Lakanen, 1999).

Definitions of Violence in Nursing Textbooks

The definitions of violent behaviour used in Finnish nursing textbooks emanate from the international literature and studies. Finnish nursing textbooks depict violent behaviour in terms of verbal aggression against a nurse, which may occasionally lead to physical violence (Iija et al, 1996). Violent behaviour is also seen as an interactive situation, where violence is not only a characteristic of a client, but rather an element of interaction resulting from of a number of factors. Violent behaviour is defined as behaviour whose purpose is to harm others and the environment physically and psychologically. Violent behaviour may, on the other hand, be directed inwards where it turns against the person him/herself resulting in self-blame and self-hatred (Vuori-Kemilä, 2000).

Another approach to violence used in textbooks (e.g. Iija et al, 1996, Latvala et al, 1996, Vuori-Kemilä, 2000) is through the concept of anger. Anger is associated with rage, aggression, hostility and aggravation and it may manifest itself in violent behaviour, destructive qualities or indirect expressions of anger (Latvala et al, 1996). Most people repress or deny their anger because it frightens them and is not as readily acceptable as other emotions. Repressed anger induces anxiety and fear, which may result in open aggression or in depression and self-destruction. The Finnish culture and educational tradition tend to eliminate and condemn anger, which may be one of the underlying reasons why depression is considered a national health problem in Finland (Iija et al, 1996).

Defining Workplace Violence

The Finnish literature does not offer an easy or unequivocal way to define workplace violence. One of the reasons for this is that in many cases the underlying definitions emanate from international perspectives on violence. Finnish studies and reports draw on the definition set out in a study commissioned by the European Commission (Wynne, 2000), defining violence as an incident where people are verbally abused, threatened or assaulted in circumstances related to their work, involving an explicit or implicit challenge to their safety, wellbeing or health. Workplace violence covers both direct violence against workers and indirect violence against members of the workers' family or friends (Piispa and Saarela, 2000).

Violence or threat of violence endangers the life, health and bodily integrity, sometimes also freedom, of others. Violent acts may also be directed against property. Violence can also be carried out through other people and even through animals or inanimate objects. In such cases, a person's act of will must nevertheless underlie the violence (Lakanen 1999, Majanen, 2000). Hakola (1992) suggested that violent behaviour refers to physical acts causing injuries to the victim and possibly loss of life.

The definition of violence may be narrow or broad. A narrow definition may include particular criteria for the occurrence of violence. The criteria may be drawn, for instance, from the Finnish Penal Code (39/1889). A broad definition may include both physical violence and intimidation, as done by Piispa and Saarela (2000) in their study of workplace violence. In their definition, violence refers to any incident involving actual, attempted or threatened physical or sexual violence. The authors also examined violence in terms of its possible consequences.

Vartia and Perkka-Jortikka (1994) defined workplace violence as psychological and physical violence or threat of violence experienced by people at work. Violence is intentional and purposeful as distinct from unintentional harm to other people, which can be classified as an accident. In its violation of bodily integrity, physical violence differs from psychological violence, which refers to repeated negative interaction. Physical violence is more frequently a one-time incident, whereas psychological violence is repeated in nature (Salminen, 1997).

Studies conducted by Finnish organisations for social and health service professionals (Majasalmi, 2001; Markkanen, 2000) defined workplace violence as physical violence or threat of violence. The violence was manifested as pushing and shoving or as punching and kicking. It could also involve physical attacks, threatening with a cutting weapon or preventing the victim from moving. Incidents of spitting and biting have also been reported. Verbal aggression took the form of swearing, criticism, intimidation and name-calling.

A survey by Aromaa and Heiskanen (2000) used interviews in which respondents were asked whether they had been exposed to violence from a known or unknown person over the last 12 months. The following eight areas, found in the study, define the way in which violence has been examined in Finland from the perspective of an average citizen's everyday life. The acts referred to are as follows: 1) threats; 2) an attempt to prevent the victim from moving, grabbing; 3) pushing or hitting; 4) punching without visible injuries; 5) punching resulting in visible injuries such as bruises, wounds or contusions; 6) stabbing, shooting or assaulting using a firearm; 7) some other type of violent behaviour; 8) grabbing or touching in a way interpreted as sexually offensive.

In keeping with the suggestion of the OECD working group, a study by Sirén (2000) identified a lost working day resulting from a violent incident as the criterion for seriousness of a violent incident. An accident or incident of violence in which the victim was confined to bed or which had otherwise interfered with his/her work performance or daily chores for at least 24 hours was defined as a case resulting in a lost working day. This definition incorporates both the subjective and objective dimension of a health hazard.

It should be born in mind that the concepts of accident and violent are subjective. Even a perceived threat of violence may result in a feeling of fear and threat. How, then, is it possible to assess the safety of working environment, say, in regard to violence? According to Sirén (2000), the problem with safety measurements is how to make incidents of violence of various types occurring to different people commensurable. Exposure to violence is often a more traumatic experience than an accident because of its premeditated nature. The nature of the injury resulting from violence characterises the seriousness of violence, although other things also matter (Sirén, 2000).

Prevalence of Violence at the Workplace

The literature has put forward conflicting views of the rise in violence in Finnish society. The prevalent view is that Finnish society has become brutalised and that violence has increased both generally and specifically in health care. Nonetheless, there is no unequivocal evidence of whether this is true. However, according to the statistics on Finnish society in general (Statistics Finland, 2001), the number of offences (attempted and actual manslaughter and homicide, assault, rape) has nearly quintupled since the 1950s. In 2000, 13.4% of citizens over 15 years of age had been subjected to sexual harassment or abuse, violence or threat of violence, intimidation and physical violence. Accidents and violence were the 20th leading cause of death in 1999.

Statistics show that premeditated violence is a much less serious health hazard than various accidents. Though many citizens have some experience of violence, the vast majority of cases involving threats did not lead to physical violence (Sirén, 2000). By contrast, mild violence and the number of threats have clearly increased in Finland between 1980 and 1997. While there were 191,000 reports of threatening incidents or attempted assaults in 1980, the number of incidents was 310,000 in 1997. Workplace violence against women has clearly increased (Aromaa and Heiskanen, 2000).

In 2000, an extensive report explored the prevalence of occupational injuries and violence in Finland. This interview study looked at the risk of occupational injuries and violent incidents among the Finnish adult population (at least 15 years of age) in 1980, 1988, 1993 and 1997. The number of interviewees was around 10,000 in 1980, 13,000 in 1988, over 4,000 in 1993 and 9,000 in 1997. The risk of occupational injury or violent incident seemed to decline at the beginning of the 1990s, whereas it started to rise again at the end of the 1990s. The study showed, however, that there was no clear change in the prevalence of serious occupational injuries and violence causing incapacity for work between 1980 and 1997 (Sirén, 2000). The leading cause of occupational injury in health and social services industries in 2000 was work overload (27%) (Federation of Accident Insurance Institutions, 1999, also Laitinen, 2000a,b).

Workplace violence is typically not distributed evenly across different occupations but tends to accumulate in particular occupations and workplaces (Piirainen et al., 2000; Saarela and Isotalus, 2000a,b). In Finland in the 1980s, private security workers tended to be more at risk from workplace violence. An increased risk of workplace violence was detected at the end of the 1980s in health care and social services occupations and in transport services (Isotalus and Saarela, 1997). A study conducted in 1993 showed that public transport workers, such as taxi drivers, bus drivers and ticket inspectors, and restaurant workers were at greatest risk of violence and threat of violence. Those working in law enforcement and guard services, in health and social services and in the retail trade experienced an above-average amount of violence and threat of violence (Haapaniemi and Kinnunen, 1997). A study covering the years 1990-1998 revealed that police officers were at greatest risk of dying from a violent injury: a police officer's risk of fatal workplace violence was 50-fold compared with the average risk. Fatal occupational injuries have also been reported in the nursing profession (Isotalus and Saarela, 1999). In health care and social services, 2 employees had died and 8 had retired as a consequence of an occupational injury in 1999 (Federation of Accident Insurance Institutions, 2000).

Between the years of 1994 and 1996, there were 1,496 violence-related occupational injuries. Forty-one per cent of these occurred among women and the number of occupational injuries among women increased with age. Most occupational injuries occurred in the services sector (40%) and in health care and social services (20%) (Piispa and Saarela, 2000). Between the years of 1994 and 1998, an average of 68 work-related occupational injuries occurred in health care settings. In 1996, the number of violence-related occupational injuries more than doubled compared with the mean of all occupations (Federation of Accident Insurance Institutions 2000).

According to the Work and Health interview survey (Piirainen et al, 1997), 4.1% of the respondents had experienced physical violence (1.4%) or threat of violence (2.7%) at work or on the way to work over the last 12 months. About 80,000 workers of the employed work-force had experienced violence or its threat at work. The survey showed that the social and health care fields were at risk of violence (10.5% of respondents had experienced workplace violence). A repeat survey in 2000 (Piirainen et al, 2000) found that catering services (16% had been exposed to physical violence or threat of violence) and health care and social services (12%) were problematic areas from the perspective of physical violence.

The discussion about violence or threat of violence at work (Saarela, 1999) has extended into health care and especially into nursing (e.g. Ahokas-Kukkonen, 1999; Keckman-Koivuniemi, 1999; Laaksonen, 2000; Laitinen, 2000a,b). In 1993, approximately 17,000 nursing professionals fell prey to violence or threat of violence. This represents 12% of all those working in the medical occupations. In 1996, the number of violence-related accidents in health care and hospital settings was more than double the average of all occupations. The proportion of violence-related occupational injuries of all occupational injuries in the health care industry was 1.4% whereas the proportion for all occupations was 0.4% (Saarela and Isotalus, 2000a).

A Finnish interview study (n = 31,500) conducted in 1999 showed that the fields most affected were health care services (nurse, psychiatric nurse, doctor, 27%) and social services (12%) (Paananen and Notkola, 2000). More than one-fifth of all violent incidents against women were directed at nursing staff. A study by Piirainen et al (2000) investigated violence-related fears and the incidence of actual violence in different occupations. Interestingly, social and health care workers differed from other occupations. They did not exhibit more fears of violence than did the other groups. However, these groups had more injuries compared with those who considered their occupations to be hazardous. This might indicate that health care workers are not prepared to face violence in their work.

Of all health care occupational groups in Finland, psychiatric nurses are at greatest risk of workplace violence: nearly half (47%) of them had encountered violence at work over the past year. Of nurses, 23% had been a victim of violence over the past year, whereas 21% of paramedics and 17% of doctors had been victims of violence in the same timeframe (Söderholm et al, 1999). A survey by the City of Helsinki found that over 60% of municipal workers within the city's social services and psychiatric facilities had experienced violent and threatening incidents over the last 12 months. In these groups, the incidents were also more serious: about half of the cases had resulted in visible injuries or work absenteeism (Saarela and Isotalus, 2000b).

The Nature of Violent Incidents

Types of Violence

Although the data on the real increase of violence at workplaces are conflicting, experiences of physical violence and its threat have increased especially in social and health care occupations over the past years (Haapaniemi and Kinnunen 1997; Markkanen, 2000; Majasalmi, 2001). A study by Markkanen (2000) found that nearly a half of the nurses involved in the study had been called names or criticised by patients at least once over the past year. One in three of all respondents had experienced various types of physical violence or threat of violence.

Physical violence or its threat was clearly more rare than verbal abuse. A study by Majasalmi (2001) yielded similar results: 83% of social and health care workers had experienced physical violence or its threat over the past year, whereas 72% had been exposed to name-calling, criticism or swearing from clients or patients to some extent.

Threatening behaviour usually takes the form of swearing, cursing or shouting. Incidents of punching, kicking and biting or pushing and shoving involving an invasion to the victim's bodily integrity have also been reported in health care (Junnila and Kytölä, 1990; Saarela and Isotalus, 2000a,b). The violence may also involve physical attacks, threatening with a cutting weapon or preventing the victim from moving (Markkanen, 2000), not to mention spitting and biting (Majasalmi, 2001). However, the commonest form of violence is verbal abuse. It involve insults and shouting, threatening gestures, criticism, intimidation and name-calling (Apo and Keskinen, 1983; Majasalmi, 2001; Markkanen, 2000; Saarela and Isotalus, 2000a,b).

The Assailant

In health care, the assailant is usually a client, that is, a patient. The risk of being victimised by a patient is high especially in mental health care. The most important psychiatric disorders increasing the risk of violence include personality disorders and schizophrenia, with the latter increasing the risk of homicide nearly tenfold compared with the rest of the population (Hakola, 1992; Tiihonen, 1999).

During the years 1954 - 1988, institutionalised psychiatric patients had committed 34 homicides in the psychiatric hospitals and the psychiatric departments of the then old people's homes. Most of the assailants had been diagnosed as having schizophrenia, and the illness appeared to be the primary cause of the act (Hakola et al., 1990). Violent incidents are often associated with client intoxication (Junnila and Kytölä, 1990; Hakola, 1992; Markkanen, 2000; Saarela and Isotalus, 2000a). Schizophrenia coupled with alcohol dependency is an important risk factor for violence: the risk increases more than fifteen-fold (Tiihonen, 1999). For instance, data collected from the Niuvanniemi hospital (a hospital for difficult-to-treat patients) showed that a typical patient hospitalised because of difficulty of treatment in 1994 was male, on average 31 years of age, psychotic, had severe substance misuse problems, was a multiple offender, exhibited violent behaviour or had a history of escape, had no awareness of illness and was non-compliant with treatment (Putkonen and Paanila, 1996).

In another hospital for difficult-to-treat patients, Vanha Vaasa Hospital, the majority (80%) of violent incidents occurring during the time of the study were accounted by five patients, four of which were diagnosed as schizophrenics and one with personality disorder. About one-third of the incidents were unpredictable while in the other cases the aggressive behaviour was anticipated on the grounds of agitation or a previous conflict. Female patients were more violent than male patients. Most of the violence occurred during daytime between 7 and 16 hours, which is the time when patients were expected to participate in various activities and between 13 and 15 hours, that is, during the change of working shifts (Weizmann-Henelius and Suutala, 2000). A study by Apo and Keskinen (1983) found that 45% of violent incidents were unpredictable with no connection to treatments or other procedures. One-third of the incidents occurred during the first 24 hours of treatment and 40% during the first week of treatment. Situations where patients were denied the care they desired or were dissatisfied with the care may also trigger violent behaviour (Markkanen 2000; Saarela and Isotalus, 2000a).

Violence against Nursing Staff

It is typical of violent incidents against nursing professionals that the assailant is nearly always a patient, whereas in industrial workplaces the assailant was usually a co-worker (Piispa and Saarela, 2000). Most of the violence perpetrated by patients is directed at nurses. Although the observation dates back to the 1980s (Apo and Keskinen, 1983), the situation remains the same today (e.g. Weizmann-Henelius and Suutala, 2000; Majasalmi, 2001). Violent behaviour by a patient's relative against nursing staff is an alarming new phenomenon (Markkanen, 2000). In a study by Majasalmi (2001), over half of the respondents had been exposed to violence or threat of violence from a patient's relative (also Saarela and Isotalus, 2000a).

Male caregivers are faced with violent incident clearly more frequently than their female counterparts. The more serious the type of violence, the more frequently male caregivers are the ones faced with it. It may be that males work more frequently in units whose patients may be more likely to exhibit violent behaviour (Markkanen, 2000). Majasalmi's (2001) report showed that permanent staff were assaulted more frequently by patients than non-permanent staff. In contrast, a report by Markkanen (2000) suggested that non-permanent staff and shift workers were more frequently exposed to a range of violent behaviours or threat of violence. Shift workers reported experiences of violence 2-3 times more frequently compared with day workers. Understaffing and working alone at night also predispose staff to violent behaviour.

Perceived violence and threat of violence was also associated with age. Respondents in the 41-50 age bracket had been subjected to more violence or threat of violence from patients than other age groups over the past year (Majasalmi, 2001). On the other hand, it has been found that younger and more inexperienced nurses are at a greater risk of violence than older nurses (Vartia and Hyyti, 1999; Markkanen, 2000).

Consequences of Violence against Health Care Professionals

Workplace violence has both practical and emotional consequences for the victim. Practical consequences involve sick absences, damage to property and various minor injuries. The majority of violent incidents at work are physically minor; nevertheless they carry psychological and social consequences for the well-being and coping of workers. Violence perpetrated by a patient may also induce psychological suffering and fears for both the victim and his/her co-workers. The commonest emotional consequences are anger and fear (Söderholm et al, 1999). Other consequences involve job dissatisfaction, loss of self-esteem and self-blame (Aromaa et al, 1994). In addition, the fear of having to face a violent and threatening client may reduce job satisfaction and motivation for work (Isotalus and Saarela, 1999).

Although victims of physical violence or its threat usually received support from their colleagues and superiors, it appears that workplaces have not taken workplace violence seriously enough, at least judging by the inadequacies in recording violent incidents. Follow-up and reporting procedures for violent incidents may be inadequate or non-existent. It is also unclear how, where and to whom violent or threatening incidents against staff should be reported (Markkanen 2000; Majasalmi, 2001). The incidents are usually reported to the first-line manager or the director of nursing and colleagues during daily reports or ward meetings. Once recorded, violent incidents are only rarely reported to the safety representative or occupational health services of the workplace (Majasalmi, 2001). It has been suggested that violence in health care workplaces may be grossly underreported, because nurses may feel that it is part of the job and therefore tend to ignore it (Söderholm et al, 1999).

Controlling a Violent Patient: Regulations Concerning a Patient's Violent Behaviour

Ethical principles of health professionals emphasise respect for human dignity and self-determination as these are seen as part of an individual's basic moral rights (e.g. Ethical Codes for Nurses 1996). In practice, while attempting to control an aggressive patient one must adhere to the Finnish law:
• Act on the Status and Rights of Patients (785/1992)

66

- Mental Health Act (1116/1990)
- Penal Code (39/1889)
- Act Concerning Health Care Professionals (559/1994)

The Act on the Status and Rights of Patients (785/1992) states that patient care must be planned in mutual understanding with the patient (§ 6) and that the care and treatment of the patient must be such that his/her human dignity is not violated and that his/her privacy is respected (§ 3). If a patient is incapable of deciding about his/her care because of mental disturbance, he/she must be given treatment that can be considered to be in accordance with his/her best interest (§ 6).

According to the Mental Health Act (1116/1990), a patient can be subjected to coercive measures and his/her self-determination can be restricted only to the extent necessary for the treatment, for the patient's safety or for the safety of others (§ 28). In Finland, particularly dangerous or difficult-to-treat patients are treated in state psychiatric hospitals (Mental Health Act 1116/1990, § 6). More concrete guidelines for the control of a patient's aggressive behaviour are to be found in hospital-specific guidelines (e.g. Suutala, 2000) and in textbooks (e.g. Tiihonen, 1999).

Finnish legislation includes a number of special regulations concerning different occupational groups for dealing with violence. There are specific regulations concerning law enforcement officers, prison wardens, customs officers, and captains of aircraft and watercraft (see Nuutila, 1997). Except for regulations concerning civil servants, Finnish law does not include special regulations concerning violent events encountered by health care professionals. In violence-related incidents, the Penal code (39/1889) on justifiable self-defence is applicable to health care professionals providing them the right to defend themselves, other people and property against an ongoing or threatening attack (3: § 6 and § 7) (Majanen, 2000).

The most important regulation concerning health care professionals is the Act Concerning Health Care Professionals (559/1994). The purpose of the act is to promote patient safety and the quality of health care. The National Authority for Medicolegal Affairs and the county governments bear the responsibility for controlling the actions of health care professionals. Patients and their relatives have the right to lodge a complaint about their care and treatment with the Parliamentary Ombudsman and the social and health department of the county government. They also have the opportunity to meet with the control authorities during workplace inspections (Suutala, 1999).

Physical Control of Violent Behaviour

The above-mentioned regulations determine what kind of control measures can be directed at an aggressive patient. Staffing and other resources should be considered when responding to violent incidents. On the basis of the Mental Health Act (1116/1990), the right of self-determination of a patient admitted for observation or referred for treatment may be limited, and coercive measures may be used only to the extent necessary for the patient's safety or for the safety of others (§ 22b and 22e).

Compared with some other countries, Finland has very few regulations concerning coercive measures used during psychiatric treatment (Kaltiala-Heino and Välimäki, 1999), and practices vary a great deal from one hospital district to the next (Tuori, 1999). Psychiatric hospitals have hospital-specific guidelines for restraint use and for monitoring and follow-up of restraint use. For instance, the guidelines adopted in the psychiatric division of Tampere University Hospital state that seclusion should be considered in situations where a patient acts in a violent and verbally threatening manner or is otherwise unpredictable or if a patient is dangerous to him/herself or extremely disorderly or agitated. The decision about seclusion is made by a physician (Kuisma, 1999).

Coercive measures during hospitalisation include seclusion (placement in a designated room or mechanical restraint), physical restraint and involuntary medication. The rate of use of seclusion as a method of treatment is relatively high in Finland (Tuori, 1999), because staffing levels rarely permit managing an aggressive patient by physical restraint. In Finland, the nurse to bed ratio in psychiatric hospitals' acute units and long-term wards for difficult-to-treat patients is 1:1, while the ratio in England and Norway is 2-4:1 (Suutala, 2000).

The majority of threatening or violent patients are not mentally ill (Arpo, 1992), which makes interaction a valid point of departure for controlling violence events. However, it is also somewhat unclear how violent patients should be handled; violent incidents rarely lead to a report of an offence (Markkanen, 2000), although it would be necessary in regard to the victim's legal protection. Professional secrecy in health care does not prevent nurses from reporting a crime as it only applies to confidential information entrusted by patients during treatment (Paanila et al, 1993).

If a violent event cannot be resolved by negotiation, the primary recommendation is to summon police assistance (Ministry of Labour, 1994). If the situation is so acute that there is no time to summon police assistance, the above-mentioned law on justifiable self-defence is applicable to the prevention of the attack. It should be noted while protecting oneself that the means of preventing the attack should be as moderate as possible. (Arpo, 1992; Majanen, 2000).

Prevention of Violent Behaviour

Serious attention should be focused on patients' aggressive behaviour and its prevention at workplaces, since the primary responsibility for the safety of patients and staff rests with the employer (Perttu and Söderholmm, 1998). This is also stated in the Occupational Safety and Health Act which requires Finnish employers to consider issues which may predispose employees to occupational accidents or may pose a heath hazard. Employees are thus entitled to as safe and healthy a work environment as possible.

However, the existing Occupational Safety and Health Act in Finland is outdated, since it primarily emphasises the prevention of physical health hazards whereas the current requirement underlines psychological, social and physical wellbeing. The draft of the new Occupational Safety and Health Act was issued at the end of 2001. The draft focuses more clearly on psychological workload and challenge to mental health at work in general. Preparing for violence and threat of violence, harassment and other types of impertinent treatment are a new feature of the law (Ministry of Social Affairs and Health, 2001b).

Prevention is the best way to control violent incidents. The prevention of violent behaviour can be examined from the perspective of risk management as a means of preparing for violent incidents in the health care unit and, on the other hand, by assessing the risks involved in particular situations and particular patients from the perspective of violence prevention (Hietanen and Henriksson, 2002). The perspective on violence prevention is primarily an occupational safety perspective while the perspective associated with individual patients is based on care assessment.

In Finland the Occupational Safety and Health Act (1132/1997) obliges employers to protect the safety and health of employees. The employer is required to monitor the working environment and to take measures to identify and prevent hazardous situations (§ 9). The Occupational Safety and Health Act dating back to 1958 has been changed several times over the years, but violence is still not mentioned as a health risk at work. The Act is currently undergoing total reformation and the report of the occupational safety committee issued last year (Ministry of Social Affairs and Health, 2001c) will serve as the point of departure for the new law which will include a separate paragraph for threat of violence. The paragraph lays out that the employer must determine whether work involves an increased risk of violence and must formulate guidelines for dealing with the possible risk of violence.

The Occupational Health Care Act (1383/2001) states that employers must determine and assess healthiness and safety of work and working conditions (§ 12). The risk of violence should be considered while planning work, work methods and premises and when altering working conditions (§ 12). The main function of occupational health services in the workplace is to conduct workplace analysis, which includes an assessment of the risk of violence. These surveys should be prepared in co-operation with the occupational safety representatives of the workplace (Centre for Occupational Safety, 1987).

The Finnish labour protection authorities became especially interested in workplace violence at the beginning of the 1990s. The Ministry of Labour (1994) issued a manual concerning violent incidents occurring between workers and clients. In regards to health care workplaces, the manual emphasises the importance of the management's and staff's joint and proactive view of safety at work as an important element of good service. The risk of workplace violence should be identified and violent and threatening incidents should be recorded. According to the manual, the most important preventive measures for workplace violence in health care include appropriate staffing, work design, security systems, promotion of the staff's knowledge and skills and planning of functional follow-up care. The latest manual outlining occupational safety in Finland was issued by the Ministry of Social Affairs and Health in 1999 (Ministry of Social Affairs and Health, 1999).

The provincial occupational safety authorities have increasingly emphasised consideration for the risk of violence at workplaces. For instance, the Occupational Safety and Health Inspectorate of Häme (2000) has issued an electronic manual urging employers and employees to devise written safety guidelines for health care workplaces. The guidelines should include issues related to the prevention of workplace violence, directives and responsibilities in case of a violent incident and information on post-incident follow-up care. In addition to this, the Occupational Safety and Health Inspectorate of Häme inspectors visited each social and health care workplace of their region during the year 2000 and provided information about the prevention and post-incident follow-up care of workplace violence (Rissanen, 2000).

A safety planning manual for social and health care units, issued by the Ministry of Social Affairs and Health (2001b), is the latest guide to occupational safety in health care. In regards to the prevention of violent and threatening events, the manual raises concerns about workplace facilities, written safety instructions and staff training. In addition to adequate staffing, attention should be paid to safety technology and equipment. The manual stresses the importance of regular safety surveys and continual development of safety at work on the basis of these. In addition, the Ministry of Social Affairs and Health (2001a) had drafted an occupational safety manual focusing on psychological wellbeing in the workplace.

Increasing violence in health care has prompted staff and the occupational safety units of individual workplaces to develop policies for violence prevention. For instance, the occupational safety unit in the municipal health centre of Vaasa City has initiated the Kauris project which aims at charting the risk of violence and taking measures to better control them. The project involves staff training in the prevention and control of violent incidents and exploration of factors related to the physical environment and security devices (Tolppanen, 2001).

Training nurses to prevent and control violent incidents is closely related to the prevention of violent incidents. The training facilitates staff in early recognition of incidents and in finding ways of resolving them (Saarela and Isotalus, 1998). In Finland, nursing education does not pay enough attention to the specifics of dealing with violent patients (Piispa and Saarela, 2000). Various supplementary training programmes have been developed to help caregivers prevent and control violent incidents. The training has mainly focused on the prevention of patient aggression and on verbal and physical means to deal with aggressive patients (Weizmann-Henelius, 1997).

Over the past years, occupational health stations in health care organisations have paid increasing attention to debriefing following traumatic events (Kuisma, 1994). The purpose of debriefing is to secure the work ability of individuals and teams. Debriefing aims to create a shared perception of the incident in the team and to provide victims of violence tools for understanding and coming to terms with their situation. Debriefing following the incident provides the opportunity to learn from the situation and to contribute to the prevention of further incidents (Suhonen, 1999). Debriefing following a violent incident should focus on the incident, not on finding the guilty party (Vartia and Hyyti, 1999).

As from 1998, the occupational health care services unit at Tampere University Hospital has had an emergency service in place for workers who have had a traumatic experience. Trained workers organise debriefing for employees exposed to violence or threats (Julin et al, 2001). It appears that debriefing following violent incidents is best organised in mental health care (Saarela and Isotalus, 2000b).

In addition to discussions at the workplace, victims should be offered an opportunity to deal with their traumatic experience and related emotions with professional helpers such as occupational health care personnel, clinical supervisors or trauma specialists. A violent incident may sometimes be so traumatic that the worker needs short-term counselling to regain psychological balance (Weizmann-Henelius, 1997).

Despite the various official guidelines for labour protection and the development of support systems for victims of violence in health care workplaces, it seems that these measures still fail to cover all nurses who have experienced violence or threat of violence at work (Markkanen, 2000; Jokimäki, 2001).

Development Prospects and Future Challenges

In Finland, a large number of changes affected the health and working environment of workers over the past decade. Haste and competition influence the work climate. The overall levels of violence in society and drug abuse have increased. The changes have also reverberated in nursing. Although there is no decisive evidence of the rise in violence at workplaces, various statistics and reports clearly point to the increase in violence in service occupations and especially in nursing.

The Finnish literature provides diverse definitions of violence which may cover concrete violent acts and verbal abuse or perceived threat of violence. Nurses are most frequently exposed to violence in mental health care where the assailant is usually a patient. Violence against nursing staff involving a patient's relative is a growing health hazard. Violence always has repercussions for the wellbeing of the victim. Violence in patient situations has been found to be related to mental fatigue, stress and motivation for work. Attention to workplace violence is important also from a quality assurance perspective.

The increase in the number of violent incidents in nursing has, however, not prompted workplaces to take proper precautions. Issues of prevention and management of violent incidents should be included in the curricula of all health care professions. Nursing staff should be aware of existing legislation and guidelines for occupational safety. Special attention should be focused on reducing the risk of violence at the workplace. Clear policies on how the victim of violence and the entire work team can be supported after a violent incident need to be put in place. With violence being a global problem in nursing, the situation also calls for international comparisons and studies of violence. Violence in the nursing workplace is one of the most important areas for future development for Finnish nursing leaders. This does not, however, remove the responsibility of individual nurses: each health care professional should attend to upgrading their skills in taking a stand against violence in the nursing workplace.

References

Act Concerning Health Care Professionals [Laki terveydenhuollon ammattihenkilöistä] 559/1994 http://www.teo.fi

Act on the Status and Rights of Patients. [Laki potilaan asemasta ja oikeuksista] 785/1992 http://www.finlex.edita.fi

Ahokas-Kukkonen, I. (1999) Potilaiden väkivaltaisuus sairaanhoitajan työn arkipäivää: onko meillä keinoja hallita väkivaltatilanteita? *Sairaanhoitaja* 72 (8), 17-18.

Apo, M. and Keskinen, E. (1983) Psykiatristen potilaiden väkivaltaisuus. *Suomen Lääkärilehti* 38, 166-168.

Aromaa, K., Haapaniemi, M., Kinnunen, A. and Koivula, A-K. (1994) Väkivalta työtehtävissä. Työssä koettua väkivaltaa koskevan tutkimushankkeen osaraportti. English Summary: Violence at work. *An interim report on a project concerning violence experienced at work.* Publications 124. National Research Institute of Legal Policy, Helsinki.

Aromaa, K. and Heiskanen, M. (2000) Väkivalta ja uhkailu. In: Heiskanen, M. et al (Eds.) Tapaturmat, väkivalta, rikollisuuden pelko. Väestöhaastattelun tuloksia vuosilta 1980-1997. Justice 2000:1. *Statistics Finland, National Research Institute of Legal Policy*, Helsinki, Finland, 115-134.

Arpo, L. (1992) Väkivaltainen potilas, lääkäri ja laki. *Duodecim* 108, 319-326.

Centre for Occupational Health [Työturvallisuuskeskus] (1987) Terveydenhuoltoalan työsuojeluopas. Helsinki.

Chappel, D. and Di Martino, V. (1998) *Violence at work.* International Labour Office, Geneva.

Ethical Codes for Nurses [Sairaanhoitajan eettiset ohjeet] (1996) *Sairaanhoitaja* 70 (7), 43.

European Agency for Safety and Health at Work. (1999) *Työturvallisuus ja työterveys Euroopassa – Mitä seuraavaksi? Väliraportti: työturvallisuutta, työhygieniaa ja työterveyttä koskeva yhteisön ohjelma (1996-2000).* Työturvallisuutta ja työterveyttä Euroopassa käsitelleen Euroopan Komission seminaarin päätelmät. Luxemburg, 11.12.6.1998. Office of the Official Publications of the European Communities, Luxembourg.

European Agency for Safety and Health at Work (2000a) *Future occupational safety and health research needs and priorities in the member states of the European Union.* Office of the Official Publications of the European Communities, Luxembourg.

European Agency for Safety and Health at Work (2000b) *Research on work-related stress.* Office of the Official Publications of the European Communities, Luxembourg.

European Agency for Safety and Health at Work (2000c) *Työturvallisuuden ja työterveyden tila Euroopan Unionissa – pilottitutkmus. Tutkimusraportin tiivistelmä.* Office of the Official Publications of the European Communities, Luxembourg.

Federation of Accident Insurance Institutions [Tapaturmavakuutuslaitosten liitto] (2000) *Työtapaturma- ja ammattitautitilasto.* Helsinki.

Haapaniemi, M. and Kinnunen, A. (1997) Muuttunut työtilanteiden väkivalta. *Työ ja ihminen* 11, 14-23.

Hakola, P. (1992) Väkivaltaisuuden ennustettavuuden ongelmia. *Duodecim* 108, 311-318.

Hakola, P., Vartiainen H., Hakola, M-L. and Jokela, V. (1990) Mielisairaalapotilaiden tekemät henkirikokset 1954-1988. *Suomen Lääkärilehti* 45, 846-850.

Heiskanen, M. Aromaa, K., Niemi, H. and Sirén R. (2000) Tapaturmat, väkivalta, rikollisuuden pelko. *Väestöhaastattelun tuloksia vuosilta 1980-1997.* Justice 2000:1. Statistics Finland, National Research Institute of Legal Policy, Helsinki.

Hietanen, S. and Henriksson, M. (2002) Kiihtynyt psykoottinen potilas. *Duodecim* 118, 279-284.

Iija, A., Almqvist and S., Kiviharju-Rissanen, U. (1996) *Mielenterveystyön perusteet hoitotyössä.* Kirjayhtymä, Helsinki.

Isotalus, N. and Saarela, K.L. (1997) Väkivaltatilanteet työssä ja keinot turvallisuuden parantamiseksi. *Työ ja ihminen* 11, 35-46.

Isotalus, N. and Saarela, KL. (1999) Väkivaltatapaturmat Suomessa. *Työ ja ihminen* 13, 137-149.

Jankola, K. (1991) *Henkinen väkivalta työelämässä.* Suomen Kaupunkiliitto, Helsinki.

Jokimäki, P. (2001) Väkivalta on arkipäivää hoitotyössä. *Super* 48 (5), 4-7.

Julin, A-M., Kuronen, M., Oksa, L., Roihankorpi, T. Sorri, P. and Yli-Koivisto, M. (2001) *Työnohjauksen koordinointi.* The Publication Series of Pirkanmaa Hospital District 4/2001. Pirkanmaa Hospital District, Tampere.

Junnila, S. and Kytölä, J. (1990) Joka toinen terveyskeskuksen työntekijä uhkailujen kohteena. *Suomen Lääkärilehti* 45, 626-632.

Kaltiala-Heino, R. and Välimäki, M. (1999) Esipuhe. In: Kaltiala-Heino, R. and Välimäki, M. (Eds.). *Rajoitetaanko rajoittamista – eristys ja lepositeet psykiatrisessa hoidossa.* Publications 2. University of Tampere, Tampere School of Public Health, Tampere, 1-3.

Keckman-Koivuniemi, H. (1999) *Jäsentutkimus -99.* Tampereen yliopisto, Politiikan tutkimuksen laitos, Suomen sairaanhoitajaliitto, Helsinki.

Keeler, L. (Ed.) (2001) Recommendations of the EU: *expert meeting on violence against women.* Reports of the Ministry of Social Affairs and Health 13. Ministry of Social Affairs and Health, Helsinki.

Kivimäki, M., Elovainio, M. and Vahtera, J. (2000) Workplace bullying and sickness absence in hospital staff. *Occupational and Environmental Medicine* 57, 656-660.

Kokko, P. (2000) Väkivaltainen potilas. Oikeudellisia näkökohtia. In: Kosken-vuo, K. (Eds.). *Lääkärintyö ja laki.* Duodecim, Helsinki, 93-99.

Kuisma, J. (1999) Eristäminen väkivallan ennaltaehkäisynä. In: Kaltiala-Heino, R. and Välimäki, M. (Eds.). *Rajoitetaanko rajoittamista – eristys ja lepositeet psykiatrisessa hoidossa.* Publications 2. University of Tampere, Tampere School of Public Health, Tampere, 68-73.

Laaksonen, K. (2000) Mitä kaikkea sairaanhoitajat jaksavat? *Sairaanhoitaja* 73 (3), 6-7.

Laine, M. and Wickström G. (2000) Sosiaali- ja terveysala. In: Kauppinen, T. et al (Eds.). *Työ ja terveys Suomessa v. 2000.* Finnish Institute of Occupational Health, Helsinki, 211-215.

Laitinen, H. (2000a) Tapaturmat ja fyysinen väkivalta. In: Piirainen, H. et al *Työ ja terveys – haastattelututkimus v. 2000.* Taulukkoraportti. Finnish Institute of Occupational Health, Helsinki, 14.

Laitinen, H. 2000b Työympäristö. Tapaturmavaarat. In: Kauppinen, T. et al (Eds.). *Työ ja terveys Suomessa v. 2000.* Finnish Institute of Occupational Health, Helsinki, 36-39.

Lakanen, T. (1999) *Virkamiehen väkivaltainen vastustaminen.* Lakimiesliiton kustannus, Helsinki.

Latvala, E., Visuri, T. and Janhonen, S. (1996) *Psykiatrinen hoitotyö.* WSOY, Helsinki.

Lehto, A-M. and Sutela, H. (1999) *Tehokas, tehokkaampi, uupunut. Työolotut-kimuksen tuloksia 1977-1997.* Labour Market 1998:12. Statistics Finland, Helsinki.

Leymann, H. (1992) *Från mobbning till utslagning i arbetslivet.* Publica, Stock-holm.

Majanen, M. (2000) Lääkäri väkivallan kohteena – lainopillisia näkökulmia. *Suomen Lääkärilehti* 55, 1757-1760.

Majasalmi, P. (2001) *Selvitys työpaikkaväkivallasta sosiaali- ja terveydenhuol-lossa.* Super ry, Helsinki.

Markkanen, K. (2000) Nimittely, uhkailu, potkiminen – hoitajan työarkea. Selvitys hoitohenkilökunnan työpaikallaan kokemasta väkivallasta ja sen uhasta. *Julkaisusarja B: selvityksiä* 3/2000, Tehy ry, Helsinki.

Mental Health Act [Mielenterveyslaki] 1116/1990 http://www.finlex.fi

Ministry of Labour [Työministeriö] (1994) *Työpaikkaväkivallan ehkäisy. Työn-tekijöiden ja asiakkaiden välisten väkivaltatilanteiden hallinnan opas.* Minis-try of Labour, Tampere.

Ministry of Labour [Työministeriö] (2001) *Employment bulletin of the Finnish Ministry of Labour.* April 2001. Helsinki.

Ministry of Social Affairs and Health [Sosiaali- ja terveysministeriö] (1999) *Occupational Safety and Health in Finland. Brochure 1999:7.* Ministry of Social Affairs and Health, Helsinki.

Ministry of Social Affairs and Health [Sosiaali- ja terveysministeriö] (2001a) *Henkinen hyvinvointi työpaikalla. Työsuojeluoppaita ja -ohjeita 24.* Ministry of Social Affairs and Health, Helsinki.

Ministry of Social Affairs and Health [Sosiaali- ja terveysministeriö] (2001b) *Turvallisuussuunnitteluopas sosiaali- ja terveydenhuollon toimintayksiköille.* [Safety planning manual for social welfare and health care functional units]. Handbooks of the Ministry of Social Affairs and Health 2001:2. Helsinki.

Ministry of Social Affairs and Health [Sosiaali- ja terveysministeriö] (2001c) *Työturvallisuuslakitoimikunnan mietintö. Komiteamietintö 2001:13.* [Report of the Committee on the Revision of the Occupational Safety and Health Act. Committee report 2001:13]. Ministry of Social Affairs and Health, Helsinki.

National Agency for Medicines and Social Insurance Institute [Suomen Lääkelaitos ja Kansaneläkelaitos]. *2000 Finnish Statistics on Medicines* [Suomen lääketilasto]. National Agency for Medicines and Social Insurance Institute, Helsinki.

National Public Health Institute [Kansanterveyslaitos] (2001) *HIV-infektio Suomessa. Tartunnan saaneiden ikä tartunnan toteamisvuonna. 8.8.2001 mennessä ilmoitettujen tapausten kertymä.* Kansanterveyslaitos. Infektioepidemiologian osasto, Helsinki. http://www.ktl.ttr/hivika

Nuutila, A-M. (1997) Rikoslain yleinen osa. Lakimiesliiton Kustannus, Helsinki.

Occupational Health Care Act [Työterveyshuoltolaki] 1383/2001 http://www.finlex.fi

Occupational Safety and Health Act [Työturvallisuuslaki] 299/1958, 1132/1997. http://www.finlex.fi

Occupational Safety and Health Inspectorate of Häme [Hämeen työsuojelupiiri] (2000) *Fyysisen työpaikkaväkivallan ennakointi ja jälkihoito.* Ennaltaehkäisyn mahdollisuuksia. http://www.doshnet.fi

Paananen, S. and Notkola, V. (2000) Summary and concluding remarks [Yhteenveto ja päätelmät]. In: Paananen, S. (Ed.). *Dangers at work – Perceived occupational diseases, accidents and violence at work in 1999.* [Työnvaarat 1999. Koetut työperäiset sairaudet, työtapaturmat ja työväkivaltatapaukset]. Labour Market 2000(Piispa and Saarela:15. Statistics Finland, Helsinki, 91-104.

Paanila, J., Eronen, M., Tiihonen, J. and Hakola, P. (1993) Virkamiehet tarvitsevat lain erityissuojaa väkivaltaa vastaan. *Suomen Lääkärilehti* 48, 1035-1041.

Penal Code [Rikoslaki] 39/1889 http://www.finlex.fi

Perttu, S. and Söderholm A-L. (1998) *Väkivaltaa kokeneiden auttaminen. Opas ammattihenkilöstölle.* Handbooks of the Ministry of Social Affairs and Health 1998:1 [Sosiaali- ja terveysministeriö. Oppaita 1998:1]. Helsinki.

Piirainen, H., Elo, A.L., Kankaanpää, E., Laitinen, H., Lindström, K., Luopajärvi, Mäkelä, P., Pohjanpää, K. and Riala, R. (1997) *Työ- ja terveys – haastattelututkimus v. 1997.* Taulukkoraportti. Finnish Institute of Occupational Health, Helsinki.

Piirainen, H., Elo, A-L., Hirvonen, M., Kauppinen, K., Ketola, R., Laitinen, H., Lindström, K., Reijula, K., Riala, R., Viluksela, M. and Virtanen, S. (2000) *Työ ja terveys – haastattelututkimus v. 2000.* Taulukkoraportti, Finnish Institute of Occupational Health, Helsinki.

Piispa, M. and Saarela, K.L. (2000) Työväkivalta. In: Paananen, S. (Ed.). Työnvaarat 1999. *Koetut työperäiset sairaudet, työtapaturmat ja työväkivaltatapaukset.* Labour Market 2000:15. Statistics Finland, Helsinki, 33-44.

Putkonen, A. and Paanila, J. (1996) *Vuonna 1994 Niuvanniemen sairaalaan lähetetyt vaaralliset ja vaikeahoitoiset potilaat.* Suomen Lääkärilehti 51, 1053-1059.

Quine, L. (1999) Workplace bullying in NHS community trust: a staff questionnaire survey. *BMJ* 318, 228-232.

Rissanen, A-L. (2000) Työpaikkaväkivalta lisääntyy – vai lisääntyykö? *Super* 47 (9), 19-21.

Saarela, K.L. (1999) Fyysinen väkivalta ja uhkatilanteet työssä. In: Huuhtanen P. et al (Eds.) *Työ vuonna 2005 – näkymiä suomalaiseen työelämään.* Finnish Institute of Occupational Health, Helsinki.

Saarela, K.L. and Isotalus N. (1998) Väkivalta uhkana työpaikoilla. *Hyvinvointikatsaus* 3, 25-30.

Saarela, K.L and Isotalus, N. (2000a) Väkivaltatilanteet ja niihin varautuminen terveydenhuollossa. *Suomen Lääkärilehti* 55, 3323-3326.

Saarela, K.L. and Isotalus, N. (2000b) *Väkivalta- ja uhkatilanteiden ehkäisy Helsingin kaupungin työpaikoilla.* Finnish Institute of Occupational Health, City of Helsinki, The Finnish Work Environmental Fund 99160, Unpublished report 29.2.2000, Helsinki.

Salminen, S. (1997) Fyysinen väkivalta työpaikoilla 1988. *Työ ja ihminen* 11, 5-13.

Sirén, R. (2000) Turvallisuusindikaattori. Tapaturman ja väkivallan vaara – fyysisen turvallisuuden indikaattoreita. In: Heiskanen, M. et al (Eds.) *Tapaturmat, väkivalta, rikollisuuden pelko. Väestöhaastattelun tuloksia vuosilta 1980-1997.* Justice 2000:1. Statistics Finland, National Research Institute of Legal Policy, Helsinki, 19-30.

Social Insurance Institute (2001) *Kansaneläkelaitoksen sairausvakuutus- ja perhe-etuustilastot 2000. Kansaneläkelaitoksen julkaisuja T11:12.* Tilastoryhmä. Kansaneläkelaitos, Helsinki.

Statistics Finland [Tilastokeskus] (2001) *Statistical Yearbook of Finland 2001.* [Suomen tilastollinen vuosikirja 2001] Otava, Keuruu.

Suhonen, H. (1999) Väkivalta- ja muiden ahdistavien tilanteiden jälkipuinti työyhteisössä. *Työterveyslääkäri* 17 (3), 312-313.

Sutela, H. and Lehto, A-M. (1998) Henkinen väkivalta on koko työyhteisön ongelma. *Hyvinvointikatsaus* 3, 18-24.

Suutala, H. (1999) Pakkotoimet ja ihmisoikeudet Euroopassa. In: Kaltiala-Heino, R. and Välimäki, M. (Eds.). *Rajoitetaanko rajoittamista – eristys ja lepositeet psykiatrisessa hoidossa.* Publications 2. University of Tampere, Tampere School of Public Health, Tampere, 25-33.

Suutala, H. (2000) Katsaus mielenterveyspotilaan hoitoa koskeviin normistoihin. In: Välimäki, M., Holopainen, A. and Jokinen, M. *Psykiatrinen hoitotyö muutoksessa,* WSOY, Helsinki, 104-119.

Söderholm, A-L, Piispa, M and Heiskanen, M. (1999) Sairaanhoitajan työssä kokema väkivalta ja häirintä. *Suomen Lääkärilehti* 54, 4257-4261.

Tiihonen, J. (1999) Oikeuspsykiatria. In: Lönnqvist, J., Heikkinen, M., Henriksson, M., Marttunen, M. and Partonen, T. (Eds.). *Psykiatria.* Duodecim, Helsinki.

Tolppanen, M. (2001) Hoitajat pelkäävät tulla töihin. *Tehy* 18, 14-16.

Tuori, T. (1999) Pakkotoimenpiteet Suomen psykiatrisissa sairaaloissa vuonna 1996. In: Kaltiala-Heino, R. and Välimäki, M. (Eds.). *Rajoitetaanko rajoittamista – eristys ja lepositeet psykiatrisessa hoidossa.* Publications 2. University of Tampere, Tampere School of Public Health, Tampere, 68-73.

Vartia, M. and Hyyti, J. (1999) Väkivalta vankeinhoitotyössä: fyysisen ja henkisen väkivallan kohtaaminen vankeinhoidossa. Oikeusministeriön vankeinhoito-osaston julkaisuja 1/1999. Ministry of Justice, Finnish Institute of Occupational Health, Helsinki.

Vartia, M. and Perkka-Jortikka, K. (1994) *Henkinen väkivalta työpaikoilla.* Gaudeamus, Tampere.

Viitanen, R. (1998) Nuorisotyöttömyys ja nuorison syrjäytymisen riskit. *Hyvinvointikatsaus* 4, 2-7.

Vuori-Kemilä, A. (2000) Uhkaavasti käyttäytyvän asiakkaan kohtaaminen. In: Saarelainen, M., Stengård, E. and Vuori-Kemilä, A. (Eds.). *Mielenterveys- ja päihdetyö: yhteistyötä ja kumppanuutta.* WSOY, Porvoo, 167-176.

Weizmann-Henelius, G. (1997) *Väkivaltaisen ihmisen kohtaaminen.* Kirjayhtymä, Helsinki.

Weizmann-Henelius, G. and Suutala H. (2000) Violence in a Finnish forensic psychiatric hospital. *Nord J of Psychiatry* 54, 269-273.

Wickström, G., Laine, M., Pentti, J., Elovainio, M. and Lindström, K. (2000) *Työolot ja hyvinvointi sosiaali- ja terveysalalla – muutokset 1990-luvulla.* Finnish Institute of Occupational Health, Helsinki.

Wynne, R. (2000) *Guidance on the prevention of violence at work.* Office for Official Publications of the European Communities. Luxembourg.

Chapter Four: Violence in Nursing in two African Countries

Leana R Uys and Rhosta S Gcaba

Introduction

The African Region of the World Health Organisation comprises 47 countries of which 29 are classified as least developed (Torquist, 1997). This means that 57% of all least developed countries of the world are found in this region. The World Health Development Report of 1997 shows that in Africa the average population per doctor is 16 659, the rate of population per nurse is 7 601. Coupled with the Primary Health Care approach that has been widely accepted as the health service delivery paradigm for the continent, this puts the nurse in the position of front line health worker in most settings.

Nurses form the bulk of health workers in entry-services which interfaces directly with the environment of health services, such as clinics, casualty department and outpatient departments. This makes them easy targets for violence spilling over from the community into health services. Nurses also work most intimately with patients for extended periods of time, in settings such as residences for the mentally ill, mentally retarded and frail old people. In such settings the potential for violence against patients are high, due to the vulnerability of the patients and the relative isolation of the services from scrutiny. Lastly, since many nurses are women, they are often the victims of violence (Ogale, 2000). Nurses therefore frequently meet with violence.

Aggression refers to all behaviour by which one person administers negative stimuli to another person with the aim of doing damage. It can be verbal or physical, direct or indirect, and active or passive. In contrast, violence refers only to behaviour which leads to actual physical damage being done to people or things (Singer, 1971). Ryan and Poster did a series of studies on the results of physical assaults on nurses, and their criteria for physical assault were physical contact, and an intention to harm (1989).

Capozzoli and McVey (1996) discuss workplace violence, its causes and prevention. They classify workplace violence according to the perpetrator (employees, former employees and non-employees), and according to where the conflict originated and was played out (originated outside the workplace, but took place inside; originated inside and took place inside; originated inside, but took place outside).

Literature Survey

In many studies violence has been shown to be an integral part of the nursing experience (Ryan and Poster, 1989). Such studies have not often been done in African countries. One can, however, expect this to be true also of nursing in Africa.

The continent is still experiencing high levels of political unrest, which spill over from communities surrounding clinics and hospitals. Yach (1992) describes the situation in South African townships during the height of the anti-apartheid struggle. Nurses in strife-torn communities had to make alternative transport arrangements due to personal danger on their way to work, and since many services did not function, the ones which were still working were overloaded by work. Gcaba (1997) took this further and showed in her survey that political violence impacted on nurses in their community settings. She found that the violence impacted negatively on the nurses' family life and work life. Some nurses lost homes, possessions and family members. Work became difficult when systems ceased to function effectively, leaving the nurse in the front line without adequate support. Zimu (1991) interviewed nurses who had been subjected to political violence over a long period of time, and found that they associated it with threat, strain, insecurity, fear and lack of concentration. She showed that the health service authorities did little or nothing to ensure the safety of nurses in dangerous areas, and had no policies to guide nurses through difficult situations.

But it is not only political violence which plays itself out in the lives of nurses. In an unpublished study by Middleton (1993) it was found that 51% of a sample of nurses working in a South African psychiatric hospital were assaulted at least once, and 6% were assaulted more than ten times. There is only one maximum security psychiatric unit in South Africa. This means that nurses are often exposed to this kind of danger. In a later study Ganga-Limando (1995) found that 36% of the aggression of violent psychiatric patients were directed against the staff, and that in 12% of the incidents a person was physically injured. Again it was found that the support and guidance given by the managers of these services were inadequate.

Research Methodology

A survey was done in two African countries to explore the types and context of violence in nursing to highlight the issue of violence and identify preventative strategies and policies to limit such incidents.

It is important to describe the extent and characteristics of violence in the nursing workplace. Without such description it is impossible to put in place preventative measures and policies for the effective handling of violence.

The specific objectives of the study were as follows:

1. Describe the settings, types and role-players in violence against nurses and patients.
2. Compare and contrast the context and components of such violence occurring in different settings.
3. Analyse the results of such violence on individuals, groups and services.
4. Describe preventative strategies and policies and procedures for handling incidents of violence.

To undertake this mail survey two questionnaires was sent and distributed on a convenient basis to rural and urban nurses. Since little is known about the prevalence and character of the problem in the African context, it was thought to be important to do an exploratory survey to describe the problem. Further studies can then be designed to explore specific aspects of violence in depth. Only Nigeria and South Africa were involved in this study, based on the availability of email contact with potential researchers in the countries, as well as the use of English. Although more than half of the African countries speak French, time and resources did not allow for all the documentation to be translated into French and for communication between researchers to take place in that language.

The questionnaires were sent only to clinical settings, although other nurses who wished to complete the questionnaires were not excluded. In each setting the nurse administrator was asked to request five to seven volunteers to complete each type of questionnaire. Every volunteer was asked to complete only one of the instruments after reading the accompanying letter explaining the research. Questionnaires were mailed directly to the researcher in each country.

Each questionnaire consists of six items dealing with demographic information, and 11 items dealing with the experience of violence and opinions about causes, results, prevention and policies. A mix of open-ended and closed items was used to ask nurses about their experience of violence. The closed items were mainly multiple-option items. The instruments were developed based on the literature, and were then discussed with a small group of research experts.

The final sample consisted of four groups, two from Nigeria and two from South Africa. The first sample refers to the two groups of nurses who completed the questionnaire on violence towards patients, and the second sample to the two groups who completed the questionnaire on violence against nurses. Sample one (n= 139) had 52% urban nurses and 22% male nurses, while in sample two (n=126) 48% were urban and 8% male. The age of sample one ranged from 22 to 64 years, with an average of 38 years, and the respondents had an average of 10 years of school, and 4 years of nursing education. Their work experience averaged 12 years, on average. Sample two ranged from 23 to 65 years, with an average of 40. They had an average of 11 years of school, 3 years of nursing education, and ten years of nursing experience.

Table one: Work settings of nurses in both samples.

SETTING	NIGERIA				SOUTH AFRICA				TOTAL	
	Patients		Nurses		Patients		Nurses			
	F*	%	F	%	F	%	F	%	F	%
Clinic or health station	8	10	9	16	14	23	20	28	51	19
Community Health Centre	10	13	10	18	11	18	7	10	38	14
Small hospital	6	8	3	6	20	32	19	27	48	18
Regional hospital	20	26	20	36	3	5	18	25	61	23
Academic, central or specialist hospital	20	26	3	6	7	11	7	10	37	14
Training institution	2	3	0	0	0	0	0	0	2	1
Central office of health services	1	1	0	0	1	2	0	0	2	1
Psychiatric hospital	10	13	10	18	5	8	0	0	25	9
TOTAL	77		55		62		71		265	

F = Frequency

The work settings in which the nurses of both samples worked, are summarised in table 1. In Nigeria sample one consisted mainly from nurses working in regional and specialist hospitals (40%), while in South Africa the majority worked in clinics or small hospitals (55%). In sample two nurses from regional hospitals dominated in the Nigerian group, and South Africa there was a spread in a number of services.

Violence against Patients

Table two: Perpetrators of Violence against Patients

PERPETRATOR	NIGERIA				SOUTH AFRICA				TOTAL	
	Patients		Nurses		Patients		Nurses			
	F	%	F	%	F	%	F	%	F	%
Senior nurses	10	15	4	8	2	5	4	9	20	10
Junior nurses	3	4	1	2	9	23	1	2	14	7
Administrative clerks	1	2	3*	6	4	10	10	23	18	9
Security guards	15	22	-	-	3	8	-	-	18	9
Doctors	8	12	7	13	3	8	3	7	21	10
Allied health professionals	1	2	-	-	1	3	-	-	2	1
Acquaintances of the pt from outside the service	16	24	9	17	7	18	6	14	38	19
People from outside who do not know pt or nurse	6	16	1	2	2	5	2	5	11	5
Patients	5	7	20	38	4	10	16	37	45	22
Health care assistants	3	4	-	-	3	8	-	-	6	3
Friends or relatives of the nurse	-	-	8	15	1	3	1	2	10	5
TOTAL	68		53		39		43		203	

* In the questionnaire dealing with violence against nurses, different subordinates of the nurse was not identified separately.

Of the 139 nurses who completed this questionnaire 97 (70%) reported having witnessed violence against patients, with 83% of Nigerian respondents and 53% of South African respondents reporting such incidents. Not all the respondents identified the perpetrators, but some listed more than one category. According to table 2, junior nurses are the main nursing culprits in South Africa, while senior nurses are more violent in Nigeria. Security guards and people from outside the service seem to be a greater problem in Nigeria, while administrative clerks are a problem in South Africa.

The qualitative descriptions of violence was classified into a number of themes. The quotes from respondents are given in italics, and the reference behind each quote refers to the country (1= Nigeria, 2= South Africa) and the second figure to the respondent.

The intolerant nurse or doctor

Doctor smacking a patient in labour who was crying loudly (2.94).
Nurse abusing geriatric patient who soiled bed linen (2.78).

These descriptions usually refer to a health worker verbally abusing a patient, and administering smacks, pushes, and pulls to patients. Respondents speculate about a number of possible causes, such as stress from overwork, substance abuse and a wrong attitude.

Because of their military style training health workers have a low tolerance for disobedience (1.13)
Some male health workers come on duty having had substances the previous day and therefore cannot tolerate any misbehaviour from patients (2.113).

The South African sample described a category of violence which was classified as negligence. Here is one example:

The doctor did not give due care to a patient who had a caesarean section under ineffective epidural anaesthesia. I (the nurse) told the anaesthetist, but he did no do anything. The patient was in severe pain for the whole operation (2.90).

This category includes behaviour that causes the patient pain or injury, even though it was done in the process of giving care or treatment. Clearly, if health professionals act without due care or respect, their actions become violent. In this regard the observations of one respondent need to be pointed out:

In this rural hospital blacks were labelled as people who tolerated any pain. Furthermore, even the matron, who was black, was so submissive to the whites who happened to be doctors, that she did not do anything (2.94).

This element of racism in the violence directed against patients, may not be peculiar to Africa, but it is still seen as a prevalent problem.

The South African respondents also referred to destruction of property and neglecting of patients during a strike. They pointed out that the strike action was sometimes related to political violence.

Patients on continuous oxygen had it discontinued, and nurses ate patient's food instead of serving it during the strike (2.96).

Administrative staff and security guards on strike threw stones at the clinic building. Patients ran and left the clinic without treatment (2.99).

The aggressive security guard

Gateman beating the patient to force him back to the ward when the patient wanted to abscond (1.2)

Security guard hitting patient on the head because the patient had been smoking dagga (marijuana) in the ward *(2.84)*.

The violence demonstrated by security staff of the hospital or policemen guarding prisoners hospitalised for treatment seemed to be of a much more serious nature. It consisted of beatings, kicking and dragging. Respondents saw the threat of this category of workers loosing their jobs, if patients absconded or were allowed to damage property, as the main cause for this type of violence. However, one incident of a security guard raping a patient was also noted.

Serious violence was also sometimes caused by nurses. One respondent described an incident of a nurse beating a patient in the face to the extent that fractures were caused.

Angry community members

A patient was shot by hired men of the underworld, then they came back to the hospital to make sure he is completely dead (1.34).

The patient's husband attacking her because she contracted HIV/AIDS. (1.14).

There were many incidents described where relatives became involved in abusing their own family members, sometimes due to a conflict that had originated outside of the hospital. Many times, however, the violence came from criminal elements. These people were either criminally involved with the patient prior to admission, or they ran criminal scams inside the hospital, such as offering to go and buy goods for the patient at the shop, without any intention of ever returning with either money or goods.

Fighting among patients were frequently mentioned. They fought about cigarettes, money and other possessions. More often though, were descriptions of mentally ill patients who became aggressive and then met with violence by the staff.

In self-defence a nurse may attack back when a patient wants to maim her (1.4).
Patient's relations were seen on several occasions beating their relation who was disturbing them or others around them (1.3).
Mental patient who was violent was restricted with shackles thereby causing him injuries (1.6).

Violence against Nurses[*]

Of the 126 nurses who completed this questionnaire, 79 (63%) had experienced violence against nurses in the workplace, with 80% of Nigerian respondents and 49% of South African respondents reporting such incidents. The main perpetrators of violence against nurses were the patients (38% on average in the two countries) (Table 2). Except for patients and their relatives, the main category of worker involved in violence in South Africa (23% of incidents), were subordinates of nurses, such as administrative clerks and security guards. In Nigeria, relatives or friends of the nurse were the next most frequent offenders (15% of incidents).

The following are typical incidents described by respondents:

Criminals: One evening a man was rushed into A&E unit. In the course of his resuscitation, even though the hospital gate was locked and people were searched before they pass through the gate, suddenly four men with guns and axes surrounded the patient's bed and wanted to take the patient with them to kill him (1.37).
People from outside handcuffed the security guard, the police officer guarding the prisoner and the nurses to get rid of the car theft evidence (2.65).
Other health workers: A house officer slapping a nursing sister due to corrections given to him over the wrong dosage of drug (1.39).
Admitting clerk hit the nurse stating that the nurse was gossiping about him (2.30).
Relatives: I was assaulted because a patients' relation said I did not set up an IV line which auxiliary nurses do in private hospitals, so I caused the mother's death (1.38).

---

[*] In the questionnaire dealing with violence against nurses, different subordinates of the nurse was not identified separately.

Patient's relatives demanded that I transfer the patient to hospital from the clinic. There was no indication, but when they started breaking the lockers and removing the fire extinguishers from their places, I just sent the patient off, since they also had guns (2.95).

Respondents saw the violence caused by doctors as being the result of a superiority complex, and differences in status between nurses and doctors. The violence coming from relatives were ascribed to their stress levels, as well as the inability of nurses to perform to the standards expected by the community in settings with too few staff and other resources.

The violence caused by psychiatric patients against nurses, other patients and property was of a very serious nature, and was often unprovoked and unexpected. These incidents of violence was mostly handled by counter-violence from nurses and security staff, or by medication. The only preventative measures mentioned by nurses consisted of appointing more male nurses in these settings, improving the training of nurses to handle such incidents and better security.

Table three: Perceived Causes of Violence

CAUSES	NIGERIA				SOUTH AFRICA				TOTAL	
	Patient		Nurse		Patient		Nurse			
	F	%	F	%	F	%	F	%	F	%
Threat to job or employment	4	5	1	2	1	2	-	-	6	3
Threat to self or others	14	16	5*	10	3	7	8	18	30	13
Interpersonal conflict: work	13	15	14	37	5	11	11	25	43	19
Interpersonal conflict: home	5	6	3	6	8	18	4	9	20	9
Substance abuse	8	9	8	15	7	16	7	16	30	13
Mental illness	2	2	11	21	3	7	10	23	26	12
Overload stress	24	28	6	12	7	16	4	9	41	18
Intolerance	10	11	1	2	6	14	-	-	17	8
Job dissatisfaction	2	2	-	-	2	5	-	-	4	2
Crime, personality, witchcraft	5	6	3	6	-	-	-	-	8	4
Negligence	-	-	-	-	2	5	-	-	2	1
TOTAL	87		52		44		44		227	

* Incidents of nurses getting hurt when breaking up a fight is included in this category.

Patient smashed the nurse's radio and beat her up to the point that she had a compound fracture (1.46)
Patient A was sleeping when patient B gave him a blow on the head (1.49).

The multiple choice item asking respondents about the causes of the violence was interpreted carefully, taking into account their description of the violence and their motivation for the cause they gave. The range of causes identified is summarised in table 3. Some respondents listed no causes, while others listed more than one.

With regard to violence against patients, overload stress is a cause often mentioned by nurses from both countries. Nigerian nurses also see the patient as a threat to him or herself or others and interpersonal conflict at work as major causes, while South African nurses see substance abuse and interpersonal conflict at home as the next most common causes.

With regard to violence towards nurses, interpersonal conflict at work was the main cause with mental illness coming a close second.

Responses and Results

The first response from the reporting nurse can be classified as doing nothing, verbal intervention, reporting and/or calling for assistance. Only the South African sample mentioned calling security to come to help.

Doing nothing: I just watched with pity (1.13).
Verbal intervention: I advised that such restraint was unnecessary (1.1).
   I pleaded with the person concerned (1.4)
   Counselled the person concerned (2.100)
   I told the doctors their behaviour was unacceptable (2.94).
Reporting: The matter was reported to the Superintendent (2.85).
   I wrote a report to the management (1.38).
Calling for assistance: Called security to help (2.84).

The response from others also included all the above categories of action. However, it also included problem solving.

In a case where a women was operated on with inadequate anaesthetic, the theatre policy was changed to make is impossible for this to happen again (1.11).

It should also be pointed out that in many cases of serious violence, such as the rape incident, no action was taken by higher authorities. When something was done, it often included using the formal disciplinary process, reporting to the regulatory body or to the police.

The incidents all left the respondents with negative feelings such as anger, fear, shock, insecurity and guilt. The only positive result was that it called for courageous behaviour from the nurses, such as reporting perpetrators of violence, and it motivated nurses to intervene in caring ways.

A nurse pulled the hair of a patient in labour and shouted at her to push harder. I did nothing the first two times, but the third time I asked the nurse to explain to the nurse supervisor how she conducted the delivery. She did not say everything and I told the supervisor what she had done (2. 93).

When nurses reported incidents, it sometimes led to victimisation.

I was black-balled by the workers and my community for reporting the doctor and making him angry(1.11).

The incidents described above show that, in almost all respects, respondents mentioned only negative results for patients and the service. However, in terms of abuse of psychiatric patients to control their behaviour, one respondent remarked:

The system seems well suited with that service. In fact, it does not seem odd to handle patients that way (1.13).

Prevention

Respondents were given a list of mechanisms suggested to prevent violence in the workplace, and they were first asked whether these were in place in their setting, and secondly whether they though the mechanisms would have helped if they had been in place during the incident. From the responses are summarised in table 4. It would seem that in Nigeria the utilisation of these mechanisms range from 16 (21%) of respondents perceiving legal steps against perpetrators to be used, to 31 (40%) perceiving screening, discipline of employees and supervisor's training to be in place. In South Africa disciplining of employees is perceived to be the most common deterrent (27 or 44%), whilst creating a crisis management team is the least common (11 or 18%).

In their qualitative answers respondents listed many avenues to be explored in order to prevent violence against patients. These included putting appropriate policies in place, measures to increase job satisfaction, improving training and security and giving adequate attention to patient welfare issues. The suggestion that improving patient welfare might help was mentioned only by the Nigerian sample, where it was indicated that patients were put out of beds forcibly because of non-payment of hospital bills.

Table four: Mechanisms to Prevent Violence in the Workplace.

MECHANISM	NIGERIA		SOUTH AFRICA	
	F in place	F useful	F in place	F useful
Screening employees more thoroughly	31	38	25	26
Providing assistance with personal problems	30	41	26	32
Discipline employees timeously	31	29	27	27
Put adequate security procedures in place	24	46	22	34
Create a crisis management plan for violent events	21	39	11	32
Train staff in violence control	20	44	16	34
Train supervisor/managers	31	34	26	32
Take legal steps against perpetrators	16	30	26	32
TOTAL RESPONSES	77	77	62	62

Policies: Policies to prevent violence should be in place (2.103).
Job satisfaction: Make sure that all that is needed to carry out duties are provided (1.24). Employ more workers when there is more work (1.27).
Training: Provide adequate training and incentives to enable nurses to handle such violent situations with wisdom (1.13).

In-service education on the patient charter and the bill of human rights (2.91). Patients should be educated on the procedures of the hospital, their rules and regulations (1.51).
Security: Employ enough security and make sure they function (1.69).

Adequate protection for the nurses such as good lighting systems, well secured doors and windows (1.56).
Patient welfare issues: Some genuinely poor patients should be accorded pauper status (1.25)

The social worker should intervene in non-payment of hospital bills (1.40).

Perceived Violence

Although the definition of violence was given, many respondents described incidents that reflected verbal aggression rather than violence. Since these incidents were clearly felt to be actions of violence by the respondents, they need to be included to give a complete picture of their experience. Some examples of verbal aggression are:

The matron shouted at the staff nurse, who continued with her work. This infuriated the matron and she rained abuse on the nurse (1.36).
The administrative clerk rained abuses on the patient for demanding receipts of payments made (1.40).

Passive aggressive behaviour to punish nurses or patients were often described.

A husband refused to pay for blood which had been given to his wife without his permission, so the nurse had to pay for it (1.13).
The patient had left his OPD card at home and had no money to pay. He was made to wait in the queue until all other patients were done. He was even left when the particular clerk went for tea and lunch (2.110).

Discussion

The study sample had a number of limitations. Firstly, the samples are too small too really represent the nurses of whole countries. For instance, in South Africa there were 90 923 nurses on the registers in 1997 (SANC). Clearly, the 126 in this sample are not representative of this group, especially since it was not a random sample. Furthermore, the two countries cannot be used to extrapolate to the rest of Africa. Both are anglophone countries, and both fall into the more developed group, which does not represent the total continent. Secondly, the samples from Nigeria and South Africa differed in terms of their work settings. The Nigerian sample were drawn more from regional, central and psychiatric hospitals, while the South African sample came mainly from primary health care settings and small hospitals. Since the samples were stratified with regard to settings, this does represent the work settings in the two countries, but the differences in settings might have influenced their experience of violence. The differences between the two countries should therefore be interpreted very carefully, and be seen as indicators for future research, rather than firm facts.

Comparing the average percentages of nurses who experienced violence (70% against patients and 63% against nurses), there is a wide difference between the two countries, with the South African sample reporting on average 30% less violence than the Nigerian sample. This might be because the South African sample is so heavily drawn from smaller hospitals and primary health care services, and there might be less violence in these settings. In primary health care settings there are usually only nurses, and this means that the categories of violence between nurses and other health workers, is limited. The Nigerians seem to be closer to the international figures. While 85% of Australian nurses have been the target of patient aggression and 76% of psychiatric nurses in the USA report similar experiences, the average in this study is rather low (Holden, 1985; Poster and Ryan, 1994).

The perpetrators of violence are mainly staff members, with senior nurses and doctors, as well as security guards and administrative clerks being almost equal contributors. Patients and people who know the patient also contribute to the violence. The situation in Nigeria with regard to security guards needs further scrutiny. Firstly, this group is heavily involved in violence against patients (Table 2), and the incidents described often involve serious violence. Seemingly, this is because they have to prevent confused patients from escaping, and are in danger of loosing their jobs if they fail (Table 3). It is also interesting to note that Nigerian respondents very rarely deal with violence by calling on the security guards to assist, while in the South African sample it happens frequently. It may be that in the Nigerian setting security guards are more often used only as "gatemen" rather than security personnel with a wider and more positive role.

The different forms of violence coming from health professionals and from other hospital workers are important. In general, nurses and doctors slapped patients, while security staff beat them up. This qualitative difference does not excuse the violence against patients, since the ethical code of health professionals makes them the guardians of the vulnerable patient. However, it does point to the urgency of giving attention to the training and supervision of other staff members in health care settings. But even with regard to health professionals respondents felt that continuous training, reminding nurses about the rights of patients, and about the ethical code of their own profession, is necessary. Currently a national project in South Africa called Batho Pele (People First) has been established. This focuses on improving service delivery to the public and tries to set clear standards for behaviour. Such initiatives and other which make behaviour standards more explicit might bring the expectations of health workers and their clients closer together..

The high levels of violence from other staff members against nurses (26% and 30% of reported incidents of violence against nurses) need further exploration. Some of this violence occurred because expectations about proper care not being met. It would seem that public education by means of posters or brochures explaining the procedures followed in health care settings, could improve the situation. For instance, if a poster in a clinic explains that more serious cases will be seen first, even when they have come last, this will assist clients in understanding what is happening and why it is happening.

It is no secret that the nurse is often given less status than other health professionals. This may be related to the fact that in Anglophone countries most nurses are women, which further contributes to their low status. However, from this study it would seem that this powerlessness of nurses invites or allows physical abuse from their colleagues. That does not only compromise the quality of care the nurse can give, but also its credibility in the society.

A high level of violence from patients are related to mental illness and substance abuse. There is evidence that there is a link between mental illness and a potential for violence, which is greatly increased if substance abuse is also present (Mulvey, 1994). To escape from this danger, some respondents recommended that the mentally ill should only be admitted to psychiatric hospitals. However, even in developed countries the integration of mental health care into general health care is now advocated (Mechanic, 1994). There is growing evidence that this improves care for this under-served population (Walkup, 1994), and it can be expected that this would be even more true in economically deprived countries. The solution to this kind of violence in health care settings therefore seems to be adequate training of staff. Such training should differ according to the role of the staff member. Security staff probably need only learn the basic causes of violence and the non-violent handling of aggressive patients. However, doctors and nurses need to know how to evaluate aggressive patients, and how to manage their care. This should include pharmacology, seclusion and restraint, environmental safety and forensic issues (Schwartz and Park, 1999).

Overload stress and associated factors such as job dissatisfaction, conflict at work and intolerance is also a major cause for concern. They are especially important since they lead the respondents to imply that the health worker in effect "could not help it", and in some cases it would seem that such violence against patients has become institutionalised and is almost accepted as "just how things are". This may also be related to the lack of intervention by many of the respondents reporting such violence. A number of them also report non-responses from higher authority when such abuse is reported and victimisation of the whistleblower. Given all these factors, one can see how such behaviour becomes accepted, if not acceptable. The difficult role of a whistleblower causes many nurses severe problems (Oberle and Tenove, 2000). It seems that managers will need to establish a range of mechanisms to ensure that a culture tolerating violence does not grow in health care settings. This should at least involve definitive action on any reported incidents, and follow-up counseling and support for the whistleblower.

Apparently, most respondents felt that very few preventative mechanisms are in place in their own workplace. They also seem to doubt that certain mechanisms, such as timeous discipline of staff members, more thorough screening of staff and training of supervisors would really prevent violence. There are a number of mechanisms that they do feel would be helpful, and these should receive more attention from health service managers. Minimally there should be a policy in place outlining how violence in their workplace can be prevented and how the organisation will respond to incidents of violence (Capozzoli and McVey, 1996). The prevention should include adequate training of staff, and the handling may include strategies such as strategically placed panic buttons and the creation of crisis management teams and post-event incident reviews.

Conclusion

Even if violence in nursing is not a phenomenon that occurs frequently, it is such a aberration of a service created for the alleviation of suffering, that it needs to be taken very seriously. One has to remember that in Africa two health services are running simultaneously; the western and the traditional. If patients are treated badly in the Western service, they often make the decision to only use the traditional system, instead of using both. This may endanger their lives or the quality of their lives.

Violence in nursing in Africa has not received much attention in the literature. In a continent which is plagued by serious health problems and a lack of resources, it can be accepted that this issue has to be addressed creatively and in a way which does not further dilute scarce resources. As it is often the case, problems in Africa are not smaller or different from those in other parts of the world, but there are just less resources to deal with them. This study has shown that lack of resources is often related to abuse or violence in the nursing situation. It is therefore pertinent to African nurses to try to implement what one African nursing school includes in their nurses' pledge:

"I will not allow my commitment to be compromised by service boundaries, lack or resources or any other limiting factor." (University of Natal, 1991).

References

Capozzoli, T. and McVey, R. S. (1996) *Managing violence in the workplace.* Delray Beach, Florida, St Lucie Press.

Ganga-Limando, R. M. (1995) A study of factors associated with incidents of aggressive behaviour within closed acute units in a psychiatric hospital. Unpublished M Nursing dissertation, University of Natal.

Gcaba, R. S. (1997) The effect of violence on Primary Health Care nurses in selected areas of he former Natal region. *Curationis,* 20 (1), 26-29.

Holden, R. (1985) Aggression against nurses. *The Australian Nurses Journal,* 15 (3), 44-48.

Mechanic, D. (1994) Integrating mental health into a general health care system. *Hospital and Community Psychiatry,* 45 (9), 893- 897.

Middleton, L. (1993) *Attitudes of nurses toward physical assaults by psychiatric patients.* Unpublished research report, University of Natal, School of Nursing.

Mulvey, E. P. (1994) Assessing evidence of a link between mental illness and violence. *Hospital and Community Psychiatry,* 45 (7), 663-668.

Ogale, R. (2000) Violence against nurses. Proceedings of the 2000 International Women's Conference, Women's status: vision and reality. in Delhi, India.

Oberle, K. and Tenove, S. (2000) Ethical issues in public health nursing. *Nursing Ethics,* 7 (5), 425-438.

Poster, E. C. and Ryan, J. A. (1993) A multiregional study of nurses' beliefs and attitudes about work safety and patient assault. *Hospital and Community Psychiatry* 45 (11), 1104-1108.

Ryan, J. A. and Poster, E. C. (1989) The assaulted nurse: short-term and long term responses. *Archives of Psychiatric Nursing,* 3 (6), 323-331.

Singer, J. L. (1971) *The control of aggression and violence.* New York: Academic Press.

Schwartz, T. L. and Park, T. L. (1999) Assaults by patients on psychiatric residents. A survey and training recommendations. *Psychiatric Services,* 50 (3), 381-383.

South African Nursing Council (1998) *Statistical returns for the calendar year 1997.* Pretoria, SANC.

Tornquist, E (ed.) (1997) *Nursing practice around the world.* Geneva, WHO.

University of Natal (1991) *Nurses' pledge of service.* Durban: University of Natal.

Walkup, J. (1994) The early case for caring for the insane in general hospitals. *Hospital and Community Psychiatry,* 45 (12), 1224-1225.

World Bank (1997) *World Development Report 1997.* Washington: The International Bank for Reconstruction and Development.

Yach, D. (1992) The impact of political violence on health and health services in Cape Town, 1986. *Critical Health,* 41, 17-19, December.

Zimu, T. E. (1991) The effects of violence on Black professional nurses working in peri-urban areas. Unpublished dissertation, University of Natal.

Chapter Five: Violence in Psychiatric Care: German Experiences

Dirk Richter

Introduction

It is only a few years since violence against nurses in health care has become an important subject of discussion. For decades the issue has evidently been underestimated, if not tabooed. Aggressive and violent behaviour of patients did not fit the image of a psychiatric reform intending to open the doors of the units and improve the treatment of difficult patients. Violence in nursing care was usually associated with nurses assaulting patients. This kind of violence has certainly not completely disappeared from nursing care (Richter and Sauter, 1997), but patient violence against nurses in clinics and health services demands at least similar attention. In any case, hospitals and their nurses feel considerably intimidated by the issue. Without doubt, this feeling results from the gap between the way the institutions and their employees see themselves on the one hand and the demands by the community on the other hand.

Contrary to a multitude of epidemiological studies on the relationship between risk of violence and mental illness there is, particularly in German-speaking countries, a shortage of surveys dealing with the phenomenon of violence taking place in psychiatric clinics. The studies which have been carried out in the medical fields on this topic in Germany after World War II can also be summarised quickly (Genz et al., 1988; Stierlin, 1956). It is only in the 1990s that research done by Steinert and colleagues (Steinert et al., 1995; Steinert et al., 1991) as well as an interpretation of the psychiatric base documentation (Spießl et al., 1998) provided results on this subject. In Anglo-Saxon countries, however, there exist both a number of empirical studies (for a summary see Davis, 1991; Whittington, 1994) and official publications issued by professional psychiatric associations (Royal College of Psychiatrists, 1998; Tardiff, 1996).

The German nursing care and nursing care science literature on the management of patient violence is sketchy, too. The research is dominated by reflections on the nurses' background and their own involvement in the origin of violent situations and in the institutional functioning of psychiatric hospitals (Gottfrois, 1995; Gottschewski, 1997; Kerres and Falk, 1996; Leichtenberger, 1992; Nagel, 1995; Schädle-Deininger and Villinger, 1996; Scharf, 1997). Primarily, German literature aims at making the nursing personnel sensitive to violence-inducing scenarios in order to take precautions. Thus, Gottfrois (1995) as well as Schädle-

Deininger and Villinger (1996) list staff behaviour that have the potential to cause violence. The list includes refusals, incorrect information and too many demands on the patients.

The small number of German studies is to be regretted especially since a sufficient empirical basis to take preventive measures against patient violence is missing. Preventive measures, however, are urgently needed. These violent acts frequently result in occupational accidents that lead to physical and psychological damage. Besides being absent from work due to accidents, the motivation of the personnel to cope with difficult patients may suffer and therefore the quality of treatment may deteriorate. It was the staff injuries following patient assaults that drew the attention of the British and American professional associations and lead to the development of guidelines (Royal College of Psychiatrists, 1998). According to an internal survey of the Regional Accident Insurance of Westphalia-Lippe patient assaults amount to almost 40 percent of all accident reports (Wehrmann-Kececiolgu, personal communication).

The void in German empirical research is unfortunate, because the scientific results from the Anglo-saxon countries can only be translated with great reservations into German conditions. Even between the USA and Great Britain considerable differences exist regarding the extent of violence within clinics and society as a whole (Davis 1991; Whittington, 1994). Basically, the USA is more prone to violence. Only limited comparisons of the organisational structures and professional qualifications in the different health care systems are possible. Looking at surveys carried out in psychiatric hospitals in the USA it is important to bear in mind that there the threshold of hospital admission is considerably higher, in many places comparable to compulsory admission in this country. Therefore, USA hospital populations are clearly smaller in numbers, but considerably more prone to an aggressive and suicidal behaviour. Naturally, the mode of admission affects the patients in the community. On average ambulatory patients, therefore, are considerably unhealthier in the USA than in Europe, because many ambulatory patients in the USA would already have become an in-patient here.

Modern social psychiatry cannot evade the obligation to treat aggressive patients. Contrary to the original expectations the massive extension of ambulatory and local forms of medical care has not reduced the number of compulsory admissions so far (Bruns, 1993). This leads to the question, how the subject of violence is currently dealt with. The aim of the discussion can only be to further reduce these incidents. To reach this end, however, violence must be made the subject of a deliberate discussion in the hospitals (Hubschmid, 1996). Evidently, it is necessary to develop professional and preventive standards for the management of violence. The object cannot be to "dominate" the aggressive patient, but rather

100

to react early and adequately to imminent signs of impending violence and to defuse the situation.

The following report presents a research project that is primarily designed for psychiatric nursing (see also Richter 1999; Richter and Berger, 2001). First, the numbers of assaults that have actually taken place were identified in several institutions of adult psychiatry and prisons. As is well known, only accidents with serious consequences such as physical impairments are reported. They hardly represent the actual situation. Second, the analysis focuses on the assessment of the resulting psychological damage suffered by the affected staff, which is the first analysis of its kind carried out in a German speaking country. Only the physical damage inflicted on staff members has been the subject of previous research. And third, the circumstances under which the assaults took place are analysed in order to be able to convert these research results into actual preventive measures. The hospitals involved in this research are institutions of the regional association Westphalia-Lippe (LWL). Finally, a prevention programme will be presented that is currently being implemented in many Northern German hospitals.

Patient Violence against Nurses: Empirical Data

During six months, all patient assaults were investigated in six hospitals in Westphalia, a region in northwest Germany. The participating clinics included four hospitals of adult psychiatry and two hospitals of forensic psychiatry. A residential home for psychiatrically ill or handicapped people associated with one of the psychiatric hospitals, was included into the sample since the problem of assaults on staff were well known in that area. The nursing management was chosen as the avenue into the institutions. A reporting system for this purpose established in the participating hospitals collected the data on the incidents.

Study Design

The staff were questioned by a nurse with experience in psychiatry by means of a self-designed interview schedule after the assault had been reported. The interviews usually took place within three days after the incident, but in a few cases within a week.

According to the research objectives several broad areas were addressed:
- socio-demographic, diagnostic and psychopathological information on the patient,
- characteristics of the ward where the incident took place,

101

- socio-demographic and professional information on the affected staff member as well as information on physical injuries and on the behaviour of the staff member after the incident,
- reconstruction of the assault with the help of the staff member by including the potential conflict between nurse and patient as well as any indication of an escalating situation and the staff members' coping with the assault,
- collection of data on the physical damage following the assaults on staff.

After the interview staff were given an anonymous questionnaire in order to collect information on a post-traumatic stress reaction. The questionnaire is the German version of the PTSD-Interview (Watson et al., 1991). The PTSD-Interview was developed along the criteria of a Post-Traumatic Stress Disorder according to DSM-III-R techniques. Anonymity was ensured because the staff of the participating hospitals expressed great reluctance to talk since they feared the state of their mental health might become known to their respective institutions.

In accordance with the DSM-III-R techniques the PTSD-Interview classifies all symptoms into three groups , namely "recollection", "avoidance" and "level of agitation". To diagnose a posttraumatic stress reaction the symptoms should last at least one month. Since the affected staff were interviewed relatively soon after the incident had happened and received the questionnaire at the same time, we could not collect the exact data. To complete the PTSD-Interview the question-naire contained items such as gender, age and the time the incident had taken place.

Frequency of Patient Violence and Patient Characteristics

Within the six months survey period the number of assaults inflicted by patients amounted to 155 in the six participating hospitals. Presumably, the figure is lower than the "true" number of incidents, but higher and more realistic than the number of official accident reports. It is interesting to note that only 8 out of 155 incidents were reported from the forensic clinics. This finding strikingly contra-dicts the image the forensic institutions have in the public. Evidently, physical fights do not play the major role that one might expect in these institutions. In-stead, staff of the forensic institutions report to be especially stressed by physical and verbal threats and verbal abuses they are regularly exposed to.

The majority of the patients involved in violent incidents had a long history of mental illness. Their biography frequently showed that they easily got into violent fights with other people such as family members or friends and neighbours, and not only with staff members from psychiatric institutions. Information on earlier incidents in the patient's biography can play an important role in developing preventive measures, since these incidents evidently indicate a risk not to be under-estimated.

The number of assaults found in our study is similar to those from other German institutions. Disregarding incidents that involve patients of forensic institutions for reasons of comparison, 132 episodes occurred during a six months period. During that time 5276 patients were admitted to the four regular psychiatric hospitals (forensic hospitals were excluded from this analysis). Hence a violence incidence rate of 2.5 % of all admissions was found over the survey period. Steinert et al., (1991) found an incidence rate of 1.9 % in Baden-Württemberg at the end of the eighties. The same figure can be found in data of physical injuries from a Bavarian hospital, which were published by Spießl et al. (1998). In comparison, our numbers are slightly higher. The difference in numbers presumably comes from the mode of access via the nurses. It also included incidents that might have been hidden from the medical personnel.

Characteristics of the Affected Staff

A total of 170 staff members were involved in the 155 incidents. In some cases several staff members were involved in a single patient assault. The incidents involved nurses and nurses' aides (like student nurses or persons rendering their civil-service duty) almost exclusively. Only two members of the medical personnel were victims of assault in this survey. This results without doubt from the fact that nurses spend more time on the ward and with the patients.

The age of the staff involved, and less so their gender was significant for the circumstances described here. Younger staff members were involved in assaults more often than was to be expected according to the age distribution of the employees in the wards of the respective institutions. The fact that inexperienced staff were victims of violence more frequently than expected was even more informative.

While the connection between age and limited experience is known from different studies (Steinert et al., 1991; Whittington, 1994), this study surprisingly shows that the risks increase again after 5 or 6 years of professional experience. This is possibly due to the fact that professional responsibility increases after having completed the training and that the nurses may overestimate their abilities to master crisis situations.

Regarding the functional groups within the staff indicates a relation between limited professional experience and the risk to become a victim of violence. Student nurses were involved in assaults in proportion to their share in staff. But sharing the same proportion in the sample this professional group clearly has a higher risk, since its temporary exposure is considerably lower. Student nurses only spend about 50 % of their training in the wards of the psychiatric hospitals. The remaining time is spent on theoretical instruction and on assignment to external institutions. Therefore, the risk to the students is twice as high. This fact should be a good reason to develop preventive measures which have hardly existed so far.

Without insinuating a conscious participation in escalating violent situations on part of the affected staff, a multitude of cases showed inappropriate reaction or behaviour by staff members toward the tense and already latently aggressive patient. Considering their poor professional experience it is hardly surprising. More experienced staff often develop a intuitive reaction to "difficult" patients. Understandably, younger and more in-experienced staff do not have such skills.

Characteristics of the Assault

After having described significant characteristics of the people involved in the violent situation the particulars of these situations are now explored. According to findings of this study patient assaults mostly take place in closed wards. Only a small part of the incidents are reported from open wards or from outside the wards. They often happen at the beginning of a hospital stay or after the patients were transferred to a closed ward. Admission and transfer to such a ward obviously demands from the affected patient an adjustment that he/she cannot make. As treatment proceeds, the frequency of such incidents decreases considerably. On admission, therefore, time is of the essence in describing risk characteristics and the resulting preventive measures, since having that information admission and transfer of patients can be arranged more suitably to them.

Against all expectations night shifts with few personnel did not incur special risks for violence. Rather, most of the incidents took place during daytime with particular emphasis on mornings, peaking between 8 and 9 hours. This was specially true for incidents that involved patients afflicted with senile dementia and mental handicaps. In the mornings these patients usually have intensive contacts with nurses that include personal hygiene and meals. Analysing the incidents reported by staff confirms the hypothesis that activities such as giving meals and washing the patient frequently gave rise to assault. Patients with schizophrenia were clearly less violent in the mornings; regarding personal hygiene these patients had usually considerably fewer contacts with the nurses.

In most cases conflict between staff member and patient preceded the violence. During the reconstruction of the assault staff members described the above mentioned care activities, but also other incidents such as refusing a request or refusing discharge. When asked which patient behaviour was observed by staff before the assault, the nurses often spoke of menacing gestures, little physical distance as well as threats and verbal abuse. This has been specially true in regard to mentally handicapped patients and patients suffering from a schizophrenia. Patients with dementia, however, often showed spontaneous and unpredictable aggressive reactions.

Shortly before the assault many patients demonstrated the expected psychopathological behaviour and symptoms, mostly attacks of irritability, non-cooperative behaviour and psycho-muscular tensions. Beyond that people with dementia were also disoriented.

Physical and Psychological Injuries Following the Assault

Out of 170 affected staff 121 (71,2 %) indicated physical injuries. Mostly minor injuries were reported such as a few hematomas, scratches, bites, excoriations, contusions, bruises, strangling marks and hair pulling. Three employees suffered from more permanent head aches. Thirteen percent of staff reported pains without evident physical injuries. Two staff members suffered more serious injuries: one person was stabbed with a knife in the face, breast, back and calves and suffered peripheral nerve injury, another person was unconscious for a short time after sustaining a blow on his/her head.

The extent of the physical injuries essentially corresponds to the distribution pattern of other well-known studies. Internationally, the classification of Fottrell (1980) has become the standard. Category one contains the invisible injuries, category two the visible minor physical injuries such as scratches, hematomas, etc. and category three the serious physical injuries such as stabbings, unconsciousness or bone fractures. Well-known studies (Noble and Rodger, 1989; Reid et al., 1989) show that two to five percent of affected staff sustain serious physical injuries. In our study two staff members (1.2 %) suffered such injuries. On the other hand we found considerably more minor injuries than did Noble and Rogers (1989) in their evaluation of 12.000 British injury reports. While in their study 37 % of all cases fell within the scope of category two, in our study 58 % did. Presumably, the difference can be explained in the way the data were collected (study versus routine documentation). Routine registration usually leaves out a significant part of the minor injuries.

Three staff members were treated in their own hospital, 12 nurses received ambulatory treatment. One nurse had to stay in the hospital for some time. Immediately, 4.1 % of staff changed their place of work. Disability was granted in 4.7 % of the cases. The period of disability could not exactly be determined, since the nurses were interviewed relatively soon after the incident had happened. Approximately, a period from two days to several weeks was reported.

On the whole, these results correspond to those of Germany's only study carried out by Steinert et al. (1991) covering the extent of injuries. The data on the injuries following the assault reported there are similar to the results of our study. Steinert et al. (1991) even report a death and during our survey an almost fatal incident took place.

Immediately after the assault the mental health of the staff was clearly affected by the incident. Looking back at the incident, almost half of the respondents disclosed that they had been shocked by it. To a smaller extent they felt stressed by fear and depression. The standardised evaluation of the posttraumatic stress reaction showed the following: of 170 staff 85 (50 %) responded to the questionnaire. The socio-demographic data of the respondents did not differ significantly from the staff interviewed before. Both the age and gender distribution of the respondents corresponded to the sample distribution of the victims of patient assaults.

None of the respondents fulfilled all the criteria necessary for the diagnosis of a Post-Traumatic Stress Disorder (PTSD) according to DSM-III-R techniques. That means that none of the 85 staff was diagnosed with PTSD, but several of the respondents suffered from considerable psychological consequences.

Over 10 % of the respondents meet the criteria for the category of "re-experience". The criteria for the category "increased arousal" were fulfilled by 3.5 %, and one respondent felt sufficiently stressed to come under the category of "avoidance". As one respondent met the criteria for two groups of symptoms, a total of 14% of the respondents suffered some aspects of the post-traumatic syndrome.

The sum of the stress factors (addition of all values) shows that the mean cumulative value hardly differs within the age groups of the respondents. The analysis of gender shows a clear, marginally significant difference. On average, the participating female staff members have a stress score of 23.9 points, male employees a score of 21.6 point (median: 21 versus 19, p = .06). For comparison: no stress at all would result in a figure of 18. The range of stress scores was 18-65 points.

The time span after the patient assault did not reduce the cumulative value of the stress factors. Thus, a group of respondents who were attacked more than 4 weeks ago and a group who was assaulted less than a week ago showed a similarly high stress factor expressed in their mean value (23.4 versus 23.5). During the intermediate weeks the mean value was slightly lower. It was, however, remarkable that some deviations adding up to 60 points happened after more than 4 weeks. This indicates that some few staff members were stressed very much and that this deterioration can last for some weeks or did even come up after several weeks.

Regarding the psychological consequences our study can claim to be the first one in the German-speaking region to have explored this subject. It also belongs to the relatively small number of international surveys carried out on this theme. This reluctance is all the more surprising since our research demonstrated that psychological damage is more prevalent than physical injuries. While about 10 % of the affected nurses were physically wounded in such a way that they needed medical treatment, 14 % of the affected staff responding to an anonymous questionnaire showed psychological symptoms that met the criteria of at least one of the three categories of PTSD according to DSM-III-R.

Compared to other surveys mentioned above it is remarkable that none of the injured staff members was diagnosed with a full-blown posttraumatic strain reaction. Caldwell (1992) discovered the complete picture of the disorder in 9 % of the interviewed psychiatric nurses. Whittington und Wykes (1992) found in 4 of the 24 (16 %) examined nurses symptoms which would have justified such a diagnosis. The differences to our results may be based on various factors. Our survey was anonymous. Therefore, it is not clear whether the respondents had experienced a distortion of the answers, however come about. Faced with comparative studies seriously stressed staff might not have participated in our research. It could also be that only those answered who felt themselves under a serious psychological stress, or only those responded who were prepared to discuss their feelings and attitudes. Because the survey was anonymous, a connection with the actual patient assault was not possible. Therefore, it is not known, how serious the assaults were and what the physical injuries inflicted on the nurses looked like. Presumably, there is an association, also not linear, between the seriousness of the assault and the resulting physical injuries on the one hand and the psychological stress reaction on the other hand.

Chances to Prevent Patient Assaults and their Consequences

The presentation of the results made evident that prevention strategies are needed. The possible preventative strategies described here have been developed in the framework of a project which is currently established in many local hospitals (Richter et al., 2001). The project specially involves the training of coaches who in turn instruct their colleagues. It focuses on training, that is the deescalation of aggressive situations and the defence from physical assaults, which will be described in more detail as follows.

To begin with, patient assaults do not happen without an early warning. The early warning signs observed in the survey such as little physical distance or threatening gestures can be perceived as just such indications in order to react appropriately. In this context training of student nurses and other in-experienced staff, who should be prepared by management to work in difficult areas and to handle tough patients, are to be considered .

The fact that a violent situation may escalate leads to the conclusion that defusing strategies employed by staff should be an essential element of prevention. In this context, de-escalation means ways of behaviour contributing to reduce the potential of danger and to render safe the aggressive situation by means of communication. The full details of the individual methods cannot be given here, but only partly described. Considering the actual prevention strategies only comprehensive behaviour training can lead to the appropriate results. This is true for both the de-escalation of a violent situation and the defence from an assault.

Effective de-escalation demands extensive knowledge of the patient, his/her medical history and his/her actual health. The more the patient's possible reactions are known the better the nurse will be prepared for them. Naturally, this is only possible if patients have been staying in the hospital for some time. In any case, no provoking by staff should be allowed. The patient should meet with empathy, respect, honesty and fairness. Sympathy and solicitude should be signalled by staff.

The predominant aim is to avoid violence. Other aspects are of secondary importance, insofar as the long-term object of treatment allows this. This means that staff make such concessions to the patient that do not give rise to conflicts at a later time. Such a concession would be to agree with a person regarding certain issues. In such a situation it is not relevant who is right. Power struggles should be avoided at all costs. Mastering the situation and not the patient is the objective.

The correct use of language, body language, miming and gestures is also important so that the patients do not feel threatened or even dominated. This strategy requires self-knowledge of how one reacts to stress and also self-control. Verbal de-escalation means not provoking the patient with statements or questions and not pushing him/her "into a corner" from which the patient can only get free by means of violence. Therefore, closed questions that can only be answered by yes or no should be avoided. Open questions integrate the patient into the decision making process. To indicate options to the patient saves time and gives him/her the feeling to be able to influence the outcome of a situation.

Not every violent situation in psychiatric institutions can be solved by de-escalation. If the defusing measures are exhausted or impossible to employ from the beginning, physical means should then be used . In this case, too, the aim is to avoid violence as far as possible. Only such means should be used, which neither injure the patients nor endanger the staff. With this in mind, for some time now training programmes aiming at defending oneself from an assault have successfully been employed in various local hospitals.

Restraining and isolating a patient, which experience shows, cannot be avoided in some cases should be used with the same objective in mind. Restraining and isolating patients certainly belong to the most disagreeable tasks of psychiatric nursing. Therefore, a professional execution of this potentially dangerous task needs careful planning which includes the respect for human dignity and safety of the participants. Only if the team has learnt to work well together and has clear rules and behaviour guidelines, can the strategies be employed as intended. These steps should be trained and not arise from the actual situation aimed at mastering the patient. The necessity of the action taken should be discussed with the patient after having been released from restraint in order to reduce the potential for further aggression. Without doubt, being restrained is one of the worst experiences that a person can have specially in terms of the therapeutic objectives of the hospital. Therefore, the patient should be given a platform to talk about the experience.

The last prevention strategy described here is the protection from the consequences of psychological damage. The survey showed a significant strain on the staff. Dealing with this strain should not be a taboo any more in the hospital. Thus, a staff member assaulted by a patient should be given the opportunity to leave the ward for some time in order to mitigate the experience. Furthermore, being socially supported by colleagues and supervisors is very important. A remark such as "Don't make such a fuss" is not appropriate in that context, but is still used here and there.

Instead, it is the task of the colleagues and of the organisation to take care that the affected staff is supported in a professional way both with regard to counselling or even therapy to avoid mental strain. Each psychiatric institution should offer addresses of specialised therapists whom the affected staff can call. Respondents in this study did not wish for treatment in their own institution, e.g. a therapy with a psychotherapist from their hospital. The risk was considered too great that their own mental health becomes known in their workplace.

Conclusions

In the past issues of violence had not been discussed in German psychiatric institutions, but for some years now the debate has increasingly turned to the subject of violence. In many institutions the issue is considered central with regard to staff satisfaction and staff performance. Real strain inflicted by aggression and violence are known to lead to significant psychological problems which, in turn, result in low job satisfaction and burn-out of affected staff.

The projects presented here are certainly only a beginning in the efforts to prevent assaults by patients in psychiatric hospitals. Further and improved empirical surveys and training projects have to follow. However, staff and management have successfully been made sensitive to the difficult issue and to providing more safety and job satisfaction. In so far, Germany is on the right track to catch up with the Anglo-Saxon countries.

References

Bruns, G. (1993) *Ordnungsmacht Psychiatrie? Psychiatrische Zwangseinweisung als soziale Kontrolle.* Opladen: Westdeutscher Verlag.

Caldwell, M.F. (1992) Incidence of PTSD Among Staff Victims of Patient Violence. *Hospital and Community Psychiatry*, 43: 838-839.

Davis, S. (1991) Violence by psychiatric inpatients: a review. *Hospital and Community Psychiatry*, 42: 585-590.

Fottrell, E. (1980) A Study of Violent Behaviour Among Patients in Psychiatric Hospitals. *British Journal of Psychiatry*, 136: 216-221.

Genz, A., E. Krüger and Dost, B. (1988) Aggressives Verhalten in der psychiatrischen Klinik. *Psychiatrie, Neurologie, medizinische Psychologie*, 40: 542-551.

Gottfrois, W. (1995) Umgang mit aggressiven Heimbewohnern. *Pflegezeitschrift*, 48: 527-530.

Gottschewski, A. (1997) Gewalt in der psychiatrischen Pflege. *Pflege aktuell*, 51: 527-530.

Hubschmid, T. (1996) Erfahrungen im Umgang mit Gewalttätigkeit in der psychiatrischen Klinik. *Psychiatrische Praxis*, 23: 26-28.

Kerres, A. and Falk, J. (1996) Gewalt in der Pflege: Sensibilisieren Sie sich für den Umgang mit den eigenen Aggressionen! *Pflegezeitschrift*, 49: 174-177.

Leichtenberger, R. (1992) Macht – Ohnmacht – Gewalt. *Deutsche Krankenpflegezeitschrift*, 45: 525-527.

Nagel, C. (1995) Gestaltung eines gewaltarmen Milieus im psychiatrischen Pflegealltag: Wunschdenken oder Möglichkeit? *Die Schwester/Der Pfleger*, 34: 1010-1015.

Noble, P. and S. Rodger (1989) Violence by Psychiatric Inpatients. *British Journal of Psychiatry*, 155: 384-390.

Reid, W.H., Bollinger, M.F. and Edwards, J.G. (1989) Serious Assaults by Inpatients. *Psychosomatics*, 30: 54-56.

Richter, D. (1999) *Patientenübergriffe auf Mitarbeiter psychiatrischer Kliniken. Häufigkeit, Folgen, Präventionsmöglichkeiten.* Freiburg: Lambertus.

Richter, D. and Berger, K. (2001) Patientenübergriffe auf Mitarbeiter – Eine prospektive Untersuchung der Häufigkeit, Situationen und Folgen. *Nervenarzt*, 72: 693-699.

Richter, D., Fuchs, J.M. and Bergers, K.-H. (2001) *Konfliktmanagement in psychiatrischen Einrichtungen.* Münster/Düsseldorf: Gemeindeunfallversicherungsverband Westfalen-Lippe, Rheinischer Gemeindeunfallversicherungsverband, Landesunfallkasse Nordrhein-Westfalen.

Richter, D. and Sauter, D. (1997) *Patiententötungen und Gewaltate durch Pflegekräfte: Beweggründe, Hintergründe, Auswege.* Eschborn: DBfK-Verlag.

Royal College of Psychiatrists (1998) *Management of Imminent Violence. Clinical practice guidelines to support mental health services.* London: Royal College of Psychiatrists. (Occasional Paper 41).

Schädle-Deininger, H. and Villinger, U. (1996) *Praktische Psychiatrische Pflege. Arbeitshilfen für den Alltag.* Bonn: Psychiatrie-Verlag.

Scharf, W. (1997) Gewalt in der Pflege In: W. Schnepp, S. Schoppmann, W. Scharf and H. Wippermann (eds.), *Pflegeforschung in der Psychiatrie.* Berlin/Wiesbaden: Ullstein/Mosby, 79-112.

Spießl, H., Krischker, S. and Cording, C. (1998) Aggressive Handlungen im psychiatrischen Krankenhaus. Eine auf die Basisdokumentation gestützte 6-Jahres-Studie bei 17943 stationären Aufnahmen. *Psychiatrische Praxis*, 25: 227-230.

Steadman, H.J., Mulvey, M.V. and Monahan, J. (1998) Violence by People Discharged From Acute Psychiatric Inpatient Facilities and by Others in the Same Neighbourhoods. *Archives of General Psychiatry*, 55: 393-401.

Steinert, T., Beck, M., Vogel, W. D. and Wohlfahrt, A. (1995) Gewalttätige Patienten. Ein Problem für Therapeuten an psychiatrischen Kliniken? *Der Nervenarzt*, 66: 207-211.

Steinert, T., Vogel, W.D. Beck, M. and Kehlmann, S. (1991) Aggressionen psychiatrischer Patienten in der Klinik. *Psychiatrische Praxis*, 25: 221-226.

Stierlin, H. (1956) *Der gewalttätige Patient: Eine Untersuchung über die von Geisteskranken an Ärzten und Patienten verübten Angriffe.* Basel: Karger.

Tardiff, K. (1996) *Concise Guide to Assessment and Management of Violent Patients.* Washington, London: American Psychiatric Press.

Watson, C.G., Juba, M.P. Manifold, V. , Kucala, T. and Anderson, P.E.D. (1991) The PTSD Interview: Rationale, Description, Reliability, and Concurrent Validity of a DSM-III-based technique. *Journal of Clinical Psychology*, 47: 179-188.

Whittington, R. (1994) Violence in Psychiatric Hospitals In: Til Wykes (Hrsg.), *Violence and Health Care Professionals*. London: Chapman and Hall, 23-42.

Whittington, R. and Wykes, T. (1992) Staff Strain and Social Support in a Psychiatric Hospital following assault by a patient. *Journal of Advanced Nursing*, 17: 480-486.

Chapter Six: Violence against Elderly People and its Prevention in Nursing Care Institutions in Germany

Rolf D. Hirsch

Introduction

While society and social sciences paid intensive attention to abuse of children and women in the 1960s and 1970s, violence against older persons has become an issue only since the 1980s. Interest varies in intensity from state to state. It is not a phenomenon of our times but was only recognised as a societal problem of considerable magnitude during the last two decades. The increase in the proportion of the elderly in the population has also made the issue a current topic internationally (Council of Europe, 1992; Kosberg and Garcia, 1995).

Looking at the previous international conventions, the problems of elderly persons are not always adaequatly considered. The Convention on the Political Rights of Women was drawn up in 1952, the Declaration on the Rights of the Child in 1959, the Declaration on the Rights of Mentally Handicapped Persons in 1971 and on The Rights of Disabled Persons in 1975.

In 1982 the World Assembly on Ageing which took place in Vienna was proposing a plan of action. It recommended that nursing care be given equal importance to therapeutic treatment and that the elderly who have to live in a nursing home have the right to live in dignity. To guarantee better nursing care there should be minimum standards (United Nations 1983 recommendations 1 and 34).

In Germany the federal government has so far predominantly focused on "domestic violence against the elderly" by means of expert meetings (BMFSFJ, 1996) as well as with a pilot project called "Violence Against the Elderly in their Domestic Environment" and carried out in Hanover from 1998 till 2001. In 2000 the "Committee on Human Rights and Humanitarian Assistance" of the German parliament held a session on " Violence against the Elderly in Nursing Homes". More recently, the "Council of Europe Committee for the Prevention of Torture and Inhuman or Degrading Treatment or Punishment (CPT)" did the same in the framework of its specific duties. So far the federal government has not yet enacted any laws against age discrimination as has been done in other countries and has hardly attended to the "state of emergency in nursing homes" which has existed for about 20 years. Only one federal state, Schleswig-Holstein, passed a resolution on " Violence against the Elderly – Prevention and Intervention" in 1998, which resulted in activities contributing to a reduction of violence. In 2002,

113

in the state of North-Rhine-Westphalia a commission of inquiry was set up to investigate the current situation and the future of nursing care. Since 1999 the "Federal Working Group on Crisis Telephone Lines, on Centres for Advice and Grievances for the Elderly" exists which constitutes a union of 15 emergency and grievance telephone lines (Hirsch and Erkens, 1999) that deals predominantly with abuse in homes for the elderly.

Associations for the care of the elderly have pointed to abuse in nursing homes for a long time. In 1987, therefore, the geriatric nurses issued a statement of professional ethics "We do not want to become accomplices" (Langkau, 1987) that was announced at a demonstration of geriatric nurses in Hanover. In 1998 the "Action against Violence in Nursing Care" was founded by five associations and societies, which published a memorandum to ensure humane nursing care that met with an overwhelming response (AGP, 1999). In 2002 the law on institutional homes was amended and a law on quality assurance in nursing care was introduced. Their effects, however, are uncertain, since even previous policies were not sufficiently applied.

Nursing Homes and their Residents in Germany

The number of homes for the elderly increased considerably in the last years. In 1999 more than 8200 institutions had been listed offering placement for almost 700 000 older persons, among them about 600 000 especially included geriatric care. It can be assumed that 70 to 80 % of nursing homes residents suffer from a mental disorder, about two third of these of senile dementia (first diagnosis). In addition, the entry age has risen considerably. It can be observed that "shunting stations" among geriatric psychiatry, geriatrics and care for the elderly have developed. The route from the hospital to the nursing home is often preprogrammed: Short stays in hospitals to curb costs resulting in more infirmity leading to nursing care instead of treatment and rehabilitation.

While at any given time only 5 % of the German population aged 65 years and older live in homes for the elderly (Wahl and Reichert, 1991; Schneekloth and Müller, 1997), in the beginning 1990s the probability of spending the last part of their lives in a home for the elderly or a nursing home amounted to 17 % for men and 37 % for women (Bickel, 1992). Faced with a growing share of older persons in the population the number of persons in need of care is expected to rise. That number is expected to increase from today's 1.8 million to 2.15 million in 2010 (Görgen, 2000).

For quite some time now there has been a serious discussion about the extent to which current care facilities meet the needs of persons requiring care. Increas-

114

ingly, these facilities have difficulties in complying with the minimal standards of care. Additionally, most residents -although technically and legally admitted of their own free will – are forced to live there, because there are no alternatives or they and the professionals do not know about existing alternatives. New approaches and different societal attitudes toward the elderly and their caregivers are necessary. In 2001, therefore, the research team "People in Institutional Care" of the University of Bielefeld supported by well-known experts and scientists urged the political administration to set up a commission titled "Inquiry into Institutional Care".

Definition and Forms of Violence in Institutions

Following the American literature, in gerontology violence is defined "as a systematic, non-unique act or neglect resulting in a distinctly negative effect on the recipient. A unique act/neglect must lead to very serious negative consequences for the recipient in order to be classified as violence" (Dieck, 1987). The resulting forms of violence are as follows: active and passive neglect as well as abuse: physical and emotional, financial exploitation, restriction of one´s freedom. All these acts of violence, however, only refer to interactions among persons. They only describe interpersonal forms of violence (table 1). Some definitions also include the care settings. Elder abuse is then defined as "harmful or distressing behaviour to an older person (aged 65 plus) by someone whom he or she should be able to trust – e.g., a family member or a paid caregiver" (Mc Creadie et. al., 2000, p. 68). The National Center on Elder Abuse (NCEA, 2000) includes in its definition the scene of violence, thereby distinguishing between domestic and institutional forms of violence.

Particularly social scientists indicate that violence does not only constitute a problem of relationship or an interpersonal incident, but is also influenced by situational and environmental factors. Terms like indirect violence are justified if these factors represent the indirect causes of violence. Examples taken from homes for the elderly are as follows: inadequate staff presence, lack of supervision to support the caregivers and of time to reflect on one´s own actions or daily rigid work rituals, which are intended to assist in mastering the amount of work involved, but instead oppose the actual needs of the residents . Such factors increase the probability of abuse. Galtung (1975) refers to them as structural factors. A comprehensive understanding of violence also needs to take into account cultural factors (figure 1). These factors are reflected for instance in the view that older persons represent a financial burden on society or that caring should fulfil the ideal of the good Samaritan (Hirsch, 2000).

Table 1: Forms of Violence against the Elderly (according to Johnson, 1991)

Physical	Mental	Social	Legal
• **Misuse of drugs** Withholding	• **Humiliation** Shame	• **Isolation** Induced with-drawel	• **Material abuse** Mismangement of property
Inappropriate and unnecessary Medication	Accusation Rejection	"Voluntary" re-treat Inappropriate supervision	Mismanagement of contracts Access to prop-erty or contracts
• **Restricions**	Ridiculing • **Torture**	• **Confusion of roles**	• **Theft**
Ignoring medical needs Lack of hygiene	Insults Intimidation	Competition Stress	Theft of property or contracts Involuntary submission
Malnutrition	Scaring	Reversal	Unnecesssary le-gal assistance
Disturbance of the rest Restriction of freedom of movement	Upsetting	Disintegration	Abuse of the professional authority
• **Assault**	• **Manipulation**	• **Interference in the living space**	• **Abuse of law**
External injuries Internal injuries	To hold back in-formation Withdrawel of stimuli	Disorganised househould Lack of privacy	Denial of con-tracts Involuntary submission
Rape	Interference in decision making	Inappropriate surroundings	Unnecessary le-gal assistance
Suicide/homicide	Restriction of the internal freedom	Giving up the familiar sur-roundings	Abuse of profes-sional authority

Including three levels of activity the triangular model or "violence triangle" determined by structural, cultural and personal forms of violence tends to regard violence as a societal issue and to consider the "perpetrator" to be a "victim" in some cases and vice versa. It strongly contradicts the crime model which incorporates delinquent personalities, criminal motives and deserved punishments. The personal responsibility of the perpetrator has to be taken into account. Health professionals need to create frameworks of action aiming at changes in the system of professional relationships. The triangular model proposes three approaches (Hirsch and Vollhardt, 2002):

116

1. To define violence as an avoidable restriction of the basic needs to people. The definition is neutral and avoids scandalising or emotionalising which frequently impedes solution;
2. To view violence as being caused by a multitude of factors and presenting dimensions that that can be the focus of intervention;
3. To avoid the dichotomy of perpetrator and victim or to regard violence simply as relationship problems. This is vital to avoid emotionalising the incidents and to identify alternatives.

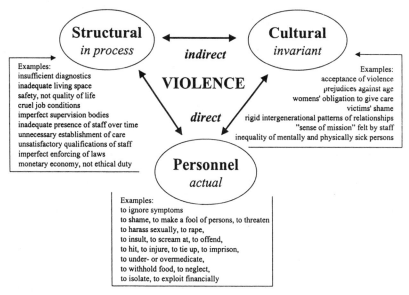

Figure 1: Triangle of Violence (according to Galtung, 1993; Hirsch, 2000)

In institutional care an older person can be affected by violence threefold: he or she can experience , perceive or commit violence, thus be a victim, witness or perpetrator of violent acts. Sometimes, the part of perpetrator or victim cannot be assigned correctly to a single person, so that the actual events may not justify the terms of perpetrator or victim.

Extent of Violence in Nursing Homes

Although the public is sensitive to scandals about elder abuse that happen from time to time in hospitals and homes for the elderly not much is known about the actual prevalence of the problem. Various factors have hampered research in this field. For example, interviews with recipients of institutional care who suffer from partial amnesia and have difficulties communicating cannot be used. Because the participating staff may distort the facts of a violent incident by glossing over the accounts, their descriptions should be assessed in a critical way. In addition, the institutions are very heterogeneous , a representative sample survey, therefore, is very difficult. The only characteristics these institutions have in common are those of a "total institution" (Goffman, 1961), that is determined by directives and standardised sequences of routines. In such institutions the lives of the recipients of care are separate from those of the care givers. As a result abuses are not noticed or are denied. Therefore, the boundaries between normal routines and abuses are not easily recognised in an individual case. In addition, "violence" as research subject is defined very differently in surveys.

While there are several studies on violence in geriatric care to be found in the United States (Goddriges et al., 1996; Hagen and Sayers, 1995; Foner, 1994), in Germany only data on the frequency of individual forms of violence exists.

In September 1999 the Medical Service of the Health Insurance (MDK) carried out a random survey in 715 nursing homes in Bavaria. Shortcomings were located in the areas of quality management (537), work organisation (467), proportion of qualified personnel (362) and model/nursing care concept (350). The MDK is carrying out a similar survey in Schleswig-Holstein at the moment. The provisional results after 116 institutions had been tested showed a similar picture: Almost one third of the recipients of care were diagnosed with nursing care unduced injuries and almost half of them lacked the necessary prophylactic nursing actions (Bruckner, 2000).

From 1996 to 1999 the Medical Service of the Health Insurance carried out inspections about 4000 services (about 1800 ambulatory and about 2200 residential ones). Almost all institutions had serious shortcomings regarding the decubitus prophylaxis and care, nutrition/liquids, incontinence care, handling of drugs and restraining measures (Brüggemann, 2000).

While evaluating the calls received by the Bonn emergency telephone service for older persons and their relations (Bonn Initiative Against Violence in Old Age, 2002) in 2001, 40 % of the violent incidents described in the emergency calls were experienced in homes for the elderly and nursing homes, in 2000 it was 51%. The victims rarely called themselves. Most of the callers were family members describing the experiences of their relatives. The majority of complaints refer to structural deficits in nursing care settings.

Hirsch and Fussek (1999) record about 60 fateful stories on elder abuse. The paper met with overwhelming response. Numerous moving reports continued and are continuing to be described to the emergency telephone staff.

Medical and Nursing Care Methods Related to Violence

Corresponding to the above-mentioned reflections on violence several medical and nursing care methods have to be considered.

Mechanical Restraining Techniques

At the latest the success of the wide-ranging anti-restraints programmes in US geriatric and nursing homes regulated by the Omnibus Budget Reconciliation Act of 1987 (OBRA) made evident that the practice of physically restraining persons used so far was used excessively. In the United States the number of mechanical restraints was reduced from formerly 40 % to 21% on average (Williams and Finch, 1997), a number that is probably still too high as the rate of 4 % of mechanical restraints applied in some homes for the elderly indicates (Neufeld et al., 1999). On condition that the characteristics of the residents are comparable, the willingness to use restraining techniques is very variable in different geographic locations and facilities (Phillips et al., 1990). The refusal to employ physical restraints corresponds to an increase in the numbers of staff and in other structural changes in the institutions (Castle et al., 1997) without the risk factors of the residents having changed.

The old justifications are still used. It is said, that restraint instruments prevents falls. However, falling cannot be prevented by using mechanical restraints, and the refusal to use those does not result in more frequent falls in appropriate anti-restraint programmes (Capezuti et al., 1996; Neufeld et al., 1999). On the other hand resorting to restraining techniques brings with them an increased risk of falling, particularly after terminating the restraining measure (Arbesman and Wright, 1999). Other frequent justifications are behavioural disorders and hyperactivity, particularly if coupled with dementia. However, practise shows that restraining is more likely to increase anxiety and agitation and result in severe suffering (Evans and Strumpf, 1989). There is no evidence of any positive effects regarding restraining measures in geriatric nursing. There is proof, however, that they go hand in hand with objective signs of intellectual decline, immobility, loss of bodily functions, increased morbidity (Evans and Strumpf, 1989) and even casualties (Parker and Miles, 1997). It has been proved that the use of restraining techniques depends less on the specifics of the elderly patients, but rather on the structures of the institutions such as staff distribution, proportion of specialists, geography and the care allowance paid per resident. In addition, cultural factors such as the philosophy of the institution and the prevailing "myths" are also significant (Evans and Strumpf, 1989; Strumpf and Evans, 1991; Phillips et al. 1996; Castle et al., 1997).

Regarding physical control techniques in Germany there exist no data except for surveys in geriatric-psychiatric hospitals (Hirsch and Kranzhoff, 1996; Hirsch et al., 1992). A survey in 26 homes for the elderly with over 3000 residents showed, that more than 2200 actions restricting personal freedom were taken on one day (Klie, 1998). The most frequent ones were bedsides and immobilising drugs. The frequency of actions taken to restrict the freedom of movement varies greatly extremely among the institutions as well as among the geriatric-psychiatric hospitals.

Hollwig (1994) investigated an open nursing care unit in six homes over a period of three months. A participating observer recorded that restrictive measures were taken involving 51% of the residents (N=110) over a 48 hours period. 10 % of the residents suffered more than one restraining measure. During that period more than 70 % of the patients were physically restrained for more than eight hours per day.

Psychopharmacological Drugs

Psychotropic drugs are frequently employed in homes for the elderly and nursing homes, as international research shows. In the United States between 17 and 78 % of the residents receive at least one prescription drug each (Llorente et al., 1998; Schmidt et al., 1998). The wrong doses of psychopharmacological drugs often given to patients, the drugs are unfavourably selected, combined in a dangerous way and taken for too long periods of time (Board of Directors of the American Association for Geriatric Psychiatry, 1992). The misuse is more common in institutions with less adequate resources (Svarstadand and Mount, 1991; Riedel-Heller et al., 1999).

The following surveys have been conducted in Germany:

- Drugs were prescribed without a diagnosis for more than half of the 108 residents of two homes for the elderly. Prescribing more than one drug at the same time was customary (about 1/3 of the patients were treated with more than four different drugs). Almost 2/3 of the elderly received psychopharmacological drugs. The so-called "prescription on demand" was common. Frequent prescribing of neurological drugs (for 42 of 108 inmates) is judged as an expression of helplessness in the face of "difficult" patients on the part of doctors and care givers.
- Another survey analysing the prescription of neurological drugs for demented elderly patients (N = 49) states that psychopharmacological drugs are pre-

scribed very frequently and neurological drugs even more frequently in spite of increased side effects for demented elderly persons (Wilhelm-Gößling, 1998). It turned out that the patients in the survey received significantly more neurological drugs in the homes for the elderly (46 - 66 % of the residents) than when discharged from the hospital (20%). The relationship therefore exists between living in a home and extensive prescription of neurological drugs. Benzodiazepines were prescribed twice as much in institutions as at home. Permanent prescriptions were customary. The survey shows that those residents received particularly high dosages of neurological drugs, whose symptoms were not influenced in a positive way by the drugs.

- An expert opinion written by the inquiry commission on "Demographic Change" (Glaeske et al., 1997) explicitly mentioned "drug misuse in homes for the elderly". It quoted surveys proving that the proportion of psychiatric drug consumers in homes amounts to about 50 % and is rising. According to another survey quoted in this report 27 % of the residents take between 6 and 11 different drugs as permanent medications, 45% at least one psychopharmacological drug. It was indicated that the more favourable the distribution of staff in the homes, particularly of qualified nurses, the less the psychiatric drugs are prescribed for the elderly there.

There are indications that conditions in Germany are similar to the United States regarding the type of psychiatric drugs used: While neurological drugs and hypnotics and specially benzodiazepines are prescribed too frequently, anti-depressive drugs are not taken often enough in spite of the well-known high prevalence of depression in homes for the elderly (Board of Directors of the American Association for Geriatric Psychiatry, 1992). The typical profile of application of psychopharmacological drugs indicates that treatment is more symptom-oriented and less specific to a diagnosis; mirroring the fact that provision of psycho-geriatric care in institutions is insufficient. Developments as the USA experienced, therefore, could also be of help to Germany.

After the prescription misuse in American care facilities had become widely known, specific guidelines under OBRA 87 were passed to regulate the use of psychopharmacological drugs. Measures taken include specific treatment according to diagnosis, firm routines in order to reduce or to go off pharmacological drugs entirely, the use of non-pharmacological treatment alternatives (such as behaviour therapy) and the banning of medication on demand. These regulations to reduce the amount of psychotropic medication were very successful, particularly, when at the time training of non-pharmacological methods of treatment was offered (Rovner et al., 1992; Llorente et al., 1998).

Decubitus sores are widely considered to be avoidable and, if found, an indication of serious shortcomings in nursing care. In spite of existing care and treatment standards some institutions do not apply the necessary risk assessment and do not take the necessary preventive steps such as regular laying and turning to a sufficient extent (Bergstrom et al., 1996, Heinemann et al., 2000). Decubitus sores are present more frequently in facilities where medication errors happen more often, ADL-loss occurs faster, behavioural disorders of patients are more frequent, the number of staff is comparably low and their fluctuations high (Rudman et al., 1993; Ooi et al., 1999).

In 1998 the Institute of Forensic Medicine at the University of Hamburg conducted a cross-section survey of 10222 post-mortem examinations in order to determine the frequency of pressure sores (Heinemann et al., 2000). It showed an overall prevalence of 11,2 % decubitus ulcers. The proportion of very serious ulcers amounted to 2 %. More than half of the serious pressure sores took place in nursing care settings, 11,5 % in hospitals and about 33 % at home. A Munich survey conducted by Pelka (1998) and called Initiative on Chronic Wounds shows that 10 % of all hospital patients and up to 30 % of nursing home residents suffer from decubitus ulcers. According to a projection it can be assumed that about 750 000 patients (hospital and nursing home) suffer from pressure sores.

Although the prevalence and incidence data reported in the relevant literature are not comparable due to different risk profiles of the sampling units indications are that the rates of incidence for decubitus sores in stage two and higher start from 0% to 15 % to more than 38%. (Bergmann et al., 1992; Rudman et al., 1993). Decubitus prevalence for all stages varies between 12 and 83 %. In as far as these deviations cannot be attributed to different characteristics of the residents, they may indicate very heterogeneous levels of quality in institutional care settings for the elderly.

These studies show how significant and important it is to point out the neglect suffered not only by nursing home residents but also by hospital patients. Martin & Behler (1999) report that more than half of the decubitus ulcers diagnosed in nursing homes originated in hospitals before the admittance to the nursing home.

Specific Aspect: Serial Killing in Nursing Homes

The serial killing of patients and nursing home residents that became known in recent years is mostly supported by the analysis of records. A respective summary written by Maisch (1997), titled "Killing of Patients" and subtitled "A

Helping Hand to Death" indicates the novel aspect of these killings. He interprets the most massive form of violence as an action that is subjectively understood by the perpetrator as an assistance to die. On the basis of actual cases he describes "rituals of denial" and "barriers to discovery" among the nursing staff and in the care facilities. Beine (1998) writes of defensive attitudes towards beginning suspicions and of grave leadership deficits in dealing with early warning signs. Although the perpetrators were convicted, the serious institutional shortcomings established in the trial were not remedied. Opinion polls amongst nurses in the USA and Australia on euthanasia assisted by nurses, which is prohibited, suggest a large twilight zone. About 20% of the respondents had participated in the active assistance to die.

Causes of Abuse: Risk Factors, Stress Factors and Characteristics of the Perpetrators

Prevalence studies indicate regular relations between incidents of abuse and numerous contextual factors. These factors are frequently called risk factors which indicate a high probability that abuse may occur when they are present. This does not imply a causal connection. A great variety and a multitude of risk indicators suggest that very different circumstances may influence abuse and a multifaceted model of explanation is needed. Jones et al. (1997) summarised 19 risk factors concerning the persons involved in an abusive situation – "victim", "perpetrator" and their relationships- and 14 risk factors describing the situational circumstances. In their research Reis and Namish (1998) were able to isolate three categories by means of a discriminant analysis: indices regarding the abuser (mental disorders, inexperience with nursing), the abused person (abuse in the past, social isolation) and finally interpersonal relations (problematic social and personal relationships, financial dependency on the care recipient, limited empathic abilities). The complex structure of different, mutually conditional factors from various spheres was summed up in a presentation by NACEA (2000) into 4 categories: nursing care stress, dependency on care on the part of the elderly, cycle of abuse and personal problems of the abuser. The actual significance of such risk indices, however, is uncertain, since with the exception of the study by Lachs et al. (1997) no long-term studies with a prospective approach exist, which could test the predicative significance of single factors. In addition, the existing surveys are based on a predominantly restrictive methodological approach which only records personal and situational parameters, but does not take into account structural and cultural variables.

Many studies that wanted to investigate risk markers were guided by existing models of explanation on the origin of abuse. The oldest model adopted from research on child abuse defines the abusive behaviour as learnt and transferred from one generation to the next. However, it did not mean that the experience of abuse inevitably leads to abusive behaviour. Originally, this hypothesis was formulated in case studies, but the relation between elder and child abuse was later proved statistically in a comprehensive population study (Jogerst et al., 2000). The family dynamics was described specially in relationships between couples, where one partner had become demented and a recipient of care (Homer and Gilleard, 1990; Coyne et al., 1993) The familiar constellation of family members, specially adult children, who were abusers has frequently been understood not as an intergenerational pattern of transmission but rather as an reaction to the aggressive behaviour of the care recipient (Pillemer and Suitor, 1992, Cooney et al., 1995). The dynamic of such a mutual abuse is not restricted to families , but is also evident in institutional nursing care where aggressive behaviour of the residents results in staff violence (Pillemer and Moore, 1989; Schneider, 1990).

An independent model of explaining the causes of abuse was based on the observation that elder abuse occurs predominantly in care giving relationships. The well established risk markers in this respect by means of prospective studies consist of the reduction of ordinary and cognitive abilities, psychiatric symptoms such as confusion and depression as well as a recent deterioration of an already existing reduction of cognitive abilities (Lachs, 1997; NACEA and Westat, 1998). Nursing care dependency as a risk marker has also been proved in larger neighbourhood studies (Pillemer and Finkelhor, 1988; Podniecks, 1990). With regard to family care of demented patients, however, it seldom becomes significant (Coyne et al., 1993), obviously, because in this setting different factors can become more important such as stress symptoms of the care givers through behaviour disorders shown by the care recipient (Paveza et al., 1992; Cooney and Mortimer, 1995). The needs of the care recipient make high emotional, physical, temporary and financial demands on the care giver; these demands are a continuous challenge to his or her tolerance. Constant stress caused by giving care and the necessity to put one´s own interest last may result in exhaustion, social isolation and psychological stress symptoms. (Coyne et al., 1995). However, in spite of these stress factors it is frequently not the nursing situation as such, but additional factors that may crucially increase an existing risk, such as a certain lifestyle, lacking support in the provision of care and financial and emotional dependencies. Situational triggers, external stress factors or illness may also be risk factors (Jones et al., 1997; Kleinschmidt, 1997). In institutional care stress also leads frequently to abuse. A particularly frequent diagnosis here is staff burn-out (Pillemer and Moore, 1989). Also stress factors originating in the personal lives

of the staff and institutional and situational factors play an important role (Görgen, 2000; Gröning, 1998; Schneider, 1991; Foner, 1994; Goodridge et al., 1996;
Glendenning, 1999).

Many studies describe the personal problems of the "perpetrator", which include besides the above-mentioned stress symptoms also alcoholism, various psychiatric disorders, social isolation, emotional and material dependency on the
care recipient (Jones et al., 1997). These factors usually co-exist with each other.
An evaluation of this factors already existed before the incident or following the
incident, is not possible by means of cross-section studies. It is evident that these
factors characterise persons who are mentally at risk themselves and are hardly
equal to the task of a difficult nursing care. This makes it clear that many abusers
are themselves fragile and therefore, it can be justified to see the "perpetrator" as
a "victim" of circumstances which he/she cannot shape actively any more.

Consequences of Abuse

The consequences of violence against the elderly, especially mental and physical
damage, are particularly grave (Whittaker, 1987), but there are hardly any empirical data. It emerges from the Bonn study that 17 out of 44 older persons suffered lasting effects from the abuse (Brendebach and Hirsch, 1999). Fifteen persons reported anxieties and 12 feelings of disrespect and humiliation. 10 persons
suffered financial losses and 6 persons physical injuries. Many persons did not
react to violence or resisted it. In the long run strategies were developed to avoid
contact or to break up ties. A study by Comijs et al. (1998) shows that most victims react with anger, disappointment and grief. At least 11 of 43 persons in this
study reacted aggressively to verbal and physical abuse. It is known from homes
for the elderly that violence, especially neglect, results in increased helplessness,
loss of interest in one's surroundings, symptoms of depression, loss of identity,
resignation, regression and suicidal tendencies (Meyer, 1998; Schneider, 1994).
Empirical studies on these subjects do not exist at present.

Considering the previous empirical, case and descriptive studies on this subject the following consequences of elder violence can be suggested:
- long-term feelings of humiliation, shame, disrespect and hopelessness and
  giving up on life,
- increasing isolation, loneliness and fear of other persons,
- pathological reaction of grief and reactive depression,
- helplessness, dependency and paralysing inaction,
- increase of chronic anxieties,
- long-term physical and mental damage after a massive physical mistreatment,

- occurrence of psychosomatic illness,
- loss of trust in relations or professionals, if these are perpetrators,
- destructive behaviour towards oneself and attempts at suicide,
- falling into poverty after financial exploitation.

The question is if experiences of violence can result in mental disorders which can be added diagnostically to the post-traumatic stress disorder (ICD-F43.0).

Naturally, many of the above-mentioned topics also apply to the nursing staff in institutions. Hierarchy, competition, division of labour as well as regression because of exhaustion and frustration silence many staff members (Rudnitzki and Voll, 1991). It is well-known that many staff members give up their profession after a short time or change the institution.

Assessment of Violence

Violence does not happen by chance and only rarely spontaneously. It usually has a long history and is influenced by numerous, particularly psychosocial factors. The efforts to prevent and reduce violence are as numerous as the sources are manifold. A condition for intervening against violence is to recognise, to experience and to evaluate a violent action as such and not to regard it as a single isolated case, but one that has multidimensional facets and is in process. The trivialisation of violent actions must not be allowed. Violent actions constitute bogus solutions to problems, result in thoughtless acts and encourage institutional totality. Violent acts committed in relationships also signify signs of communication or contact, even if it is of a rather desperate kind marked by fear, helplessness, dependency, and destruction. Violence damages, insults or injures not only the victim, but also the perpetrator and, beyond that, the social environment where the violent actions takes place. Violence stimulates violence in return. It is "contagious". Therefore, it is necessary not to dismiss violence uncritically as "necessary", "sensible", etc., when confronted by it. Violent actions are not "normal", "everyday" and "usual" interactions.

The clarification concerning if and how a violent action can be influenced demands a multi-layered process (Figure 2). If suspicion is aroused, it has to be followed up. In principle, an intensive physical examination (for injuries, decubitus sores and/or malnutrition) is needed and over-medication has to be checked for. Information from third parties has to be taken into account. So far, physical changes as indications of a violent action has been neglected. Unfortunately, objective criteria, such as are known for the abuse of children and women, are missing, bruises are easily overlooked by doctors or are declared to be normal for the

126

elderly. A further step towards clarification is to include the "perpetrator(s)" and to study both the pathological patterns of relationships and the situational factors. Further steps are to find out how motivated the affected person is, if he or she can imagine his- or herself changing and to what extent that person is willing to actively participate in the necessary changes. In some relationships, outside assistance is refused, since it is feared that the affected person will suffer more violence. If a further process of clarification is possible, more differentiated investigations concerning the person, the situation and the respective environment must follow. It must also be explored what type of assistance to change is really possible. The interventions that can sometimes result in a charge are based on these investigations.

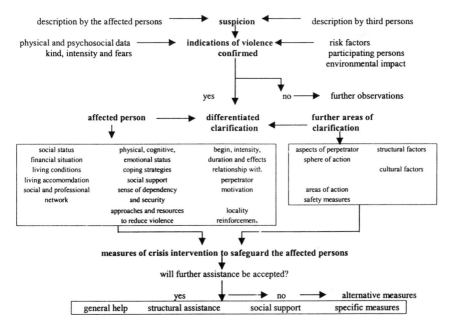

Figure 2: Assessment of Violence (according to Hirsch and Vollhardt, 2002)

Prevention

The precondition for all preventions is the social ostracism of violence and the protection for weaker groups by the community. The present laws concerning protection in the institutional area in Germany are insufficient. The existing controls, such as the supervision of homes and the medical service of the health insurance agencies, seldom lead to a reduction of violence. The certainly meaningful support of quality control is still in the beginning stage in the institutions. Also, the people who are implementing it are not always accepted to the extent necessary to carry out their role. Thus, their influence on the reduction of violence is still too limited. The discussion about anti-discrimination laws for the elderly is not yet concluded. If the obligation to notify about and report incidents were discussed, then it would be understood as a sign that the punishment for abuse of the elderly cannot be ranked lower than that for the abuse of women and children. However, every member of a community is responsible for reducing the abuse. Existing laws state that all people must look after both their own and others' safety. However, these laws cannot replace the individual responsibility of every citizen for his or her behaviour.

If one considers the sources of violence against the elderly, and considers that these include many things that are taboo, then appropriate measures could contribute to the prevention or reduction of abuse (see Table 2). Of course, one should not reach the false conclusion that with optimal prevention, freedom from violence would be achievable.

Preventative measures in institutions depend on the employees, their social support for each other and from their superiors, team supervision as well as on the form of the organisation, the way the superiors interact with the employees, the clarity of the work areas, the work atmosphere, the kind of work regulations, the institutional philosophy and the opinions of the people on which it rests. It is also decisive that, according to the needs and the extent of care needed by those living in the home, adequate care personnel is there. Another imperative is that the personnel must be given enough time to reflect on their work and that the enjoyment of their job should not be diminished by chronic overwork and unpredictable working times.

Education, including continuing and further education, is especially meaningful for all professionals who work with the elderly. This helps them to understand their own impulses to abuse, the situations of abuse, its causes and consequences as well as means for its active prevention or reduction. Only a few learning aids and textbooks about medicine and care deal with this theme. Therefore, it is all the more important for each professional to find the opportunity for further education. Currently, besides the specialist literature, there are also training manuals,

Table 2: Possibilities to Influence Violence

Institution	"philosophy"
	structure
	working conditions
	support of staff
	qualification of staff
	quality assurance
	nursing care management
	adequate staff presence at all times
	continuous training (also supervision)
	mental hygiene
	sufficient medical provision
	division of rooms, etc.
	architecture
	working materials
Personnel:	team meeting
	documentation
	mutual social support
	professional expertise
	solution of relationship problems (proximity and distance)
	motivation to work
superiors:	social support
	encouragement of independence and teamwork
	"help" instead of "punishment"
	raising the awareness of problems
	development of alternatives to violence
local area:	"round table"
	advice and crisis centre
	"grievance/crisis telephone lines"
	public events
society:	recognition of work with the elderly
	de-stigmatising of "violence"
	attitudes towards age and ageing
	equal treatment of the physically and mentally disabled
science:	interdisciplinary research on "violence"
	study of alternatives
	establishment of guidelines on the handling of violence

structured curricula and challenging continuing education possibilities (Hiss et al., 2000; Kemshall and Pritchard 1998, MASGV, 2000, 2002; Münchenstift, 2002; Pritchard 1996, 1990; Piantanida 1990 a & b; .Pritchard 1996, 1990).

Interventions

Every institution has its rules, regulations and institutional philosophy. The staff suffer from structural violence in institutions (for example, bad or unfavourable working conditions, unspecific work regulations, the encouragement of a general sense of anxiety about sanctions, lack of inclusion in important decisions, unreasonable structural conditions) as much as the patients or the residents living in a home (not being included in decisions about the times to wake up or to eat, a reduction in competence, the loss of the privacy). In addition, there are the socially negative judgements about psychiatry, homes and elderly people. One-sided and sometimes biased perceptions by those in charge of the institutions concerning such factors as ethics and social requirements are not helpful. If violent phenomena occur in the interactions of patients or people living in homes and the younger personnel, in order to reduce violence, more levels (directors of the institutions, institutional management, employees in the stations, patients or people living in homes and their relatives) must be included in order to be able to bring about changes (Hirsch, 1998). A change is necessary in the way people are employed or given responsibility (direct or indirect) in the care industry. It is important to allow the people living in homes to have freedom in their actions, movements and planning that is oriented to the outside world and to ensure their optimal conditions so that they can make their own decisions. A precondition for this is that a corresponding freedom is also made possible for the care personnel.

In the interaction with the elderly, there is a spectrum of psychodynamic aspects that can be extremely powerful. Therefore, it is important for everyone who works with the elderly to be aware of these difficulties and aspects of counter projections (mostly subconscious feelings and perceptions that are released in young people by the elderly). To handle the everyday situations in a place where the elderly are cared for, a certain self respect and an ability to maintain both closeness and distance in relationships are necessary.

Possible measures to reduce violence are, for example: (1) team discussions about the management of violence, (2) admitting one's own feelings of powerlessness, anger and helplessness as well as frustration about the lack of social support, (3) presentations (documentation) of violent situations and a search for sources, (4) working out and implementing alternatives, (5) the inclusion of superiors and others, (6) the reduction of burn-out symptoms, (7) continual team su-

130

pervision (quality indicator for an establishment and a necessary work method) and (8) working on relationships in the form of a Balint group (Hirsch, 2002). Examples for the reduction of indirect violence are:

Structural:

- the analysis of work regulations and "grey zones"
- the inclusion of legal assistance for questions about the employer's obligation to provide for the welfare of the employees
- increasing personnel and their professional competence
- care management
- to introduce care standards and ensure quality
- to study and standardise alternatives to violent actions
- support from superiors and doctors
- reduction of feelings of helplessness of the employees by the inclusion of decision-making processes
- the encouragement of continuing and further education, including supervision
- the reduction of hierarchical structures and the encouragement of team work and emancipation as well as of a self-responsible way of working
- encouragement of contentment with work and life as well as social support
- violence-free shaping of the milieu
- optimise the working material, the set up of the station and the structural conditions
- examine the balance of the composition of the people living in the homes (clinic patients or people living in homes who are physically and mentally chronically sick)

Cultural:

- discussing the issue of being the "Samaritan"
- the encouragement of the equalisation of the physically and mentally sick
- the encouragement to think of the whole person, not just the organic medical problem
- raising consciousness about ageism
- It also needs to be tested, for example, to what extent the milieu of a ward encourages orientation, friendliness and self assurance and reduces anxiety for both the patients and the employees.

Social Reorientation

In spite of many individual activities of associations, communal establishments, political bodies and initiatives – for example, emergency telephones and complaint centers (Hirsch and Erkens, 1999), there still needs to be an analysis to see if violence in homes for the elderly is not more sanctioned than opposed by society.

Although our general perceptions of norms ostracise violence, there are many indirect, hidden messages that arouse the readiness for violence, make it possible and strengthen it, including a tendency to play it down, to excuse it or even to consider it necessary and justify it. Especially those institutions with their own regulations, taboos and models, their own world and a tendency to "ghettoisation" are vulnerable to violence.

For years it has been observed that extremely old people are increasingly coming into nursing homes with very bad mental and physical illnesses. Because of changes in the health services, the time spent on treatments is declining. The number of insufficiently treated elderly patients as well as the number of forced moves into nursing homes are increasing. Because of the variety of partial responsibilities and the different cost carriers, who are mainly worried about reducing the costs, ultimately, no one feels responsible. This deplorable state of affairs is legally safeguarded and socially sanctioned. Today, whoever is old, mentally ill and in need of care seems to have only a very limited right to existence.

The many and diverse burdens placed on the employees in a nursing home are well known. The low level of respect accorded to these people by society is a reality. Sickness, burnout and changing or quitting jobs are the consequences (Zimber and Weyerer, 1998; Becker and Meifort, 1998). Not only the relatives of people living in nursing homes but also the experts in the field criticise the completely unsatisfactory ratio of personnel to patients and the paucity of qualified employees in the institutions. In addition to this, the employees protest the unsatisfactory mental health measures (e.g. professional supervision). It is shocking that there seems to be no time for reflection about what professional behaviour is. These deplorable conditions lead to the hidden forms of violence and are responsible when employees in nursing homes become emotionally hardened, avoid professional relationships with the people living in the homes and become violent.

Laws in Germany, such as the home law, should guarantee the protection of people living in homes from infringement on their rights by the institutions, an as-high-as-possible quality of life and the right to live in dignity. However, reality is often different. The range of interpretations of these laws is so broad that they can even be used against the protection of the elderly. A variety of complaints are heard by the emergency and complaint centres in Germany. Society feels little responsibility in this, having the impression that everything is taken care of by the laws. It is forgotten that the application of the laws and their implementation are dependent upon all participants bring sincerely interested in seeing that the dignity also of the elderly is inviolable.

Supervision of the homes and the medical service branch of health insurance carry out the function of controls. Reading the laws and instructions pertaining to these branches, one could feel secure. But the reality is completely different. Observing the small number of people supervising the homes and who are responsible for a region, their previous experience (mostly with management personnel), their ability to get things accomplished as well as their reports of home supervisions, one reaches the conclusion that society is not at all interested in having violence against the elderly in nursing homes punished thoroughly and without reservations.

Conclusions

Also this review has not been exhaustive, it is enough to allow us to conclude that violence against people in nursing homes is at least tolerated by society. But we must consider that every participant is also a member of society and carries responsibility. This cannot be delegated. Social ostracism of violence against the elderly is not enough. If there is a consensus that violence is not a humane method, then there should be no question of cost in the measures against it. Addressed here are the ethical principles that bind a society together and are expressed in the question: "What is an elderly person worth to us?"

Violence against the elderly is a social problem that can only be reduced through the efforts of all participants. The various images of violence, such as physical, mental, social, structural and cultural, make clear how complex a violent situation can be and how necessary a differentiating perspective is. It is decisive that no violent action be trivialised or excused; rather, alternatives must be found. This is also true for situations in which the care personnel become the victims of violent elderly people. It is also necessary for care personnel to finally be granted the right to a humane work place in the institutions. In addition, doctors should not just overlook emerging violent situations but should assist in their reduction. There are still too few possibilities for those affected (people living in homes, their relatives and those working in the field of helping the elderly) to be taken seriously and to be helped.

References

Aktion gegen Gewalt in der Pflege (AGP) (1999): Memorandum. *Für eine menschenwürdige Pflege.* Bonn, Eigendruck.

Arbesman, R.C. and Wright, C. (1999) Mechanical restraints, rehabilitation therapies, and staffing adequacy as risk factors for falls in an elderly hospitalized population. *Rehabilitation Nursing,* 24, 122-128.

Beine, K.-H. (1998) *Sehen Hören Schweigen.* Freiburg, Lambertus.

Becker, W. and Meifort, B. (1998): *Altenpflege-Abschied vom Lebensberuf.* Bielefeld: Bertelsmann.

Bergstrom N., Braden, B. Kemp, N., Champagne, M. and Ruby E. (1996) Multi-site study of incidence of pressure ulcers and the relationship between risk level, demographic characteristics, diagnoses, and prescription of preventive interventions. *Journal of the American Geriatrics Society,* 44, 22-30.

Bickel, H. (1992) Zur Inanspruchnahme von stationärer Pflege und Versorgung im Altersverlauf. *Gesundheitswesen* 65, 363-370.

Board of Directors of the American Association for Geriatric Psychiatry (1992) *Position Statement.* Psychotherapeutic Medications in the Nursing Home.

Brendebach, C. and Hirsch, R.D. (1999) Gewalt gegen alte Menschen in der Familie. In: Hirsch, R.D., Kranzhof, E.U. and Schiffhorst, G. (ed.) *Untersuchungen zur Gewalt gegen alte Menschen.* Bonner Schriftenreihe „Gewalt im Alter" Band 2 (pp. 83-108), Bonn, HsM.

Bruckner, U. (2000) *Erste Erfahrungen und Ergebnisse der Qualitätsprüfungen.* Statement. Pressekonferenz des Kuratoriums Deutsche Altershilfe (KDA) vom 2. Februar 2000. Köln: KDA.

Brüggemann, J. (2000) Korrekturbedarf. *Pflegen ambulant* 11, 4, 33-40.

Bundesministerium für Familie, Senioren, Frauen und Jugend (1996) *Gewalt gegen Ältere zu Hause.* Fachtagung 11. Und 12. März 1996 in Bonn. Broschüre. Bonn, BMFSFJ.

Capezuti, E., Evans, L., Strumpf, N. and Maislin, G. (1996) Physical Restraint Use and Falls in Nursing Home Residents. *Journal of the American Geriatrics Society,* 44, 627-633.

Castle, N.G., Fogel B. and Mor, V. (1997) Risk factors for physical restraint use in nursing homes: pre- and post-implementation of the Nursing Home Reform. *Act. Gerontologist,* 37, 737-747.

Comijs, H., Pot, A. M., Smit, H.H., Bouter, L. M. and Jonker, C. (1998): Elder abuse in the community: Prevalence and consequences. *Journal of the American Geriatrics Society,* 46, 885-888.

Cooney, C. and Mortimer, A. (1995) Elder abuse and dementia - a pilot study. *International Journal of Social Psychiatry,* 41, 276-283.

Council of Europe (1992) *Violence against elderly people*. Report prepared by the Study Group on Violence against Elderly People. Council of Europe Press, Strasbourg.

Dieck, M. (1987) Gewalt gegen ältere Menschen im familialen Kontext – Ein Thema der Forschung, der Praxis und der öffentlichen Information. *Zeitschrift für Gerontologie*, 20, 305-313.

Evans, L.K., and Strumpf, N. E. (1989) Tying Down the Elderly. *Journal of the American Geriatrics Society*, 37, 65-74.

Foner, N. (1994) Nursing Home Aides: Saints or Monsters? *The Gerontologist*, 34, 245-250.

Galtung, J. (1975) *Strukturelle Gewalt*. Rohwolt, Reinbek.

Galtung, J. (1993) Kulturelle Gewalt. In: Landeszentrale für politische Bildung Baden-Württemberg (ed): *Aggression und Gewalt*. Stuttgart, Kohlhammer.

Glaeske, G., Graalmann, J., Häussler, B., Keller, S. and Stillfried, V.S. (1997) Ursachen für den überproportionalen Anstieg der Gesundheitskosten im Alter. Gutachten für den Deutschen Bundestag – Enquete-Kommission Demographischer Wandel. Bonn

Glendenning, F. (1999) Elder Abuse and Neglect in Residential Settings: The Need for Inclusiveness in Elder Abuse Research. *Journal of Elder Abuse and Neglect* 10, 1-11.

Goffman, E. (1961): Asylums: Essays on the Social Situations of Mental Patients and Other Inmates. Anchor, Garden City, N.Y.

Goodridge, D. M., Johnston, P. and Thompson, M. (1996) Conflict and Aggression as Stressors in the Work Environment of Nursing Assistants: Implications for Institutional Elder Abuse. *Journal of Elder Abuse and Neglect*, 8, 49-67.

Görgen, Th. (2000): Gewalt gegen alte Menschen in stationären Pflegeeinrichtungen. *In:* Jacob, R. and Fikentscher, W. (eds): *Korruption, Reziprozität und Recht*. Schriften zur Rechtspsychologie, Band 4. Stümpfle, Bern, S. 157-178.

Gröning, K. (1998) *Entweihung und Scham*. Mabuse, Frankfurt.

Hagen, B.F. and Sayers, D. (1995) When Caring Leaves Bruises. *Journal of Gerontological Nursing* 21(11), 7-16.

Heinemann A., Lockemann U., Matschke, J., Tsokos M. and Pueschel, K. (2000) Dekubitus im Umfeld der Sterbephase: Epidemiologische, medizinrechtliche und ethische Aspekte. *Deutsche Medizinische Wochenschrift*, 125 (3) 45-51.

Hirsch, R.D. (1998): Gewalt in der Gerontopsychiatrischen Klinik. In: Hirsch, R.D., Vollhardt, B.R. and Erkens, F. (eds): *Gewalt gegen alte Menschen*. 1. Arbeitsbericht, Bonn, HsM, S. 33-56.

Hirsch, R.D. (2000) Definition und Abgrenzung von Gewalt und Aggression. *In*: Hirsch, R. D., Bruder, J. and Radebold (eds): *Aggression im Alter*. Bonn, HsM-Bonner Initiative gegen Gewalt im Alter, 15-43.

Hirsch, R.D. (2002) *Supervision, Teamberatung, Balintgruppe*. München, Reinhardt.

Hirsch, R.D. and Erkens, F. (1999) (eds) *Wege aus der Gewalt. Notruftelefone, Beschwerdestellen, krisenberatungs- und interventionsangebote für alte Menschen und deren Helfer in der Bundesrepublik Deutschland*. Bonner Schriftenreihe „Gewalt im Alter", Band 5. Bonn, HsM-Bonner Initiative gegen Gewalt im Alter.

Hirsch, R.D. and Fussek, C. (1999) (eds) *Gewalt gegen pflegebedürftige alte Menschen in Institutionen. Gegen das Schweigen*. Bonner Schriftenreihe „Gewalt im Alter", Band 4. Bonn, HsM-Bonner Initiative gegen Gewalt im Alter.

Hirsch, R.D. and Kranzhoff, E.U. (1996) Bewegungseinschränkende Maßnahmen in der Gerontopsychiatrie. Teil I u. Teil II. *Krankenhauspsychiatrie*, 7, 99-104 u. 155-161.

Hirsch, R.D. and Vollhardt, B.R. (2002) Elder maltreatment. In: Jacoby, R. and Oppenheimer, C. (eds*) Psychiatry in the elderly*. University press, Oxford (3. Ed.), 869-918.

Hirsch, R.D., Wörthmüller, M. and Schneider, H.K. (1992) Fixierungen: Zu viel, zu häufig und im Grunde genommen vermeidbar. *Zeitschrift für Gerontopsychologie und –psychiatrie* 5, 127-135.

Hiss, B., Rufer, F., Ruthemann, U., Schmitt, R., Schneider, H.-D., Schüpbach, B. and Wattendorf, I. (2000) Fallgeschichten Gewalt. Vincentz, Hannover.

Hollwig, T. (1994) Freiheitsbeschränkung und Freiheitsentziehung in *Altenpflegeheimen*. Unveröff. Diplomarbeit, Universität Marburg.

Homer, A. C. and Gilleard, C. (1990) Abuse of elderly people by their carers. *British Medical Journal*, 301, 1359-1362.

Jogerst ,G.J., Dawson, J. D., Hartz, A.J., Ely, J.W. and Schweitzer, L.A. (2000) Community Characteristics Associated with Elder Abuse. *Journal of the American Geriatrics Society*, 48, 513-518.

Johnson, T. (1991) *Elder mistreatment: deciding who is at risk*. Greenwood Press, Westport CT.

Jones, J. S., Holstege, C. and Holstege, H. (1997) Elder Abuse and neglect: Understanding the Causes and Potential Risk Factors. *American Journal Of Emergency Medicine 15*, 579-583.

Jones, J. S., Veenstra, T.R., Seamon, J.P. and Krohmer, J. (1997) Elder Mistreatment: National Survey of Emergency Physicians. *Annals of Emergency Medicine*, 30, 473-479.

Kemshall H. and Pritchard J. (1996) *Good Practice in Risk Assessment and Risk Management*. London et al., Kingsley Publishers.

Kleinschmidt, K. C. (1997): Elder Abuse: a review. *Annales of Emergency Medicine*, 30, 463-472.

Klie, Th. (1998) Zur Verbreitung unterbringungsähnlicher Maßnahmen im Sinne des § 1906 Abs. 4 BGB in bundesdeutschen Pflegeheimen. *Betreuungsrechtliche Praxis*, 7, 2, 50-53.

Kosberg, J.I. and Garcia, J.L. (1995) *Elder Abuse: International and Cross- Cultural Perspectives*. New York, Haworth Press.

Lachs, M.S., Williams, C., O'Brien, M. S., Hurst, L. and Horwitz, R. (1997) Risk Factors for Reported Elder Abuse and neglect: A Nine-Year Observational Cohort Study. *The Gerontologist*, 37, 469-474.

Langkau, G. (1987) Wir wollen nicht mitschuldig werden. *Altenpflege*, 9, 566-567.

Llorente, M.D., Olsen, E.J., Leyva, O., Silverman, M.A., Lewis J.E. and Rivreo, J. (1998) Use of Antipsychotic Drugs in Nursing Homes: Current Compliance with OBRA Regulations. *Journal of the American Geriatrics Society*, 46, 198-201.

Maisch, H. (1997) *Patiententötungen*. Kindler, München.

Martin, U. and Behler, R. (1999) Duisburger Modell – intensivierte Heimaufsicht des Gesundheitsamtes in Zusammenarbeit mit dem Sozialamt. *Gesundheitswesen* 61, 337-339.

Mc Creadie, C., Bennett, G., Gilthrope, M. S., Houghton, G. and Tinker, A. (2000) Elder abuse: do general practitioners know or care? *Journal of the Royal Society of Medicine*, 93, 67-71.

Meyer, M. (1998) *Gewalt gegen alte Menschen in Pflegeeinrichtungen*. Bern, Huber.

Ministerium für Arbeit, Gesundheit und Soziales des Landes Schleswig-Holstein (2000) (ed) *Gleich nehme ich ihr die Klingel weg. Eine Arbeitshilfe für die Aus-, Fort- und Weiterbildung*. Kiel, MAGS.

Ministerium für Arbeit, Gesundheit und Soziales des Landes Schleswig-Holstein (2002) (ed) *Da kann man doch nur noch durchgreifen, oder...?*. Eine Arbeitshilfe für die Aus-, Fort- und Weiterbildung. Kiel, MAGS.

Münchenstift (2002) (ed) *Pflege ohne Gewalt*. Schulungsordner. München, Eigendruck.

National Council On Elder Abuse in collaboration with Westat Inc. (1998) The National elder abuse incidence study: Final report September. Adminstration on Aging. Available: www. aoa. gov /abuse /report /Cexecsum.html.

National Council On Elder Abuse: The Basics. Available: NCEA Web site www. gwjapan. com/ NCEA /basic /index.html (visited August 26, 2000).

Neufeld, R.R., Libow, L., Foley, W.J., Dunbar, J. M., Cohen, C. and Breuer, B. (1999) Restraint reduction reduces serious injuries among nursing home residents. *Journal of the American Geriatrics*, Society 47, 1202-1207.

Ooi, W. L., Morris, J. N., Brandeis, G. H., Hossian, M. and Lipsitz, L.A. (1999) Nursing home characteristics and the development of presure sores and disruptive behaviour. *Age and Ageing*, 28, 45-52.

Parker, K. and Miles, S.H. (1997) Death Caused by Bedrails. *Journal of the American Geriatrics Society*, 45, 797-802.

Pelka, R.B. (1998) Expertise zur Kostensituation bei chronischen Wunden. München, Manuskript.

Phillips, C.D., Hawes, C., Mor, V., Fries, B.E., Morris, J.N. and Nennstiel, M.E. (1996) Facility and area variation affecting the use of phsical restraints in nursing homes. *Medical Care*, 34, 1149-1162.

Piantanida M. (1990 a) *Basic Training in protective services. Part 1: Protective Services Regulations*. Harrisburg, Pennsylvania Department of Aging.

Piantanida M. (1990 b) *Basic Training in protective services. Part 2: Protective Services Casework*. Harrisburg, Pennsylvania Department of Aging.

Pillemer, K. and Finkelhor, D. (1988) The Prevalence of Elder Abuse: A Random Sample Survey. *The Gerontologist*, 28, 51-57.

Pillemer, K. and Moore, D.W. (1989) Abuse of patients in nursing homes: Findings from a survey of staff. *The Gerontologist*, 29, 314-320.

Pillemer, K. and Suitor, J.J. (1992) Violence and Violent Feelings: What Causes Them Among Family Caregivres? *Journal of Gerontology*, 47, 165 - 172.

Podnieks, E. (1990) *National survey on abuse of the elderly in Canada, The Ryerson Study*. Toronto, Ryerson Polytechnic Institute.

Pritchard, J. (1996) *Working with elder abuse. A training manual for home care, residential and day care staff.* London, Kingsley Publishers.

Reis, M. and Nahmish, D. (1998) Validation of the Indicators of Abuse (IOA) Screen. *The Gerontologist*, 38, 471 - 480.

Riedel-Heller, S.G., Stelzner, G., Schork, A. and Angermeyer, M.C. (1999) Gerontopsychiatrische Kompetenz ist gefragt. *Psychiatrische Praxis*, 26, 273 - 276.

Rovner, B.W., Edelman, B.A., Cox, M.P. and Shmuely, Y. (1992) The Impact of Antipsychotic Drug Regulations on Psychotropic Prescribing Practices in Nursing Homes. *American Journal of Psychiatry*, 149, 1390-1392.

Rudman, D., Mattson, D. E., Alverno, L., Richardson, T.J. and Rudman, I. W. (1993) Comparison of Clinical Indicators in Two Nursing Homes. *Journal of the American Geriatrics Society*, 41, 1317-1325.

Rudnitzki, G. and Voll, R. (1991) Institutionen als Tagungsveranstaltung. *Gruppenpsychotherapie und Gruppendynamik*, 27, 141-152.

Schmidt, I., Claesson, C.B., Westerholm, B., Nilson, L.G. and Svarstad, B.L. (1998) The impact of regular multidisciplinary team interventions on psychoactive prescribing in Swedish nursing homes. *Journal of the American Geriatrics Society* 46, 77-82.

Schneekloth, U. and Müller, U. (1997) *Hilfe- und Pflegebedürftige in Heimen: Endbericht zur Repräsentativerhebung im Forschungsprojekt Möglichkeiten und Grenzen sebständiger Lebensführung in Einrichtungen.* Schriftenreihe des BMFSFJ, Band 147.2. Stuttgart, Kohlhammer.

Schneider, H.J. (1994) *Kriminologie der Gewalt.* Stuttgart, Hirzel.

Schneider, H.-D. and Sigg, E. (1990) Gibt es das: Gewalttätigkeit in Alters- und Pflegeheimen? *Forschungsgruppe Gerontologie, Universität Freiburg/ Schweiz.*

Schneider, H.D. (1990) Bewohner und Personal als Quellen und Ziele von Gewalttätigkeit in Altersheimen. *Zeitschrift für Gerontologie*, 23, 186-196.

Strumpf, N.E. and Evans, L.K. (1991) The Ethical Problems of Prolonged Physical restraint. *Journal of Gerontological Nursing*, 17, 27-30.

Svarstad, B.L. and Mount, J.K. (1991) Nursing Home Resources and Tranquilizer Use among the Institutionalized Elderly. *Journal of the American Geriatrics Society,* 39, 869-875.

United Nations (1983) *Wiener Internationaler Aktionsplan zur Frage des Alterns. Weltversammlung zur Frage des Alterns, 26. Juli - 6. August 1992,* Vienna, New York.

Wahl, H.W. and Reichert, M. (1991) Psychologische Forschung in Alten- und Pflegeheimen in den achziger Jahren. Teil 1: Forschungszugänge zu den Heimbewohnern. *Zeitschrift für Gerontopsychologie und –psychiatrie,* 4, 233-255.

Whittaker, T. (1987*) Elderly Victims.* U.S. Department of Justice. Rockville/Md.

Wilhelm-Gößling, C. (1998) Neuroleptikaverordnungen bei demten Alterspatienten. *Nervenarzt*, 69, 999-1006.

Williams, C.C. and Finch, C.E. (1997) Physical Restraint: Not Fit for Woman, Man, or Beast. *Journal of the American Geriatrics Society*, 45, 773-775.

Zimber, A. and Weyerer, S. (1998) (eds) *Arbeitsbelastung in der Altenpflege.* Göttingen, Verlag für angewandte Psychologie.

Chapter Seven: Physical Restraint in Gerontology in Ireland

Róisín Gallinagh

Introduction

It has been discussed in previous chapters how and why nurses may encounter violence from those they serve. However, the converse is also true. Nurses can are also be the perpetrators of control and violence towards one of the most vulnerable groups in society – older people. Common methods of impeding an older person's freedom under the premise of safety is now facing greater scrutiny. A physical restraint constitutes any device that is applied directly or indirectly to an individual with the purpose of impeding freedom (Molassiotis, 1995). Relating this definition to practice, it can mean that commonly used and accepted devices in the care of the older person can be deemed to be a physical restraint. This includes and is not limited to; side rails, screw on table tops, immobilisation of furniture, reclining chairs, means of immobilisation the limbs and or torso and removal of mobility aids. It should be clarified from the outset that whilst many devices have the potential to be physical restraints, their categorization is dependent on the individual's physical and cognitive ability and the outcomes for him/her (Gallinagh, 2002).

This chapter will identify the negative outcomes associated with physical restraint, trace it's roots in history and discuss the complex decision making that nurses must face in achieving a balance between patient protection and patient safety. Increasing physical and mental frailty should not be an indicator for the indiscriminate use of physical restraints and an individualised approach to their use is advocated. Finally an overview of a recent study on physical restraint use in the care of the older person setting is presented.

Institutional Abuse

Indiscriminate physical restraint in gerontology can be regarded as a form of institutional abuse. Hindmarch (1999) regards institutional abuse as being conducted in a registered facility by individuals who have a legal or contractual obligation to care for the older person. It is regarded that it is particularly difficult form of abuse to eradicate as it becomes entrenched in the accepted practice of the institution (Hindmarch, 1999).

Physical restraints when used in an indiscriminate fashion can aggravate or even instigate the very problems that they are designed to prevent. As well as affecting problems associated with prolonged immobilisation and increased dependency on staff, they can also cause falls (Cohen-Mansfield and Billig, 1986; Magee et al., 1983), serious injury from falls (Hanger et al., 1999), patient entrapment (Todd et al., 1997; Food and Drug Administration, 1995), and even death as a result of asphyxia (Powell et al., 1989; Miles and Irvine, 1992; Parker and Miles, 1997; Paterson et al., 1998).

The psychological repercussions have also been isolated. Strumpf and Ellis (1988) interviewed 20 patients who had been subjected to physical restraint. They categorised their feelings in terms of fear, anger, resistance, humiliation and resignation. Patients' perceptions (n=25) of physical restraint use was also investigated by Hardin et al. (1993). Overall the majority of patients were negative about their use and some likened their experience to being 'caged' or 'jailed' and 'powerless'. Both these studies are from the USA, where it must be highlighted that more limiting devices such as Posey vest restraints and limb restraints are used compared with the UK. This must be borne in mind when interpreting the findings of the study. However, a comparable study by Gallinagh et al. (2001a), in the UK found similarly negative feelings expressed by 17 older patients. Furthermore, families dislike the use of restraint and they associate their use with loss of dignity, deterioration as well as posing safety hazards (Hardin et al., 1993; Newbern and Lindsay, 1994; Gallinagh et al., 2001b).

It has been long assumed that physical restraint type measures are employed to prevent harm to the older person (Hardin et al., 1993; Lee et al., 1999). However, research studies indicate that this is no longer the sole motivating force. Now it is more commonly accepted that a factor in nurses' decision includes non compliance with therapy and this is reinforced by the greater acuity of conditions, the typically more invasive therapies and confounded by shorted inpatient stays (Minnick et al., 1998; and Terpstra et al., 1998). Those who present with confusional type manifestations are also associated with the likelihood of having their freedom impinged upon by the use of mechanical restraints (O'Keefe et al., 1996; Ludwick and O' Toole, 1996; and Hantikainen, 2001).

Historical Perspectives

The use of physical restraint is linked to the societal era. For example, the Greeks practised a benevolent form of care with little use of impeding devices. Comparatively, during the Middle Ages a more sinister ethos prevailed towards the more vulnerable in society. Those with mental health problems were incarcerated in institutions with the use of shackles. They were regarded by their warders as being in need of behaviour management and were subjected to unquestioned acts of brutality, neglect and seclusion. This model became widely accepted throughout Europe and subsequently spread to the Americas. Religious fervour also did not ease their plight as there was then an accepted association between mental health manifestations and the forces of evil.

Restraint reduction was aided radically by the underlying humanitarianism philosophy of the French Revolution. Dramatic changes were made by Phillipe Pinel a distinguished and prolific physician in Paris, who is credited with the removal of physical restraints in 1794. Levine (1996) quotes Pinel as saying: 'to detain maniacs in constant seclusion... and to load them with chains; to leave them defenceless to the brutality of underlings.... is a system more distinguished for its convenience than for its humanity or its success....'

His writings influenced the practice of the day and his textbooks became standard material for psychiatry. He was subsequently made chief physician to Napoleon (Levine, 1999). This milieu of institutional care continued to improve. A cornerstone of psychiatric care in the UK was the passing of the Lunatic Asylum Act in 1842. This saw the first regulation of basic standards inclusive of restraints use and deportment of care workers within the mental health setting.

Strumpf et al. (1991) consider it curious that while that there was a reduction in restraint use in mental health in the twentieth century there was a concomitant increase in the apparent use of physical restraint within the gerontology setting. They are unclear as to when this surge took place. Certainly, the twentieth century did pose new challenges to care workers in the sense that that there were an increasing number of older people living longer and requiring long term care.

Up until the early 1970's it was generally accepted that the older person could be restrained at the care giver's discretion to prevent falls or the interruption of therapy. The ethos of 'protection at all costs' prevailed and issues such as patients rights, physiological and psychological repercussions were viewed as secondary. Families agreed to various restraint practices as they and the clinicians were acting in the best interests of the patient (Kane et al., 1993). From a litigation point of view, American courts tended to value paternalism of the older person and to punish institutions that deviated form the then accepted practice. It could be suggested then that they did an injustice to honouring patient's freedom and dignity. It should also be noted that while the UK did not use the array of physical restraints that were used in the USA, nonetheless, there was a dearth of professional guidelines and literature governing the use of devices that impeded freedom of the older person. The absence of directives may thus have unwittingly protracted the unquestioned use of freedom limiting approaches.

In the Western world in the late 70's and early '80s more credence was given to patients rights and philosophies of care. The development of the study of bio-ethics had a strong role to play in this. There was a subsequent surge in government and legislative directives reflecting this radical approach. Care of the older person in both the acute and long term care setting gradually began to embrace societal demands of patient autonomy. This principle of autonomy included self-determination for both those with active involvement in their care and those who were passive recipients. Partnership in care and quality of life issues became core of standard setting in national and local professional guidelines.

The use of physical restraint and its repercussions on the individual came under scrutiny. There was no quantifiable evidence linking their use to positive patient outcomes. In the USA, a key legislative document in 1990, the Nursing Home Reform Law, part of the Omnibus Budget Reconciliation Act (OBRA) 1987 sought to mandate the use of both physical and chemical restraints. Prior to the OBRA recommendations, physical restraint use was deemed to be 41% and afterwards to be on average 21% (cited in Cohen et al., 1998). To date there has been no specific British legislative directive on the use of physical restraints in gerontology.

Pan cultural comparisons on physical restraint rates is difficult given the variation in what constitutes a physical restraint. For example, in the UK, side rails have long being classed as a physical restraint particularly if they prevent the patient leaving the bed voluntarily. Comparatively, in the USA, side rails have only been regarded recently as a physical restraint and this may affect their prevalence rates. In the UK, the prevalence of restraint use (inclusive of side rails) in gerontology is 68% (Gallinagh et al., 2002). Side rails are commonly used in the British setting with Ramprogrus and Gibson (1991) finding that the incidence of their use was 100%. While it would be naïve to presume that a totally restraint free environment is possible, it is still notable that the prevalence of physical restraint use is high in the gerontology. Reasons for continued restraint use reflect conflicts that nurses have between the interplay between organisation of care and professional/personal knowledge. These are now discussed in light of recent literature.

Organisation of Care

This reflects factors such as the degree of emphasis on historical practice, national and local policy, fear of litigation, staffing levels, influence of peers, patients and families and how they might impinge on a nurse's decision to use a physical restraint.

Policy for an Individualised Approach

Professional guidelines for restraint use on the older person are provided by the RCN (1999). Physical restraint use should be directed by a local management policy that balances elements of risk taking vs. outcomes of the devices for the patient (Winston et al., 1999). Glanville et al. (1998) purports that these guidelines need to be evidence based and the origins and type of review highlighted. A good policy should encourage caregivers to search for alternatives to the patients needs without resorting to control measures. It should have emphasis on individuality and quality of life. Core issues to be addressed include the least physical restraint approach, patient/family involvement, alternatives to physical restraints, a framework for an interdisciplinary decision-making tree, physical restraint assessment and documentation pro-forma, approved devices per directorate, review times as well as addressing the concern of checking the device before and during use for safety and suitability (Gallinagh, 2002). Patients and families need also be made aware of the risks associated with the use and without the use of physical restraints.

Furthermore, to prevent administrator ambivalence, as highlighted by Mc Hutchion and Morse (1989), it could be suggested that such policies should be written and approved by the inter-professional team who have both the research, legal and working knowledge of the equipment. Once agreed upon they can be endorsed by the hospital administrators and lawyers. This will ensure that nurses are not forced to work with a policy that is vague, in conflict with hospital loyalties or of no support in a legal case. It could be surmised that if a local policy had involvement from nursing and other colleagues, was reflective of national and professional guidelines, sanctioned by the hospital, this would go a long way towards decreasing the prevalence of physical restraint use.

Peers

While the traditional influence of physical restraint use has been highlighted, it still plays an important role in gerontological nursing. Physical restraints are viewed as a routine in nursing (Rubenstein et al., 1983; Donius and Rader, 1994; Gallinagh et al., 2001 b). Tradition needs not be spoken, it can be procured by unquestioned, repeated acts. Examples include indiscriminately putting up side rails on the older patient in bed or installing screw on table tops on the older patient who is in a seating position. It is commonly known that once physical restraint have been put in place, their use is unquestionably perpetuated. It is un-

145

derstandable that it may be difficult for the reflective practitioner to mitigate against a system that does not have individualised care as a true foundation.

The decision to restrain ideally involves the multidisciplinary team, the patient and the family. However, as nurses are 24 hour care providers, initial restraint measures is often taken by them and the family with subsequent ongoing involvement from the multidisciplinary team. It thus cannot be suggested that nurses in the UK are pressurised by the multidisciplinary team to restrain the behaviourally challenged older person. Comparatively, in the USA, nurses require an order by the physician to instigate physical restraint use. Thus it seems that in the UK, decision making for physical restraint rests heavily on the nursing team and does not appear to be influenced by colleagues or family members. It could be suggested that if the nurses are autonomous to instigate a restraint then in light of their ongoing evaluation and discussions with others, they are also autonomous to cease its use.

Litigation

Fear of litigation also plays a part in defensive practice and the use of physical restraints (Brennan, 1999). Physical restraint can be viewed as a form of imprisonment as it disempowers the patients. Denying an individual's right to move at will is unlawful unless justified by consent or is a temporary measure (Dimond, 1995). Creighton (1982) claims that ruling on clinical practice is based on how closely the action adheres to accepted professional standards. The standards for physical restraint use should embedded in research and not on their custodial function. However, Rubenstein (1983) asserts that the law does not always differentiate between professional standards and those that reflect routine. Creighton (1982) and Rubenstein et al. (1983) highlight that earlier court decisions have favoured the use of freedom limiting devices in gerontology. The ethos of these rulings may have protracted the use of impeding devices. Methods of overcoming this tendency is to have sound professional practice rooted in research and reflect nursing assessment, planning, implementation, monitoring and ongoing evaluation (Evans and Strumpf, 1990). More recent cases such that in the Court of Appeals in Minnesota in 2000, upheld a nurse's decision to not use side rails. The verdict was based on the nurse's assessment of the patient and efforts made to maintain a safe environment (Anonymous, 2000).

Staffing Shortage

Physical restraints may also be used as a measure during staffing shortages (Jehan,1999; Royal College of Nursing, 1999). Evans and Strumpf (1990) claim that application of physical restraints does not require a lot of training, have immediate effect and are thus appealing when the patient case load is too high. However restraint use requires regular monitoring and their prolonged or inaccurate use causes a myriad of negative effects. Thus while their impact may seemingly relieve nursing pressures instantaneously, in the interim and long term the nursing workload is increased.

Patients and Families

As previously highlighted, patients and families express negative feelings pertaining to the use of physical restraints (Strumpf and Evans, 1988; Hardin et al., 1993). So, while there is evidence that patients and families usually do not value restrictive devices, nurses must be basing their reasons to restrain on other factors. Therefore, it can be surmised that patients and families are not requesting restraints.

Knowledge

Carper (1978) has isolated 4 sources of knowing in nursing. These include empirics, ethics, aesthetics and personal knowledge. The use of restraints on older people will now be examined from the perspective of these four sources of knowledge.

Empirics

Empirically, physical restraints contribute negatively both physically (Powell et al. 1989; Karlsson et al., 1997; Hanger et al. 1999; MDA, 2000) and psychologically towards the individual (Strumpf and Evans, 1988; Gallinagh et al., 2001 a&b)). In the literature, physically restraint use in gerontology is regarded as a routine (Rubenstein et al., 1983; Lee et al., 1999). It could thus be surmised that their continued use is in breech of clinical directives such as Health Advisory Service (1999) and the principles of clinical governance. Chalifour (1997) is of the opinion that the use of these restrictive devices does not reflect rationalised nursing care since the preventative function of therapeutic mechanisms is not proven. It is important that nurses as accountable professionals are familiar with the untoward affects and be able to counsel clearly against their use. (See also the previous discussion and other chapters).

Ethics and Professional Knowledge

Nurses may be opposed to using restrictive devices on older people from both an ethical and professional stance, they nonetheless persist in the activity (Marangos-Frost and Wells, 2000). A cross-cultural study by Molassiotis and Newell (1996) investigated perceptions of restraint use among 50 nurses form Britain and Greece. It was revealed that the nurses disagreed with the principle of restraint use, but 17 (44%) of the British nurses and 11 (100%) of the Greek nurses did assert that they used these approaches within their practice. A UK study by Brennan (1999) highlighted that 53 % (n=170) of UK gerontological nurses admitted to personally restraining a patient. Sullivan-Marx identifies that nurses need to consider potential harm caused by application of restraints as well as issues such as their use in the absence of informed consent. Furthermore, giving information to families about a patient's possible need for a restraint measure, needs to be impartial and not influenced by the desire for custodial management. Families should be provided with details of the institutional policy, a thorough assessment, assurance of regular monitoring activities and multidisciplinary evaluation and a consent form.

As literature assuages that physical restraint use has negative consequences for patients, it is still surprising that their use permeates in many institutions. A possible reason for this is that this information is not widely disseminated. Many researchers have demonstrated a decrease in physical restraint use in the care of older people by having patient-centred educational programmes for staff, combined with organisational consultation (Strumpf et al., 1992; Cohen et al., 1998; Stratmann et al., 1997). These programmes have a reflective ethos and advocate behavioural measures as opposed to physical methods to manage patients. Alternatives to physical restraints include re-examination of ward layout and changes to it, organisational changes such as various recreational and alternative therapies as well as a general patient centred approach with active involvement of family and friends.

Given the recent shift in emphasises from nursing being the protectors of patients to patients/families being informed risk takers, Kane et al. (1993) assert that an erroneous dichotomy has developed in the nursing literature on the repercussion for nurses to trade on their autonomy for patient safety. They disregard

148

this claim and assert that there is no choice to make i.e. informed risk taking leads to better quality of life for patients.

Aesthetics and Personal Knowledge

It is considered that aesthetics and personal knowledge reflect the therapeutic use of self, and empathy with the patient and family and the consequences of their use, (Sullivan-Marx, 1996). It could also be added that as nurses often use 'intuition' as a form of knowing. While intuition may influence a nurse to restrain or not, the decision cannot be based solely on this subjective feeling. The logic of the judgement needs to reflect a decision making tree approach as outlined in any good policy and be documented as such.

Aim

Compared with North America or Sweden, the issue of the use of physical restraint use is less explored and debated in the UK. The focus of my study was to identify the magnitude of the problem within a typical gerontological setting and to explore the relationship of physical restraint use to other variables such as age, gender, medical diagnosis, nursing rationales, drug therapies and nursing staffing levels.

Method

The definition used to categorise restraints was that of Molassiotis (1995). A modified version of Magee et al.'s (1993) Research Observation Sheet was used. An observational approach was used. Rigour was incorporated into the tool by having its content checked for quality, adequacy and accuracy and inter-rater reliability was established. Patients' nursing notes were then examined to identify whether or not patients had sustained falls in the previous month, what drugs they were on and whether the nursing care plan indicated the use of restraint. A pilot study was also conducted. Data was analysed using the Statistical Package for the Social Sciences (SPSS) and descriptive and inferential tests (parametric and non parametric).

Setting and Sample

All patients from five wards in two acute care hospitals in Northern Ireland were included in the study. These were all gerontology/rehabilitation wards and had shared philosophies of care. One hundred and two patients were observed yielding 1224 observations. The observations took place on the same day and on the same weekend day. Each patient was observed four times over a three day period. Data were collected over a five week period by three observers. To prevent sensitisation, staff were only officially told that the researchers were examining an aspect of care.

Results and Discussion

Profile of Restrained Patients

The average age of the restrained patient was 77 years (n=33) and 75 years (n=69) for the non restrained. A chi square test confirmed that there was no significant difference between males and females in relation to restraint and non restraint use: x^2 (df=1)=0.024 (p>0.05). Most of the patients who were restrained (69.9%) were very dependent on nursing staff for their care (n=48). In comparison, only a small number of those not restrained (6.1%) were very dependent (n=2). This corroborates Tinetti et al.'s finding (1991) demonstrating a link between restraint use and patient dependency levels.

The most common diagnosis for restrained patients were stroke and fractures (n=27) and n=10 respectively. A chi square test confirmed that there is a significant difference in the number of stroke diagnosis between restrained and non restrained patients.

Presumably, nurses are using physical restraints as positional support for stroke patients (e.g. Screw-on table tops). Whilst this is a rationalised measure, nursing documentation would need to reflect this as there is no legislative support for prolonged use of physical restraints.

Type and Prevalence

Most patients 69 (68%) were subjected on at least one occasions to some form of restraint over the three day period. The most commonly used devices were side rails, reclining chairs and screw on table tops. Side rails were also frequently were found to be frequently used in Australian studies by Retsas (1997), and Ret-

150

sas and Crabbe (1997) as well as in the UK settings by Ramprogus and Gibson 1991 and O'Keefe et al. (1996).

Nurses' Rationale

At the end of the observations, the nurses were asked to choose more than one category for using physical restraints. The nurses cited patient wandering as the main reason for using a restraint. This indication is generally not supported in the literature. Wandering is regarded as a natural process of searching for security and familiarity and as having benefits for individuals (Coltharp et al., 1996). It could be suggested that many other patient centred approaches exist to manage wandering as opposed to limiting the persons freedom. Patient confusion was also regarded to be a determining factor for using a restraint, again similar to studies by Magee et al. (1993) and Ludwick (1999).

Falls

A review of patients' charts showed no association between falls and physical restraint. For example, those not restrained had a reported incidence of previous falls of 20 (61%) compared with 28 (41%) who had recently fallen and were restrained. There does not appear to be a link here between falls and the likelihood of restraint use. This is similar to that reported by Magee et al. (1993) and Karlsson et al. (1997)

Prescribed Drugs

Restrained patients received more drugs (benzodiazepines, opioids, diuretics, laxatives and anti-psychotics). This is similar to Magee et al.'s study. It is unclear whether the patients presenting conditions influenced the drug use or whether their use is an affect of the increased agitation and side effects from prolonged immobilisation. Furthermore, the use of many of these drugs will cause immobility problems in the older person, thus perpetuating the cycle of physical and chemical restraint.

Care planning

Only 23 (35%) of the 45 (65%) who were restrained had reasons for its use documented in their care plan. Furthermore, only 20 (30%) of care plan entries cited evidence of patient/family involvement in the decision. Malpractice suits on restraint use have been settled due to inadequate documentation (Rubenstein et

151

al., 1993). Nursing decision making, and care planning needs to reflect sound institutional policy.

Proximity to Nurses' Station and Staffing Levels

It was assumed that those not situated in the vicinity of the nurses' station would be more likely to be restrained. However, this was not statistically supported: Chi square test; 2(df=1) = 0.336 (p>0.05). There is a small difference between the groups, but this is not statistically significant (9.1% who were visible and 13% who were concealed). Any relationship between staffing levels and restraints was only tenuous and this is similar to Magee et al.'s study (1993).

It can be concluded from this study that the use of physical restraint in a gerontology setting is high. Nurses appear to restrain patients who have had a diagnosis of stroke and fractures, those who wander and are confused and these patients seem to be more dependent on staff for their care. Those who do have their freedom impinged upon also receive more drugs than those who are mobilising at will. No association was found between restraint use and the incidence of falls or staffing levels. On the whole, nursing documentation of the decision making process, implementation, and evaluation and involvement of others was inadequate.

Recommendations

Whilst a totally restraint free practice would be impossible to achieve, there are many steps that nurses can take to ensure that patients who present with challenging behaviour do not suffer abuse as a result of the 'quick fix' physical restraint. Immobilising the patient under the premise of safety is no longer an acceptable part of professional practice. Practice recommendations include:
- The development of detailed 'least restraint policy' policy emphasising a holistic inter-professional assessment and incorporating a decision making tree, outline of available creative alternatives, monitoring arrangements and frequency of inter-professional evaluation.
- The use of an individualised validated assessment tool for side rails and physical restraint use
- The use of sensor bed and chair alarms
- Practice updates for qualified and non qualified staff
- Implementation of a fall risk assessment and prevention programme
- Sound nursing documentation reflecting the institutional policy

Conclusion

Increasing frailty, mobility problems and confusion present everyday challenges to the nurse in the gerontology setting. It is apparent that decision making in physical restraint use is complex and influenced by various competing issues such as policy, tradition, legal issues, as well as research and the nurses innate value system. A change in philosophy has taken place that places choice with the patient and demand their involvement in decision making. The onerous task of patient protection needs to be rooted in an inter-professional policy that is patient and family centred, is evidence based and outlines the decision making process and protocol. This does not override the autonomy or accountability for nurses but indeed add to it, in the sense that vulnerable adults and their families are being given maximum input into their care.

References

Anonymous (2000) Bed rails up or down; court says when it is a professional nursing judgement. *Legal Eagle Eye Newsletter for the Nursing Profession* 8 (7) 1.

Brennan, S. (1999) Dangerous liaisons. *Nursing Times*, 95 (3) 30-32.

Chalifour, R. (1997) Implementing a non restraint environment. *Canadian nurse*, 93 (6) 46-47.

Carper, B. (1978) Fundamental patterns of knowing in nursing. *Advances in nursing Science*, 1 13-23.

Cohen-Mansfield, J. and Billig, N. (1986) Agitated behaviours in the elderly Part 1.a conceptual review. *Journal of the American Geriatrics Society*, 34 (10) 711-721

Cohen, C., Neufeld, R., Dunbar, J. Pflug L, Breuer B (1998) Old problem, different approaches; alternatives to physical restraints. *Journal of Gerontological nursing*, 22 (2) 23-29.

Coltharp, W., Ritchie, M. Kaas, M. (1996) Wandering. *Journal of Gerontological nursing*, 22 (11) 5-10.

Creighton, H. (1982) Are side rails necessary? *Nursing Management*, 13 (6) 45-48.

Dimond, B. (2002) *Legal Aspects of nursing.* Prentice Hall, London.

Donius, M. and Rader, J. (1994) Use of side rails: rethinking a standard practice. *Journal of Gerontological Nursing*, 20 (11) 23-27.

Evans, L. and Strumpf, N. (1990) Myths about elder restraint. Image: *Journal of Nursing Scholarship*, 22 (2) 124-128.

Evans, L., Strumpf, N., Taylor, L., Capezuti, E., Maislin, G., Jacobsen, B. (1997) a clinical trial to reduce restraints in nursing homes. *Journal of the American Geriatric Society,* 43 (6) 675-681.

Food and Drug Administration (1995) *FDA Safety Alert: Entrapment Hazards with Hospital Bed Side Rails.* Rockville, USA.

Gallinagh, R., Slevin, É. and Mc Cormack, B. (2002) Side rails as physical restraint in the care of older people: a management issue. *Journal of Nursing Management* (in press)

Gallinagh, R., Nevin, R., Campbell, L., Mitchell, F. and Ludwick, R. (2001b) Relatives' perceptions of side rail use on the older person in hospital. *British Journal of nursing,* 10 (6) 391-399.

Gallinagh, R., Nevin, R., Mc Aleese, L. and Campbell, L. (2001a) Perceptions of older people who have experienced physical restraint. *British Journal of Nursing,* 10(13) 852-859 in text

Gallinagh, R., Nevin, R., Mc Ilroy, D., Mitchell, F., Campbell, L., Ludwick, R. and Mc Kenna, H. (2001) The use of physical restraints as a safety measure in the care of older people in four rehabilitation wards: findings form an exploratory study. *International Journal of Nursing Studies,* 39 (2002) 147-156.

Glanville, J., Haines, M. and Auston, I. (1998) Getting research into practice. Finding information on clinical effectiveness. *British Medical Journal,* 317 (7152) 200-203.

Hanger, H. ,Ball, M., Wood, L. (1999) An analysis of falls in the hospital: can we do without bed rails? *Journal of the American Geriatrics Society,* 47(5) 529-531.

Hantikainen, V. (2001) Nursing staff perceptions of the behaviour of older nursing home residents and decision making on restraint use: a qualitative and interpretative study. *Journal of Clinical nursing,* 10(2) 246-256.

Hardin, S., Magee, R., Vinson, M., Owen, M., Hyatt, E., Stratmann, D. (1993) Patient and family perceptions of restraints. *Journal of Holistic Nursing,* 11(4) 383-397.

Health Advisory Service 2000 (1999) *Not because they are old-an independent. Inquiry into the care of older people on acute wards in general hospitals.* HAS 2000, London.

Hindmarch, V. (1999) Elder Abuse. *Professional Nurse.* 14(4) 249-252.

Jehan, W. (1999) Restraint or protection? *Nursing Management,* 6(2) 9-13.

Kane, R., Williams, C., Williams, T. and Kane, R. (1993) Restraining restraints: changes in a standard of care. *Annual Review of Public Health 14,* 545-584.

Karlsson, S., Nyberg, L., Sandman, P.O. (1997) the use of physical restraints in elder care in relation to fall risk. *Scandinavian Journal of Caring Sciences* 11(4) 238-242.

Lee, D., Chan, M., Tam, E., Yeung, W. (1999) Use of physical restraints on elderly patients: an exploratory study of the perceptions of nurses in Hong Kong. *Journal of Advanced Nursing* 29(1) 153-159.

Levine, J. (1996) Historical notes on restraint reduction: the legacy of Dr. Phillipe Pinel. *Journal of American Geriatrics Society*, 44(9) 1130-1133.

Ludwick, R. (1999) Clinical decision making: recognition of confusion and application of restraints. *Orthopaedic Nursing*, 18(1) 65-71.

Ludwick, R. and O'Toole, A. (1996) The confused patient: nurses knowledge and interventions. *Journal of Gerontological Nursing* 22(1) 44-49.

Mc Hutchion, E. and Morse, J. (1989) Releasing restraints: a nursing dilemma. *Journal of Gerontological Nursing*, 15(2) 16-21.

Magee, R., Hyatt, E., Hardin, S., Stratmann, D., Vinson, M. and Owen, Mm (1993) Use of restraints in extended care and nursing homes. *Journal of Gerontological Nursing* 19(4) 31-39.

Marangos-Frost, S., Wells, D. (2000) Psychiatric nurses' thoughts and feelings about restraint use: a decision dilemma. *Journal of Advanced Nursing*, 31(2) 362-369.

Medical Devices Agency (2000) *Bed Side Rails (Cotsides): Risk of Entrapment and Asphyxiation*. Hazard Notice HN9711, MDA, London

Molassiotis, A. (1995) Use of physical restraints 1: Consequences. *British Journal of Nursing*, 4(3) 155-157.

Molassiotis, A. and Newell, R. (1996) Nurses' awareness of restraint use with elderly people in Greece and the UK: a cross-cultural pilot study. *International Journal of Nursing Studies*, 33(2) 201-211.

Miles, S. and Irvine, P. (1992) Deaths caused by restraints. *The Gerontologist* 32(6) 762-766.

Minnick, A., Mion, L., Leipzig, R., Lamb, K. and Palmer, R. (1998) Patterns and prevalence of physical restraint use in the acute care setting. *Journal of Nursing Administration*, 28(11) 19-24.

Newbern, N., Lindsay, I. (1994) Attitudes of wives toward having their elderly husbands restrained. *Geriatric Nursing* 15(3) 135-8.

O'Keefe, S., Jack, C., Lye, M (1996) Use of restraints and bedrails in a British hospital. *Journal of American Geriatric Society*, 45(7) 1086-1088.

Parker, K., Miles, S. (1997) Deaths caused by side rails. *Journal of the American Geriatrics Society*, 45(7) 797-808.

Paterson, B., Leadbetter, D., Mc Comish, A. (1998) Restraint and sudden death from asphysxia. *Nursing Times*, 94(44) 62-64.

Powell, C., Mitchell-Pedersen, L, Fingerote, E., Edmund, L., (1989) Freedom from restraint: consequences of reducing physical restraints in the management of the elderly. *Canadian Medical Association Journal*, 14, 561-564.

155

Ramprogus, V. and Gibson, J. (1991) Assessing restraints. *Nursing Times* 87(26) 45-47.

Retsas, A. (1997) The use of physical restraints in Western Australian nursing homes. *Australian Journal of Advanced nursing*, 14(3) 33-39.

Retsas, A. and Crabbe, H. (1998) Breaking loose: use of physical restraints in nursing homes in Queensland. *Australia Collegian*, 4(4) 14-21.

Rubenstein, H., Miller, F., Postel, S., Evans, H. (1983) Standards of medical care based on consensus rather than evidence: the case of routine bedrail use for the elderly. *Law, Medicine and Health Care,* 11, 272-276.

Royal College of Nursing (1999) *Restraint Revisited-Rights, Risk and Responsibility. Guidance for Nurses Working with Older People.* RCN, London.

Stratman, D., Vinson, M., Magee, R., Hardin, S. (1997) the effects of research on clinical practice: the use of restraints. *Applied Nursing Research*, 10(1) 39-43.

Strumpf, N., Evans, L., Wagner, J., Patterson, J. (1992) Reducing physical restraints: developing an educational program. *Journal of Gerontological Nursing* 18(11) 21-27.

Strumpf, N., Evans, L. and Schwartz, D. (1991) Physical restraint of the elderly. *In:* Rader, I. (ed.) *Clinical Gerontological Nursing: a Guide to Advanced Practice.* W.B.Saunders Company, Philadelphia.

Sullivan-Marx, E. (1996) Restraint –Free Care. How does a nurse decide? *Journal of Gerontological Nursing*, 22(9) 7-14.

Tinetti, M., Liu, W., Marottoli, R., Ginter, S. (1991) Mechanical restraint use among residents of skilled nursing facilities: prevalence, patterns and predictors. *Journal of American Medical Association*, 265(4) 468-471.

Terpstra, T., van Doren, E. (1998) Reducing restraints: where to start. *The Journal of Continuing Education in Nursing* 29(1) 10-16.

Todd, J., Ruhl, C., Gross, T. (1997) Injury and death associated with hospital bed side rails: reports to the US Food and Drug Administration from 1985-1995. *American Journal of Public Health*, 87(10) 1675-1677.

Winston, P., Morelli, P., Bramble, J., Friday, A., Browb-Sanders, J.(1999) Improving patient care through implementation of nurse-driven restraint protocols. *Journal of Nursing Quality*, 13(6) 32-46.

Chapter Eight: Violence against Caregivers in Nursing Homes in the USA

Donna M. Gates

Introduction

Workplace violence is a major public health concern; many employees and employers are dealing with incidents of threats, harassment and assaults. Most experts agree that violence against workers includes both overt and covert behaviours that range from verbal harassment to murder and include four major types of violence, based on the intent of the violence, the victim and the perpetrator. The first type includes violence committed during a robbery or other crime. Most workplace homicides are due to this type of violence. The second type of violence involves customers who become violent during the course of a transaction; the perpetrator is a customer of the victim. This risk is routine and common in health care settings where patients and families are abusive to nurses, nurse assistants, physicians and other healthcare workers. The third type of violence includes worker-on-worker violence. The perpetrator is an employee or former employee who strikes out during a work or interpersonal related dispute at the workplace. The fourth type of violence results from the spill-over of domestic violence from the home. Perpetrators are usually boyfriends or husbands of employees at work. Although caregivers are at risk for all four types of violence, this chapter will focus on the second type, the violence encountered from residents.

There are approximately 1.5 million residents living in 17,176 nursing facilities in the United States (American Healthcare Association, 2001a). In 1999, there were 34.5 million persons 65 years of age and older. The elderly population in the United States will grow dramatically as the "baby boomers" reach 65 years of age between the years 2010 and 2030. The proportion of elderly population is expected to increase by 17% from 1995 to 2010 and 75% from 2010 to 2030 (Administration on Ageing, 2000). Even if the proportion of elderly who resides in nursing homes remains constant, the number of nursing home beds is expected to increase because almost 90% of nursing home residents are over 65 years of age. In addition, the number of persons over 85 years of age will increase by 56% and this population represents those who are most likely to live in nursing homes (Administration on Ageing, 2000).

Although there are approximately 643,080 Nursing Assistants (NAs)[1] working in nursing homes in the United States, many of these facilities suffer from a shortage of NAs. Caregivers who work in nursing homes are not highly regarded by society and often receive lower wages and benefits than those working in hospitals and home care. The turnover rate for NAs working in long-term care ranges from 40 to 400% annually (American Healthcare Association [AHCA], 2001). Large turnover rates in nursing homes have dramatic negative effects on workers, residents and organisations. It is estimated that it costs nursing homes $7,000 to replace a registered nurse and over $2,200 to replace a nursing assistant (Caudill & Patrick, 1991; Cohen-Mansfield, 1997). High turnover rates therefore, substantially contribute to pressures the industry is currently experiencing.

The Blue Ribbon Panel, assembled under the auspices of the University of Illinois in the U.S calls for immediate action to avoid a severe crisis in 2010 due to the severe shortage of healthcare workers (University of Illinois, 2001). The panel reports that there will not be enough nursing care providers for the ageing population. Their recommendations include the need for increased wages and benefits, improved work environment, adequate training and education for providers, and research related to healthcare labour issues. The report emphasises that more money by itself will not solve the labour shortage. The panel also stresses that unlike years ago when attention was focused on Registered Nurses (RNs), today we need to realise that Licensed Practical Nurses (LPNs)[2] and nurse assistants are an important and integral part of the healthcare team. A report by the United States General Accounting Office (2001) states that the demographic changes are likely to worsen the current shortage of nurse aides in hospitals, nursing homes and home health care. With the ageing population, the demand for nurse aides will grow dramatically. The report states that the difficulty recruiting and retaining nurse aides is related to the low wages and benefits, physical demands of the work, and aspects of the work environment. Yet, they state that few studies have evaluated the effect of these factors on recruitment and turnover.

The largest group of workers in nursing homes is NAs, who represent 43% of the employees and 70 to 90% of the nursing personnel (AHCA, 2001b; Hagan and Sayers, 1995; Wunderlich et al., 1996). NAs, who are most likely to be in direct contact with residents (patients) in nursing homes, will continue to be the largest group of workers in nursing homes and the primary providers of direct care. In the U.S more than 90% of NAs working in nursing homes are women.

---

1 "Nurses Assitants" work under the control and guidance of Registered Nurses. They have a limited training focusing on basic care

2 Trained for two years

Approximately 17 percent are less than 25 years of age and 44% are between 35 to 54 years of age. The proportion of blacks is 29% and nearly 75% did not complete high school and many come from low-income families. These healthcare workers currently have the least amount of education and training of all healthcare professionals working in nursing homes. Yet, the care of residents in nursing homes is difficult and challenging because of the prevalence of sicker patients, often with mental disorders, Alzheimer's type dementia, and physical limitations.

While NAs are exposed daily to many physical and emotional stressors on the job; however, little is known about how these stressors are related to occupational strain in these workers. The author, along with Evelyn Fitzwater is currently conducting research to explore the working conditions for nurse assistants (NAs) working in long-term care and their relationships to the high rate of absences, injuries and turnover in this industry. One of the many negative exposures experienced by NAs in nursing homes is the violence they experience from residents on a daily basis. Nursing assistants (NAs), who work in hospitals and nursing homes ranked second only to truck drivers and labourers in the incidence of injuries and illness that involved loss of workdays. In addition, NAs in nursing homes have the highest incidence of non-fatal workplace assault among all workers in the U.S. NAs provide 90% of the direct care to residents who reside in nursing homes.

A series of research studies have been done over the past seven years by the author and different collaborators to examine work conditions for caregivers in nursing homes. Results from two of those studies, a focus group study and an intervention study will be described throughout this chapter, along with the findings from other researchers.

The research into nursing home violence by residents started with focus groups in seven nursing homes (Gates, Fitzwater, and Meyer, 1999). The focus group method was used to capture the feelings and beliefs regarding violence in nursing homes. This was done because administrators and experts in the nursing home industry expressed the opinion that nursing assistants would not consider aggression from a resident toward a caregiver as "violence". Thus, the research aimed at determining whether staff would consider resident aggression to be violence and if it was bothersome to them. Focus groups started by asking the NAs to "describe what they consider to be a violent episode in their workplace". Then they were asked to describe "what happens after they are physically or verbally assaulted". The discussion continued with the questions "what they thought increases the violence" and "what their employer currently does to keep them safe at work". The investigators also met with the nursing directors at the seven homes to determine how they describe violence in the nursing home setting and to explore policies, procedures and safety precautions in place to decrease the incidence of violence.

The intervention study was done to test the effectiveness of an intervention to increase the NAs' self-efficacy to prevent violence, increase NAs' violence prevention skills and decrease the incidence of assaults. At initiation of the intervention study (3 experimental and three control groups) the nursing homes where the study was done were similar in size, location, types of residents, and nursing assistants. The 134 NAs carried an Assault Log for 10 working days (80 hours) to capture the incidence and context of the assaults. NAs also participated in a simulation exercise so that we could evaluate their use of violence prevention skills with an actress who portrayed a resident. In addition, the NAs completed demographic and employment surveys, an occupational stress survey and an anger survey. Measurements were done before and after the intervention.

Scope and Types of Violence

Nursing personnel are frequently subjected to abuse by patients and the occupation at greatest risk for non-fatal assault is the NA working in long-term care (Bureau of Labor Statistics [BLS], 1994; BLS, 1996; Toscano and Knestaut, 1998).

Long-term care facilities were found to be the healthcare setting where most non-fatal assaults occur and the perpetrator is most often the resident. Violence research, and in particular nursing home violence, is in its infancy. In a study of 101 nursing homes Winger et al. (1987) found that 84% of nursing home residents displayed behaviours that endangered staff.

Ryden et al. (1999) found that 51% of aggressive behaviour was physical, 48% verbal and 4% sexual. Several studies describing NAs and their experiences with violence in nursing homes found that these workers often experienced harassment, threats and assaults from patients (Ryden et al., 1991; Gates et al., 1999; Lusk, 1992). In addition, a study by Gates et al. (2002) found that 10.1 % (14 of 138) of subjects responded that a co-worker had physically assaulted them and 4.3% (6 of 138) responded that a family member had physically assaulted them.

In the focus group study (Gates et al., 1999) the majority of caregivers overwhelmingly described workplace violence as including verbal and physical assaults, which they stated occurs daily. They stated that the violence from the residents was by far the most common type of violence. They also discussed employee-to-employee violence, family to employee violence, and family to resident violence but stated that these do not occur frequently. They described physical violence by residents as grabbing, pinching, hitting, poking, pulling hair, spitting and throwing objects. Verbal violence included threats of harm, cursing, yelling, demeaning remarks and racial slurs. The NAs were particularly concerned about episodes when residents spat at them or grabbed their genitals. It was sad to hear several NAs state "it is really upsetting when a resident that I thought really liked me hit me when I tried to take care of them". This was true even for demented residents, supporting our belief that many NAs truly do not understand the effect of dementia on the residents' behaviour. Every NA in the focus groups had experienced verbal and physical violence from residents at least once while working in a nursing home.

Assaults against caregivers by elderly residents are common and occur primarily during basic care activities, such as dressing and changing (43%), turning and transferring (26%), bathing (19%), feeding (12%), and toileting (9%). During an intervention study the NAs recorded a total of 624 assaults that were experienced by 71% of the nursing assistants over the period of 80 hours. Twenty nine percent of the NAs did not encounter any assaults. The mean number of assaults was 4.52 for NAs and 6.64 for those who encountered at least one assault. The number of assaults per caregiver ranged from 0 - 64 and the mean number of assaults per nursing home ranged from 1.57 to 8.42. Five percent of the assaults resulted in an injury. This wide range of assaults between nursing assistants and between nursing homes supports our belief that the violence is multi-factorial.

For each assault during the 80 hours the NAs recorded on the Assault Log the type of assault and the care-giving activity being performed when assaulted. Listed below are the types of assaults and the activities by percentages for the 624 assaults. Percentages do not add up to 100% since several assaults included more than one type and included more than one activity. The types of assaults described were:

Hitting or punching	51%
Grabbing, pinching or pulling hair	40%
Kicking	27%
Scratching or biting	23%
Spitting	11%
Throwing or hitting with object	9%

Effects of Violence

Workplace violence can seriously impact the employer, the employees and the clients. Effects include the costs of medical care for injuries such as black eyes, eye injuries, headaches, sore or broken jaws, lacerations or bruising, fractures, bite wounds, and temporary hearing loss. There can be additional costs related to psychological care, increased absenteeism, property damage, decreased productivity, increased security, litigation, increased workers' compensation and personnel changes. In addition there may be costs related to personnel changes from employee burnout and turnover. Studies have found that healthcare workers who experience physical assault experience both short-term and long-term emotional reaction, including anger, sadness, frustration, anxiety, irritability, fear, apathy, self-blame, and helplessness (Gage and Kingdom, 1995; Gates et al., 1999; Lanza, 1992). The emotional toll that occurs to caregivers when they are physically abused on a daily basis is certain to have an impact on the quality of care provided to nursing home residents. A secondary effect is that NAs who are not able to effectively cope with the daily emotional and physical stressors related to resident care are more prone to respond with aggressive and abusive response toward residents (Pillemer and Hudson, 1993; Pillemer and Moore, 1989; Pillemer and Bachman-Prehm, 1991). There is a reciprocal relationship between the violence that occurs against the caregiver and the violence that occurs against the resident. Either type of occurrence has the potential to cause the victim to retaliate, thus resulting in two victims of abuse (Pillemer and Moore, 1989). NAs who do not have adequate coping skills to deal with daily verbal and physical abuse by residents are more likely to respond with aggression.

Results from our focus groups also indicate that many NAs do not receive adequate support from their supervisors related to the violence they are experiencing. These workers believe their employers should make more efforts to protect them from violence. While the majority (56%) reported they always report assaults to supervisors, 15% reported they seldom report assaults. Reasons given for not reporting include "a lack of concern about the NAs well-being", "supervisors do not want to fill out incident reports", "violence is considered part of the job", and "NAs are blamed for poor care-giving skills". Thus, reports of assault incidence against NAs are likely to be underestimated. Sixty-two percent of subjects reported they had received training to deal with aggressive residents and 45% had received this type of training at their current work place.

Conceptual Model for Violence

Results from the focus group study (Gates et al., 1999) suggest that the NAs and Nursing Directors in the nursing homes agree and differ on the variables that increase the risk of caregiver violence (Table 1).

Two common themes were noted throughout all the focus groups with the caregivers. First, caregivers were very disgruntled in their perception that residents and families have rights but they do not. Secondly, many caregivers felt that their administrators and supervisors did not appreciate and respect them.

162

Based on the focus group results, our expertise and the literature, we developed and currently use the following conceptual model (Figure 1) to describe the violence that occurs against caregivers in nursing homes. The model is useful in understanding the multi-factorial nature of the violence against caregivers and to plan interventions to decrease the violence. Characteristics of the caregiver, the resident and the nursing home environment all interact to increase or decrease the risk of violence against the caregiver.

Table 1. Variables Related to the Violence Against Caregivers

	Nursing Assistants	Nursing Directors
Approach of the caregiver		X
Lack of knowledge	X	X
Lack of training	X	X
Characteristics of the NAs		X
Resident's dementia		X
Resident's anger	X	X
Resident's mental illness		X
Resident's loss of control	X	
Sundowner syndrome	X	
Nursing home regulations	X	X
Inadequate staffing	X	X
High staff turnover		X
Family guilt and anger	X	X
High stress	X	X
Acceptance of violence	X	X
Societal violence		X
Full moon	X	
Hectic routines	X	
Lack of employee rights	X	

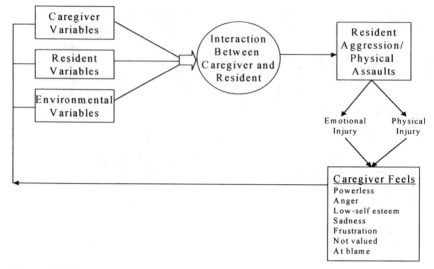

Figure 1. Violence Against Caregivers: A Conceptual Model

Caregiver Risk Factors

NA characteristics that are commonly cited in the literature as being related to the risk of violence from residents in nursing homes include the following:

- Unfamiliarity with the resident
- Limit setting
- Time pressures
- Lack of violence prevention knowledge and skills
- Personal characteristics, such as age, anger, stress and attitudes

Unfamiliarity with the residents can be a problem for several reasons. When caregivers do not know the residents they are not able to incorporate into their plan of care those routines that are important to persons who may be confused or anxious. In addition, a caregiver who does not know a resident will not be alert for specific cues or triggers for agitation and aggression. Caregivers who set limits on patient behaviours, especially with those with dementia or organic brain disorder, may unknowingly increase their chances of being assaulted (Lanza, 1991). Ditasio (1994) explains that some caregivers put a lot of effort into the maintenance of the nursing homes routine and feel under pressure to complete these activities in the allotted time period. This type of pressure on the caregiver is likely to result in a care-giving approach that is hurried, impersonal and lacking in concern about the resident's feelings, desires and choices.

Even though we found that many NAs had participated in violence prevention training, many believe they lack the knowledge and skills to prevent the violence (Gates et al., 1999). As part of the intervention study, we collected data about how NAs felt about their violence prevention knowledge and their ability to prevent assaults from residents. They expressed feeling the most knowledgeable about "why residents become aggressive" and "how to recognise when a resident is agitated or becoming aggressive". They feel the least knowledgeable about how to keep residents from becoming agitated or aggressive and how to decrease a resident's agitation or aggressive behaviour once they become agitated or aggressive. Similarly, the NAs felt the most confidence (self-efficacy) in their ability to recognise when a resident is agitated or becoming aggressive. In contrast, they had the least confidence (self-efficacy) in their ability to keep residents from becoming agitated or aggressive and decrease a resident's agitation or aggressive behaviour. Whereas perceived knowledge was significantly related to the incidence of assaults ($p<.05$), there was no relationship between perceived self-efficacy and the incidence of assaults (Gates et al., 2002c)

A list of violence prevention skills was identified that would be important for caregivers to use in preventing aggression and assaults by residents (Gates et al., 2002a). These violence prevention skills were chosen based on the literature, the authors' expertise, and the need to choose skills that could be observed and measured during a simulation experience. The twelve skills that eventually made up the Violence Prevention Checklist included skills that are important to keep residents from becoming agitated, skills that de-escalate agitation when they recognise that resident is becoming agitated, and skills that prevent them from being assaulted (Gates et al., 2002b). During simulation exercises with a standardised simulated patient it was noted that the caregivers demonstrated more skills in the area of keeping residents from becoming agitated and less skills required to the de-escalate the resident's agitation and prevent assault. In particular, few of the NAs used validation to recognise the resident's feelings or used distraction methods or time-outs. A majority of them did not move out of the resident's personal space when the resident began to become physically aggressive. Some NAs actually commented that they "did not want the resident to think they were backing down". This shows that many NAs do not understand dementia, over-estimating the degree of insight and control of such patients.

During the intervention study, we found interesting results regarding the incidence of assaults and the following NA characteristics: age, training, duration of employment, number of assigned residents, anger, role stress and occupational strain (Gates et al., 2002a). Each of these characteristics and their relationship to the assaults against caregivers will be discussed below. Age was significantly ($p<.001$) related to the incidence of assaults; as age increased incidence of assaults decreased. It is possible that older caregivers have a different approach when taking care of their residents. Maybe they work more slowly or are more flexible, or maybe they are more patient or empathetic in their approach to the elderly patients.

Surprisingly, we did not find any significant relationships between incidence of assaults and previous training, either at the current facility or the previous facility where they worked. Many experts believe that the training related to preventing aggressiveness and assaults would result in decreased incidence. It is possible that the training that is provided does not meet the needs of the caregivers. As discussed earlier, during a simulation exercise caregivers were able to identify and perform behaviours that keep residents from becoming agitated, such as their initial verbal and physical approach to residents. The NAs were less skilled in how to perform when the resident's actions or anger is escalating. In fact many caregivers state that they take these aggressive responses personally even when the resident is demented and become "hurt" or angry. Many caregivers state that although they have had violence prevention training, they often feel that the training does not meet their needs since it is too didactic and "over their heads". Training should provide caregivers the opportunity to practice learned skills through role modelling and demonstration. A problem solving approach to dealing with challenging residents is also helpful. It is important that administrators and nursing directors examine their programs to determine if the training they are providing is actually useful in making changes in their caregivers' behaviours (Gates et al., 2002b).

Many experts, as well as caregivers and supervisors believe that a high turnover rate is directly related to the violence against caregivers. It was thought that the longer a caregiver was employed at a facility the greater the chance that he or she would know the residents' moods, triggers for aggression and that this increased knowledge and familiarity would result in less assaults. This study, however, found that there was no significant relationship between duration of employment at the facility and the incidence of assaults.

NAs often care for a large number of residents during a day. In the intervention study 83% of NAs report that they were responsible for more than 10 residents each per shift and that the average number of residents per shift for each NA was 13. As expected there was a significant relationship between ($p<.05$) between incidence of assaults and number of residents assigned. Most probably this is related to care-giving that becomes hurried, pressured and even assembly like. Such an approach is likely to result in an aggressive response from a resident, especially those suffering from dementia or other mental health disorders. Most long-term care experts believe that one of the greatest problems plaguing nursing homes is the staffing issue, with quality of care being the most important outcome of interest.

We found a significant relationship between the incidence of assaults and the following variables on the Occupational Stress Inventory-2; a) role insufficiency stress (p<.05), b) role ambiguity stress (p<.05), c) vocational strain (p,>05), d) physical strain (p<.05), e) state anger (p<.001), and f) trait anger (p<.001) (Gates et al., 2002a). Role ambiguity stress measures the extent to which the individual's priorities and expectations about work are clear to the individual. Workers who have high role ambiguity may report they are experiencing conflicting demands from supervisors (Osipow, 1999). Role insufficiency stress measures the extent to which the individual's education, skills and experience are appropriate to job requirements (Osipow, 1998) As discussed earlier NAs often feel that they are inadequately prepared to meet the needs of the their residents. In addition, they often feel that they lack the support and direction they would like from their supervisors and administration. Workers who have high vocational strain may state that they have poor attitudes toward their work and that they make errors in their work or have accidents. They may even feel that their quality of work is suffering due to concentration problems. They often have high absenteeism rates. Persons who have high physical strain at work may report that they have frequent health problems, such as colds, headaches, stomach-aches and heart palpitations. These workers may also overuse alcohol or drugs, or experiencing sleep problems or depression. Healthcare workers who are suffering from vocational and physical strain may be experiencing burnout. Maslach (1982) defines burnout as a condition of emotional exhaustion, depersonalisation and reduced personal accomplishment. Burnout occurs when a motivated and dedicated employee loses their joy in providing a service to their clients. Burnout in healthcare professions results in decreased job performance, increased accidents, absences and tardiness, and increased turnover.

Using the State-Trait Anger Expression Inventory with NAs, we found a significant, positive relationship (p<.05) between both state and trait anger and incidence of assaults against NAs in nursing homes (Gates et al., 1999; Gates et al., 2002a). Anger is a subjective emotional state and this emotional state may give rise to aggression, which is a verbal or physical act of violence. Spielberger (1999) states that whereas persons with high State Anger are currently experiencing relatively intense angry feelings, persons with high Trait Anger frequently experience angry feelings and often feel that they are treated unfairly by others. Spielberger's Trait Anger scales correlate significantly with Hostility Scales, including the Buss-Durkee Hostility Inventory and the Minnesota Multiphasic Per-

167

sonality Inventory (Spielberger, 1999). Persons with a high Trait Anger score are often more easily frustrated and such frustration is likely to result in how and when care is delivered. For example, frustrated and hostile people might be loud, their movements might be rougher or they might disconnect from and neglect their residents. When encountering anger and aggression from residents, hostile caregivers might have a tendency toward physical retaliation, depending on their propensity to aggression and their ability to cope with their intense feelings. Studies have found that nurses become angry when they feel they are treated unfairly, unjustly accused, blocked in task completion, and when experiencing fear, anxiety and frustration (Smith and Hart, 1994).In addition, nursing assistants, who have minimal education, training and coping skills may have difficulty depersonalising the verbal and physical assaults they encounter from residents who are demented or angry.

Resident Risk Factors

Resident characteristics commonly cited in the literature as being related to the risk of violence from residents in nursing homes include the following:
- Medical diagnoses of dementia, organic brain syndrome, schizophrenia, and temporal lobe epilepsy
- Medication toxicity
- Past history of assaultive behaviour
- Other factors such as hallucinations, poor impulse control, regressed behaviour, disorientation, restlessness, agitation
- Upset about restrictions, death of a significant person, and violation of personal space
- Feelings of powerlessness

Several investigators have found that the incidence of assaults was highest with those patients with dementia and organic brain syndome (Colenda and Hamer, 1991; Gates et al., 2002a;.Tardiff and Sweillam, 1979). It is commonly believed that such illnesses result in a loss of control and confusion. Colenda and Hamer (1991) also found that elderly persons with schizophrenia and bipolar affective disorders committed a large number (20% and 10% respectively) of the assaults. Medication toxicity from benzodiazepines and psychotropic drugs has been reported to cause assaultive behaviour in the elderly (Jacobs, 1983).

The best predictor for violence is a past history of violence (Jones, 1985; Lanza, 1988). Other behaviours that are often precursory to violence include hallucinations, poor impulse control, regressed behaviour, disorientation, restlessness, agitation. It is important to consider that powerlessness may also be related to aggression. Elderly residents often perceive that others are controlling their fate with decisions about restraints, transfers to facilities, medications, and the strict daily routines of eating, bathing and sleeping.

Environmental Risk Factors

Environmental characteristics can be related to the immediate physical environment that surrounds the resident or the culture of the entire organisation. As for the resident, it is important to recognise that the space around violence-prone individuals needs to be much larger than those who are not violent. When space is limited it may provoke anxiety. In addition, any unpredicted movement of the caregiver can result in a resident attempting to protect his space, often in an aggressive manner. Assaults often happen when the caregiver physically prompts the resident to eat, dress, or move. The unpredicted actions or behaviour of other persons in the environment can also provoke anxiety and aggression. This occurs when new residents or caregivers are brought into the facility or when there are environmental changes such as furniture or equipment. The anxious resident may assault others in an attempt to defend his space or personal belongings (Bridges et al., 1994).

Excessive stimuli, particularly noise, can also provoke violence prone individuals. It as been found that assaults are more common during times of high activity, such as between 7 AM and 11 AM, between noon and 2 PM and between 4 and 7 PM. Assaults on Monday were found to be double that of on Sunday. It is not clear whether this is related to the difference in activity level or in response to a relative's visit or lack of such visits over the weekend (Carmel and Hunter, 1989; Carmel and Hunter,1993; Gates et al., 2002a). Many NAs state that residents often become upset after family visits due to their anger of being placed in the nursing home. Although there is a lack of empirical studies regarding the organisational variables that are related to the incidence of assaults against caregivers, the list below includes those cited in the literature and in the two studies mentioned as risk factors for violence in healthcare settings:
- acceptance of violence as "part of the job"
- beliefs that violence cannot be decreased
- a high caregiver-resident ratio
- lack of violence policies and procedures
- lack of record-keeping about violent incidents
- lack of support after a violent episode
- employees are blamed for a violent incident
- lack of appreciation of the employees

- no screening process for violence
- lack of communication about violent prone individuals
- a hostile work environment

Healthcare facilities must eliminate the belief that violence is part of the job. Although all violence against caregivers in nursing homes cannot be eliminated, it can be decreased. In addition, caregivers will vary in their ability to cope and deal with violence from residents. Whereas some caregivers will be particularly bothered by sexual harassment, others will be offended more by biting. Just because an assault does not result in an injury, does not mean the event is not upsetting. Supervisors need to talk with their employees about the violence and find ways to show support and appreciation for the work they do in often difficult situations.

All facilities need to have a definition of violence and communicate this to all employees. There should be zero tolerance for worker against worker violence and violence from families. Family members who are abusive to staff should be reported to authorities and not be allowed in the facility. Caregivers who are abusive to other staff or residents should be reported to authorities. Administration needs to work with the physicians and families of residents who are not demented and are abusive. If the behaviour does not change, the facility should have the individual removed from the facility. With residents who are demented it is important that the supervisor and administration work closely with the physician, residents and caregivers to decrease the problem. Violence, whether intentional or not should never be expected, tolerated and accepted as part of the job.

In addition to those factors listed above there are additional security measures that facilities should consider. These include the use of video cameras, curved mirrors in isolated hallways or rooms or isolated rooms, areas and hallways. There needs to be clear policies and procedures regarding restraining and medicating residents, as well as a plan to respond to any weapons. When new residents are admitted to the facility, a supervisor should carefully screen for any history of verbal or physical aggressiveness. This information should be used to plan for room location, furnishings in the room, assignment of staff and training of staff. It is imperative that information regarding the resident's propensity toward aggression be communicated to all caregivers, as well as a plan to minimise triggers for aggression and what to do in case of escalation of aggression.

Interventions

A search of the literature provides minimal information regarding interventions that have demonstrated success in increasing violence prevention skills and decreasing violent incidents against nursing home caregivers. Most of the published, violence intervention studies in nursing homes measured changes in knowledge, beliefs about safety or self-efficacy to prevent violence (Feldt et al., 1992; Mentes and Ferrario, 1989; Cohen-Mansfield et al., 1997).

Interventions should be planned and implemented to prevent all four types of violence. These efforts include interventions to improve the organisational culture, as well as actions for the staff to take with residents. Primary prevention strategies with residents are aimed at keeping the resident from becoming agitated. These activities include:

- assign caregivers who are familiar with residents to take care of residents. If unfamiliar with resident, caregiver and supervisor make efforts to learn about resident's likes, dislikes, triggers for aggression and history of violence. Always introduce yourself to the resident and call resident by name.
- provide quiet and non-crowded surroundings
- give simple and concrete directions to the resident
- involve residents in care as much as possible
- provide care in a non-hurried, gentle manner
- always tell the resident what you plan to do before you do anything or before you touch them
- help the resident to recognise and express feelings
- be cognisant of the resident's space and how you enter their space
- be aware of any signs that the resident is becoming agitated
- minimise change in the resident's immediate environment and be prepared when changes are inevitable

Once a resident becomes agitated, the caregiver should make efforts toward the following aims:

- prevent resident from becoming increasingly fearful or anxious
- reduce any outbursts of anger
- decrease agitation

To prevent fear and anxiety the caregiver should communicate in a soft, calm, caring tone aimed at establishing trust and reducing any sense of powerlessness. At the same time the caregiver needs to recognise increasing anger and be prepared to respond to angry outbursts. The caregiver needs to use active listening skills to defuse anxiety. Encourage the resident to express any feelings of frustration, fear, sadness or anger and validate those feelings. If appropriate the caregiver needs to set limits for the resident, use distraction, provide other outlets for anger or offer solutions. As agitation increases, the resident may be experiencing increased frustration and vulnerability. This may result in blaming the caregiver and losing ability to control the anxiety. The resident may exhibit behaviours such as pacing, flaying of arms, becoming loud, and pounding of fists. When the caregiver observes these behaviours it is important that the caregiver notify her supervisor. It is important that the supervisor and caregiver be prepared to respond with the least restrictive approach that includes:

- de-stress the caregivers
- use de-escalation techniques to decrease the agitated behaviour
- allow ample interpersonal space between caregivers and resident
- provide clear, simple, and calm communication aimed at increasing the residents self-esteem and decreasing anxiety
- administration of anxiolytics
- continue de-escalation when the resident's anxiety has decreased

If the psychological approach does not work and the resident becomes assaultive, the supervisor should decide whether to use a physical and/or pharmacological approach. The physical approach involves the use of restraints or seclusion. The pharmacological approach includes the administration of sedatives, benzodiazepines, or short-acting barbiturates followed by de-escalation and continuous monitoring until stable.

Interventions aimed at the organisational level should include the following interventions by administration:

- institute a zero tolerance for violence against residents or co-workers
- demonstrate beliefs that violence from residents can be reduced
- demonstrate beliefs that ALL violence can have serious emotional and physical effects
- develop a support system for persons that are victims of violence
- demand that violence, including that from demented residents be reported
- institute a communication system to report violence and update staff on violent residents and families
- develop strategies to minimise caregiver turnover and use of agency personnel
- provide on-going training in violence prevention and violence reporting for ALL staff that comes in contact with residents
- develop procedures for screening new residents for violence
- develop protocols for when residents become agitated and assaultive

Conclusion

Violence, which is common in nursing homes, includes the following types: residents assaulting caregivers, caregivers assaulting residents and caregivers assaulting co-workers. Caregivers who are physically and verbally abused by residents experience both short-term and long-term emotional reactions, including anger, sadness, frustration, anxiety, irritability, fear, apathy, self-blame, and helpless-ness. The emotional toll that occurs to caregivers when they are abused on a daily basis is certain to have an impact on the quality of care provided to nursing home residents. A secondary effect is that NAs who are not able to effectively cope with the daily emotional and physical stressors related to resident care may be more prone to respond with aggressive and abusive response toward residents. There could therefore be a reciprocal relationship between the violence that oc-curs against the caregiver and the violence that occurs against the resident. Either type of occurrence has the potential to cause the victim to retaliate, thus resulting in two victims of abuse. For nursing homes to be a positive environment to live and work, it is imperative that administrators take immediate steps to improve the culture of the environment. Such changes will require policies and procedures that recognise that all types of violence can have serious psychological and physical effects on the residents and the workers.

References

Administration on Ageing (2000) *Profile of older Americans: 2000* [On-line], Available:
wysiwyg://74http:www.aoa.dhhs.gov/aoa/STATS/profile/default.htm.
American Healthcare Association (2001a) *Facts and trends series* [on-line], Available: http://www.ahca.org/research/nfbook.htm.
American Healthcare Association (2001b) *Nursing shortage creates growing consensus to begin problems solving.*[on-line], Available http://www.ahca. org/brief/nr010320.htm.
Bridges- Parlet, S., Knopman, D., and Thompson, T. (1994) A descriptive study of physically aggressive behaviour in dementia by direct observation, *Journal of the American Geriatrics Society*, 42, 192-197.
Bureau of Labor Statistics (1994) Issues in labor statistics: *Violence in the work-place comes under closer scrutiny* (Summary 94-10). Washington, DC: United States Department of Labor.
Bureau of Labor Statistics (1996) *Characteristics of injuries and illnesses result-ing in absences from work* 1994, USDL-96-163, Washington, DC: United States Department of Labor.
Carmel, H. and Hunter, M. (1989) Staff injuries from inpatient violence. *Hospital and Community Psychiatry*, 40(1), 41-46.
Carmel, H. and Hunter, M. (1993) Staff injuries from patient attack: five years data, *Bulletin of the American Academy of Psychiatry and the Law*, 21, 485-93.

Caudill, M.E. and Patrick, M. (1991) Costing nurse turnover in nursing homes. *Nursing Management*, 22 (11), 61-64.

Cohen-Mansfield, J. (1997) Turnover among nursing home staff. *Nursing Management*. 28 (5), 59-64.

Cohen-Mansfield, J., Werner, P., Culpepper, W J., and Barkley, D. (1997) *Journal of Gerontological Nursing*, 23, 40-7.

Colenda, C.C., and Hamer, R.M (1991) Antecedents and interventions for Aggressive behavior of patients at a geropsychiatric hospital, *Hospital and community Psychiatry*, 42, 287-292.

Ditasio, C.A. (1994) Violence in healthcare: Institutional strategies to cope with the phenomenon, *Health Care Supervisor*, 12, 1-34.

Feldt, K.S. and Ryden, M.B. (1992) Aggressive behavior: educating nursing assistants. *Journal of Gerontological Nursing* 18 (5) 3-12.

Gage, M. and Kingdom, D. (1995) Breaking the cycle of aggression. *Journal of Nursing Administration*, 25 (12), 55-64.

Gates, D., Fitzwater, E. and Deets, C. (in press) .Testing the reliability and validity of the assault log and violence prevention checklist, *Journal of Gerontological Nursing*.

Gates, D., Fitzwater, E. and Meyer, U. (1999) Violence against caregivers in nursing homes: expected, tolerated and accepted. *Journal of Gerontological Nursing*, 25 (4), 12-22.

Gates, D., Fitzwater, E., and Succop, P. (2002a) Predicting assaults against nursing home caregivers, *Journal of Occupational Psychology*, submitted for publication.

Gates, D., Fitzwater E. and Telintelo, S. (2002b) Using simulations to assess skill performance, *Clinical Nursing Research* 10 (4), 387-400.

Gates, D., Fitzwater, E., Telintelo, S., Succop, P. and Sommers, M.L. (2002c) Preventing assaults by nursing home residents: Caregivers' knowledge and confidence. *Journal of the American Medical Directors' Association*. Submitted for publication.

Hagen, B. and Sayers, D. (1995) When caring leaves bruises; the effects of staff education on resident aggression. *Journal of Gerontological Nursing*, 21 (11), 7-16.

Jacobs, D. (1983) Evaluation and management of the violent patient in emergency settings. *Psychiatric Clinics of North America*, 6, 259-269.

Jones, M.K. (1985) Patient violence. Report of 200 incidents. *Journal of Psychosocial Nursing*, 23, 12-17.

Lanza, M.L. and Campbell, D. (1992) Patient assault: a comparison study of reporting methods. *J Nurs Qual Assur*, 5 (4), 60-68.

174

Lusk, S.L. (1992) Violence experienced by nurses' CNAs in nursing homes: An exploratory study. *AAOHN Journal* 40, 237-241.

Maslach, C. (1982) Understanding burnout: definitional issues in analyzing a complex phenomenon. In: S.Paine (Ed) *Job stress and burnout*. Sage: Beverly Hills, CA.

Mentes, J. and Ferrario, J. (1992) Disruptive behavior in elderly nursing home residents: a survey of nursing staff. *Journal of Gerontological Nursing*, 18 (10), 13-17.

Osipow, S.H. (1998) *Occupational Stress Inventory revised edition* (OSI-R). Odessa, FLA: Psychological Assessment Resources, Inc.

Pillemer, K. and Hudson, B. (1993) A model abuse prevention program for nursing assistants, *Gerontologist*, 33, 128-131.

Pillemer, K. and Moore, D. (1989) Abuse of patients in nursing homes: Findings from a survey of staff. *The Gerontologist* 29 (3), 314-320.

Pillemer, K. and Bachman-Prehm, R. (1991) Helping and hurting, predictors of maltreatment of patients in nursing homes. *Research on Ageing* 13 (1), 74-95.

Ryden, M.B., Bossenmaier, M., and McLachlan, C.(1991) Aggressive behavior in cognitively impaired nursing homes, *Research in Nursing and Health*, 14 (2), 87-95.

Shaw, M.M. (1998) Nursing home resident abuse by staff: Exploring the dynamics, *Journal of Elder Abuse and Neglect*, 9, 1-21.

Smith, M.E. and Hart, G.(1994) Nurses' responses to patient anger: From disconnecting to connecting, *Journal of Advanced Nursing*, 20, 643-51.

Spielberger, C.D. (1999) *State-Trait Anger Expression Inventory-2*. Odessa, FLA: Psychological Assessment Resources, Inc.

Tardiff, K. and Swiellam, A. (1979) The relationship of age to assaultive behavior in mental patients. *Hospital and Community Psychiatry*, 30, 709-710.

Toscano, G.A. and Knestaut, A. Summer, (1998) Work injuries and illnesses occurring to women. *Compensation and Working Conditions*, 16-23.

University of Illinois (2001) *Who will care for each of us? America's coming health care labor crisis*. [on-line].
Available:
http://www.uic.edu/nursing/nursinginstitute/policy/finalreports/finalreport.pdf

United States General Accounting Office (2001) *Nursing Workforce: Recruitment and Retention of Nurses and Nurse Aides is a Growing Concern*, statement by Scanlon, W.J. , Washington, DC.

Winger, J., Schirm, V., and Stewart, D. (1987) Aggressive behavior in long-term care. *Journal of Psychosocial Nursing and Mental Health Services*, 25 (4), 28-33.

Wunderlich, G.S., Sloan, F.A, and Davis, C.K. (1996) *Nursing Staff in Hospitals and Nursing Homes, Is It Adequate?* Washington, D.C.: National Academy of Press.

Chapter Nine: Identifying and Reducing Nurse-Nurse Horizontal Violence and Bullying through Reflective Practice and Action Research in an Australien Hospital

Bev Taylor

Introduction

Violence happens in many forms, often in contexts where it is least expected and where caring practices are espoused, such as in hospitals. Nursing in hospitals involves negotiating complex interpersonal relationships, and working in a social and political context within economic constraints, while balancing a multiplicity of tasks and roles. Nurses are busy practitioners who need to have a broad range of clinical knowledge and skills, and they are accountable to many people (Benner, 1984; Benner and Wrubel, 1989; Taylor, 1997). Authors agree on the chaotic nature of nursing practice (Holmes, 1992; Pearson, 1989) and the constraints nurses face everyday in delivering quality care (Cox, Hickson and Taylor, 1991; Taylor, 1994, 2000b; Street, 1995). Given the complexity of nursing practice and the constraints in work settings, to some extent it is unsurprising, that nurses may try to cope by lashing out against one another laterally in forms of horizontal violence.

This chapter describes an action research project undertaken in Australia, through which research participants identified nurse-nurse horizontal violence and bullying in their workplace. At the outset, the aims of the project were broad, to facilitate reflective practice processes in experienced registered nurses, in order to: raise critical awareness of practice problems they face everyday; work systematically through problem solving processes to uncover constraints against effective nursing care; and improve the quality of care given by hospital nurses in light of the identified constraints and possibilities. As the action research project progressed, the nurses identified dysfunctional nurse-nurse relationships and they used the project time to address some of these behaviours through an action plan they negotiated collaboratively. This chapter relates the story of the action research methods and processes and the relative success of the resultant action plan, in reducing horizontal violence and bullying.

Literature Review

This review examines the origins of action research, reflection in nursing and workplace violence, with special reference to horizontal violence and bullying in the nursing profession.

Action Research

Action research is a cyclic series of planning, acting, observing and reflecting phases, in which co-researchers work together on areas of mutual concern (Roberts and Taylor, 2001). Although the action research approach is being used as a methodology for qualitative research across various disciplines, it is not new. It was introduced as a method for social science research by Kurt Lewin (in Hart and Bond, 1995) in the 1940's. The purpose was to bring about change in the social status quo during the postwar years within industry through improved management which, in change, would lead to increased output. These steps included general fact-finding, resource statements and planning, planning courses of action to achieve the objectives, and, finally, reflecting on the degree of success achieved as a result of the actions. This reflection on action then led to a new 'planning about further action' stage. Thus an important aspect of Lewin's action research was to reflect on or evaluate the result of the action taken. Despite the fact that present-day action research is defined variously depending on the discipline and purpose for which it is used, the latter aspect of reflection on action is regarded as central to all action research, and the aim of such reflection is to determine whether an improvement has resulted from the action.

Carr and Kemmis (1986) point out several areas in which contemporary action research diverges from the Lewinian approach, namely, they do not regard group democracy and decision-making simply as a technique for social change, but rather as part and parcel of committed group participation. Action research should not merely be a tool for achieving social change, but it should be seen as a research method which endorses democracy and individual freedom to participate in, collaborate with, critique and influence processes towards social change, particularly where social conditions allow exploitation and inequality. Moreover, because action research is participatory and collaborative, the researcher does not set the agenda, but allows it to grow out of the group process itself. The latter leads to self-awareness and empowerment. Thus, the Lewinian positivist stance toward engineered change in social groups or situations has been replaced with a qualitative philosophical tradition (Hart and Bond, 1995; Reason, 1988).

Action Research in Nursing

A major problem in nursing has been the so-called theory-practice gap. It seems that expert knowledge resulting from the research of academics has been difficult to integrate or translate into practical hands-on knowledge and expertise on the part of nurses. Action research emphasises the blending of the role of researcher and practitioner, to provide the conditions which enable genuine self-reflection. As Kemmis et al. (1982, in Hart and Bond, 1995) point out: its power for change lies in the use of action research to develop a critically reflexive practice, in which theory and practice are integrated and in which theory emerges from practice (p. 31).

Schon (1983) focused his thoughts on individual reflection and Adelman (1993) suggests that action research could become truly participatory if Schon's reflexive emphasis and Lewin's emphasis on organisational and group development were brought together. Thus, action research which entailed reflection on action could become reflexive in that it changed and improved practice through the practice of reflection within the context of a participatory group, within a wider social group or community.

Action research in nursing has been varied, and it includes studies aimed at changing work conditions for nurses, helping them reclaim their authority, organising themselves to be more effective in their practice and to clarify their roles and their status. It has facilitated self-directed learning (Owen, 1993) and provides them with a means of dealing with problem-solving, planning and evaluating (Hart and Bond, 1995; Nichols, Meyer, Batehup and Waterman, 1997; Waterman, 1998). Action research does not only aim at change and improvement in practice, but it also has the result of empowering participants, by allowing them to acknowledge who they are as persons and having a sense of self-determination (Reason, 1988). As action research entails working in a collaborative group, all participants are involved actively, and it allows individuals to take responsibility for themselves and the group. Thus, action research is also holistic, in the sense that knowledge development is not fragmented or separated from practice and experience.

Hart and Bond (1995) identify 7 criteria in action research which distinguish it from other methodologies, namely, that it: is educative; deals with individuals as members of social groups; is problem-focused, context-specific and future orientated; involves a change intervention; aims at improvement and involvement; involves a cyclic process in which research, action and evaluation are interlinked; and it is founded on a research relationship in which those involved are participants in the change process (p. 38). Action research includes types of action research that range from a Lewinian style to participatory and co-operative research in which the barriers between researcher and participants are removed (Rolfe, 1996).

Reflection and Reflective Practice

Taylor (2000a, p.3) defines reflection as 'the throwing back of thoughts and memories, in cognitive acts such as thinking, contemplation, meditation and any other form of attentive consideration, in order to make sense of them, and to make contextually appropriate changes if they are required. This definition allows for a wide variety of thinking as the basis for reflection, but it is similar to many other explanations (Mezirow, 1981; Boyd and Fales, 1983; Boud et al., 1985; Street, 1992) by the inclusion of the two main aspects of thinking as a rational and intuitive process which allows the potential for change.

One important aspect of action research with nurses has been 'systematic self-reflection, reflective discourse and critically oriented change' (Kim, 1999, p. 1206). Donald Schon advanced the concept of reflective practice in education and it has gathered momentum in nursing research and practice. It is, in effect, an extension of action science and it acknowledges that nursing practice is more than an application of theories or models to practice but is a complex, content-, person-, and situation-dependent process. Schon (1991) maintains that reflective practice encompasses reflection-in-action (the reflection on the way knowledge is used in action) and reflection-on-action (the reflection on experiences and the way practitioners can gain additional knowledge from these experiences to improve future practice). Reflective practice thus facilitates learning during practice, learning from practice and learning from past experience, and it acknowledges nurses as people within their contexts of past, present and future. In this critical self-reflection, change and improvement in practice is generated and theories of practice can be generated and maintained. However, such research in action is neither intended for generalisation nor external validation and often remains personal knowledge.

Argyris and Schon (1974) and Argyris, Putnam and Smith (1985) have suggested that practitioners such as nurses often practice at less than effective levels because they follow routine. Furthermore, their actual practice does not necessarily coincide with their 'better knowledge' or espoused theories about good practice. In fact, as Kim (1999) suggests, they may not even be aware of this divergence. Action research which includes reflective practice is, therefore, a way of determining why nurses' perception of their practice diverges from 'good practice'.

Self-emancipation is the crucial aspect which enables change in practice. Where groups are involved in such research, emancipatory change on a larger scale would ideally be the outcome (Kim, 1999; Johns, 1996a). Kim suggests that critical reflective inquiry can have benefits in knowledge development, improvement of individual practice and shared learning among nurses, perhaps during clinical conferences.

Learning through reflection on experience has been defined in different ways in the nursing literature since the 1980's and was adopted by nurses and nurse researchers as a tool for understanding and improving nursing practices. Johns (1995b) refers to this type of learning as a process of enlightenment, empowerment and emancipation. "Enlightenment refers to understanding oneself within one's practice context; empowerment allows the nurse to change herself in order to change her practice; emancipation enables nurses to liberate themselves from previous practice and as a consequence, to take congruent action ... toward desirable practice" (Johns, 1995b, p. 2).

Horizontal Violence in Nursing in the Form of Bullying

It has been found that workers' sense of safety in a group and the degree to which they will interact with one another, take (personal) risks and be innovative, depends on their level of participation. Within a non-threatening and supportive working environment, workers will be more committed and productive (West, 1996). Unfortunately the reality often is that nurses' work environments are often fraught with workplace violence in the form of horizontal violence (also known as bullying or mobbing). Bullying in the workplace can be investigated from perspectives such as determining its incidence, understanding its process and determining the effects of bullying behaviours on victims and organizations. Such investigations could draw on a wide range of social psychology, health-related and legal literature (Rayner and Hoel,1997). Alternative research approaches to quantitative projects are possible and Smith (1997) suggests that more qualitative studies are needed to investigate the effects of bullying and possible ways of preventing recurrences. For the present study, workplace violence and bullying was defined in terms of dysfunctional nurse-nurse relationships and explored through the qualitative approaches of action research and reflection.

Bostock (1998) performed a study in a community health setting in Australia using phenomenology as a method for determining negative communication patterns in the workplace. She identified three groups into which themes resulting from the research could be placed, namely, the individual context, the group context and the organisational context. The individual context encompassed themes such as powerlessness, stress, absenteeism, bullying, impact on well-being and creativity. She equates negative communication patterns with abuse and suggests intervention strategies such as education to combat the high incidence of workplace violence. Education would include a clear definition of bullying and its effects on organisational functioning, an understanding of personal rights, training in empowerment and dealing with despotic behaviour. Further to education, policy development, counselling and changing 'meeting culture' were seen as strategies towards intervention.

Literature about bullying in the workplace derives mainly from non-health arena publications. Australian literature about workplace violence in the health context is largely anecdotal with the exception of the work by authors such as Glass (1994, 1997, 1998), Serghis (1998) and Farrell (1997, 1998, 1999). Recently, however, organisations such as Nurses' Unions, the Online Nurse Advocate, and the Queensland Women's Service have released statements and accounts about bullying in the health sector on the Internet, and the problem of horizontal violence in nursing is becoming more familiar.

As a result of rising numbers of complaints about bullying amongst nurses, the Queensland Nurses' Union (QNU) in association with the Australian Nurses' Federation has released a statement on workplace violence. It defines workplace bullying as 'less favourable treatment of a person by another in the workplace, beyond which may be considered reasonable and appropriate workplace practice'. It points out that the effects of bullying can lead to mental and physical illness and overall loss of productivity. Ultimately patient care becomes more costly and less effective.

According to the QNU, bullying amongst nurses in Australia remains largely unreported because of the disposition of its victims who often have low selfesteem, feel responsible for the abuse, and have a sense of powerlessness. Spring and Stern (1997) report that horizontal violence can occur in the physical and psychic areas and suggest that it would possibly be more appropriate to use the term horizontal 'abuse' because the inflicted damage is often invisible, degrades and injures the dignity and worth of the individual.

The reasons for the prevalence of horizontal violence in nursing have been investigated from various perspectives. Spring and Stern (1997) comment that nurses enter their profession after having been educated to be caregivers. This means that they take on the role of carer and advocate for their patients whose needs always have priority. As a result, nurses' humanity and their needs are often not acknowledged. In addition, nurses, traditionally female, have undergone socialisation into the female role or otherwise grown up in situations where they learned to be caregivers (Valentine, 1995; Spring and Stern, 1997). Furthermore, nurses are outer-focused due to their daily exposure to human illness and tragedy.

182

According to Spring and Stern this leads to a desensitisation about the effects these daily experiences have on themselves. Finally, as largely women, nurses remain an oppressed professional group. A sense of powerlessness and helplessness often turns into oppressed person behaviour which is turned against colleagues. In reality, such behaviour is adaptive in that it consists of displaced attempts at gaining power in helpless situations. Lastly, nursing has a long tradition of hierarchical power-structure in which the young and less experienced are the targets of victimisation. Nurses themselves maintain the status quo through denial, minimisation and ritualization and thereby overlook the effects of horizontal abuse. Not only are there personal consequences of abuse but also for the profession as a whole.

In an editorial of 'Nurse Advocate online' it is stated that world wide only 20% of workplace related violence incidents are reported. This under-reporting as stated previously, is due to the belief that violence is 'part of the job', lack of policies and guidelines about reporting incidents and helplessness and powerlessness perceived by nurses (International Council of Nurses, in Lybecker, 1999). Australian nurses are believed to experience a sense of self-blame, lack of support and denial (Lybecker, 1999) in situations of horizontal violence. Fear for their jobs is also a strong motivator for denial. On a world wide level, nurses are under-supported by management, they are often blamed, the event is minimised, invalidated and reprisals are common. This is particularly the case if the offender is a doctor. Lybecker points out that the absence of clear definitions of terms such as horizontal violence, abuse, assault and harassment contributes towards the under-reporting of events.

Regarding the need for anti-bullying policies and guidelines, Oughtibridge (1998) suggests that an over-emphasis on rules and regulations reinforces nursing's history and leads to a lack of independent judgement on the part of individual nurses. The nurse-doctor relationship has often been blamed as the source of much of the disempowerment experienced by nurses. This sense of being oppressed is believed, then, to manifest itself in horizontal violence. While the nurse-doctor relationship is beyond the scope of this review, Oughtibridge (1998, p. 2 context) sums up some of the major concerns in this area by saying: because doctors have an established and prestigious place in health care, nursing as a profession is overshadowed by medical professionalism. It would seem that attitudes which have become entrenched within the health care system are the biggest barrier to nurses introducing innovation and change, and that the process of attitude change will be gradual. According to Farrel's (1998) study, 34% of nurses tended to have scores on the General Health Questionnaire (GHQ) which indicated that they were in emotionally ill health and which indicated distress. The sample of nurses was drawn from medical and psychiatric units. While the detrimental negative stress may derive from various sources in nurses' lives, workplace violence would certainly increase the likelihood of long-term ill effects. Nurses found colleague aggression to be the most distressing aspect of their work. While varying forms of aggression occurred at differing rates of frequency, nurses found nurse-nurse aggression as the most difficult to deal with. On the other hand, nurses who were victims of abuse most often sought support from friends and colleagues. Thus, collegiality amongst nurses is of prime importance not only as a resource for support but also a preventative of horizontal violence (Farrell, 1999; Lees, 1999). Garland (1999) suggests that personal empowerment through increased knowledge about bullying, bullies and victims in conjunction with policies may prove helpful in dealing with this problem. Furthermore, mentoring and counselling could be facilitative.

Factors which could make certain people more susceptible to bullying have been examined. Quine (1999) says that because bullying is usually defined in terms of the negative effects on the recipient it becomes subject to the recipient's perspective and experience. Bullying is often reported by staff who have low job satisfaction and high job-induced stress. Furthermore, these nurses are more likely to be depressed, anxious and wanting to leave. While bullying can be responsible for the ill health and low job satisfaction, it is possible that a person with a more pessimistic nature is more likely to report bullying. Alternatively, being in poor physical and emotional health could make certain people prime targets for bullies. Depression and anxiety in themselves can lead people to perceive certain behaviours as more hostile and threatening. Nevertheless, despite these subjective aspects of bullying, it is evident that many incidents are, in fact, witnessed by others. There is also greater likelihood of younger, less qualified staff to be victims. Thus, organisational climate appears to play a role also.

Summary

Action research and reflection are complementary inquiry processes, requiring nurses to think carefully on their practice experiences in order to make sense of them, and bring about changes if necessary. The literature suggests that the problem of workplace violence is multifaceted and not easily solved. Various possible avenues for attacking the problem have been suggested and nurse empowerment and emancipation through various means appear to be foundational steps toward creating a more positive work environment for nurses and, hence, improved patient care. Therefore, this project used the facilitative processes of action research and reflection to identify and reduce horizontal violence and bullying in nursing practice.

184

The Research Plan

Given the collaborative nature of the project, a qualitative approach was chosen, informed by reflective practitioner concepts and the technical, practical and emancipatory intentions of action research (Taylor, 2000a). Full ethical clearance processes through Southern Cross University and the Northern Rivers Areas Health Service preceded the commencement of the project. It was intended that the research would be for a 12 month period, from January to December 1999. However, difficulties in recruiting participants necessitated a change of setting, therefore the project began in August and finished in late December 1999.

Participants

Convenience sampling was used to target intentionally those research participants who were interested in reflecting on their practice in order to improve it. Twelve experienced female Registered Nurses (RN) working in a large local rural hospital, with an age range of 25 to 50 years, agreed to participate on a one hour per week basis for 16 weeks. The number of participants was appropriate for a qualitative project because of the potential of the research to generate rich data sufficient to bring about changes in work practices. The number of participants was also congruent with the assumptions of qualitative research, which emphasise the context-dependent quality of process, experience, and language. Therefore, this project did not seek high numbers to generalise results or use them for predictive purposes. Also, in collaborative research of this nature, the process becomes as important as the potential outcomes, because the focus is on what people learn as they experience the research itself (Roberts and Taylor, 2001).

Methods and Processes

The nurses met weekly for one hour to discuss clinical problems raised by them in their journal writing and discussion. The researcher acted as a group facilitator, and as a guide in the research processes, keeping meeting notes, writing up minutes, preparing agendas and contributing as appropriate. Introductory sessions allowed group members to become familiar with some reflective practitioner and action research literature and with the activities outlined in the project materials. Processes to enable effective reflection included coaching and practice in writing and speaking descriptively, in confidential and facilitative group meetings. Confidence was bolstered in undertaking reflection in practice (during practice) and reflection on practice (after practice) through individual and collective storytelling, journalling, critical analysis and discussion.

The methods of action research involved a four stage problem solving approach of collectively planning, acting, observing and reflecting. This phase led to another cycle of action, in which the plan was revised, and further acting, observing and reflecting was undertaken systematically, to work towards solutions to problems. The planning and acting phases included keeping a journal as a method of gathering and analysing data. The non-confidential parts of journals were shared with peers in the weekly group meeting. Participant observation occurred during practice in clinical areas. Notes and/or journal entries were made after the nursing activities, given the immediacy of clinical situations.

The data analysis method included an analysis of journal experiences by individual and group critical reflection and problem solving strategies. Group discussion also identified the specific nature and determinants of problems, the most appropriate methods to investigate problems further, and the most practical and useful plan of action. Descriptions of participant observation were analysed individually using a reflective analysis method and collectively by group discussion. In each action research cycle the findings were pooled and discussed and the appropriate action was planned and taken. Successive observation of the effects followed, before further reflection led to further action and analysis.

Findings and Discussion

In this project there were three discernible action research cycles. The first cycle (Weeks 1-3) involved the development of group processes, becoming familiar with the research aims and action research and reflective processes. The second cycle (Weeks 4-7) involved using reflective processes to locate individual and collective practice issues. Difficulties with nurse-nurse relationships were identified as important, specifically dysfunctional behaviours such as bullying and horizontal violence. The third cycle (Weeks 8-16) involved working together on this common practice issue to generate and act and reflect on an action plan. The activities within the three action research cycles were documented in the group's minutes, written by myself as facilitator and confirmed weekly as faithful accounts by the group members, to represent the analysis and interpretation processes of individuals and the collective.

The First Cycle (Weeks 1-3)

In the first meeting I introduced myself as a facilitator and co-researcher and gave out packages containing a meeting agenda, a summary of action research, a summary of reflective practice, an exercise book to be used as a journal and two articles to read on action research and reflective practice respectively. We agreed to introduce ourselves using a 'round the table' approach, and participants told where they work and why they decided to join the group. We moved through the agenda at a relatively relaxed pace, as I explained that we could use next week also to get through the introductory ideas. I explained my expectations for co-researchers' involvement, including keeping and sharing a journal, being involved in discussion and being involved in action research cycles.

A co-researcher expressed her concern that the group would need to agree on certain 'rules' and dynamics in order to preserve individual's privacy and confidentiality. This led to a discussion of the areas that were important to the group. Co-researchers described the kind of group dynamics they wanted to foster so that trust, openness and confidentiality could be established and maintained. These included applying the general rules of professional confidentiality as practised already in work settings to the group, a respect for co-researchers' feelings, informing the group if an area being shared was confidential as sensitivities may vary, listening carefully, acknowledging the person speaking if only with attention and a nod of the head, refraining from criticism and unnecessary advice, and withholding the desire 'to fix things' except in cases where that was the explicit intention.

I reiterated the point that reflective disclosures should only be made at a level with which individuals were comfortable. If any group member experienced profound catharsis or was in need of emotional support it would be offered by the group members immediately and appropriately (given they were registered nurses and midwives), and if further help was required, names of counsellors were available. Also, journals were to be the private domain of individual co-researchers (with the exception of my meeting process notes). When co-researchers read from their journals it would only be those excerpts they chose to share with the group.

In the second and third meetings, we continued to discuss and practice group processes. I explained that I would maintain meeting notes, adjusted for anonymity, as research data and to assist us to ascertain our progress over time. I introduced the agenda topic of how we could manage power influence differences in the group and these areas were discussed. Strategies included making sure everyone had a voice, encouraging co-researchers who were not speaking while being sensitive to their need to be quiet at times, and accepting speakers in non-judgemental ways. We recognised that power comes from different amounts of knowledge and for everyone to feel equal we needed to respect one another's knowledge to empower one another.

I used an action research summary sheet handed out previously to explain the data collection (planning, acting, observing) and data analysis (reflecting) ideas in action research. I also read from a summary sheet on reflection I prepared for the meeting, describing the reasons why it was useful to reflect on childhood experiences and 'rules of living'. I read an example of my own childhood memories and encouraged co-researchers to write their own reflections in their own unique way. Some discussion followed about what the task was about, why it was important, and hints for how to reflect spontaneously.

Many co-researchers shared their experiences 'from the heart' and generously offered their insights into themselves as people and practitioners. The group discussed some of the ideas raised and supported one another as sensitive and precious disclosures were made. Most co-researchers indicated that they found the reflective writing task useful and enjoyable. One co-researcher shared that she has difficulty speaking her ideas, but found writing them so easy that she had written many pages in her journal and that she really enjoyed the experience. I guided co-researchers through a summary sheet for writing a practice reflection and reiterated that we would have at least four weeks of sharing practice stories to decide on a thematic concern to work on together using action research and reflection.

The Second Cycle (Weeks 4-7)

In the second cycle, the group located individual and collective practice issues within participants' stories. For each story, I guided the storyteller through the reflective process of locating the bases of her actions, and of looking at all of the determinants and constraints of the situation. Two co-researchers shared from their journal and responded to the group questions, comments and other contributions. The first story had an underlying theme of advocacy – of wanting to speak up in situations where it is difficult, because of doctor-nurse relations and professional expectations about roles. The story also sparked discussion about horizontal violence in nursing and how 'nothing changes' in some respects, when it comes to some negative aspects of professional relationships. The second story contained a theme of professional victimisation and the group discussed many issues relating to this story, including a sense of betrayal by peers, fear of powerful hierarchical figures, problems about clinical incompetence in peers, doctor-nurse relations, nurse-nurse relations, the need for fearful obedience and the message to not complain. For many of the stories, co-researchers acknowledged similar circumstances and responses.

When locating and collating issues in practice reflections, one by one co-researchers talked about the issues they had noted in their journals and the meeting discussions. These included many issues that grouped into two main areas: professional relationships and professional identity. Professional relationships included the doctor/nurse, patient/nurse, and nurse/nurse relationship. Within these relationships there were issues of gender, hierarchy, communication, peer pressure in decision-making, power, advocacy, and recognition as professionals. Professional identity included issues such as guilt, regret, 'feeling I haven't performed', 'not really knowing my work peers', lack of confidence and self esteem, blaming the past instead of learning from it, feeling responsible, needing to be invincible and perfect, having pride in work, needing to achieve and accountability. We discussed the two categories and realised that they were related, in that if the professional identity issues were remedied, professional relationships would most probably benefit also. We decided to focus on professional relationships firstly and see if some of the other issues from professional identity are also addressed along the way.

The Third Cycle (Weeks 8-16)

The third cycle (Weeks 8-16) involved working together on a common practice issue to generate and act and reflect on an action plan. The group members decided that they wanted to stay as one large group, rather than divide into two smaller groups. At this point appreciation was expressed for the process thus far and co-researchers acknowledged how much they had derived from the trusting and open dynamics the group had evolved over the time they had been meeting.

As nurse/nurse relationships were being discussed, it sparked analogies for other co-researchers who related similar issues. The conversations were very direct and the stories were risky in terms of anonymity and confidentiality. At this point a co-researcher asked how we could be sure that we were doing research and not engaging in a 'witch hunt' for certain unfavoured individuals. We realised that we needed to discuss issues directly, clearly and with a very high degree of confidentiality, if we were to get to a place in which we felt we were focussed on issues in relationships and strategies with which to approach them effectively.

The statement was repeated that we were focussing on nurse-nurse professional relationships, as they were ones we could probably fix. At that point, a co-researcher located an article in a professional magazine 'Lamp' entitled: 'Those who can, do – those who can't, bully' (1999). The article related to the incidence

189

of bullying in workplaces, and its prominence in nursing. We agreed that while we were grateful for the insights the article provided us, we needed to be careful to avoid assuming that all nurse-nurse professional relationships that do not work well are based on some kind of bullying.

The planning phase continued as we looked at 'filling in the gaps' in the participants' stories to find commonalities and general principles about how to manage nurse-nurse professional relationships. We looked at how each situation came about, and what could be done about it. For example, in one story the issues were about devious behaviour, bullying by proxy, betrayal and being let down, and problems that happen when events are twisted out of context. Professional jealousy and the use of power in a manipulative way, may have been determinants in the situation, related to perpetuating the culture of horizontal violence.

When we looked at the sheet prepared for analysis of the scenarios to find commonalities and principles for action, we noted that the common issues and feelings were all of a negative, unfair, unprofessional and disempowering nature. The common determinants could be linked to the historical progression of nursing, cultural norms in roles and relationships, and political and personal aspects of interpersonal communication in nurse-nurse encounters in the hospital setting. For example, co-researchers identified the possibilities of low self esteem in the person causing the problem, gender issues of 'tittle tatting', undermining and horizontal violence, bullying by proxy, attempts to carry out a 'put down', professional jealousy and the use of power in a manipulative way.

The list of common strategies from the previous meetings was varied and contained numerous suggestions, with the addition of a review of job descriptions to ensure that persons had acted within the boundaries of work activities and responsibilities. The next step was to look at the list of strategies and prioritise them into a plan of action, which needed to be flexible to allow for unforeseen effects and constraints, take account of the social risks involved and recognise the material and political constraints in the situation, and allow us to go beyond our present constraints to empower us to act more effectively in the situation.

Using the white board to post our decisions, we discussed and subsequently eliminated those ideas that were too non-specific, idealistic and unlikely to be of practical use in the four or so weeks remaining in the project. The strategies retained in the action plan included:

- start a culture of positive strokes and acknowledgement;
- deal with the nurse directly and immediately and through recourse to policies and procedures;
- provide strong leadership ourselves;
- look carefully at the determinants of situations and try to 'turn them around';
- engage in conflict resolution;

- raise the possibility that maybe nurses are in need of recognition, acknowledgement and involvement in creating practice policies;
- encourage nurses to support one another; use evidence and documentation, such as professional journals, incident forms, annual reviews, and Occupational Health and Safety procedures;
- use the line of command; build skills to deal with situations directly, and/or ask for facilitation as soon as possible;
- and use 'people power' and a 'united front' to senior staff in the line of command.

We agreed that this list of strategies had many ideas within it which begged the question: 'How?!' For example, how can we handle issues directly, provide strong leadership and deal with conflict resolution? I made the point that all of the co-researchers in the group had experience and varying degrees of training in interpersonal communication skills. The group discussed how it would be necessary to approach situations directly with a tentative and gentle attitude, seeking to clarify the situations. Reflective listening would be needed, and organisation of face to face meetings between the key people in the situation, with strict attention to confidentiality. Also, specific skills such as statement of one's own feelings and paraphrasing were necessary. Knowing the difference between aggression and assertiveness was important, so that direct approaches in conflict resolution used the attitude and skills discussed in such a way that all parties felt they were being heard, so that they could negotiate fair and reasonable solutions to nurse-nurse relationship problems.

The research intention from then, was to use whatever skills in the action plan deemed appropriate to directly manage nurse-nurse professional relationship problems which arose in the weeks ahead. Observations of the effectiveness or otherwise of the strategies would be written in journals. Stories would be shared in meetings as to the success of the actions, and adjustments would be made along the way to make them as effective as possible.

When we began sharing the effectiveness of the action plan, an opening comment was: 'It feels good to be positive'. Two stories were shared relating to the use of the action plan. The first story was about a situation in which the co-researcher felt reactive, recognised her feelings and turned it around so that it was no longer an issue for her. After group discussion the co-researcher said she might speak with the nurse to clarify her position. The co-researcher felt that she had begun to establish a culture of positive strokes by her action in being self reflective and non reactive.

If one analyses this incident, it is clear that the co-researcher's action was not one of those listed explicitly in the action plan. What she actually used, was the reflective process inherent in the action research process the group had adopted.

The increased self-awareness empowered her to feel more in control, and that changed the situation for her, without anything changing externally. It would also seem that creating a culture change can include more than just giving positive strokes or acknowledgement. It can also include being less reactive, and thereby lowering the "temperature" in the situation.

The second story involved a co-researcher's use of many of the strategies in the action plan, which turned out to be of little use, given further events over time, which exacerbated nurse-nurse relationships. Co-researchers were aware of the situation and provided other perspectives on the same situation. As the perspectives unfolded, it became apparent that the situation was very complex and that it involved nurses' unequal willingness/ability/preparedness to communicate openly and directly. It also showed that it takes courage to communicate effectively, there are perils inherent in trying to be everything to everyone, and difficulties can ensue with an unclear and broad job description. Thus, the first try of the action plan resulted in stories with different outcomes. We discussed how it was important to realise there were no quick fix remedies, that nurse-nurse relationships were complex and required lots of work in acting, observing, and reflecting in the goal of improving them.

In this description the importance of having a support group to which she could come for ventilation and understanding seemed to be important. In many situations things cannot be changed, at least not in the short term, and it would seem that the support that the research group provided became increasingly important in such situations.

As we continued to explore the benefits of the action plan for improving nurse-nurse relationships, one co-researcher said she found herself communicating directly more often. For example, if someone came up to her 'for a whinge' she checked whether she should regard the interaction as 'just a whinge' or something which should be taken further. The discussion then turned to what to do when you do your best to communicate directly and with all the ideas in our action plan, and the other party is unwilling/unable to do likewise. Suggestions offered resembled the action plan, for example, to provide strong leadership in how to communicate, recognise the person's lack of skills/willingness, use direct one to one approaches and then resort to the line of command if necessary. After many anecdotes, we came to the conclusion that nurses from various backgrounds face multiple constraints in their practice and they are often thwarted in giving ideal care and communicating with one another. This being so, we all needed to recognise our part and the contribution of constraints, forgive ourselves our imperfections, and work towards identifying and remedying the constraints.

192

We reviewed the progress of the previous few weeks, pointing out that the action plan had been used with some success, co-researchers being able to get to the basis of their interactions with other nurses. Also, we noted that we had been able to look at some of the economic, sociocultural and political reasons for problems in nurse-nurse professional relationships.

During the informal last meeting, that served as a group farewell and Christmas celebration, co-researchers agreed that there was a need for ongoing connections so that the spirit engendered in the meetings could continue. I suggested that this was possible if co-researchers gathered together for regular conversations and support and that I had intended to coach co-researchers in maintaining their own group processes for any problems they may have. While co-researchers agreed the processes had been very helpful, they also acknowledged the need for the role of an 'outside' facilitator, who could guide the co-researchers through 'delicate situations'. Unfortunately, the group did not continue in a self-supporting fashion the following year, although I am still receiving positive feedback about the processes.

Conclusion

This chapter described an action research project undertaken in Australia, through which research participants identified nurse-nurse horizontal violence in form of bullying in their workplace. At the outset, the aims of the project were broadly emancipatory, to identify constraints and to free the nurses to other possibilities in their nursing practices. As the action research project progressed, the nurses identified dysfunctional nurse-nurse relationships and they used the project time to address some of these behaviours through an action plan they negotiated collaboratively. This chapter related the story of the action research methods and processes and the relative success of the resultant action plan, in reducing horizontal violence known as bullying.

References

Adelman in Hart, E. and Bond, M. (1995) Action Research for Health and Social CareBuckingham: Open University Press.

Argyris, C. and Schon, D. (1974) in Kim, H.S. (1999) Critical reflective inquiry for knowledge development in nursing practice. *Journal of Advanced Nursing* 29, 5: 1205-1212.

Argyris, C. Putnam, R. and Smith, D.M. 1985 in Kim, H.S. (1999) Critical reflective inquiry for knowledge development in nursing practice. *Journal of Advanced Nursing* 29, 5, 1205-1212.

Benner, P. (1984) From Novice To Expert: Uncovering The Knowledge Embedded. In: *Clinical Practice*. Addison-Wesley, California.

Benner P. and Wrubel J. (1989) *The Primacy Of Caring : Stress And Coping In Health And Illness*. Addison-Wesley, California.

Bostock, J. (1998) *Communication patterns in the workplace: a study of perceptions held by health professionals at a community health service.* Masters Thesis Charles Sturt University: Australia.

Boud, D., Keogh, R. and Walker, D. (1985) *Reflection: Turning Experience into Learning*. Kagan Page, London.

Boyd, E.M. and Fales, A.W. (1983) Reflective learning: key to learning from experience. *Journal of Humanistic Psychology* 23, 2, 99-117.

Carr, W. and Kemmis, S. (1986) *Becoming Critical: Education, Knowledge and Action Research*. Falmer Press, Lewes.

Cox, H., Hickson, P. and Taylor, B.J. (1991) Exploring Reflection: Knowing and Constructing the Practice of Nursing. In: Gray, G. and Pratt R. (Eds) *Towards a Discipline of Nursing*, Churchill Livingstone, London, 373-389.

Farrell, G. (1997) Aggression in clinical settings: Nurses' views. *Journal of Advanced Nursing*. 25, 3, 501-508.

Farrell, G. (1998) The mental health of hospital nurses in Tasmania as measured by the 12-item General Health Questionnaire. *Journal of Advanced Nursing* 28, 4, 707-712.

Farrell, G. (1999) Aggression in clinical settings: Nurses views - a follow-up study. *Journal of Advanced Nursing* 29, 3, 532-541.

Garland, A. (1999) Beware of the bully. *Nursing Standard* 13, 23, 65-67.

Glass, N.E. (1994) Women's disruptive voices: registered nurses and tertiary qualifications. *Journal for Social Justice Studies*. 5, 61-84.

Glass, N.E. (1997) *Moving on from horizontal violence: celebrating conscious healing strategies for women nurse academics*. NSW Nurses Research Interest Group, 13th Annual Conference Sydney, July 25th.

Glass, N.E. (1998) The contested workplace: reactions to RN's doing degrees. *Collegian* 5, 1: 24-31.

Hart, E. and Bond, M. (1995) *Action Research for Health and Social Care*. Buckingham. Open University Press.

Holmes, C. (1992) The drama of nursing. *Journal of Advanced Nursing*. 17, 954-960.

Johns, C. (1995) Framing learning through reflection within Carper's fundamental ways of knowing in nursing. *Journal of Advanced Nursing.* 22, 2: 226-234.

Johns, C. (1996a) Using a reflective model of nursing and guided reflection. *Nursing Standard.* 11, 2, 34-38.

Johns, C. (1996b) Visualizing and realizing caring through guided reflection. *Journal of Advanced Nursing* 24, 6, 1135-1143.

Kim, H. S. (1999) Critical reflective inquiry for knowledge development in nursing practice. *Journal of Advanced Nursing* 29, 5, 1205-1212.

Lees, C. (1999) *A description of some incidents of horizontal violence within the nursing profession: identification of the type of support provided throughout the incident, and the victim's resultant attitude towards nursing.* Masters Thesis Charles Sturt University, Australia

Lybecker, C. (1999) *Violence against nurses: a silent epidemic.* Nurse Advocate: nurses and workplace violence. Available: http://www.nurseadvocate.org. guestbook.html.

Mezirow, J. (1981) A critical theory of adult learning and education. *Adult Education,* 32, 1, 3-24.

Nichols, R., Meyer, J., Batehup, Z.L. and Waterman, H. (1997) Promoting action research in health care settings. *Nursing Standard,* 11, 40: 36-38.

Oughtibridge, D. (1998) Under the thumb. *Nursing Management,* 4, 8: 22-24.

Owen, S. (1993) Identifying a role for the nurse teacher in the clinical area. *Journal of Advanced Nursing,* 18, 816-825.

Pearson A. (1989) *Translating rhetoric into practice: theory in action.* National Nursing Theory Conference, School of Nursing Studies, Sturt, South Australian College of Advanced Education.

Queensland Nurses (1997) *Union Statement on Workplace Bullying 1997.* Available: http://www.qnu.org.au.

Rayner, C. and Hoel, H. (1997) A summary review of literature relating to workplace bullying. *Journal of Community and Applied Social Psychology,* 7, 3, 181-191.

Reason, P. (1988) *Human inquiry in action: developments in new paradigm research.* London: Sage Publications.

Roberts, K. and Taylor, B. (2001) *Nursing Research Processes: An Australian Perspective 2nd ed.* Nelson ITP, Melbourne.

Rolfe, G. (1996) Going to extremes: Action research, grounded practice and the theory-practice gap in nursing. *Journal of Advanced Nursing,* 24, 6: 1315-1320.

Schon, D. (1991) in Kim, H. S. (1999) Critical reflective inquiry for knowledge development in nursing practice. *Journal of Advanced Nursing* 29, 5, 1205-1212.

Schon, D. A. (1983) *The Reflective Practitioner: How Practitioners Think in Action.* Basic Books, New York.

Schon, D.A. (1987) *Educating the Reflective Practitioner.* Jossey-Bass, London.

Serghis, D. in Bostock, J. (1998) *Communication patterns in the workplace: a study of perceptions held by health professionals at a community health service.* Masters Thesis Charles Sturt University, Australia.

Smith, P.K. (1997) Bullying in life-span perspective: what can studies of school bullying and workplace bullying learn from each other? *Journal of Community and Social Psychology*, 7, 3: 249-255.

Spring, N. and Stern, M. 1997-2000 *"Nurse abuse? Couldn't be!."* Nurse Advocate: Nurses and Workplace Violence Online, Available: http://www.nurse advocate.org.guestbook.html.

Street, A. (1995) *Nursing Replay: Researching Nursing Culture Together.* Churchill Livingstone, Melbourne.

Street, A.F. (1992) in Farrell, G. (1997) Aggression in clinical settings: Nurses' views. *Journal of Advanced Nursing*, 25, 3: 501-508.

Taylor, B.J. (1992) From helper to human: A reconceptualisation of the nurse as person. *Journal of Advanced Nursing*, 17, 1042-1049.

Taylor, B.J. (1994) *Being Human: Ordinariness in Nursing.* Churchill-Livingstone, Melbourne.

Taylor, B.J. (1997) Big battles for small gains: A cautionary note for teaching reflective processes in nursing and midwifery. *Nursing Inquiry*, 4, 19-26.

Taylor, B.J. (1998) Locating a Phenomenological Perspective of Reflective Nursing and Midwifery Practice by Contrasting Interpretive and Critical Reflection. In: Johns, C. and Freshwater D. (Eds) *Transforming Nursing Through Reflective Practice*, Blackwell Science, Oxford,134-150.

Taylor, B.J. (2000a) *Reflective Practice: A Guide for Nurses and Midwives.* Allen and Unwin, Melbourne.

Taylor, B.J, (2000b) Being Human: Ordinariness in Nursing. Adapted for Southern Cross University Press, Lismore.

Those who can, do – those who can't, bully (1999) In: '*Lamp*' October, New South Wales.

Valentine, P. (1995) Management of conflict: do nurses/women handle it differently? *Journal of Advanced Nursing*, 22,1, 142-149.

Waterman, H. Embracing ambiguities and valuing ourselves: issues of validity in

West, M. and Bostock, J. (1998) *Communication patterns in the workplace: a study of perceptions held by health professionals at a community health service,* Masters Thesis.

Chapter Ten: The Content and Development of Management of Violence Policies in Inpatient Psychiatric Settings

James Noak and Steve Wright

Introduction

Policies provide the framework for working practices in any organisation. As such, they are credible and useful to the extent that they provide practical, relevant, and clear guidance on practice, which makes explicit the organisation's expectations of how staff should act when faced with certain situations arising from the course of their work. Conversely, the absence of clear policy guidance and training can result in poor practice and dysfunctional responses by staff, which may result in harm to staff or others present in the workplace, thereby rendering the employer vulnerable to litigation. Of course, the absence of clear policy guidance and training might also actually precipitate the very problems that the organisation wishes to avoid.

This chapter is predominantly concerned with the content and development of management of violence policies in inpatient psychiatric settings in the UK, which reflects the experience and interests of the authors. However, the content will be of international interest, as violence towards health care staff (and nurses in particular) is a problem that does not recognise international boundaries. Although the needs of community-based workers are also considered, the particular needs of health care professionals working in non-psychiatric specialities have not been addressed. However, it is hoped that some of the points raised will be relevant and applicable to other settings.

Violence as an Occupational Hazard in Healthcare.

Violence is an increasingly serious problem, and has become so common that it has been described as a public health problem in its own right (Shepherd and Farrington, 1993; Golding, 1996). It is therefore unsurprising that violence in the workplace has also increasingly become a topic of major academic, legal, managerial and governmental concern. Not only does violence in the workplace represent a threat to the physical and psychological wellbeing of its victims (whether employees or others present in the workplace), but the negative impacts upon organisational functioning (in terms of such considerations as assault-related sick leave, staff recruitment and retention, litigation, and associated financial costs) are also recognised within the literature (e.g. Lanza, 1983; Lanza and Milner, 1989; Poster and Ryan, 1994; Barling, 1996; Alderman, 1997).

Healthcare workers of all disciplines are at increased risk of being assaulted at work, and this is an international problem (Flannery, 1996). In the UK, the Health Services Advisory Committee (HSAC) survey (1987) found health care sites to have the greatest risk for verbal abuse and threats to staff of all worksites. This is worrying, given the suggestion that verbal aggression is not separated from physical aggression, but forms a continuum with it (McNeil and Binder, 1989). Furthermore, Adams and Whittington (1995) found that high levels of anxiety and traumatic stress were reported by a sample of psychiatric nurses who had been exposed verbal abuse and threats. In the UK violence in healthcare settings is particularly common in psychiatry and in Accident and Emergency departments (HSAC, 1987; Ryan and Poster, 1993; Gournay et al., 1998; Nolan et al., 1999; Cembrowicz and Shepherd, 1992), it has also been found to be prevalent in medical wards in general hospital settings (Whittington et al., 1996; O'Connell, 2000) and in general practice (Hobbs, 1991). While all healthcare workers are at increased risk, it is well established that the major risk is experienced by nurses working in all areas of health care (HSAC, 1987; Carmel and Hunter, 1989; Flannery et al., 1994).

Why should violence be a particular occupational risk in the healthcare professions? Beale et al. (1999a) propose that violence occurs when conflict situations escalate into manifest hostility or physically exhibited aggression. Given that healthcare staff (and particularly nurses) frequently deal with people whose history they do not know, and who are often in pain, anxious, and uncertain as to what is happening or what the future holds, where their clinical interventions in themselves can often be painful or otherwise aversive, and considering the frustration and resentment that can be borne of long waiting times for outpatient treatment and the loss of autonomy and subjugation to institutional routine on becoming an inpatient, the potential for violence becomes readily understandable. Since violence is an unintended and undesirable by-product of the work undertaken by healthcare professionals, the reduction of the likelihood and impact of violence in the workplace should be viewed as an organisational problem, requiring an organisational approach to its prevention and management.

The Role of Policy in an Organisational Approach to Violence.

Cox and Cox (1993) view work-related violence as similar to more tangible occupational hazards (such as toxic chemicals or dangerous machinery), and suggest that the problem can be most effectively managed within the framework of practice that has been proven successful in managing such workplace hazards. Essentially, this entails a problem-solving approach to hazard control and risk management (Cox and Tait, 1991). This same approach is in fact set out in various statutory regulations, such as the Health and Safety at Work Act 1974, the Regulations for the Control of Substances Hazardous to Health 1988 (COSHH), and the Management of Health and Safety at Work Regulations (Health and Safety Executive, 1992) in the UK, and the Occupational Safety and Health Act 1970 in the USA. Not only does such legislation direct that employers adopt hazard-specific standards, but it also mandates that employers have a responsibility to provide employees and others who might be present with a workplace that is as free from recognised hazards likely to cause death, injury, or harm as is reasonably possible. Such legislation obliges employers to undertake an assessment of risk within the workplace, and to assess the effectiveness of existing systems for minimising exposure to and harm resulting from such hazards. With regard to mental health care in the UK, the Mental Health Act 1983 Code of Practice (Department of Health and Welsh Office, 1999) specifically states that all providers of inpatient psychiatric care should have clear policies on the management of violence[1]. In fact, nurses in the UK who agree to work in settings where risk assessments have not been performed and safe systems of work have not been put in place to address hazards identified by such assessments (which includes violence at work), not only put themselves at risk, but also fail to comply with Section 10 of the United Kingdom Central Council for Nursing, Midwifery, and Health Visiting Code of Professional Conduct (1992), which addresses safe standards of practice.[2]

The occupational health and safety legislation discussed above specifies the need for systematic and proactive management of risks and hazards. A method for achieving this is depicted in Cox and Cox (1993), who describe a 'control cycle', a six-step method for systematic problem solving and organisational learning. This cycle of activities aims to ensure that the development of safe work environments is a continuous process, and consists of the following stages:

1. Problem or hazard identification, and the analysis and assessment of risk.
2. Design of intervention strategies.
3. Planning and implementation of strategies.
4. Implementation.

---

[1]   The Mental Health Act 1983 is the legislation that covers the care of the mentally disordered in the UK.

[2]:   The UKCC is the statutory body which regulates the professional practice of Registered Nurses in the UK. It is due to be superseded by the Nursing and Midwifery Council in 2002/3.

5. Evaluation and monitoring.
6. Feedback to earlier stages.

Cox and Cox (1993) point out that the whole range of actions for controlling a hazard need to be integrated into a coherent programme. With regard to work-related violence, Cox and Leather (1994) describe three types of intervention or control which can be employed by organisations:

1. *Preventative strategies*, which focus upon reducing the number of identifiable 'triggers' for violence in the workplace, with particular regard to work procedures and social interactions. Implementation strategies here focus upon employee training, work design, and environmental change.

2. *Timely reactive strategies*, which enable managers and staff to cope with violent or potentially violent incidents as they arise in such a way as to prevent them from occurring or to minimise their impact.

3. *Rehabilitative strategies*, which aim to offer support to employees to help them to cope with the aftermath of their direct or indirect involvement in the incident. (In the healthcare setting, of course, this might be expanded to include the assaultive patient, patient victims or witnesses, and relatives and visitors to clinical areas where such events have occurred.)

To be effective, specific interventions applicable to each set of strategies must be addressed at each level of management structure, with different strategies being implemented at individual, team, and organisational levels to provide a truly integrated and holistic approach.

The key element of this is the organisation's policy or code of practice on the management of violence, because it translates the organisation's strategy into the procedures whereby it is applied in practice to ensure as safe a working environment as is reasonably possible. While it is unrealistic to expect policies to provide exhaustive detail about how staff should act in all possible circumstances, they should provide staff with sufficient guidance to allow staff to respond to the demands of their work in ways that are logically, ethically, and legally justifiable. A good policy specifies the arrangements, resources, and organisation to support prevention, timely reaction, and rehabilitative strategies, and sets basic standards against which the development of such strategies can be monitored and evaluated. Leather et al. (1999) suggest that, at a minimum, the policy or code of practice should:

1. Communicate a clear statement of zero tolerance for work-related violence.
2. Encourage employees to report incidents swiftly and fully.
3. Inform employees of the structures and arrangements established to combat violence, including training, support from the line manager and other welfare and support functions, how and to whom incidents are to be reported, and what rehabilitation or aftercare facilities are available.

4. State unequivocally that no reprisals will be taken against an employee who reports or experiences work-related violence.
5. Assign resources and authority to those responsible for the various elements of the programme.

Unfortunately, the implementation of the legislative recommendations discussed above concerning risk assessment and the planning and implementation of safe systems of work has been slow in the British healthcare system. For example, a Royal College of Nursing (RCN) survey of community nurses (1994) found that just under 17% of employers had a policy on violence and aggression, while a later survey conducted in 1991 by the National Union of Public Employees (NUPE) discovered that only 40% of hospitals had a policy on violence[3]. More recently, studies of management of violence policies in National Health Service (NHS) Trusts which offer regional secure units (RSUs) and psychiatric intensive care units (PICUs) (Wright et al., 2000) and acute inpatient care (Noak et al., 2002) have found considerable shortcomings in such documents, which will be discussed below[4].

The only guidance on content for policies addressing the prevention and management of violence in the UK is that offered by Kedward's (1990) survey of violence in UK social services and probation settings. While these suggestions are comprehensive, sensible, and largely compatible with the suggestions of Leather et al. (1999) described above, they do not provide advice that is specifically relevant to inpatient settings (particularly inpatient psychiatric settings), which have been identified as the most risky work sites (e.g. HSAC, 1987; Flannery, 1996). Furthermore, a conspicuous absence among Kedward's (1990) suggestions is any reference to training in and the use of physical interventions in the management of violence. The Mental Health Act 1983 Code of Practice specifically states that staff working in inpatient psychiatric units who are ordinarily likely to encounter situations where physical restraint is necessary should attend an appropriate course taught by a qualified instructor.

---

3   The Royal College of Nursing is the professional body and one of the trade unions for Registered Nurses in the UK. NUPE is also a health care workers' union in the UK.

4   Regional Secure Units in the UK are mental health units for inpatients who require treatment in a secure environment (RSUs usually also have a perimeter fence). Psychiatric Intensive Care Units are inpatient units which deal with disturbed patients who cannot be safely managed in an acute ward, usually on a temporary basis. The UK also has Special Hospitals, which provide treatment in a highly secure environment for patients who have dangerous or violent propensities.

Shortcomings in Management of Violence Policies and their Application in British Inpatient Psychiatry

Various shortcomings in management of violence policies and failures in their application have been noted in the literature, particularly in relation to inpatient mental health care units. Atakan (1995) draws attention to the need for clear management of violence policies to increase staff awareness of their role during violent incidents. Pereira et al. (1999) conducted a nation wide study of good practice issues in PICUs, and found that a significant minority of PICUs surveyed did not have a policy for the use of physical interventions in the management of violent or disturbed behaviour, or for seclusion. Both of these shortcomings have obvious implications for practice in care environments which typically have a high risk of violence, and where the methods used to deal with such a risk have the potential to cause harm or to be counter-therapeutic in inexperienced hands.

As part of the research underpinning a Standing Nursing Midwifery Advisory Committee (SNMAC) report (Department of Health, 1999), a team from the Institute of Psychiatry in London reviewed the content of management of violence policies in 33 Trusts which operated RSUs and PICUs. This study (Wright et al., 2000) took the previously mentioned policy content suggested by Kedward (1990) as a starting point, and then expanded them to make them more applicable to inpatient psychiatric settings. The original items suggested in Kedward (1990) are:

1. A definition of violence.
2. A statement of responsibility on the part of the employer (thereby demonstrating a commitment to an organisational approach to the prevention and management of violence).
3. Some account of the incidence of threats and violence (to give an idea of the scale of the problem).
4. A statement of the aims of the policy preferably expressed in measurable terms which will allow the policy's effectiveness to be determined).
5. A statement of the expectations and responsibilities of staff.
6. A commitment to appropriate training for all staff.
7. A description of measures employed to prevent violence.
8. A description of warning signs of increased risk of violence (i.e. verbal and behavioural cues, etc.).
9. A description of risky working practices and situations that should be avoided.
10. Methods of coping with violence (such as de-escalation, self-preservation and physical restraint).

11. Details of reporting methods (including an example of the reporting instrument).
12. Instructions to line managers.
13. Details of post-assault support available (e.g. from counselling, occupational health, or other welfare organisations).
14. Information about financial and legal help.

An adequate definition of violence is essential for the accurate monitoring of incidents which enables policies and the procedures that they specify to be evaluated, and can help to set the parameters for course training standards. Consistent definitions of violence and aggression are quite elusive (see Rippon, 2000, for a discussion of this complex topic), and Haller and Deluty (1989) comment that the differences in the operational definitions of assault used by different studies, and the lack of distinction between different levels of assault seriousness make comparisons between studies on the nature and correlates of violence in psychiatry very difficult. In the interests of clarity, policies should therefore distinguish between *aggression* (a willingness to inflict emotional or physical harm to another, whether or not this is sustained), *violence* (the unlawful and intentional use of force, in physical irrespective of whether it results harm and/or injury), and *verbal abuse* (expressed aggression or hostile verbal attack directed against a victim) (see Turnbull and Paterson, 1999; Wondrak, 1999).

Kedward's (1990) guidelines were expanded to address certain other issues that are pertinent to inpatient psychiatric settings. These included mention of training in physical interventions in the management of violence and other considerations concerning physical restraint, post-incident care for patients, complaints procedures for patients, summoning police assistance, and procedures for evaluating and developing policies.

An area of major concern in the management of violence in inpatient psychiatry is the issue of physical restraint. Researchers examining the issue of management of violence have emphasised the need for appropriate staff training in this area (e.g. Ritchie et al., 1985; Powell et al., 1994; Walker and Siefurt, 1994), and a variety of training systems are available in the UK (see Paterson and Leadbetter, 1999, for a review). However, since concerns have been voiced regarding the possibility of the abusive use of such methods by staff (e.g. Blom-Cooper et al., 1992; Allen and Harris, 2000) and about delays in receiving training (Lee et al., 2001), items were added concerning the situations under which physical restraint should be used and the purpose of it, and unacceptable methods of restraint (derived from the recommendations in the Mental Health Act 1983 Code of Practice). Because training in physical skills needs regular refresher training to maintain competence and to ensure safe application (see Grimley and Morris, 2001), policies were also examined to see if the need for such training and the time interval for it were specified. Examination of policies for any mention of post-incident analysis and support for staff and patients was also included, because the Mental Health Act 1983 Code of Practice advises that post-incident analysis and support should be developed for both staff and patient, the provision of which should be included in a clear, written operational policy on all forms of restraint. Patient complaints procedures was also looked for, because of the concerns mentioned above regarding the possible abuse of physical restraint by staff, and because patients can view physical restraint as oppressive (see Kumar et al., 2001). The Mental Health Act 1983 Code of Practice also advises that the Hospital Managers should appoint a senior officer[5] with the responsibility for seeing a patient who has been restrained for a protracted period, and who should ascertain whether the patient has any concerns or complaints, and if so, to assist the patient in putting them forward.

The issue of summoning police assistance was also included since the team were aware of situations where ward staff had been faced with dangerous situations which were developing beyond their safe control and had been uncertain as to whether police assistance should be requested. This issue was particularly highlighted because of concerns regarding the use of CS incapacitant spray by police officers (which has been in operational use since 1996) to subdue resistive mental health service users who required physical restraint, both in the community and in inpatient units (see Bell and Thomas, 1998; Police Complaints Authority, 2000). Finally, it was thought necessary to examine policies for various features concerning their ratification, monitoring, and review. Burke et al. (1990) recommended that each clinical policy and guideline document should record a clear indication of its authors, the date of its completion, and a specified date for its review.

Wright et al. (2000) found considerable shortcomings in the content of the policies reviewed. Regarding basic aspects of the administration, review and evaluation of policies, while 67% of policies stated that they should be regularly reviewed, only 42% actually specified how frequently this should be undertaken. Over a quarter (27%) of the policies were undated (rendering it impossible to tell if they were still current), and 9% were definitely out of date. Those responsible for the ratification and updating of the policy were only identified in a third of the policies.

A commitment to appropriate training for all staff was specified in 76% of the policies, but the period within which training should be undertaken after appointment was specified in only 8%, and while the need for refresher training was

---

5   The term 'officer' refers to a senior member of staff, with responsibility for the welfare of detained patients.

mentioned in just over half (52%) of the policies, the frequency with which this training should be undertaken was only specified in 46%. This might partially explain Lee et al.'s (2001) findings concerning uptake of training in the management of violence in RSU and PICU staff in the Trusts which participated in the Wright et al. (2000) study. Lee et al. (2001) report that only 39% of respondents reported receiving training within three months of appointment, and 21% still had not been trained within a year of being appointed. Worrying findings regarding the standard of staff training in physical restraint are also reported in Dowson et al.'s (1999) evaluation of the management of violence in general psychiatric units (GPUs) and learning disability units (LDUs) in the Anglia region. It was found that, where two or more staff were involved in physical restraint, none of the LDU staff and only 27% of the GPU staff had received appropriate training within the previous 12 months. While physical restraint was accomplished without injury to the patient in nearly all incidents, staff received injuries in 40% of the GPU incidents and in 33% of the LDU incidents. More worrying still, a relationship between lack of staff training and the probability of staff injury during restraint was found, with 61% of the restraint incidents where staff received injuries not meeting the standard for staff training.

Regarding the prevention of incidents, Wright et al. (2000) found that, while most policies (79%) emphasised prevention, only 54% mentioned specific preventative strategies, and descriptions of behavioural cues of possible immanent violence and of risky working practices and situations (themselves vital aspects of prevention) were only mentioned in 33% and 27% of the policies respectively. While most policies (94%) mentioned the use of physical restraint as a method of managing violent incidents, important aspects concerning its use were often ignored. Less than half of the documents mentioned justifiable reasons for initiating restraint, the need to use minimal or reasonable force, inappropriate methods of restraint, the need to protect the patient's dignity during the procedure, or the need to visually check for weapons beforehand. Advice on when to summon police assistance was included in only 27% of policies, and no policy gave any guidelines concerning the use of CS incapacitant in clinical areas, the treatment of persons exposed to it, or the decontamination of the environment following its use.

All the policies detailed how incidents were to be reported, but only 9% of the documents included the report form within the policy. Under-reporting of violent incidents is a common problem; the Health and Safety Executive (1989) found that only 20% of violent incidents were reported. Even where incidents are reported, the quality of information recorded can be poor. Dowson et al. (1999) found serious deficiencies in the standard of reporting of violent incidents which had required the application of physical restraint. Overall, the standard for reporting of these incidents was only achieved in 3% of incidents which were recorded in GPUs, and in 15% of those recorded in LDUs. Omissions included failure to identify the staff members involved and in recording the roles undertaken by them, and failure to note all injuries that had resulted from the incident. This lack of reporting and poor standard of reporting has obvious implications, both for any attempt to evaluate a policy and from the point of view of protecting both staff and employer from subsequent litigation. Stark and Kidd (1995) suggest the following reasons for poor incident reporting:

- Lack or available guidelines or operational policy, or lack of knowledge about such guidelines and policies.
- No (or inadequate) incident recording form.
- Time and effort required to complete the incident recording form.
- A perception that violence is 'part of the job', and therefore insufficiently unusual to report.
- Concern that violent incidents represent professional failure.
- Fear of litigation.

It follows therefore that reporting can be improved by convincing staff of the benefits of reporting incidents, and by stating within the policy that blame will not necessarily be attached for incidents recorded. It might also be necessary to introduce training in how to complete the form. The document used should also be easily understandable, and not too long or cumbersome. Beale (1999a) suggests the following features:

- It should record hard factual information (e.g. who was involved, when and where the incident occurred, whether a weapon was used, what injuries were sustained).
- It should describe how the incident occurred and what the outcome was.
- It should allow staff to make suggestions or comments to management.

In terms of post-incident actions, while the need for a review or support meeting for staff was mentioned in 85% of the policies, the need for such a meeting with patients (perpetrators, victims, or witnesses) was only mentioned in 55%, 58% of documents did not mention any need for a physical examination of the patient to be conducted following the application of physical restraint. And only a third of documents mentioned any need for a review of the patient's care plan following a violent incident. More worrying still in the light of the concerns discussed above regarding the possible abuse of physical restraint, only *one* document described the procedure by which a patient who had been physically restrained could make a complaint. Aspects of post-incident care for staff were also poorly represented in the policies, with the line manager's responsibilities being specified in 24% of the documents and the role of occupational health and other welfare organisations and information concerning financial and legal assistance each only being mentioned in a third. Again, Dowson et al. (1999) found evidence of poor policy guidance and practice in relation to post-incident support for victims (support for witnesses was not considered). It was found that only four out of the 15 participating sites (i.e. 27%) had policies which mentioned the provision of post-incident support for victims. Of staff who had been assaulted, 16% from GPUs and 24% from LDUs considered that the support that they had received had been inadequate.

Wright et al.'s (2000) study was expanded by Noak et al. (2002), who examined management of violence policies in 40 Trusts providing acute inpatient psychiatric care throughout the UK. These policies were more likely to be definitely up-to-date (in 39% compared to 9%), to identify those responsible for monitoring and updating the policy (39% compared to 33%), to define violence (76% compared to 64%). Other instances where policies examined in Noak et al. (2002) were more likely to contain information than those examined by Wright et al. (2000) include:

- The need for a post-incident review of the assaultive patient's care plan (52% compared to 33%).
- Advice regarding when police assistance should be sought (52% compared to 27%).
- The role of occupational health and other welfare support for staff (45% compared to 33%).
- Advice regarding financial and legal help (45% compared to 33%).
- Patient complaints procedures (61% compared to 3%).
- Emphasis on minimum or reasonable force (67% compared to 48%).
- The need for a post-incident review of the patient's care plan (52% compared to 33%).

However, the policies reviewed by Noak et al. (2002) were less likely than those reviewed by Wright et al. (2000) to include:

- The need for refresher training (45% compared to 52%).
- Emphasis on prevention (55% compared to 79%).
- Frequency of refresher training (30% compared to 54%).
- A requirement for a staff support or debriefing session (64% compared to 85%).
- A requirement for a support, debriefing, or review session for patients (15% for patient witnesses and 12% for the assaultive patient, compared to 55%).
- The expectations and responsibilities of staff (64% compared to 82%).

Once again, no guidance was offered regarding the use of CS incapacitant spray, or for the treatment of those concerned or for decontamination of the area where it has been deployed.

Finally, it should also be recognised that staff might be unaware of the presence of management of violence policies, despite the Mental Health Act 1983 Code of Practice stipulation that all providers should have clear, written policies on the use of restraint, of which all staff should be aware, and Burke et al.'s (1990) recommendation that all relevant policy documents should be readily accessible on each ward. This is a serious problem, because policies can only guide practice if staff are aware of their existence and if they are to hand. Dowson et al. (1999) found that while such policies were available on almost all GPUs and LDUs where incidents occurred, staff who physically intervened in these incidents were aware of them in only 56% of those occurring in GPUs and in 67% of those occurring in LDUs.

Community-based Workers

Health care services in the community have undergone considerable expansion in the UK over the last two decades (particularly in relation to mental health and learning disabilities) which has implications for the prevention of violence and for policy development. While healthcare workers in the community generally experience lower levels of physical violence (HSAC, 1987) they have been found to be exposed to higher levels of non-physical violence (HSAC, 1987; Beale et al., 1999b). Furthermore, because the work of community staff is usually quite isolated, they are at greater risk should an incident occur (Whittington, 1997).

As discussed above, The RCN (1994) discovered that fewer than a fifth of community nurses surveyed reported that their employer had a policy on violence. The most commonly stated fears by the survey's respondents were those of working alone or during the hours of darkness. Since then a number of publications have pointed out the specific needs of isolated community workers in relation to the risk of assault (e.g. Department of Health and Social Security, 1988), although employers have been slow in implementing suggested strategies. The RCN (1998) stated that Trusts needed to include community workers in their policies, encompassing travelling, lone working, and home visits. Galloway (2002) recommends several essential components of a lone worker policy. These include:

1. The identification of a 'responsible person' (e.g. a consultant's secretary) who is aware of the intended whereabouts of lone workers and who can raise the alarm should any of them either fail to return to base or report in by telephone at a prearranged time. This responsibility may need to be passed on to an out-of-hours service manager or a ward manager at the end of normal working hours.

2. The responsible person should have access to the following details:
   - Make, model, colour, and registration number of the worker's car.
   - Mobile telephone number.
   - Home telephone number.
   - Names, addresses, and home telephone numbers of service users being visited.
   - Approximate times of visits.
   - Agreed time for worker to ring back after visits.
3. If a worker fails to make contact the responsible person should:
   - Telephone the mobile number.
   - If no reply, telephone the home number.
   - If still no reply, telephone the home numbers of service users visited, in reverse order.
   - If contact has still not been made, the previously arranged period should be allowed to elapse and the police should be informed.

Of course, where there are concerns regarding the risk posed by an individual client, home visits should not be conducted, but appointments for the service user to attend the team base should be arranged. Where the client is unlikely to attend such appointments, or if it is considered that a home visit would actually still be preferable (e.g. to check for neglect), then joint visits should be considered. If this is decided against or is not practicable, a suggestion by Turnbull (1999) is for the worker to arrange for a colleague to telephone either the worker's mobile phone or the client's home number during the visit, to allow the caller to be alerted or reassured.

Conclusion

The issue of violence in health care as a major issue of international concern for nurses and nursing practice has been explored throughout this book. Nurses do not operate in isolation from the organisation within which they work, and so both nurses and employing organisations have a responsibility to ensure a safe working environment for all. Policies play a key role in helping to provide a safe environment by providing staff with guidance concerning appropriate working practices and emergency procedures, and by specifying the training and resources necessary to allow staff to carry out the courses of action specified within the policies. Despite their pivotal role in defining the organisation's response to violence, management of violence policies have been found to have major shortcomings, which seriously compromise their utility as guidelines to practice. This has serious implications, not only for the health and well-being of staff, visitors, and patients, but also for the protection from litigation of the employer. It would therefore be prudent for health care providers to examine their policies from a legal standpoint in the light of the shortcomings detailed above, given the increasingly litigious climate within which health services operate.

There are two possible remedies for this situation. Firstly, the development of minimum mandatory standards for policy content would be valuable. In the British context, this should be informed by reference to guidance and good practice currently available in the Mental Health Act 1983 Code of Practice, or as has been established by the Royal College of Psychiatrists (1998). Further guidance in Britain will be available in the near future from the forthcoming UKCC initiative on the prevention and therapeutic management of violence, and the forthcoming guidelines from the National Institute for Clinical Excellence. Similar guidance on the development of professionally acceptable practice in the prevention and management of violence in healthcare in other countries should be provided by the relevant regulatory and professional organisations. Secondly, pains should be taken to ensure that policies are informed from professional, health and safety, legal, tactical (operational), and human rights perspectives within the context of the health care environment. This can be facilitated by developing policies in consultation with clinical and audit staff, trainers, and carers and service users and/or their advocates to ensure that they are comprehensive, understandable, practical, and explicitly state the responsibilities of management and staff as well as the rights of staff and patients.

References

Adams, J. and Whittington, R. (1995) Verbal Aggression to psychiatric staff: traumatic stressor or part of the job? *Psychiatric Care*, 2, 171-174.

Alderman, C. (1997) Bullying in the workplace: a survey. *Nursing Standard*, 11 (35), 22-25.

Allen, D. and Harris, J. (2000) Abuse by any other name: a critique of some current approaches to behaviour management. *Mental Health Care*, 3, 188-189.

Atakan, Z. (1995) Violence on psychiatric in-patient units: what can be done? *Psychiatric Bulletin*, 19, 593-596.

Barling, J. (1996) The prediction, experiences and consequences of workplace violence. In: G.R. VandenBos and E.Q. Bulatao (eds.) *Violence on the Job*, Washington DC: American Psychological Association.

Beale, D. (1999) Monitoring violent incidents. In: P. Leather, C. Brady, C. Lawrence, D. Beale, and T. Cox (eds.) *Work-related violence: assessment and intervention* 69-86. London: Routledge.

Beale, D., Lawrence, C., Smewing, C. and Cox, T. (1999a) Organisational and environmental measures for reducing and managing work-related violence. In: P. Leather, C. Brady, C. Lawrence, D. Beale and T. Cox (eds.) *Work-Related Violence: Assessment and Intervention*, London: Routledge.

Beale, D., Leather, P., Cox, T., and Fletcher, B. (1999b) Managing violence and aggression towards NHS staff working in the community. *Nursing Times Research*, 4 (2), 87-99.

Bell, F. and Thomas, B. (1998) Police use of CS spray: implications for NHS mental health services. *Mental Health Care*, 1, 402-404.

Blom-Cooper, L., Brown, M., Dolan, R. and Murphy, R. (1992) *Report of the Committee of Inquiry into Complaints About Ashworth Hospital*. London: HMSO.

Burke, J., Crossfield, E., Gordon, E., Higgins, J. and Taylor, A. (1990) *Report of the Panel of Inquiry Appointed by the North Staffordshire Health Authority to Investigate the Death of Alma Simpson*. Birmingham: West Midlands Regional Health Authority.

Carmel, H. and Hunter, M. (1989) Staff injuries from inpatient violence. *Hospital and Community Psychiatry*, 40, 41-46.

Cembrowicz, S.P. and Shepherd, J.P. (1992) Violence in the Accident and Emergency department. *Medicine, Science and the Law*, 32, 118-122.

Cox, S.J. and Tait, N.R.S. (1991) *Reliability, Safety, and Risk Management*. London: Butterworth-Heinemann.

Cox, T. and Cox, S. (1993) *Psychosocial and Organisational Hazards at Work: Control and Monitoring*. European Occupational health Series No. 5. Copenhagen: WHO Regional Office for Europe.

Cox, T. and Leather, P. (1994) The prevention of violence at work. In: C.L. Cooper and I.T. Robertson (eds.) *International Review of Industrial and Organisational Psychology* (Vol. 9). Chichester: Wiley and Sons.

Department of Health and Social Security (1988) *Violence to Staff. Report of the DHSS Advisory Committee on Violence to Staff*. London: HMSO.

Department of Health (1999) *Standing Nursing Midwifery Advisory Committee Addressing Acute Concerns*. London: Department of Health.

Department of Health and Welsh Office (1999) *Mental Health Act 1983 Code of Practice*. London: The Stationery Office.

Dowson, J.H., Butler, J., and Williams, O. (1999) Management of psychiatric inpatient violence in the Anglia region. *Psychiatric Bulletin*, 23, 486-489.

Flannery, R.B., Hanson, M.A., and Penk, W.E. (1994) Risk factors for inpatient assaults on staff. *Journal of Mental Health Administration*, 21, 24-31.

Flannery, R.B. (1996) Violence in the workplace, 1975-1995: a review of the literature. *Aggression and Violent Behaviour*, 1, 57-68.

Galloway, J. (2002) Personal safety when visiting patients in the community. *Advances in Psychiatric Treatment*, 8, 214-222.

Golding, A. (1996) Violence and public health. *Journal of the Royal Society of Medicine*, 89, 501-505.

Gournay, K., Ward, M., Thornicroft, G. and Wright, S. (1998) Crisis in the capital: in-patient care in inner London. *Mental Health Practice*, 1 (5), 10-18.

Grimley, M. and Morris, S. (2001) The training of NHS staff in non-mental health settings in the recognition, prevention and management of violence and aggression and conflict management. In: A. Bleetman and P. Boatman, *An Overview of Control and Restraint Issues for the Health Service*. London: Department of Health.

Haller, R.M. and Deluty, R.H. (1988) Assaults on staff by psychiatric in-patients: a critical review. *British Journal of Psychiatry*, 152, 174-179.

Health and Safety Executive (1989) *Violence to Staff*. (IND (G)189 M100). London: HMSO.

Health and Safety Executive (1992) *The Management of Health and Safety at Work Regulations*. Sudbury, Suffolk: HSE Books.

Health Services Advisory Committee (1987) *Violence to Staff in the Health Services*. London: HMSO.

Hobbs, F.D.R. (1991) Violence in general practice: a survey of general practitioners' views. *British Medical Journal*, 302, 329-332.

Kedward, C. (1990) Current practice and policy with regard to violence in social services departments and probation services in the UK: the University of Sussex study. In: D. Norris, *Violence Against Social Workers: Implications for Practice*. London: Jessica Kingsley.

Kumar, S., Guite, H. and Thornicroft, G. (2001) Service users' experience of violence within a mental health system: a study using grounded theory approach. *Journal of Mental Health*, 10, 597-611.

Lanza, M.L. (1983) The reactions of nursing staff to physical assault by a patient. *Hospital and Community Psychiatry*, 34, 44-47.

Lanza, M.L. and Milner, J. (1989) The dollar cost of patient assault. *Hospital and Community Psychiatry*, 40, 1227-1228.

Leather, P., Beale, D., Lawrence, C., Brady, C. and Cox, T. (1999) Violence and work: introduction and overview. In: P. Leather, C. Brady, C. Lawrence, D. Beale and T. Cox (eds.) *Work-Related Violence: Assessment and Intervention*, London: Routledge.

Lee, S., Wright, S., Sayer, J., Parr, A.-M., Gray, R. and Gournay, K. (2001) Physical restraint training in English and Welsh psychiatric intensive care and regional secure units. *Journal of Mental Health*, 10, 151-162.

Noak, J., Wright, S., Sayer, J., Parr, A.-M., Gray, R., Southern, D. and Gournay, K. (2002) The content of management of violence policy documents in United Kingdom acute inpatient mental health services. *Journal of Advanced Nursing*, 37, 394-401.

National Union of Public Employees (1991). *Violence in the NHS*. London: NUPE.

Nolan, P., Dallender, J., Soares, J., Thomsen, S. and Arnetz, B. (1999) Violence in mental health care: the experiences of mental health nurses and psychiatrists. *Journal of Advanced Nursing*, 30, 934-941.

O'Connell, B., Young, J., Brooks, J., Hutchings, J. and Lofthouse, J. (2000) Nurses' perceptions of the nature and frequency of aggression in general ward settings and high dependency areas. *Journal of Clinical Nursing*, 9, 602-610.

Paterson, B. and Leadbetter, D. (1999) Managing physical violence. In: J. Turnbull and B. Paterson (eds.) *Aggression and Violence: Approaches to Effective Management*. Basingstoke: Macmillan.

Pereira, S., Beer, M.D. and Paton, C. (1999) Good practice issues in psychiatric intensive-care units. *Psychiatric Bulletin*, 23, 397-404.

Police Complaints Authority (2000) *CS spray: increasing public safety?* London: Police Complaints Authority.

Poster, E.C. and Ryan, J. (1994) A multiregional study of nurses' beliefs and attitudes about work safety and patient assault. *Hospital and Community Psychiatry*, 45, 1104-1108.

Powell, G., Caan, W., and Crowe, M. (1994) What events precede violent incidents in psychiatric hospitals? *British Journal of Psychiatry*, 165, 107-112.

Rippon, T.J. (2000) Aggression and violence in health care professions. *Journal of Advanced Nursing*, 31, 452-460.

Ritchie, S., Higgins, J. and McLoughlin, C. (1985) *Report to the Secretary of State for Social Services Concerning the Death of Michael Martin at Broadmoor Hospital*. London: DHSS.

Royal College of Nursing (1994) *Violence and Community Nursing Staff: a Royal College of Nursing Survey*. London: RCN.

Royal College of Nursing (1998) *Safer Working in the Community. A Guide for NHS Managers and Staff on Reducing the Risks from Violence and aggression*. London: RCN.

Royal College of Psychiatrists Research Unit (1998) *Management of Immanent Violence: Clinical Practice Guidelines to Support Mental health services*. (Occasional Paper OP41). London: Royal College of Psychiatrists.

Ryan, J. and Poster, E. (1993) Workplace violence. *Nursing Times*, 89 (48), 38-41.

215

Shepherd, J.P. and Farrington, D.P. (1993) Assault as a public health problem: a discussion paper. *Journal of the Royal Society of Medicine*, 86, 89-92.

Stark, C. and Kidd, B. (1995) The role of the organisation. In: B. Kidd and C. Stark (eds.) *Management of Violence and Aggression in Healthcare*, London: Gaskell.

Turnbull, J. (1999) The role of the manager. In: J. Turnbull and B. Paterson (eds.) *Aggression and Violence: Approaches to Effective Management.* Basingstoke: Macmillan.

Turnbull, J. and Paterson, B (1999) Introduction. In: J. Turnbull and B. Paterson (eds.) *Aggression and Violence: Approaches to Effective Management.* Basingstoke: Macmillan.

United Kingdom Central Council for Nursing, Midwifery, and Health Visiting (1992) *Code of Professional Conduct.* London: UKCC.

Walker, Z. and Siefert, R. (1994) Violent incidents in a psychiatric intensive care unit. *British Journal of Psychiatry*, 164, 826-828.

Whittington, R. (1997. Violence to nurses: prevalence and risk factors. *Nursing Standard*, 12 (5), 49-54.

Wondrak, R. (1999) Verbal abuse. In: J. Turnbull and B. Paterson (eds.) *Aggression and Violence: Approaches to Effective Management.* Basingstoke: Macmillan. In: J. Turnbull and B. Paterson (eds.) *Aggression and Violence: Approaches to Effective Management.* Basingstoke: Macmillan.

Wright, S., Lee, S., Sayer, J., Parr, A.-M. and Gournay, K. (2000) A review of the content of management of violence policies in in-patient mental health units. *Mental Health Care*, 3, 373-376.

Chapter Eleven: Education for Violence Prevention – A Danish Example

Vibeke Sjøgreen; Anne Jensen, and Pia Kielberg

Introduction

Being exposed to violence and threats of violence is in itself a profound experience. Being exposed to violence and threats from a person you are nursing can make this experience even more intense. However, today violence and threats of violence is a well-known part of reality in mental hospitals and in mental nursing. A study of victims of violence (Balvig, 1998) shows that 35% of all violent episodes in Denmark takes place at work. A major part of these episodes happens within the social- and health sector.

Only a few years back in Denmark violence and threats of violence were regarded as part of the "agreement" – meaning that it was an inevitable part of the job. One still comes across this attitude towards violence and threats of violence but fortunately there has been a considerable change in attitude through recent years and a substantial interest for working with this problem. This has focused the attention on the prevention of violence. In mental nursing this is a major and complex area consisting of a number of multifaceted areas which influence each other.

For a number of years the authors have provided courses in managing conflicts and preventing violence within the mental health services in the County of Aarhus. In 1994 the present training course was developed, based on the model illustrated below (Figure one). The course is compulsory for the majority of professionals employed in the mental health services in the county.

All areas included in this model are equally important and depend on each other but the importance of each factor varies from time to time and from workplace to workplace, depending on the actual situation and needs. Dialogue and co-operation are placed at the centre of the figure as these are central and bind the various parts together. Within all areas dialogue and co-operation between patients, staff and management is necessary in order to create a workplace with as few episodes of violence as possible. A workplace where you are sure to be taken care of if violence should occur (Sjøgreen, 1999).

Areas of importance for prevention of violence and other workrelated strains

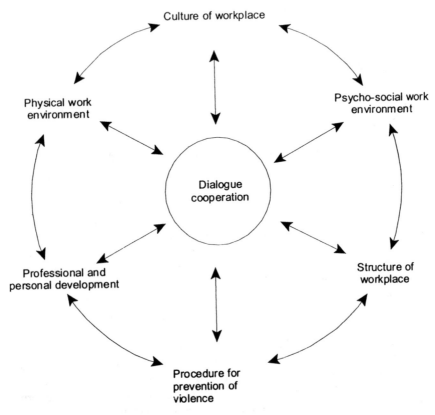

Culture of workplace

Physical work environment

Psycho-social work environment

Dialogue cooperation

Professional and personal development

Structure of workplace

Procedure for prevention of violence

Figure one: Model for Prevention of Violence, Area of Importance

Conflict and Violence Prevention

Definition of Conflict

The definition used is based on the Dutch psychologist van de Vliert's work in a simplified form (Van de Vliert, 1998) " A situation where at least one party feels restricted or frustrated by another party".

This means that a conflict arises whenever an individual feels restricted and/or frustrated – whether real or not. This definition is very applicable both in relation to conflicts with patients and in relation to conflicts among staff.

Any conflict has an issue – the facts which constitute the conflict – as well as a relationship between the parts of the conflict. Underlying the issue and the relationship are a cognitive and an emotional element. The cognitive element could for instance be that one party might feel restricted from obtaining a goal, for instance a conflict of interests. The emotional element could be frustration followed by feelings such as anxiety and/or anger. This could for instance be caused by a feeling of being ignored and/or rejected.

The development of the conflict depends on various things. Firstly it depends on how important the issue is to the parties involved. Then it depends on the relationship between the parties – are they compatible or not? Both issue and relationship are important for the way in which the parties choose to handle the conflict. Finally the culture of the workplace is essential – what are the traditions for conflict management and which opportunities do the staff and patients have for handling the conflict?

The Principles of Understanding Violence

It is essential that the staff has knowledge of conflicts with special focus on definition, types, sources, origins as well as possible actions.

Violence and threats of violence can be prevented. One of the conditions for this prevention is adequate care and nursing for mental health patients. Another necessary condition is to recognise that working with people who are in a difficult situation is to navigate in a conflict-ridden sphere. When working with prevention of violence and conflict management it is important to recognise that a conflict has existed prior to any episode with threats and/or violence – sometimes without the staff being aware of this.

Conflict cannot be controlled. Earlier on the concept "conflict control" was used in the Aarhus courses, but it has now been recognised that the mere assumption that staff must be able to "control" conflicts in itself can bring conflict. Thus the current approach is focused on how conflict can be used constructively as an opportunity for development both for patients and staff. It is therefore important, by means of lectures and training that staff be empowered to develop a joint language for and a joint consciousness about working in a sphere of conflict.

Conflict is situational, not personal. One of the main ideas in the work with conflicts, threats and violence is to change the focus from seeing conflicts as an individual problem between people, to an understanding that the environment and working conditions form part of the situation for patients and staff. When the focus is moved from the individuals and put into a larger perspective, a different set of constructive possibilities for action is created. Thus working with conflict and prevention of violence becomes a collective responsibility and challenge. It becomes a collective matter for the workplace and a task equal to any other task.

Conflict is based on differences, and differences cannot be eliminated. Another main ideas is that people (patients or staff) are different, but they basically have identical emotions when experiencing differences and conflicts. The intensity of the emotions of course varies according to who you are and which situation you are in (Bastian, 2002). Differences are part of life. Working life is full of differences, both for staff and patients. When people meet, opposites meet. This can be an enrichment for the co-operation and the quality of work can be improved when differences are seen as a resource. Differences are necessary in working life in order to create life and it is a basis for all development. Differences only become conflicts when they are incompatible – when there is a clash of contrasting interests. It is often when you are in opposition to somebody you start finding fault and the basis for a conflict is laid (Rosenberg, 1995).

People are different and therefore the basis for any conflict management must be that each individual makes his/her own perceptual version of an experienced situation. At the level of experience no version is right or wrong. Both patients and staff continuously pick up signals from themselves, from each other and from the surroundings. These signals are normally interpreted automatically. This interpretation often becomes "reality" for the individual and this will dictate the next move.

Conflicts within mental health are unique due to quite special conditions. First of all, the patients suffer from a mental illness which means that they might read signals differently and apparently react unpredictably due to internal and/or external conflicts. In many cases they get agitated and anxious more quickly and they might react strongly with loss of control in stressed situations.

Besides, due to their mental illness the patients are vulnerable and depend on the help of the staff in one way or the other. This might create an in-balance in power which in itself can cause conflicts. It could be said that the patients are "one down" in relation to the staff. Or you could say that the staff holds the "power" whereas the patient holds the "powerlessness" – they are subject to a system and a structure that creates this in-balance in power. Often discussions about this power are taboo. For many staff the word power is negative, something the staff would rather avoid talking about. However, power is a reality, and staff must take responsibility in full and apply the legitimate power they have properly before it can be turned into the care and nursing which is so essential for the patients and consequently it could also prevent violence.

Finally, staff members may become "the special one" for many patients, while the patient may only be "one of many" to the staff. This could mean that the patients build up expectations from the staff which cannot be full-filled and thus these expectations contribute to creating frustrations.

These characteristic conditions could provide a breeding ground for conflicts – especially if the staff is unaware of this and for instance induces the patients to believe that they are equal partners. The patient and staff are of course equals as human beings but they are not equal in the situation. Thus it is vital that the staff has a thorough professional knowledge of the various mental illnesses so that the patients are not exposed to unnecessary stressful situations caused by these extraordinary conditions.

Concentrate on the feelings, and the message. The task of the staff is to check how the descriptions, explanations and understanding of the individual have developed and how to get on from where they are. This applies both to prevention and management of conflicts and in relation to both patients and colleagues. By means of curiosity about their perceptions and experiences, and adequately provocative questions a staff member can stimulate people who are locked in a problem to change and develop. If people are exposed to something unusual, a change might take place. However, disturbances that are too massive, both in relation to colleagues and patients, could keep the situation at a deadlock or even make it escalate possibly resulting in violence and threats of violence. In this context violence and threats of violence can be seen as a means of communication – an expression of anxiety, helplessness and powerlessness that might result in loss of control.

Therefore an important tool when communicating with troubled people is to be able to concentrate on the underlying emotions and frustrations. It is vital that the staff practise on not seeing the aggression as personal even if they are directed towards them. When a person feels personally affected it is very difficult to avoid contributing to the escalation of the situation. Therefore the staff must pay attention to the person behind the message – the attention must be on the emotions and needs of this person so that the aggression can be labelled positively as a message.

Types of Conflict

It is extremely important that mental health staff are trained in prevention and management of violence and understand that conflicts can be used as a tool for development. The problems and conflicts which the staff face today are results of yesterday's choices. Tomorrow is based on the choices made by the staff today

(Lang, 1998). Therefore the staff must realise that what they do – or don't do – has consequences. It is also necessary that they possess various professional and personal tools to help them from escalating the conflict unintentionally.

One of these tools is the knowledge of various types of conflicts. This knowledge of various types is an important condition in the work with conflicts as the various types demand different approaches.

- *The classic conflict* – conflict of interests – is the kind of conflict where for instance several staff members require the same experience. This could be a certain course, a day off or a holiday and it is impossible to meet everybody's request. In relation to patients it could be the young schizophrenic man hearing voices. He is able to live with the voices if he plays loud music. His neighbours/other patients are unable to sleep because of the loud music he plays at night. The way to approach a classic conflict could for instance be by means of compromise.
- *The pseudo-conflict* is the kind of conflict which is caused by misunderstanding and/or lack of communication. This kind of conflict can be solved rather easily by means of explanations or apologies.
- *A conflict of issue* is the kind of conflict where parties disagree on a certain matter. For instance different staff groups might disagree whether a patient will be granted leave or not. Or if it is appropriate as professionals openly to discuss a patient's treatment in front of the patient. A conflict of issue might be solved through dialogue.
- *Displaced conflicts* are conflicts that take place elsewhere, but reflects in a different relationship or setting. There are many indications that unsolved conflicts in the staff group will show as conflicts between the patients or between the patients and staff. When a displaced conflict occurs it is necessary to identify the real conflict site and deal with it.
- *Personalised conflicts* are the conflicts which have shifted focus from the issue to the person. Instead of disagreeing on the right treatment for a patient, you start seeing the other party as stupid, professionally incompetent etc. This kind of conflict might be solved by means of mediation.

Identification of the conflict type can be of help to find possible actions as there are various possible actions according to the various conflict types.

The following is another way of classifying types of conflicts (Lennéer-Axelson, 1998):

Individual conflicts which are internal conflicts such as remorse, aggression, inhibitions and ambivalence. People often keep this kind of conflicts to themselves but sometimes they result in interpersonal conflicts.

222

Interpersonal conflicts are conflicts between people. These conflicts may be caused by opposite intentions and perceptions but can also be caused by human chemistry with likes and dislikes.

System conflicts are conflicts caused by uncertainty/disagreement on goals, roles, structure and distribution of resources. They can originate from malfunctioning organisations and show as interpersonal conflicts.

Often each individual conflict contains elements from all three areas. Classification of conflict areas can be of help both as a prevention tool and in working with conflicts trying to analyse the cause of and reason for disagreements.

Reactions to Conflict and Conflict Management

Violence prevention is dependant on a culture in the workplace in which the staff see conflicts, violence and threats of violence as a theme to be worked on collectively. A way to build up this culture is for the staff to work on creating an environment where conflicts, violence and threats of violence are discussed, and where staff work together to find new ways of acting. A condition for this is to find time and space for dialogue about issues such as attitudes, ethics and views of human nature. Another condition is the intention and wish to discuss the more complicated and emotional sides of differences and conflicts as well as violence and threats of violence in working life. The aim must be to create a work environment and culture characterised by dialogue, co-operation, appreciation, respect and an adequate degree of safety.

It is vital for mental health nursing staff to be aware of conflict in order to react professionally and appropriately. Thus it is important that the staff has a general knowledge about conflicts and at the same time know their own reactions in conflict situations. A professional must have insight into and understanding of the reasons behind the patients' reactions, so they are able to pay attention to the patients' needs. It is important to find time daily to solve minor disagreements and on a regular basis have space and time to work with major conflicts which are the conflicts that are threatening to essential values. If there is no space and time for these discussions, an accumulation of conflicts could easily take energy from the work with patients.

Conflict management is also about the way the parties choose to treat the conflict and each other. There are many possibilities and studies have shown many different options which largely are related to the personality. In practise it will be most appropriate to distinguish between 5 options (Van de Vliert, 1998 p. 355):
- Avoidance or withdrawal due to indifference in relation to the other party
- Adaptation in order to maintain a good relationship

- Compromise, where both parties are partially satisfied
- Problem solving so that both parties overcome the frustrations
- Fight in order to win and beat the other party

Successful conflict management takes place when the way a person chooses to handle the conflict minimises or solves the conflict. In some situations it is best to avoid the conflict, in other situations it must be actively suppressed to be handled at a later time. In a situation where a person is not receiving attention on an important issue, it might be helpful to exaggerate the conflict to highlight the problem. Conflicts can be useful when they open up possibilities for professional and personal development. In that case disagreements can be discussed openly and constructively and the parties work together to find a satisfactory solution. Each person is allowed to show their emotions but in the end rationality wins. In this respect one could say that development demands tensions and conflicts.

Conflicts are negative when they cause situations to deadlock and prevent development, because emotions rule instead of rationality. The feeling of being in control of the situation might disappear causing dominant feelings of anxiety and anger both in patients and staff. There is often a discrepancy between the things people say they do and what they actually do in relation to disagreements. It actually seems that most people in reality are more concerned with winning instead of learning, with protecting themselves instead of developing and of getting their own way instead of co-operating. If this is correct it is very likely that disagreements under such conditions can lead to a locked conflict. It is important to help staff to identify these choices in conflict situations.

When working with very vulnerable patients such as mental health patients these locked conflicts might provoke violence and threats of violence. During an episode of violence the primitive instinct and the entire physiological alert of fight or flight automatically takes over. When working within mental health settings staff can find themselves in dangerous situations which they cannot just leave (flight), but where they can also not fight. It is important that the staff acknowledge their own fear and are able to contain this fear in order to handle the situation. Just as the mountain climber hanging high up on a steep mountain slope who is suddenly overwhelmed by fear. If he gives in to his fear he might fall. If he has the right equipment and training he will be able to control his fear. Self-confidence based on training and skill is the only way to deal with realistic fear.

Another tool also relating to the above is the staff's knowledge of potential origins of conflicts. People have an inclination to personify conflicts. But conflicts may stem from many other sources than the individual person or the interaction of individuals and groups. When we try to understand what lies behind conflicts we have tried to identify various areas of importance (Figure 1), as will be described in the following portion.

The following six areas have dialogue and co-operation as the central focus. To have successful co-operation and conflict management the staff must be willing to take on responsibility and make demands on themselves and each other and the organisation must function appropriately. Lack of dialogue and co-operation can in itself be a source for growing conflicts.

As mentioned earlier the <u>culture of the workplace</u> – the atmosphere and tone created by the management and staff – is an important element in working with conflicts. The way people treat each other determines if the conflict is solved or will be at a deadlock with possible violence or threats of violence as a result. A workplace with a continuous tense atmosphere will be a sure source of conflicts.

The <u>psycho-social work environment</u> is important. The work must be organised and planned providing balance between demands, expectations and resources. There should be staff participation, the work must be meaningful and support from colleagues and management is vital. A strained psycho-social work atmosphere for instance with uncertain tasks and a heavy workload will also be a sure source of conflicts.

A third important area is the <u>structure of the workplace</u>. The overall framework determines the possibilities and restrictions for the staff on the particular workplace. The staffing determine the extend of activities and the quality of the work. If the quality of the work is reduced continuously it could result in the staff being worn out and this might increase the risk of conflicts, violence and threats of violence.

A fourth major area is the <u>violence prevention policy</u> of the workplace. This policy must be adapted in order not to create unnecessary uncertainty and insecurity which could provoke conflicts, violence and threats of violence. Each workplace should work out efficient action plans which are discussed, evaluated and, if necessary, adjusted on a regular basis. The action plans should contain procedures for handling violent situations as safety precautions such as alarms and escape routes are inefficient in themselves without clear guidelines for use. Efficient conflict management and follow-up on conflicts, violence and threats of violence demand action plans which contain a well-known definition of conflicts, threats of violence and violence so that everybody knows when the policy must be applied, what has to be done and who is responsible for what. The staff's familiarity with the policy is in itself a prevention of violence as knowledge and a collective understanding may ensure more security and the willingness for activresponse.

A fifth area are the <u>opportunities for professional and personal development</u> available to staff. The staff must have the professional and personal competences which are necessary for a quality work performance. This includes professional knowledge and ability in relation to patients and mental health nursing, personal competences such as sufficient communication skills and empathy. Training in conflict management and an interest in continuing training and development together with colleagues also qualify the work. Insufficient knowledge and experience can contribute to escalation of conflicts resulting in violence and threats of violence.

The last major area which plays a part is the <u>physical work environment.</u> For instance narrow space and a loud noise level might cause stress symptoms in the staff and affect vulnerable patients to such a degree that they lose control resulting in conflicts, violence or threats of violence.

Coping with Violence

Working in a mental hospital involves the risk of violence and threats of violence. There is a distinct connection between nursing and the risk of violence. The staff can be exposed to serious assaults and emotional trauma. It is important to take the risk seriously and know which reactions might occur during and after a violent episode.

In working with staff, fear should be minimised and control maintained both for the benefit of the victim and colleagues. The assumption is that people who are overwhelmed by fear lose control over the situation and consequently they will lose their professionalism and ability to act appropriately in the situation. This applies both to the person directly involved in the situation and to the witnesses of the situation. Conflict management also involves colleagues "interfering" in order to prevent the situation from escalating.

Likewise suppression of fear is a condition for maintaining the ability to communicate both with the patient and colleagues in the situation. Experience show that many conflict situations between patients and professionals could be "talked down" before they result in violence or threats of violence. It is also essential to communicate with colleagues during conflict openly and clearly even though might be extremely difficult.

The Violence Process

Conflict management and the prevention of violence can be based on an understanding of the progress of a conflict – before, during and after, as illustrated in figure two. Before a conflict turns into a violent episode there are a number of

226

signals which can be acted on and which might possibly minimise or solve the conflict. At the instant when the conflict progresses and go beyond the personal stress level, the fight/flight mechanism will go into action. After the violent episode there are a number of cognitive, behavioural and emotional reactions which gradually decrease.

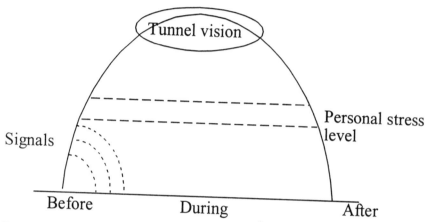

Figure 2. The Violence Process

Signals

Before a conflict turns into a violent episode there are a number of signals which can be acted on and which might possibly minimise or solve the conflict.

Signals are here seen as the stimuli which are received from internal and external sources. Signals are also received from ourselves: from our body, our thoughts and our emotions. Signals are also received from our surroundings, the physical settings, the arrangements, sounds, smells etc. Finally we receive signals from each other, both verbally and non-verbally.

People create meaning and understand themselves and their surroundings by means of interpretation of the signals they receive. There is a constant interpretation, often quite automatically, of signals received. This interpretation becomes "reality" to the individual and will determine our next action. But as a professional it is essential to know that our own interpretation is one out of many interpretations and "realities". Colleagues and patients might interpret situations differently from oneself and therefore it is necessary as a professional constantly to

227

consider the basis of our own interpretations. Dialogue with colleagues and patients is an important tool which qualify our interpretations as professionals.

An important element in working with signals is to draw attention to the differences that exists in our interpretations of reality. A patient regarded as threatening by one staff can be regarded as appealing by another staff. Consequently the two staff members will act differently in the situation. There is no right or wrong perception of the situation. The individual acts on his/her perception of the situation.

The staff should not be trained in identical interpretations but should be able to acknowledge the different interpretations and perceptions of the situation. Usually the acknowledgement of the different interpretations helps people to understand the actions and reactions of both colleagues and patients.

Warning Signals

Experienced mental health staff can give numerous examples of signals from the patients which draw the attention of experienced staff to a conflict taking place. They know they have to be particularly aware when the signals of a certain patient changes, for instance in speech or behaviour; the patient that gets agitated, the eyes that turn black, dialogue that stops etc.

The ability to read behavioural changes in patients increases with experience. It is evident that newly qualified staff, students and temporary staff are more exposed to threats of violence and violence, due to their inability to read the signs. Certain ways of behaviour should warn the staff. Almvik and Woods have worked out the following list – The Bröset Violence Check list (BVC) (Almvik and Woods, 1998):

- Confusion
- Irritability
- Noisy behaviour
- Verbal threats
- Physical threats
- Blows, kicks etc. aimed at furniture

The study shows that there is a considerably risk of violence if only two of these behaviours are present. It is hardly surprising to anybody that physical threats and blows and kicks aimed at furniture might increase the risk of violence but many are surprised by the fact that a confused and irritable patient also presents a major risk.

228

The Signals of the Nursing Staff

As described people send out and interpret signals all the time – patients as well as staff. Thus it is important that the staff is aware of their own signals and of how to use this knowledge in order to minimise a conflict.

Especially discrepancies between the spoken words and body language is an important element in professional training regarding own signals. Nursing of mentally ill patients also consists of limit settings and this can be a source of conflicts. It is important to be precise and firm in situations where it is necessary to set limits, both verbally and non-verbally. Vague messages and unclear limit setting can play a part in escalating a conflict.

If a situation turns violent it is important for the staff to know how they can use their behaviour to subdue aggression. To a large extent mental health staff already possess the competences used for subduing aggressions, for instance not getting angry, containing strong emotions, speaking calmly etc. But as mentioned earlier, it is a condition for being able to use these tools to prevent being overwhelmed by fear.

The Personal Stress Level

The personal stress level which is shown in figure 2 expresses the total stress one is under – both privately and at work. The connection between stress and violence is well-known. Breakwell (1989) explains that the risk of being involved in violent situations increases accordingly with the stress level because: "Increased stress heightens the general possibility that the staff will resort to violence as stress tends to produce emotional instability and reduced self-control". (Breakwell, 1989, p. 34). "Increased stress will reduce the staff's possibilities of anticipating patient violence and handling the violence appropriately as stress tends to reduce the cognitive efficiency and control over emotions". (Ibid, p. 34).

An important tool to deal with personal stress is dialogue between colleagues about daily stress factors and how to manage these factors or at least be aware of them. Another important element is to create a culture where vulnerability is legitimate – for the staff as well as patients. On an individual level staff should have knowledge of their own stress/vulnerability levels and thus have a possibility of avoiding conflict situations, and should avoid being worn- and burnt-out. On an organisational level the necessary staffing should be provided to enable staff members to withdraw from a conflict situation, to initiate dialogue on a general level and to create a caring environment.

During a Violent Episode

In a violent situation perceptions are concentrated on what is dangerous – the person facing you or the weapon in the hand of the assaulter – tunnel vision and in some cases tunnel hearing. This means that the person can see or hear only the anxiety provoking stimuli, and not what is happening around that. Staff at the mental hospital in Risskov, Denmark who have been exposed to a violent episode tell that in the situation they did not realise that there were colleagues present, that the emergency team had arrived or what else went on in the room. Cognition becomes fragmented and thoughts are locked and short-termed (Berliner, 1995, p. 110). The emotional reactions are surprise, fear, desperation and irritability, and the physical reactions are an increased adrenaline production and hypertension (Ibid, p. 110).

Some violent episodes occur suddenly and with only few warning signals or no warning signals whatsoever. But as mentioned earlier many conflicts/violent episodes within mental health occur in connection with limit settings. However, one is able to prepare for a potential violent episode no matter if there are warning signals or not.

It might sound paradoxically to prepare for the unexpected violent episode but preparation does not mean to make strategies for any imaginable situation but instead to be aware of the ever present risk and to consider the available possibilities for action. The awareness of risks and possible actions induces a mental robustness which will be a resource in a violent episode.

An exercise which helps many staff to handle their fear is to tell each other about the worst possible situation. Available strategies and possible actions are then discussed collectively. Apart from minimising the fear, the exercise also increases the understanding of each other.

Besides the general wish to minimise the fear of the staff there is an element of prevention in preparing for a limit-setting which could turn into violence. Preparation for limit-setting can be done in a way which can help the limit-setting from escalating into a conflict.

A thorough preparation for a possible conflict situation might contain the following elements:

Reason for the initiative: Why are we setting limits?
What are our professional motives?
Is limit setting possible – can it be carried out?

How to do it: What is the best method for this particular patient given his/her pathological picture, personality etc.?
What do we say?

230

Where to do it:	What is best for the patient?
	Safety of the staff?
	Safety of the other patients?
When to do it:	Is the patient's condition best at specific times during the day?
	Are we enough staff present?
Who should do it:	Should it be the person in daily contact with the patient or a "neutral" person?
Possible actions:	Plan A – if everything goes according to expectations
	Plan B – known deviations
	Plan C – the worst possible situation

As can be seen especially the last "possible actions" can minimise fear in a violent situation. Preparation for possible actions in the worst possible situation with the patient gives staff a better chance of maintaining control.

Reactions after a vViolent Episode

Professionals should be fully aware of the possible reactions after a violent episode. It is very helpful for the victim to know that his/her reactions are normal and to be expected. Staff should make a point of normalising the reactions, stressing that people do not act rationally in critical situations but are subject to primitive instincts. Besides helping the victim, open talks about the anger or fear one feels can be a help in creating a culture at the workplace where violence or threats of violence is taken seriously. Only when people are able to have a dialogue about violence and threats of violence is it possible to show the victim the necessary care which enables him/her to remain at the workplace and/or return to work.

This also applies in relation to the violent patient. Staff that work with their reactions and emotions, for instance by means of supervision is to a considerable extent more capable of helping the patient in a professional manner.

As colleagues to a person who has been exposed to violence or threats of violence professionals have to "know what they cannot see". A nurse may not necessarily be able to see if a colleague is undergoing a crisis and therefore s/he has to be aware of the possible reactions. It is the colleagues' responsibility to help the victim and the patient, for instance by means of mental first aid (see later).

Witness reactions need special attention. Witnesses to a violent episode identify strongly with the victim. They show many of the same reactions as the victim directly involved. A way of making sense and regaining control after the situation is to find the reasons behind the violent episode – unfortunately often blaming the victim. As Lanza explains: "Witnesses do blame the victim as a way of distancing themselves from the assault situation and in an attempt to protect themselves from the strong identification with the victim" (in Vandenbus and Bulatao, 1996, p.192).

To know that witnesses can react to violent episodes experienced by others is helpful not only to the witness but the victim as well. But especially the knowledge that blaming the victim is a defence against ones own fear will help not to stigmatise the victim. This knowledge positively changes the attitude towards violence and threats of violence from being the problem of an individual to being a collective work environment problem.

The effects of a violent episode can be extremely serious for nurses, for instance prolonged absence due to illness, reduced quality of life and early retirement (Jensen and Riis, 1998, p. 4). It is therefore of the uttermost importance to relieve the serious effects by means of competent and adequate support to the staff being exposed to violence.

Knowledge of crisis reactions is necessary in order to give support. The reactions after a violent episode are varied and differ from individual to individual. No individual will get all the reactions at the same time and the intensity and duration varies from person to person.

The reactions can be divided as follows:

Physical reactions: headache, stomach ache, dizziness, difficulty in breathing, lack of sleep, nightmares etc.

Emotional reactions: unmotivated crying, emotional withdrawal, irritability, burst of anger, flashbacks, self-reproach, sense of guilt etc.

Behavioural reactions: rushing around, passivity, tendency of isolation, fear of being alone

Cognitive reactions: lack of concentration, feeling of emptiness, difficulty in decision-making, reduced motivation, reduced general valuation ability, changed sense of time etc.

As can be seen a person who has been exposed to a violent episode will have a number of serious reactions. Nobody reacts in the same way as the reactions to a violent episode depend on various factors:

Personal factors such as: stress level, previous untreated crisis/trauma, mental problems, coping strategies

Situation factors such as: seriousness of incident, unexpectedness, level of control, role and possible actions of the staff

Work environmental factors such as: social support, culture of the workplace in relation to violence

It is important to stress the diversity in reactions. A person does not necessarily show signs of being in a crisis and one cannot expect the person to be able to express this verbally. Thus it is important that the staff in the various workplaces discuss and find a collective definition of violence and threats of violence for their workplace. This definition should make it clear when a colleague must give mental first aid to a team member who has been exposed to a violent episode.

Mental first aid is given by colleagues and is the immediate support given on the spot. The list below shows the mental first aid at the Mental Hospital in Risskov, Denmark:

1. A calm and kind appearance
2. Make sure the person is not left alone
3. Provide a peaceful setting and something to drink
4. Ask about the person's condition
5. Listen
6. Talk about the situation
7. Accept emotions
8. Do not reproach
9. Be aware of your own reactions to the episode and the influence they might have on the conversation

Mental first aid given by colleagues is the most important help for the staff who has been exposed to violence or threats of violence. The support from the workplace is crucial for the way the victim overcomes the effects of the violent episode just as the support is crucial for the victim's return to the workplace (Jensen and Riis, 1998, p. 14).

Most hospitals and institutions in the County of Aarhus have a policy on violence prevention, and practically all employees are aware of the policy and the mental first aid. But even if the formal policy has been stipulated, it is still extremely difficult for colleagues to give first aid to each other. It seems that what makes it difficult to give a colleague mental first aid is the fact that a person has to take on a professional role in relation to a colleague. The relationship between the victim and the colleague giving mental first aid changes from being equal to being asymmetrical which might make it difficult to be colleagues on equal terms again. This problem has to be addressed in training in order to counter the participants' difficulties and worries in relation to mental first aid. The purpose is to demystify the mental first aid which as can be seen in the above simply consists of ordinary care. Ordinary care for another person can be given from colleague to colleague without resulting in asymmetry or harming the relationship.

A Violence Prevention Course

The course offered at Aarhus consists of three main elements – theory, control and restraint techniques and role-play. Within each of these elements we focus on preliminary preparation, response to specific situations and supplementary work. Participants attending courses express an increased understanding of their own and others' roles, and that the tools acquired are useful in their future work with conflict management and prevention of violence.

1.Theory: The first main element consists of imparting knowledge and sharing experience in the form of lectures followed by dialogue and assignments. All the topics outlined in theoretical framework are covered thoroughly.

2. Control and restraint techniques: The second main element of the program is a training component where we work closely with a group of psycho-physical consultants. The consultants have developed a number of control and restraint holds which enables the staff to maintain the respect for and care of the patient and at the same time ensure staff safety. These very simple holds do not require great strength, only the use of proper techniques. These are taught to the participants who are then given the opportunity for daily repetition and training. Apart from physical techniques we also consider: body language, boundaries, co-operation, communication.

These verbal and non verbal aspects of communication between patient and staff are very important. We specifically consider the relationship between words, body and tone. All these factors play a role in defusing violent or threatening incidents.

3. Role Play: The third element is role play which is based on work situations. The role play mimics realistic situations and some participants undergo strong emotions such as anger, fear or anxiety. Some have described experiencing palpitations or tunnel vision. Of course one has to be careful not to push participants either too far or too little. Learning situations are created which can then be discussed and reviewed. Nevertheless participants should be confronted by sufficiently difficult challenges to develop their skills.

After the role play the events are discussed; what went well, what was difficult and how the situation might have been handled differently. Many participants come to recognise how different their interpretation of signals are and how their reactions vary to the same incident. In staging conflict situations participants are therefore given a chance to test themselves in difficult situations within secure settings. There is particular emphasis on verbal communication to enable participants to understand their use of language and what they could say in various situations. The aim of the role play is thus to give each participant a chance to work with his or her own behaviour in difficult situations and improve their ability to respond to conflict while maintaining as much of their self esteem and dignity as possible.

The success of the course lies in its ability to create a learning environment where the participants can work, learn and develop in an atmosphere of appreciation and respect. This environment allows people to achieve a better understanding of themselves, gain insight into their own and other people's motives, signals and reactions in conflict situations.

One example of how role play is used in the training is related to the topic of preparation, reactions and possible actions during a conflict. A situation is constructed where the participants are put under stress. We provide them with a patient's anamnesis and a briefing on the actual problem and give them 10 minutes to prepare how to handle this situation. The patient which they meet in the role play is an unknown person. The participants report that they do not react as intensely as in a real situation but they get a rapid pulse, tremble, tunnel vision and experience fear and anger etc.

The role play provide instructors with a possibility of working realistically with signals, interpretations, preparation, co-operation, communication, reactions, possible actions etc. The role play is an educational tool which greatly increases the understanding of the essential areas within conflict management and prevention of violence.

Conclusion

Generally professionals working within mental health have a wish to provide qualified nursing and care for the patients. However, it is a fact that the professional work with mentally ill people involves a risk of being exposed to violence and threats of violence. Being exposed to violence and threats of violence from a person one is nursing is a profound experience. In the past too many staff have had to face this problem on their own. During recent years focus has been on workplace violence as a collective problem, which has to be dealt with collectively.

The Educational Department, Psychiatry in the County of Aarhus, Denmark has focused on this area for several years by means of courses emphasising teaching, training and subsequent reflection and dialogue. In this chapter the theoretical framework for the work with prevention of violence and conflict management in relation to professionals within mental health care was described. The work is based on the assumption that prior to any episode of violence or threats of violence there has been a conflict. Thus violence and threats of violence can be an expression of helplessness, frustration and despair – an expression of not being heard or understood.

It is extremely important for this work that the management leads the way. The management should continuously focus on conflicts, violence and threats of violence as a possibility for development. Management should create the space for both knowledge, reflection and practise. In this way the quality of the mental health nursing will increase to the benefit of the patients and the professionals will get a better and more secure work environment.

References

Almvik, R. and Woods, P. (1998) The Bröset Violence Checklist (BVC) and the prediction of inpatient violence: Some preliminary results. *Psychiatric Care,* 5 (6): 208-211.

Balvig, F. (1998): *Vold på gaden, i hjemmet og på arbejdet. Oversigt over resultater fravoldsofferundersøgelsen 1995/96.* Rigspolitichefens trykkeri, Kbh.

Berliner, P. (1995). *Vold og trusler på arbejdet, G.E.C* Copenhagen: Gads forlag.

Breakwell, G.M. (1989) *Facing physical violence.* Viborg: Hans Reitzels forlag

Jensen, C. and Riis, J.O. (1998) *Krisehjælp hvordan?* Copenhagen: Kommunernes Landsforening.

Lennéer-Axelson, B. and Thylefors, I (1998) *On conflicts – at home and at work.* Copenhagen: Hans Reitzel.

Rosenberg, M. (1995) Words are windows or they are walls, a presentation of nonviolent communication. (Video).

The County of Aarhus (2000) *Voldspolitik og vejledning om vold.* Aarhus: County Press.

Vandenbus, G.R. and Bulatao, E.Q. (1996) *Violence on the Job.* Washington: American Psychological Association

Van de Vliert (1998) Conflict and conflict management. In Drenth, P.D., Thierry, H. de Wollf, C.J. (Eds.) *Handbook of work and organizational psychology.* Hove: Psychology Press Ltd.

Editors and Authors

Róisin **Gallinagh**
Lecturer in Nursing Science, School of Health Sciences, University of Ulster, Ireland

Donna **Gates**
EdD,MSPH,MSN,RN, Associate Professor College of Nursing, University of Cincinnati, Cincinnati,OH. USA

Rhosta S. **Gcaba**
M Nursing , RN and RM, and Advanced Midwife, and currently Depute Director for Nursing at the Provincial Department of Health, KwaZulu-Natal, Pietermaritzburg, South Africa

Monika **Habermann**
Dr. phil., Nurse, Social Anthropologist. Professor for Nursing Science, International Study Course of Nursing Management, Hochschule Bremen, Germany

Rolf **Hirsch**
Dr. med., Dr. phil. Specialist in psychotherapy, neurology and psychoanalysis. Director of the Gerontopsychiatric Center and Department of the Rheinische Hospital, Bonn. Honorary Professor of the University Nürnberg-Erlangen, Germany

Anne **Jensen**
Master of Science, Psychology (1998) and Educational. Consultant employed at The Educational Department in the County of Aarhus since 2001, Denmark

Pia **Kielberg**
Master of Science, Psychology (1984) and educational consultant. Educational Department in the County of Aarhus, Denmark

James **Noak**
Robert Baxter Research Fellow, Health Service Research Department, Institute of Psychiatry, and Nurse Consultant West London Mental Health Trust, London, United Kingdom

Anneli **Pitkänen**
MNSc(c), RN. University of Tampere, Department of Nursing Science/Tampere University Hospital, Finland

Penny **Powers**
PhD, RN Department Head, Graduate Nursing Programmes South Dakota State University, College of Nursing, South Dakota, USA

Dirk **Richter**
PhD, Nurse, Sociologist. Quality Manager at the Westphalia hospital for Psychiatry and Psychology Münster. Part-time Lecturer at the department of Sociology, University Münster, Germany

Vibeke **Sjøgreen**
Nurse, Master of Science (Psychology). Educational consultant employed at Educational Department in the County of Aarhus, Denmark

Johanna **Taipale**
MNSc, RN, University of Tampere, Department of Nursing Science, Finland

Bev **Taylor**
PhD, Professor of Foundation Chair in Nursing, School of Nursing and Health Care Practices, Southern Cross University, New South Wales, Australia

Leana R **Uys** D
Soc Sc (Nursing), RN and RM. Professor at the School of Nursing, University of Natal, Durban. Director of the World Health Organization Collaborating Centre for Nursing and Midwifery Development. South Africa

Maritta **Välimäki**
PhD, RN, Senior Assistant Professor. University of Tampere, Department of Nursing Science/Tampere University Hospital, Finnland